Medicine

Mark C. Fishman, M.D.

Department of Medicine
Massachusetts General Hospital
Boston, Massachusetts

Andrew R. Hoffman, M.D.

Department of Medicine
Massachusetts General Hospital
Boston, Massachusetts

Richard D. Klausner, M.D.

Department of Medicine
Massachusetts General Hospital
Boston, Massachusetts

Stanley G. Rockson, M.D.

Department of Medicine
Massachusetts General Hospital
Boston, Massachusetts

Malcolm S. Thaler, M.D.

Medicine

J. B. Lippincott Company
Philadelphia • Toronto

The authors and publisher have exerted every effort to ensure that drug selection and dosage set forth in this text are in accord with current recommendations and practice at the time of publication. However, in view of ongoing research, changes in government regulations, and the constant flow of information relating to drug therapy and drug reactions, the reader is urged to check the package insert for each drug for any change in indications and dosage and for added warnings and precautions. This is particularly important when the recommended agent is a new or infrequently employed drug.

Library of Congress Cataloging in Publication Data

Main entry under title:

Medicine.

Includes bibliographical references and index.
    1. Internal medicine.   I. Fishman, Mark C.   [DNLM:
1. Medicine.   WB 100 M4892]
RC46.M4758   616   80–27875
ISBN 0–397–50436–5

Printed in the United States of America

Contents

I. Cardiology

II. Pulmonary Disease

III. Renal Disease

IV. Endocrine Disease

V. Gastrointestinal Disease

VI. Rheumatology

VII. Hematology/Oncology

VIII. Infectious Disease

IX. Neurology

Foreword

To the beginning student of medicine and the physician commencing residency training, the information needed for optimal care of patients seems almost infinite—as in fact it is. When placed in the stressful situation of having initial experiences in management of patients' medical problems, the neophyte must have some organized conceptualization of the bare knowledge base from which to function. This book is an attempt to provide that basis in a condensed, practical manner so that the beginner will be able to acquire the necessary facts without a time-consuming search of the pertinent literature. Yet the volume is not a cookbook to be followed by rote. It gives a sketch of the underlying pathophysiology which allows the reader to think constructively about his patients' problems.

This book should be a reassuring companion on the ward or beside the pillow—ready for quick reference. The experienced specialist is likely to be critical of the superficial nature of the book in its coverage of his own field and find the other chapters to be superior. But that is what the authors planned. The book is written not as a definitive treatise in internal medicine today but rather as a guide to the beginner working in a hospital whether he be student, resident, nurse or other health worker, or as a refresher to the seasoned practitioner on topics outside of his speciality. It does not replace the more detailed and scholarly treatises on medicine. It complements them but provides a useful, practical function without relieving the physician of the obligation to build his fund of knowledge beyond the confines of this practical summary.

Alexander Leaf, M.D.
Boston, Massachusetts
February 1981

Preface

There is certainly no lack of medical literature. The great outpouring of information ranges from the esoteric case report to the exhaustive review, and includes countless journal articles, manuals, and textbooks. We have undertaken this book in the hope of incorporating this information into a clear perspective on patient care in today's modern hospital. Because the multitude of new technical developments can only complement the patient interview and physical examination, we have attempted to integrate them in that context.

This book is intended for anyone directly involved in patient care, and assumes a rudimentary knowledge of medicine. It should appeal to medical students, house staff, and physicians and other practitioners concerned with in-hospital patient care. In addition, it should be of benefit to nurses as they move into positions of greater responsibility.

This book begins with the assumption that the hospital is a dangerous place. It is the unusual patient who escapes without at least one scar: a phlebitis from an intravenous line, a miserable morning undergoing a poorly thought-out barium enema, anxiety over the when and why of the next blood drawing, the emptiness of disenfranchisement from decisions affecting his own integrity and sanity. One must therefore be sure the hospitalized patient belongs in the hospital; as soon as the patient can function at home safely and comfortably, let him go.

In order to maximize the benefit a patient can derive from the hospital, there must be a hierarchy of concern: life-threatening remediable problems must be addressed with alacrity, and only subsequently should the nature of the underlying illness and associated problems become the focus of attention. The key to patient care, therefore, is clinical judgment, and this is a major theme of this book. However, appropriate judgment entails a familiarity with the details of therapy and diagnostic evaluation, and we have therefore included concise descriptions of relevant drugs and procedures, along with their side-effects. At the end of each chapter, we have included references to major reviews and key articles.

We hope that MEDICINE will prove to be easily readable and will engender some of the excitement that we have derived from medicine.

Mark C. Fishman
Andrew R. Hoffman
Richard D. Klausner
Stanley G. Rockson
Malcolm S. Thaler

Acknowledgments

We are grateful to our families and close friends for remarkable patience and continued support throughout the preparation of MEDICINE. As they can attest, it turned out to be far more time-consuming than we had anticipated!

We would like to thank Dr. A. Fishman for the chest x-rays, Dr. M. Austin for the hematology slides, Dr. R. Birdwell-Rockson and Dr. H. Abrams for their selection of radiographs, Dr. A. Pruitt for the CT scans, Dr. F. Maloof for the thyroid scan, Roger Webb for his excellent illustrations, Beth Rosenberg for her impeccable typing of the manuscript, and Dr. K. Bridges for suggestions about hematology slides.

We also would like to thank our friends at Lippincott for guiding the book's preparation, especially the indefatigable Lisa Biello and the dapper Stuart Freeman.

Medicine

Cardiology

1

Sudden Death

Under circumstances less frenetic than those encountered in an emergency room, one might haggle over the precise definition of "sudden death." To the emergency medical team, however, the expression sudden death refers to a patient who is unconscious, apneic and without blood pressure, and whose death was unexpected, nontraumatic, and instantaneous (or, at most, evolving within minutes).

Despite the existence of critical care ambulances and highly trained personnel, more than 300,000 adults succumb to "sudden death" each year in the United States. Although these deaths are often classified as "heart attacks," this is an oversimplification. Evidence of an acute coronary occlusion or myocardial infarction is frequently, but by no means invariably, present. Identification of the precise etiology of an episode of sudden death is important both for immediate therapy and for prevention of recurrence.

MECHANISMS OF SUDDEN DEATH

Some sudden deaths are presumed to be due to respiratory failure (which may very rarely occur in asthmatics) or to a neurologic disorder (subarachnoid hemorrhage), but most are car-diovascular in origin. At least four cardiovascular mechanisms can cause sudden death:

1. _Anatomic catastrophes_ are rare. The most common among these are a ruptured ventricle, a ruptured aorta, and a massive pulmonary embolus. Even in these seemingly clear-cut instances, however, the actual cause of death may be complex. Thus, experimental evidence suggests that the extreme hypotension associated with a massive pulmonary embolus may derive more from cardiovascular reflexes than from the mass effect of the embolus.

2. _Arrhythmias_ are the most common cause of sudden death. Although any tachyarrhythmia or bradyarrhythmia can theoretically compromise the cardiac output sufficiently to cause death, ambulance monitoring within minutes of collapse indicates that ventricular fibrillation is present in 75% of these patients. Sinus and junctional bradycardias, idioventricular rhythms, and asystole are present less frequently. Underlying coronary arteriosclerosis is usually present, but evidence of a new infarction is often lacking. Myocarditis and cardiomyopathy also predispose to arrhythmic sudden death, as do anomalies of the cardiac conduction system. An overdose of a cardiotoxic drug, such as

one of the phenothiazines, can also cause arrhythmic sudden death, as can electrolyte imbalances.

3. A third mechanism of sudden death is *electromechanical dissociation*. In the laboratory, it can be shown that heart tissue that is perfused with a calcium-free solution continues its regular electrical activity although it no longer contracts. Mechanical activity is then said to be uncoupled, or dissociated, from electrical activity. An identical phenomenon has been described during cardiac catheterization following the injection of angiographic contrast agents into the coronary arteries, because these dye materials chelate calcium. Electromechanical dissociation has come to refer to the presence of continuing electrocardiographic activity in the absence of a detectable blood pressure. It can occur with global myocardial ischemia or infarction, or may appear secondary to mechanical obstruction, for example, in patients with pericardial tamponade, tension pneumothorax, cardiac rupture, papillary muscle rupture, critical aortic stenosis, or massive pulmonary embolus.

4. *Vasodepressor death* results from an inappropriate reflex decrease of the heart rate, contractility, and peripheral vascular tone. The result is precipitous hypotension. Receptors that trigger such reflexes are located in the coronary sinus and at the base of the heart. This mechanism may be involved in deaths from a hypersensitive carotid sinus baroreflex or from pulmonary thromboembolism.

EPIDEMIOLOGY

Any disease involving the myocardium predisposes to sudden death. Most cases of sudden death are associated with coronary artery disease. Clinical postresuscitative and postmortem examinations reveal that 30% of sudden death victims have evidence of a new my-ocardial infarction, and another 50% have an acutely ruptured coronary arterial plaque or a new thrombosis. The majority of patients have a past history of myocardial infarction and angina pectoris, and many have experienced chest pain or dyspnea within a month prior to death. The risk factors for sudden death and myocardial infarction are similar, and include hypertension, smoking, diabetes mellitus, and hypercholesterolemia.

A second group of patients prone to sudden death includes those who are under severe psychological stress (grief, anxiety, triumph, fear, and so on). Underlying heart disease is not always found. Although Western medicine has failed to define a precise pathophysiologic mechanism and has thus failed to accept such concepts, superstitious populations accept "voodoo" death without question. Reliable Western observers have described such events:

"The man who discovers that he is being boned by an enemy is indeed, a pitiable sight. He stands aghast, with his eyes staring at the treacherous pointer, and with his hands lifted as though to ward off the lethal medium which he imagines is pouring into his body. His cheeks blanch and his eyes become glassy and the expression of his face becomes horribly distorted . . . he sways backwards and falls to the ground and after a short time appears to be in a swoon . . . after a while he becomes very composed and crawls to his wurley . . . unless help is forthcoming in the shape of a counter-charm administered by the hands of the Nangarri, or medicine man, his death is only a matter of a comparatively short time."

The physiological pathways to such occult deaths probably involve the central nervous system. In animal experiments, stimulation of parts of the central nervous system or of the sympathetic nerves to the heart can dramatically lower the threshold for ventricular fibrillation.

PREVENTION

Many sudden death victims visit their physicians shortly before death, although often with only vague and ill-defined complaints. It is at present nearly impossible to identify patients at risk for sudden death who might therefore be hospitalized as a preventive measure.

In theory, one group at risk for sudden death that should be most easily identified is that comprising young athletic patients with structural lesions of the heart, such as hypertrophic cardiomyopathy, congenital coronary anomalies, or aortic stenosis. These diagnoses, however, are frequently quite subtle and missed on routine physical examination. It would clearly be impractical to submit all healthy youngsters to a more rigorous search, which would necessarily include screening with electrocardiography (EKG) and echocardiography.

One group of patients that is known to be at an increased risk for sudden death is comprised of those who have recently suffered a heart attack, and it is therefore imperative to utilize antiarrhythmic prophylaxis to reduce the incidence of ventricular fibrillation early in the evolution of a myocardial infarction (see Chap. 3). Ventricular ectopy *per se* in most other settings, however, is not an indication for antiarrhythmic medication. With ambulatory monitoring, the majority of the middle-aged population would be found to have ventricular premature beats. It is prudent, nevertheless, to treat patients empirically with antiarrhythmic drugs if monitoring reveals frequent ventricular ectopy (5–10 beats per minute) or ventricular tachycardia, especially if these arrhythmias are accompanied by a history of syncope, dizziness, or palpitations. Some evidence suggests that this group of patients has an increased risk of sudden death, presumably arrhythmic in origin. Patients who have such symptomatology,

but who do not evidence arrhythmias on routine EKG and in whom physical examination does not reveal alternative causes, should be monitored as outpatients with a portable electrocardiographic machine (a Holter monitor) for 12 to 24 hours to look for bursts of ventricular ectopy. Remonitoring after therapy has been instituted allows evaluation of the effectiveness of the drug.

It is still unknown whether empirical treatment will prove to be effective in the long run in preventing sudden death. Experimental techniques, in which the patient's susceptibility to ventricular arrhythmias is directly measured in the cardiac catheterization laboratory, are available in some centers and permit direct comparison of the effectiveness of various drug regimens.

Patients who experience frequent and multifocal ventricular premature beats during the late hospital phase of recovery from a myocardial infarction are especially prone to sudden death during the year following the infarction. It has become common practice to treat these patients with quinidine or procainamide, although the effectiveness of long-term antiarrhythmic prophylaxis in preventing sudden death in these patients is only now under study.

CARDIOPULMONARY RESUSCITATION (CPR)

Following an episode of sudden death, adherence to the basic precepts of cardiopulmonary resuscitation offers the patient the best chance for survival.

The airway must be cleared and the head extended to assure proper air flow. (The head should *not* be extended if a neck injury is suspected.) Mouth-to-mouth breathing is then begun. Exhaled air has an oxygen tension of greater than 100 torr and is therefore sufficient to maintain adequate arterial oxygenation.

If the arrest is witnessed, a brisk chest thump may defibrillate a heart in ventricular fibrillation and should be tried once. If this is unsuccessful, external cardiac massage should be given at a rate of about 60 compressions per minute. The sternum should be depressed firmly and then slowly released, so that compression is maintained for 50% of the cycle. The most common mistakes include massaging too rapidly or shallowly, and providing a flaccid back support. Thoracotomy for direct cardiac massage is usually inappropriate and only negligibly enhances the cardiac output over that attained with external massage. *At no time other than during electrical cardioversion should CPR cease.*

When the patient reaches an emergency room, he should immediately be intubated. A central venous catheter is inserted and sodium bicarbonate is administered to combat acidosis. Lactic acidosis is invariably present and interferes with the response to catecholamines and with cardiac contractility.

Electrical cardioversion, lidocaine, procainamide, and bretylium are used to treat ventricular fibrillation and ventricular tachycardia (see Chap. 4).

Atropine and isoproterenol are used to treat bradycardia and heart block. *Atropine* blocks the action of acetylcholine, the transmitter of postganglionic parasympathetic nerves. Atropine therefore blocks secretion of salivary and sweat glands, causes pupillary dilatation, blocks contraction of the urinary bladder, and inhibits motility of the GI tract. Its most important action, however, is to block the effects of the vagus nerve on the heart. Thus, injection of atropine causes tachycardia and hastens conduction through the A-V node. *Isoproterenol* stimulates β-adrenergic receptors. It is a powerful inotropic and chronotropic agent. β-adrenergic stimulation also causes relaxation of smooth muscle, thereby lowering peripheral resistance. Isoproterenol is therefore an appropriate drug to use for

elevating the heart rate, but should not, in general, be used as the sole agent to reverse hypotension.

When severe hypotension is present despite an adequate pulse rate, norepinephrine can raise the blood pressure by stimulating α receptors and thus cause vasoconstriction. The catecholamine *dopamine* stimulates α, β, and dopamine receptors. In low doses, the net effect of dopamine is to stimulate cardiac contractility, but it does so with less vasoconstriction than norepinephrine and thus protects some sensitive vascular beds, including those of the kidney.

If the EKG reveals a "flat line," inotropic agents, such as *calcium* and *epinephrine*, can be tried. These agents are believed to stimulate an electrically inactive heart to become more excitable.

If electromechanical dissociation is present, that is, if there is no detectable blood pressure despite electrocardiographic activity, treatable causes for the uncoupling should be sought and treated. Foremost among these are tension pneumothorax, pericardial tamponade, and massive pulmonary emboli. The first two disorders are treated by inserting a needle and aspirating the air or fluid. It is still uncertain whether pulmonary embolectomy (opening the pulmonary artery and removing the clot, referred to as a Trendelenburg procedure) is helpful.

Sometimes, as a last resort, an attempt is made to rescue an electrically inexcitable heart by insertion of a pacemaker. It is extremely unusual for a pacemaker that is inserted in the midst of CPR to capture and drive the heart effectively. Because insertion must be accomplished with alacrity, it is done by direct puncture of the myocardium through a trans-thoracic approach. Either of two insertion sites may be used: one from next to the left side of the xiphoid process angling toward the right scapula, the other through the fourth or fifth intercostal space at the left sternal border. Complications of such insertion procedures include coronary or mammary artery laceration and pneumothorax.

Mortality and Prognosis

Given the swift arrival of critical care ambulances and appropriate intervention, perhaps one-third of patients can be resuscitated from episodes of out-of-hospital ventricular fibrillation and will survive to the end of hospitalization. Even with empirical antiarrhythmic prophylaxis, however, one-third of those leaving the hospital will die soon after.

The long-term prognosis is bleakest for the patient whose episode of sudden death is arrhythmic but unrelated to myocardial infarction. Perhaps because an irritable cardiac focus (*i.e.*, a source of ectopic rhythms) is not infarcted, these patients suffer recurrent episodes of sudden death, and 50% die within two years.

Transient neurologic deficits and even coma commonly follow resuscitation from sudden death, but if the resuscitation is immediate these defects generally disappear within the first day. If, however, coma persists for longer than 12 hours, the patient's chances for survival are very poor, and those who do survive can be expected to manifest severe neurologic impairment. Other signs that bode poorly for

survival when present 12 hours after resuscitation include nonreactive pupils, absent corneal reflexes (or absent ice water caloric reflexes), and absent deep tendon reflexes.

BIBLIOGRAPHY

Cannon WB: "Voodoo" death. American Anthropologist 44:182–190, 1942

Caronna JJ, Finklestein S: Neurological syndromes after cardiac arrest. Stroke 9:517–520, 1978

Engel GL: Psychologic stress, vasodepression (vasovagal) syncope, and sudden death. Ann Intern Med 89:403–412, 1978

Engel GL: Sudden and rapid death during psychological stress: Folklore or folk wisdom? Ann Intern Med 74:771–782, 1971

Liberthson RR, Nagel EL, Hirschman JC et al: Pathophysiologic observations in prehospital ventricular fibrillation and sudden cardiac death. Circulation 49:790–798, 1974

Lown B: Sudden cardiac death: The major challenge confronting contemporary cardiology. Am J Cardiol 43:313–328, 1979

Maron B, Roberts W, McAllister H, Rosing D, Epstein S: Sudden death in young athletes. Circulation 62:218–229, 1980

Moss AJ: Clinical significance of ventricular arrhythmias in patients with and without coronary artery disease. Prog Cardiovasc Dis 23:33–52, 1980

Pruitt RD: Death as an expression of functional disease. Mayo Clin Proc 49:627–634, 1974

[handwritten notes:]

Adrenerg.
atrop → ↑HR agonist
isoprot → β₁, β₂ → ↑H.R. ↓Bp
NE → ↑HR ↑Bp
dopamine → ↑HR + − Bp.

2

Cardiac Catheterization and Hemodynamic Measurements

Human cardiac catheterization was introduced by Werner Forssman in 1929. Ignoring his department chief, and tying his assistant to an operating table to prevent her interference, he placed a ureteral catheter into a vein in his own arm, advanced it to the right atrium, and walked upstairs to the x-ray department where he took the confirmatory x-ray film. In 1956, Dr. Forssman was awarded the Nobel Prize.

The major applications of catheterization can be separated into two categories:

1. Catheterization of the right heart and pulmonary circulation is performed routinely in many intensive care units to monitor cardiac function.

2. Catheterization of the left heart and coronary arteries is performed in specialized catheterization laboratories, often in anticipation of cardiac surgery.

RIGHT HEART CATHETERIZATION (SWAN-GANZ CATHETERS)

A Swan-Ganz catheter can be introduced into any large peripheral vein and maneuvered under fluoroscopic control into the venae cavae, the right atrium, the right ventricle, and then out into the pulmonary artery. Pressures in the pulmonary artery, right ventricle, and right atrium can be measured during insertion or removal of the catheter. Figure 2–1 shows the normal contours of pressure tracings obtained in this way. Once the catheter is within the central circulation, a small balloon located near the catheter tip can be inflated, and the catheter will float and be carried by the flow of blood until it is wedged in a small pulmonary artery, occluding its lumen. Because the wedged catheter blocks blood flow through the artery, it measures pressures downstream, in the left atrium. This is called the *wedge pressure*.

There are several indications for inserting a Swan-Ganz line:

1. **To resolve any uncertainty about the filling pressures of the left heart, especially in patients with hypotension.** A high pulmonary capillary wedge pressure suggests pulmonary edema; a low wedge pressure suggests hypovolemia. Measuring the wedge pressure can therefore guide the clinician in modulating a patient's fluid balance. It is especially valuable in a patient with a compromised left ventricle, who may require a high filling-pressure to maintain cardiac output, but who is treading dangerously close to pulmonary edema. Swan-

fluid-balance

8

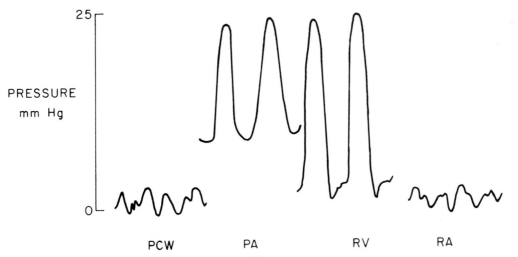

PRESSURE
mm Hg

PCW PA RV RA

FIG. 2–1. Pressures recorded from a Swan-Ganz catheter during a "pull-back" from pulmonary capillary wedge (PCW) position to pulmonary arterial position (PA), to right ventricular (RV) position, and finally to right atrial (RA) position. (The recorded pressures in this patient are normal.)

Ganz catheters are therefore routinely inserted in patients in shock, in many patients with large myocardial infarctions, and in patients with heart and lung disease in whom it is unclear how much of their hypoxemia derives from lung disease and how much from pulmonary edema.

The jugular venous pressures, measured in the neck veins, measure pressures only on the right side of the heart. They do *not* measure pressures on the left side of the heart. Thus, the jugular venous pressures may be normal in patients with left ventricular failure as long as the right ventricle continues to function well. The jugular venous pressures are elevated in patients with cor pulmonale or tricuspid valvular disease regardless of the state of the left ventricle.

2. **To measure the cardiac output.** The amount of blood ejected during systole can be measured with a Swan-Ganz line. Water

cooled to 4° C is injected through a side hole in the catheter; after dilution in the warm blood it is ejected from the right ventricle where it reaches a thermister at the end of the catheter. The measured rate of change in blood temperature at the catheter tip can be used to predict the volume in which the water was diluted and, hence, the stroke volume. Cardiac output represents the sum of the stroke volumes for one minute. The cardiac index equals the cardiac output divided by the total body surface area and is a standardized measurement that permits comparisons among people of different sizes.

3. **To measure the pressures in the right heart.** The Swan-Ganz catheter can be used to evaluate the severity of pulmonary hypertension. In addition, the contour of the pressure tracing from the right ventricle can be diagnostic in the evaluation of pericardial disease (see Chap. 9).

4. **To evaluate left-to-right shunts.** Blood can be removed from the superior vena cava, right atrium, and right ventricle by the Swan-Ganz catheter, and the oxygen saturations measured. Ordinarily, the right atrial and right ventricular oxygen saturations are virtually

the same. However, if the oxygen saturation of the right atrium or ventricle is higher than that of the vena cava, one should suspect intracardiac shunting of oxygenated blood.

Complications. Complications from placing a Swan-Ganz catheter are unusual. Occasionally, the balloon tip may become stuck in the wedge position and thereby cause a pulmonary infarction. The catheter tip may perforate the pulmonary artery. Ventricular ectopy or right bundle branch block may sometimes occur as the catheter passes through the right ventricle.

LEFT HEART CATHETERIZATION

A catheter can be passed from a brachial or femoral artery in retrograde fashion into the aorta and left ventricle. Pressure measurements and angiographic dye injection permit evaluation of aortic and mitral valvular disease (see Chap. 5). The injection of dye can also outline abnormalities of the aortic wall (dissection), the ventricular cavity (ventricular aneurysm), and the septum (ventricular septal defect). Surgery for complex congenital cardiac anomalies was made feasible by the introduction of cardiac catheterization.

A selective injection of dye into the left or right coronary artery can outline the coronary arterial tree for diagnosing the extent of coronary artery disease and in preparation for coronary artery bypass surgery. (Indications for coronary arteriography are discussed in Chap. 3.)

Complications. Complications of left heart catheterization include vascular damage at the insertion site, arterial thromboembolism, dye anaphylaxis, myocardial infarction, stroke, and even death. In good catheterization laboratories, however, the incidence of such complications should not exceed 1%. Transient hypotension or arrhythmias commonly result from catheter placement and dye injection. The volume and osmotic load of the dye may rarely cause intravascular expansion and pulmonary edema.

BIBLIOGRAPHY

Buchbinder N, Ganz W: Hemodynamic monitoring: Invasive techniques. Anesthesiology 45:146–155, 1976

Conti CR: Coronary arteriography. Circulation 55:227–237, 1977

Forrester JS, Diamond G, Chatterjee K et al: Medical therapy of acute myocardial infarction by application of hemodynamic subsets. N Engl J Med 295:1356–1362, 1976

3

Coronary Artery Disease

ANGINA PECTORIS

The distinct variety of chest pain called angina pectoris results when the myocardium is starved of oxygen and nutrients because of inadequate coronary circulation. By far the most common cause of angina pectoris is the progressive narrowing of the coronary vessels by atherosclerotic plaques.

Plaque formation often begins as early as adolescence. The lesions are composed of foamy intimal cells and disorganized medial cells surrounded by an interstitium filled with cholesterol. The relatively bountiful coronary circulation provides a large margin of safety, and, with arteriodilation, adequate flow can be maintained in a vessel until the cross-sectional area of the lumen is reduced by more than 85%. However, if myocardial oxygen demand is increased, as occurs with exercise, blood flow may become inadequate even with lesser degrees of obstruction.

A significant reduction of coronary blood flow interferes with myocardial cellular function. Affected areas of the heart become non-contractile and may even bulge outward when the rest of the heart contracts. Abnormalities of the cellular membrane pumps and ionic permeabilities alter·the cellular membrane potentials, and these changes are reflected on the electrocardiogram (EKG) as alterations in the ST segment and T wave. A shift from aerobic to anaerobic metabolism is apparent in the increased amounts of lactate leaving the heart.

Curiously, the quantity and nature of angina are inadequate indicators of the extent of underlying coronary disease. Patients may have no pain despite a frighteningly tenuous vascular supply, or they may complain of intractable discomfort despite evidence of completely patent vessels on a coronary angiogram. Not surprisingly, however, the degree of vascular obstruction correlates closely with the risk of death from heart disease.

The Coronary Vasculature

Two coronary arteries leave the aorta just above the aortic valve. The right coronary artery swings around the right side of the heart, and in 90% of people supplies the atrioventricular node. The left coronary artery divides into two vessels; the left anterior descending artery travels in front of the heart, and the circumflex artery winds around the left lateral segment. In 10% of individuals the circumflex artery continues to supply the

11

atrioventricular node. Thus, in general, the left coronary system supplies most of the left ventricle, and the right coronary system supplies the right ventricle, the A-V node, and a small part of the back of the left ventricle.

Diagnosis and Clinical Manifestations

The diagnosis of angina pectoris should not be made casually, since the stigma of heart disease can adversely affect employment, insurability, and the emotional well-being of the patient and his family. On the other hand, the diagnosis should not be overlooked, since medical or surgical intervention is available that can greatly improve the quality of the patient's life.

The diagnosis of angina is often clear from the characteristic constellation of symptoms and physical findings, and can readily be confirmed by electrocardiographic changes during episodes of pain and by the rapid amelioration of pain with nitroglycerin. If, however, the pain is atypical, the electrocardiogram nonspecific, the patient's response to therapy not convincing, and the etiology of the pain not apparent, further evidence of coronary artery disease must be sought with exercise tests, radionuclide scans, and, eventually, angiography. These studies, however, cannot confirm that the patient is suffering the pain of angina, but only whether he has anatomic coronary disease or physiologic ischemia.

Classically, angina originates in the midchest. It radiates to both arms and down to the fingers or up to the neck. In some patients, the pain may be limited to the chest or to a single area of radiation. Patients often describe anginal pain as a squeezing, tightening pressure, often using a clenched fist in their description. It typically lasts seconds to minutes and is relieved by rest or nitroglycerin. Sharp, stabbing, intermittent, or tingling pain is not as likely to be angina. In its mildest form, angina is infrequent and is precipitated only by activities or emotional states that markedly increase the need of the myocardium for oxygen: e.g., anxiety, exercise, or sudden exposure to the cold. At its worst, angina can incapacitate patients even when they are at rest. Secondary symptoms may accompany the pain, including anxiety, diaphoresis, dyspnea, and nausea.

Certain populations have a disproportionately high risk for coronary artery disease, and the presence of risk factors lends weight to the diagnosis. Most important in the diagnosis of angina are a personal history of smoking, hypertension, high serum cholesterol levels, or diabetes, and a family history suggestive of premature atherosclerosis. The incidence of coronary artery disease in women is low until menopause, but increases dramatically thereafter.

Despite the clear identification of risk factors, attempts to retard the progression of coronary artery disease in adult life by modifying these risk factors have met with little success. The one exception is the patient who can be convinced to stop smoking. It is possible that intervention during adolescence would prove to be more effective in modifying the risk factors of coronary artery disease.

During an anginal episode, physical examination reveals evidence of reflex hemodynamic changes as well as direct detrimental effects of myocardial ischemia. Hypertension and tachycardia are typical. Ischemia of the left ventricle results in a new S_4 gallop. Abnormal splitting of S_2 may also occur. Sometimes a dyskinetic segment of the myocardium becomes palpable and can be distinguished from the apical impulse. A transient mitral regurgitant murmur can be caused by papillary muscle dysfunction. The EKG may reveal ST segment depression and T wave inversion. After the pain is relieved, physical examination usually shows a reversion to normal, and the electrocardiogram may also normalize.

Differential Diagnosis

All chest pain is not ischemia. Some of the more common sources of pain that can be confused with angina include the following.

1. Hyperventilation syndrome occurs in anxious patients who hyperventilate and thus induce symptoms such as sharp chest pain, tingling fingers, tingling lips, and lightheadedness. T wave inversion on the electrocardiogram is common.

2. Tietze's syndrome is an arthritis of the chest wall that especially affects the costochondral joints. The pain can be mimicked by pressure over the offending joint, and it can be relieved by aspirin or other anti-inflammatory agents.

3. Reflux esophagitis causes heartburn owing to laxity of the lower esophageal sphincter, which allows acidic contents to reflux from the stomach, especially when the patient is lying flat. In some patients, *esophageal spasm* causes chest pain following meals. This pain may be especially difficult to distinguish from angina because it can sometimes be relieved by taking nitroglycerin.

4. Aortic dissection is a rare disorder in which the aortic intima tears and blood shears along the vessel wall (Chap. 10). The ripping pain can project to the back and abdomen. The dissection may advance to occlude vessels or cause aortic insufficiency. A chest x-ray may reveal a widened aortic shadow.

Other conditions causing angina-like pain include diseases of the lung (pulmonary embolism), pericardium (pericarditis) and abdomen (peptic ulcer disease and cholecystitis).

Diagnostic Tests

Other diagnostic tests are available and have ancillary roles. Many patients with angina will never need any of these.

Exercise Tests. The patient runs on a treadmill, which varies in speed and in the angle of incline. Symptoms, heart rate, blood pressure and the electrocardiogram (for ST segment depression and arrhythmias) are monitored. In a patient with chest pain, characteristic changes, such as hypotension or persistent depression of the ST segments, indicate with fair accuracy significant underlying coronary disease. False negatives (*i.e.,* a normal test result despite high-grade coronary obstruction) are not infrequent. The exercise test is therefore more useful for confirming the diagnosis of ischemic heart disease than for rejecting it. As might be expected, the predictive value of the test is even less when applied to populations of asymptomatic patients.

Although one might reasonably argue that an exercise test would be unnecessary in a patient with known significant coronary disease (classic angina, prior myocardial infarction, or positive findings on a cardiac catheterization), it can nevertheless help to quantitate the patient's exercise capability and response to surgical and medical intervention. It can also be used to define further a patient's risk profile when either the patient or the physician has reason for concern about coronary artery disease, but not sufficient concern to proceed to the more invasive technique of cardiac catheterization.

Radionuclide Cardiac Imaging. The use of radioactive tracers is becoming popular for noninvasive testing of cardiac function and ischemia. The role of these tracers relative to exercise tests and cardiac catheterization has not been fully evaluated.

Perfusion Scans. Thallium 201 is a photon-emitting substance with biologic properties similar to potassium. It is concentrated inside cells that are functioning normally. Regions of the myocardium that are not perfused or that are ischemic or dead do not concentrate thallium and appear as cold spots on the scan. Reversible ischemia, such as that induced by exercise, is marked by a cold spot that later "warms up" and concentrates the thallium.

Infarct Labeling. Technetium 99 stannous pyrophosphate labels acutely damaged tissue. By 24 to 48 hours following injury, it is rare for a large infarct to be missed by a technetium scan. It has been especially helpful in diagnosing infarction in situations in which serum enzymes or an electrocardiogram can be confusing; for example, when the infarct is limited to the right ventricle, in a patient with a prior left bundle branch block on the electrocardiogram, or following cardiac surgery. It can also be helpful in diagnosing myocardial contusions following blunt trauma. False positive scans, however, are not infrequent, especially in patients with other cardiac disease, such as an aneurysm or valve calcification. The recent development of antibodies to cardiac myosin may soon permit even more precise identification of areas of infarction.

Ventricular Function. Technetium-labeled albumin remains inside the vasculature and highlights the interior of the cardiac chambers. The ejection fraction (percent of diastolic volume ejected during systole) is calculated from a comparison of end-diastolic volumes with end-systolic volumes. Pictures are taken at the same part of sequential cardiac cycles by gating the camera shutter by the electrocardiogram; hence it is called a *gated cardiac scan.* Cycles are superimposed on top of one another to simulate a ventriculogram, so that a repetitive movie of the cardiac cycle can be generated and used to demonstrate aneurysms and intra-atrial masses, and to distinguish local areas of dysfunction and their degree of reversibility.

Differential Diagnosis

(The method and its risks are discussed in Chap. 2). A catheter is advanced from an artery in retrograde fashion into the heart and positioned near a coronary ostium. Radiopaque dye is then injected. Despite large variability in interpretation among observers, the resultant picture is the best antemortem method for diagnosing the severity of coronary atherosclerosis. Lesions that obstruct more than 75% of the cross-sectional area of the lumen of a coronary vessel are felt to be physiologically significant and capable of causing ischemia. Indications for coronary angiography are currently under intense debate, and are discussed in the section on coronary artery bypass surgery.

Therapy

Two types of medicines are available that can dramatically improve the quality of life of patients with angina: nitrates, including nitroglycerin, and β-blockers.

Nitroglycerin (TNG). Nitroglycerin has been employed in the therapy of angina pectoris for nearly a century. It acts (1) by dilating veins, pooling blood, and decreasing venous return (preload), (2) to a lesser extent by dilating peripheral arteries and thereby reducing the afterload, and (3) by increasing coronary collateral flow. More blood can therefore be delivered to the ischemic region while, at the same time, the oxygen needs of the myocardium are diminishing. Nitroglycerin is absorbed within minutes from under the tongue and its effects last up to 20 minutes. Pain relief within one to three minutes is almost—although not completely—diagnostic of the presence of angina. The major side-effect of nitroglycerin is a pounding headache thought to be secondary to dilatation of the meningeal vessels. The headache often abates with continued use of the drug. Although tolerance to some of the hemodynamic effects of nitroglycerin develops in time, its anti-anginal effects do not diminish with continued use. However, failure of a formerly stable patient to respond to nitroglycerin may reflect a loss of tablet potency; this is usually accompanied by the patient's failure to note sublingual burning as the tablet dissolves. Recently, longer-acting nitrate preparations have been developed for oral use. Patients experiencing frequent anginal pain can take *isosorbide dinitrate* every four to six hours or apply nitroglycerin paste as prophylaxis against angina. The use of intravenous nitroglycerin is discussed in the following section on myocardial infarction.

β-Blockade. Specific actions of the sympathomimetic amines (epinephrine, norepinephrine, and isoproterenol) are initiated by their binding to cellular receptors. These receptors have not yet been completely isolated, but have been classified into two broad categories—alpha and beta. Vasoconstriction in the skin is mediated by an alpha receptor on the surface of vascular smooth muscle. Cells of the myocardium and the myocardial conduction system have beta receptors, called β_1, to distinguish them from the β_2 receptors on bronchial and vascular smooth muscle.

Administering β-adrenergic agents or providing a direct stimulation to the sympathetic nerves to the heart increases the heart rate and contractility. These effects can be prevented by a β-blocker; the one most frequently used is *propranolol.* Propranolol decreases the metabolic requirements of the heart by decreasing rate and contractility. Blood pressure and cardiac output generally decrease somewhat as well. Through these effects, propranolol is able to decrease the frequency of anginal attacks.

Propranolol is metabolized mostly in the liver. A large percentage of an oral dose is therefore metabolized before it reaches the systemic circulation. Intravenous administration requires much smaller dosages. Variability in systemic availability and response necessitates titration on a patient-to-patient basis. The dosage is increased until either a good therapeutic response is achieved, side-effects supervene, or maximal β-blockade is achieved (as measured by the prevention of exercise-induced tachycardia).

Most of the side-effects of propranolol follow predictably from the blockade of beta receptors. The diminished contractility can precipitate congestive heart failure in patients with borderline cardiac function. Propranolol can induce A-V block in patients with conduction system disease, and must be used carefully in these patients. The symptoms of hypoglycemia are blunted by propranolol, and the drug therefore removes a valuable warning sign of insulin overdose in diabetics. Propranolol may precipitate bronchospasm in patients with asthma by means of its effects on the bronchial smooth muscle. Recently developed β-receptor antagonists selected to act specifically on the heart (β_1 antagonists) may help to circumvent such pulmonary problems. Abrupt withdrawal of β-blockade in patients with coronary artery disease may precipitate a worsening of angina or even myocardial infarction.

UNSTABLE ANGINA PECTORIS

When the severity or frequency of angina increases precipitously, or when angina begins to appear at rest or during sleep, it is termed unstable angina. The first clue to the onset of unstable angina may be the patient's increased reliance on nitroglycerin. The pain is almost always crippling to the patient, and hospitalization is mandatory. Considered as a group, these patients have significant coronary artery disease and thus a high mortality rate from myocardial infarction. Precipitants of angina, such as congestive heart failure and thyrotoxicosis, must be sought. Patients with unstable angina are not in danger of immediate death, at least with present therapy, but unstable angina does require aggressive treatment. Nitrates (especially isosorbide dinitrate) and β-blockers can almost always relieve the pain. Coronary artery bypass graft surgery relieves pain even more effectively over the long run, but long-term mortality is at present identical with that achieved by medical therapy alone (discussion follows).

As more coronary vessels become involved in the disease process, the prognosis for a patient with unstable angina worsens. Patients with disease of a single vessel (left anterior descending, right coronary, or circumflex artery) do well, and more than 95% survive two years after the diagnosis is made with or without therapeutic intervention. Prior to modern medical and surgical therapy, however, only 70% of patients with three-vessel disease survived two years. The only other reliable prognostic sign is the presence of heart failure, which is a poor sign for the patient's survival.

PRINZMETAL'S ANGINA

Prinzmetal's (variant) angina is a clinical syndrome distinguished by the occurrence of angina at rest with accompanying ST segment elevation and a high frequency of accompanying arrhythmias. Transient coronary artery spasms are probably responsible for many of these episodes. In the catheterization laboratory, patients with Prinzmetal's angina frequently are found to have diffuse coronary artery disease, but may have entirely patent vessels until spasm occurs spontaneously or is pharmacologically provoked (with ergonovine maleate). Prinzmetal's angina can be difficult to control with the usual medical regimen of nitrates and propranolol. In patients with fixed stenoses of the vessels, bypass surgery may be helpful. Nifedipine, an agent that inhibits the influx of calcium into cells, has been demonstrated to prevent coronary spasm and is used in Europe for that purpose.

CATHETERIZATION AND CORONARY ARTERY BYPASS GRAFT (CABG) SURGERY

The CABG is a surgical procedure that complements medical treatment with propranolol and nitrates. The precise indications for the procedure remain the center of heated debate.

The technique was introduced by Favaloro. A saphenous vein is stripped from the leg, its side branches tied off, and the vein connected from a side hole made in the aorta to a coronary artery beyond the site of occlusion. The saphenous vein thus bypasses the occlusion and delivers blood to the distal part of the coronary vessel, enhancing myocardial oxygenation.

The procedure has an operative mortality of 1.5%. At least 90% of the veins remain patent for one year. Nearly 90% of patients experience dramatic relief from their pain. The operation is so effective that angina which is unresponsive to medical therapy is an absolute indication for cardiac catheterization to determine if a CABG is feasible.

Whether the CABG actually prolongs life remains controversial. In patients with disease of the left main coronary artery, the CABG does reduce the 3-year mortality from the 40% expected with medical therapy alone to 17%. In patients with disease of the right coronary artery, circumflex artery, or left anterior descending artery, the procedure appears to have little effect on longevity, and in patients with two- or three-vessel disease the data is still inconclusive.

Coronary artery catheterization is performed to outline the anatomy of disease, to help choose between medical and surgical therapy, to facilitate surgery, and to obtain a prognostic index. In more than 40% of patients with angina who undergo catheterization, the question of whether to operate is settled to everyone's satisfaction: 10% will have disease of the left main artery (and therefore undergo CABG), 20% will have insignificant disease or disease of only one vessel, and 10% will have lesions that appear to be surgically inoperable.

Despite the potential value of the information obtained, the decision to perform catheterization should not be made lightly, since the procedure is uncomfortable for the patient and carries the risk of stroke, myocardial infarction, and even death. The most conservative cardiologists choose to perform catheterization only in patients with refractory angina and to operate only for relief of pain. Others study any patient with evidence of coronary artery disease and bypass any approachable lesion. Probably the most reasonable approach lies somewhere between these extremes. One is more apt to perform catheterization in younger patients, in patients with diffuse anterior electrocardiographic changes or hypotension that appear with angina or during exercise testing (although these changes correlate only poorly with the extent of disease), and in patients whose symptomatology is that of unstable angina. A CABG should be reserved for those with refractory symptoms or with left main artery disease. However, if a single tenuous vessel supplies the entire left ventricle, and the other vessels are occluded to the extent that one hemorrhage into a plaque could lead to destruction of the whole anterior wall, many believe that vessel should be bypassed.

A new therapy that is now undergoing investigation and producing some exciting results is *coronary angioplasty*. In this procedure, a small balloon is inserted into a coronary vessel by means of a catheter and inflated within the lumen directly beneath the obstruction. The balloon flattens the plaque into the vessel wall and restores vessel patency. Coronary angioplasty can be performed in the cardiac catheterization laboratory and, when successful, obviates the need for surgery.

MYOCARDIAL INFARCTION

When myocardial cells are deprived of their blood supply, they lose the ability to contract and soon die. The result is a myocardial infarction, or "heart attack." Atherosclerosis underlies virtually all cases of myocardial infarction. The precipitating event is often an acute occlusion of a coronary vessel from thrombosis of, or subintimal hemorrhage into, an atherosclerotic plaque. Permanent total vessel occlusion is not necessary for infarction to occur.

The size of the infarct depends upon the location of the occlusion, the extent of collateral blood supply, and the oxygen requirements of the heart. Oxygen demands increase with tachycardia, increasing contractility and systolic pressure, and increasing the diameter of the heart (because of additional tension on the chamber walls). In some cases, the vessel may be only intermittently occluded; arterial spasm is often more important than thrombosis early in a myocardial infarction.

Anterior Myocardial Infarction

Infarction of the anterior wall of the left ventricle is caused by occlusion of the left coronary system—either the left main coronary artery, the left anterior descending artery, the circumflex artery, or their major branches.

The hemodynamic problems that the patient will encounter depend upon the extent of the myocardium that is compromised. If the infarct affects 20% to 25% of the left ventricle, the ventricle can no longer empty adequately. As the infarct enlarges, end diastolic pressures rise with resultant pulmonary edema. With loss of 40% of the left ventricle, significant pump failure supervenes, blood pressure falls, and usually the patient dies. This last state, marked by the combination of low blood pressure and pulmonary edema, is called *cardiogenic shock*. As the size of the infarct increases, so does the incidence of arrhythmias.

Inferior Myocardial Infarction

Infarction of the inferior, diaphragmatic myocardium is caused by occlusion of the right coronary artery. Because the right coronary artery supplies most of the right ventricle and only a small part of the left ventricle, the syndrome of inferior myocardial infarction is very different from anterior infarction. Left ventricular function is usually maintained without pulmonary edema or cardiogenic shock, and the right ventricle may become transiently or sometimes permanently dysfunctional. The right ventricle usually generates such small pressures, however, that even when the right ventricle is reduced to a passive conduit, blood pressure can be maintained by providing volume infusions and thereby improving venous return. Venous blood can then reach the lungs without the need for an actively pumping right ventricle.

The patient with an inferior myocardial infarction and right ventricular involvement is thus said to have *volume-dependent* blood pressure, and requires infusions of saline despite elevations in venous pressures; this is clearly in contrast to the patient with a large anterior infarction who can develop pulmonary edema if given too much fluid, and who may require catecholamines to support his blood pressure.

In 90% of people, the right coronary artery also provides the blood supply to the A-V node, and A-V nodal ischemia and edema can cause frequent transient episodes of heart block. Patients with an inferior myocardial infarction frequently progress from first degree heart block to second degree block and even to complete heart block (see Chap. 4). A temporary pacemaker may be required if the heart block is hemodynamically significant and fails to respond to atropine. Usually, however, heart block is only transient and poses little danger to the patient.

Parasympathetic reflexes are triggered in patients with right ventricular myocardial infarctions, manifested by cholinergic symptoms, often referred to as "vagal" symptoms. The patient frequently appears pale and pasty and complains of nausea and vomiting. Bradycardia is often severe and should be treated with atropine. Cells responsible for the initiation of these reflexes are thought to lie in the distribution of the right coronary artery.

An inferior myocardial infarction cannot, however, be distinguished from an anterior myocardial infarction either by the nature of the pain or by the incidence of ventricular ectopy, ventricular fibrillation, atrial arrhythmias, or cardiac enzyme levels.

Subendocardial Myocardial Infarction

The inner third of the myocardium, nearest the ventricular cavity, is called the subendocardium. The subendocardium is especially susceptible to ischemia, because its nutrient vessels are completely occluded during systole by the high intramuscular pressures generated by the contracting heart. With coronary atherosclerotic narrowing, the situation is exacerbated. Infarctions are therefore frequently not transmural (*i.e.*, across the full thickness of the myocardium), but are often limited to the more vulnerable subendocardium.

Subendocardial infarctions are just as dangerous as transmural infarctions. The incidence of arrhythmias is identical, and shock can ensue if the area of necrosis is large enough or if the myocardium has been compromised by previous infarcts. Electrocardiographic localization of the infarct is difficult, because the electrocardiogram only poorly reflects subendocardial electrical activity.

Signs and Symptoms of Myocardial Infarction ↑BP ↑HR S₃/S₄

Myocardial infarctions may be accompanied by pain similar to that of angina. If preceded by chronic angina, the pain of infarction may be identical, more prolonged and severe, in a different distribution, or distinguished by unresponsiveness to nitroglycerin. The patient may complain primarily of non-specific anxiety or dyspnea. Inferior myocardial infarctions may be accompanied by evidence of heightened parasympathetic activity: bradycardia, nausea, and vomiting.

Not infrequently, myocardial infarctions are silent. The diagnosis of infarction can be especially difficult in the elderly patient. Syncope, confusion, agitation, or pain suggestive of abdominal disease can be the presenting complaint.

The distinction between a myocardial infarction and an acute episode of angina without infarction can be difficult to make solely on clinical grounds, and may ultimately depend on an evaluation of the EKG and cardiac enzyme abnormalities (see following sections).

On physical examination, the blood pressure and heart rate are usually increased, and diaphoresis may be noted. Bulging of the neck veins suggests chronic or acute right ventricular failure; the neck veins do not accurately reflect left ventricular function. Auscultation may reveal a soft S_1 that is not sharp. S_3 and S_4 gallops may be present. The infarcted myocardium may bulge dyskinetically and can

then be felt as a rocking motion distinct from the apical impulse.

Other findings reflect the development of complications: an irregular pulse suggests ectopic beats, an apical murmur may reflect mitral regurgitation from papillary muscle dysfunction, rales may indicate pulmonary edema, and vasoconstriction may presage hypotension and cardiogenic shock.

Electrocardiogram

Clinicopathological correlation has shown that focal myocardial infarctions are best reflected in specific leads: Inferior infarctions are visible in leads II, III, and aVF, extensive anterior wall infarctions in leads V_1 through V_6, and high lateral wall infarctions in leads I and aVL.

Classic electrocardiographic evidence of infarction has three components:

1. **Q waves:** the progressive loss of R waves, with the eventual appearance of a QS complex, suggests transmural death of myocardium. However, the correlation between pathologic evidence of transmural infarction and the electrocardiographic appearance of Q waves is far from perfect.

2. **ST segment changes:** ST segment elevation, with the segment bowed like a hill, suggests injury. It is thought to be secondary to the loss of normal myocardial cell membrane ion pumps. ST segment elevation classically has been taken to suggest a transmural infarction, and ST segment depression to reflect ischemia or subendocardial infarction.

3. **T wave changes:** the first evidence of myocardial infarction is the peaking of T waves. Later, they become inverted. If a patient's T waves are inverted chronically, the peaking may make them look normal, a process referred to as "pseudonormalization."

Because ischemia, injury, and infarction occur in neighboring regions of the heart, ST segment and T wave changes and the appear-

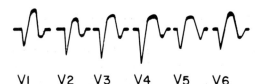

VI   V2   V3   V4   V5   V6

FIG. 3–1. The chest leads to an electrocardiogram taken on a patient during an acute transmural, anterior myocardial infarction. Note the presence of Q waves, elevated ST segments, and inverted T waves.

ance of Q waves often occur together. In general, ST segment and T wave changes appear over the first minutes to hours of infarction, and Q waves appear over days. Thus, an evolving myocardial infarction might first manifest peaked T waves, followed by ST segment elevation and T wave inversion. Eventually, Q waves would appear. In a large anterior wall infarction, these changes would be most noticeable in leads V_1 through V_6 (Fig. 3–1). Inferior leads might show a mild ST depression; this is not believed to represent additional disease, but rather to be caused by reciprocal electrical changes.

In many cases, however, the EKG is unreliable in diagnosing and localizing a myocardial infarction. This is because: (1) some regions of the heart are electrocardiographically silent; (2) previously undiagnosed myocardial infarctions may modify or even cancel any acute changes; and (3) many nonischemic events (hyperventilation, anxiety, certain drugs, pulmonary emboli, pericarditis, and abdominal pathology) can mimic a myocardial infarction on the EKG, especially by causing ST segment and T wave alterations. In addition, the electrocardiogram cannot always accurately predict whether the infarction is transmural or subendocardial.

Cardiac Enzymes

The dying myocardial cells release their contents into the cardiac lymphatics and the bloodstream, and the increased concentration of myocardial enzymes can be measured in the peripheral blood after a myocardial infarction. These include the SGOT (serum glutamic oxaloacetic transaminase), LDH (lactic dehydrogenase), and CPK (creatine phosphokinase). Their concentrations peak at different times after an infarct. CPK rises within hours, and SGOT and LDH appear later during the first 24 hours. By three to four days, the CPK and SGOT have decreased to normal, whereas the LDH diminishes more slowly over the next two weeks.

Since these enzymes are not restricted to myocardial cells, their elevation may represent damage to other organs. For example, SGOT and LDH are released during liver necrosis, and CPK during skeletal muscle ischemia. The structure of the protein CPK varies among different organs, and a specific myocardial subgroup (the MB isoenzyme) can be distinguished. LDH isoenzymes have also been identified. The recognition and measurement of isoenzymes has enhanced the specificity of the diagnosis of myocardial infarction.

If the blood is drawn at appropriate times, all myocardial infarctions are accompanied by an elevation of these enzymes, and the extent of elevation roughly correlates with the size of the infarction.

Course and Management of Myocardial Infarction

Three components are used to make the diagnosis of infarction: medical history, EKG, and cardiac enzymes. Usually, only a history and EKG are immediately available when the patient reaches the emergency room, and these are often nondiagnostic. Enzymatic confirmation awaits repeated blood sampling.

Initiation of therapy does not require absolute confirmation of an infarction. If a brief history raises any serious suspicions of an infarction, an intravenous catheter should be inserted and electrocardiographic monitoring should be started even before the decision is made to admit the patient to the hospital. Even in the absence of a confirmatory electrocardiogram, patients with a convincing history deserve admission.

If a myocardial infarction seems likely, the next step is to institute pain relief and begin prophylaxis against arrhythmias. Morphine should be given intravenously or subcutaneously to relieve pain; an intramuscular injection will cause a misleading rise in the CPK that can only be resolved by isoenzyme determinations. If a prolonged bout of angina, rather than infarction, is suspected, sublingual nitroglycerin may be effective. A constant intravenous infusion of lidocaine should be started, whether or not the patient manifests ventricular ectopy. This should be preceded by a loading dose. The risk of sudden death from ventricular fibrillation or ventricular tachycardia is extraordinarily high, and is one of the reasons that many patients with myocardial infarctions die before reaching the hospital. A lidocaine infusion continued for two days decreases the incidence of ventricular fibrillation.

Previously, antiarrhythmic therapy was delayed until the appearance of *malignant irritability*. (Malignant irritability is defined as [1] several premature ventricular beats in a row, [2] more than five premature ventricular beats in a minute, or [3] beats deriving from multiple origins of ectopy.) Continuous monitoring has revealed, however, that the majority of patients have short periods of malignant irritability, and that many patients have ventricular fibrillation without preceding ventricular ectopy. There is, therefore, no reason to delay lidocaine therapy.

Once the steps previously described have been carried out, the patient should be admitted to an intensive care unit. If, after two days, daily electrocardiograms and enzymes have not revealed an infarction, the patient may go home. Unstable angina requires further in-hospital evaluation. If the patient has an infarction, he should remain in the hospital for approximately two weeks. The first three days should include enforced bed rest; then the patient should progress to sitting and gradual ambulation. Standard orders include a stool softener and milk of magnesia to prevent constipation and straining, and a mild sedative to decrease some of the anxiety associated with confinement to an intensive care unit. Continuous low flow oxygen and antihypertensive medicines are given for reasons that will be discussed in the following section.

Next, steps are taken to prevent and treat complications. The risk of the two serious complications of myocardial infarctions— ventricular arrhythmias and cardiogenic shock—is proportional to the size of the infarct.

In the early hours of coronary occlusion, the region of the myocardium that is threatened by ischemia is not completely infarcted. The viability of some cells can be salvaged by decreasing their oxygen requirements. Thus, hypertension, tachycardia, and the cardiomegaly of congestive heart failure, all of which increase the need for oxygen, should be treated. Blood pressure should not be brought below what is normal for the patient's age, or else the coronary flow may be compromised. Hypoxemia and anemia reduce oxygen delivery, and both should be corrected. Enhancement of the Pa_{O_2} to supranormal levels by nasal-prong delivery of oxygen-enriched air may also be of some benefit.

In some centers, more aggressive attempts have been made to restore some blood flow before the infarction is completed. This therapy includes intravenous nitroglycerin, the assistance of an intra-aortic balloon pump (described later in this chapter), or emergency surgical revascularization. At present, such techniques are experimental, and it is not known whether these efforts to reduce infarct size improve long-term mortality.

Complications

Arrhythmias. Most deaths from myocardial infarction occur within the first hours and are due to arrhythmias. The majority of such deaths occur at home. Early monitoring has shown that these arrhythmic deaths are due to both bradyarrhythmias and tachyarrhythmias.

Ventricular Arrhythmias. Ventricular tachycardia, and especially ventricular fibrillation, are lethal arrhythmias. Prophylactic lidocaine administration appears to diminish their incidence. It is probably wise to add quinidine and procainamide to the regimen of patients who present with ventricular tachycardia or ventricular fibrillation, or who continue to have malignant ventricular premature beats (VPBs) on lidocaine therapy.

Therapy must then be reassessed toward the end of hospitalization. The one-year mortality for patients with myocardial infarctions following hospital discharge is about 10%. This mortality appears to be unrelated to the arrhythmic complications that occur early in the course of the infarction. However, the mortality is substantially higher in patients who at discharge manifest malignant VPBs or who have evidence of heart failure. These deaths sometimes occur as a result of a new infarction, but many die a purely arrhythmic and sudden death. Evidence has begun to accumulate that long-term mortality after infarction can be decreased by the chronic use of appropriate antiarrhythmic medications.

Supraventricular Arrhythmias. Many patients with an inferior myocardial infarction manifest sinus bradycardia, usually from heightened parasympathetic tone. Sinus bradycardia is usually well tolerated by the patient. Sinus tachycardia is usually a secondary rhythm disturbance associated with anxiety, fever, or heart failure. Significant supraventricular tachycardias occur in about 10% of patients with myocardial infarctions, regardless of the site of infarction. Some of these arrhythmias derive from concomitant pericarditis, and others probably from atrial infarction. Most supraventricular tachycardias are transient, consisting only of a burst of paroxysmal atrial tachycardia, and are often so brief that they require no therapy. The ventricular rate of atrial fibrillation or atrial flutter can usually be controlled with digoxin. If these arrhythmias are associated with recurrent ischemia or hypotension, electrical cardioversion will be required.

Heart Block. In patients with inferior myocardial infarctions, A-V nodal block is due to ischemia of the A-V node. Nodal dysfunction may progress from first degree to third degree A-V block, but is almost always transient. The escape rhythm usually manifests a narrow QRS complex, suggesting an origin above or high in the bundle of His. Such heart block is usually hemodynamically insignificant and can be remedied with atropine. The heart rate occasionally decreases to less than 45, and a temporary pacemaker is required.

On the other hand, complete heart block during an anterior myocardial infarction implies extensive damage to the ventricular septum with destruction of the right bundle and both fascicles of the left bundle of His. Complete heart block may appear abruptly. The rate may be slow and the QRS may widen, because the escape pacemaker lies below the damaged bundle of His. A transvenous pacemaker can prevent syncope that is due to the slow escape rate. It is prudent to insert such a pacemaker in a patient with an anterior myocardial infarction who has electrocardiographic evidence of damage to both the right bundle and even just one fascicle of the left (*i.e.*, right bundle branch block and left anterior hemi-block), or evidence of involvement of all three branches (Mobitz type 2 heart block), since these patients may progress to complete heart block. Therapy may be futile, however, since patients with complete heart block and an anterior myocardial infarction frequently die of cardiogenic shock.

Cardiogenic Shock. As an infarct expands, systolic function progressively deteriorates and cardiac output diminishes. Left ventricular end-diastolic pressures rise and pulmonary edema may result. Selective arterial beds are vasoconstricted to support the blood pressure. Aggressive therapy during this preshock stage may salvage some ischemic, noninfarcted myocardium and may make the patient more comfortable. Pulmonary edema must be treated with oxygen, morphine, and diuretics, and the left ventricle must be unloaded (see Chap. 7).

Once the sum of past and recent infarctions has destroyed 40% of the left ventricle, the syndrome of full-blown cardiogenic shock may supervene with hypotension, pulmonary edema, oliguria, clammy skin, confusion, and agitation. Patients with these symptoms have a cardiac index below 2.2 liters/m² and a pulmonary capillary wedge pressure above 18 torr. The majority of patients in cardiogenic shock die.

Effective and accurate therapy necessitates rapid placement of arterial and Swan-Ganz catheters to allow hemodynamic monitoring and measurement of the cardiac output (see Chap. 2). It is possible that there may be some reversible components—hypovolemia, arrhythmias, or the effects of drugs with myocardial depressant effects—that can be aggressively remedied.

Hypotension may require the use of inotropic agents. *Dopamine* directly enhances cardiac contractility and dilates some critical vascular beds (especially the renal), but the drug also increases myocardial oxygen re-

quirements. *Norepinephrine* is a more potent peripheral vasoconstrictor. It has less effect on the myocardium and may dramatically raise the blood pressure. Unlike dopamine, however, it may exacerbate the regional (especially renal) hypoperfusion. Norepinephrine may therefore be preferred early in an infarction when some of the myocardium may still be salvageable, and dopamine can be used later when persistent low cardiac output threatens the patient with multi-organ failure.

In some instances, refractory shock has been reversed by mechanical assistance with an intra-aortic balloon pump. The balloon is introduced through the femoral artery and advanced to the aorta. It inflates during diastole, when the aortic valve is closed, thereby pumping blood to all vascular beds, including the coronary vessels. The balloon collapses during systole, and thus helps to suck blood out of the compromised left ventricle. In most patients, the balloon is able to reverse shock, but death will eventually occur unless emergency surgical revascularization can be accomplished.

Ventricular Rupture. Ventricular rupture is a catastrophic event. Rupture may occur through the free wall or the ventricular septum, especially during the early days following infarction when the myocardium has not yet had time to scar. Ten per cent of deaths from myocardial infarction are caused by ventricular rupture. Free wall rupture presents as sudden hypotension with continued electrical activity (electromechanical dissociation; see Chap. 1) and often with renewed chest pain. *SYMPT.* A pericardiocentesis will reveal blood. A ventricular septal rupture presents as a new systolic parasternal murmur with accompanying hemodynamic deterioration. The diagnosis can be confirmed by catheterization of the right side of the heart. Immediate surgical repair is mandatory.

Recurrent or Persistent Ischemia and Pain. Certain components contributing to new or refractory ischemia, including arrhythmias, congestive failure, and hypertension, may be treatable. The aggressiveness of further therapy must be tempered by the age of the patient and the availability of facilities. Four therapeutic steps should be attempted in the following order:

1. Narcotics can be given in an attempt to relieve pain.

2. Nitrates should be tried. They reduce both venous return and peripheral resistance, thereby decreasing the work of the heart. In addition, they redistribute coronary blood flow. Sublingual nitroglycerin or isosorbide dinitrate (and, eventually, intravenous nitroglycerin) may be given. The blood pressure should be monitored continuously. Amelioration of ischemia may be marked by a return to the baseline of elevated ST segments.

3. Intra-aortic balloon pumps are often effective if medical therapy fails to relieve the pain.

4. Myocardial revascularization (coronary artery bypass graft surgery) is a last resort and can be performed even in the throes of infarction. At present, evidence suggests that myocardial revascularization may be helpful in patients who cannot be weaned from intravenous nitrates or the intra-aortic balloon pump.

Emboli. Pulmonary emboli, originating from thrombi in the deep veins of the legs or from the right ventricle, and systemic emboli originating from the left ventricle are common complications of infarction. Anticoagulation cannot be universally recommended, but its use seems prudent in patients with congestive heart failure, evidence of deep venous thrombosis, or ventricular aneurysm. Low dose, subcutaneous heparin is a sensible prophylaxis for most patients at bed rest.

Mitral Regurgitation. An apical murmur of mitral regurgitation can frequently be heard following infarction, but it is usually hemodynamically insignificant. Mitral regurgitation is due to dysfunction of the ischemic papillary muscles or the subjacent myocardium. The murmur often disappears after the first few days. Rarely, the papillary muscle infarcts and ruptures. This is a catastrophic event, and few patients survive long enough to undergo surgical repair.

Pericarditis. Pericarditis is a common accompaniment of the early days of a transmural infarction. It can present with an auscultatory rub, pleuritic or position-dependent chest pain, or elevation of the ST segment. Pericarditis can be confused with recurrent ischemia, but does not usually pose a danger to the patient.

Dressler's Syndrome. Approximately 3% of patients exhibit a complex syndrome of clinical findings within days to months following a myocardial infarction. They present with evidence of pericarditis, pleuritis, myalgias, arthralgias, fever, leukocytosis, and an increased erythrocyte sedimentation rate. If these patients are anticoagulated, there is a significantly increased risk of hemorrhage into the pericardium.

Home Care Versus Hospitalization

The final firm scar does not form until about six weeks after the infarction. Although, in the past, six weeks was mandated as the length of hospital stay, it now appears that a two-week hospital sojourn is equally safe. Evidence from a large study in England further suggests that patients with uncomplicated myocardial infarctions who have survived the first hours of an infarct may fare as well at home as in the hospital.

Bibliography

Braunwald E, Maroko PR: Limitation of infarct size. Curr Probl Cardiol 3, No. 1:10–51, 1978

Borhani NO: Primary prevention of coronary heart disease: A critique. Am J Cardiol 40:251–259, 1977

Cohn JN, Guiha NH, Broder MI et al: Right ventricular infarction: clinical and hemodynamic features. Am J Cardiol 33:209–214, 1974

Dellipiani AW, Colling WA, Donaldson RJ et al: Teeside coronary survey—Fatality and comparative severity of patients treated at home, in the hospital ward, and in the coronary care unit after myocardial infarction. Br Heart J 39:1172–1178, 1977

Fortuin NJ, Weiss JL: Exercise stress testing. Circulation 56:699–712, 1977

Gordon T, Castelli WP, Hjortland MC et al: High density lipoprotein as a protective factor against coronary heart disease: The Framingham Study. Am J Med 62:707–714, 1977

Johnson AD: Management of variant angina and coronary spasm. Hosp Pract 13:57–64, 1978

Julian DG: Towards preventing coronary death from ventricular fibrillation. Circulation 54:360–364, 1976

Lie KI, Wellens HJJ, Downar E et al: Observations on patients with primary ventricular fibrillation complicating acute myocardial infarction. Circulation 52:755–759, 1975

Schulze RA, Strauss HW, Pitt B: Sudden death in the year following myocardial infarction: Relation to premature ventricular contractions in the late hospital phase and left ventricular ejection fraction. Am J Med 62:192–199, 1977

McNamara JJ, Molot MA, Stremple JF et al: Coronary artery disease in combat casualties in Vietnam. JAMA 216:1185–1187, 1971

Strauss HW, Pitt B: Evaluation of cardiac function and structure with radioactive tracer techniques. Circulation 57:645–654, 1978

Unstable angina pectoris: National cooperative study group to compare medical and surgical therapy. II. In-hospital experience and initial follow-up results in patients with one, two and three vessel disease. Am J Cardiol 42:839–848, 1978

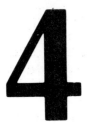

Cardiac Arrhythmias

Sinus Rhythm

Normal sinus rhythm is generated by specialized pacemaker cells located in the sinus node of the right atrium. When these cells are removed into a Petri dish, they depolarize spontaneously about once every second. In the atrium, they serve as the locus of initiation of the heartbeat. A wave of depolarization spreads outward from the pacemaker cells along specialized conducting tissue of the atria to reach the A-V node. This wave causes atrial contraction, and is marked by the P wave on the electrocardiogram (Fig. 4–1). After a delay of about 100 milliseconds in the A-V node, the wave continues down the Purkinje fibers of the His bundle and depolarizes the myocardium, inscribing the QRS complex on the electrocardiogram, and causing ventricular contraction. Repolarization of the myocardial cells follows and is reflected as the T wave on the electrocardiogram.

Nonsinus Pacemakers

The sinus node is not the only pacemaker tissue, but it is generally the fastest pacer, and under normal circumstances the fastest pacer runs the heart, overdriving all other potential renegade pacemakers. The normal sinus rate is between 60 and 100 beats per minute. However, if the sinus dies or slows excessively, cells located near the A-V node may begin to drive the heart at their intrinsic rate of 45 to 60 beats per minute. If these cells fail, cells within the ventricle may take over at what is often an inadequately slow rate of 35 to 45 beats per minute.

There are other situations in which a nonsinus mechanism can run the heart:

1. If one of the slower pacers accelerates, it can outrun the sinus and take over the heart. Such foci are said to be *ectopic.*

2. Under abnormal circumstances, when neighboring muscle cells are not simultaneously depolarized, a *re-entry loop* can form. Normally, two neighboring pieces of muscle tissue (A and B) are depolarized simultaneously (Fig. 4–2). But if path B conducts impulses in only one direction (retrograde), and if antegrade conduction in path A is slowed, the wave of depolarization will rush down path A and then return along path B, by which time path A will have recovered from its refractory period and be able to conduct again. Thus, a continuous, autonomous loop is formed. Impulses can leave the loop and drive the heart.

26

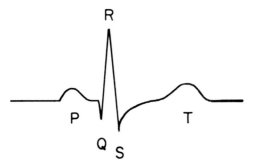

FIG. 4–1. The normal electrocardiogram.

rate or rhythm. There are three steps in the interpretation of any arrhythmia:

1. Determine whether the heart is beating too rapidly (tachycardia, greater than 100 beats per minute), too slowly (bradycardia, less than 60 beats per minute), or irregularly.

2. Locate the pacemaker that is driving the heart. (That is, is it the sinus node, the A-V node, or extranodal tissue?)

3. Search for any underlying illness that may have precipitated the arrhythmia.

SINUS NODE ARRHYTHMIAS

Interpreting Arrhythmias

An arrhythmia is any abnormality of cardiac

Determining the site of origin of an arrhythmia can be difficult. If P waves of normal contour precede each QRS complex, the mech-

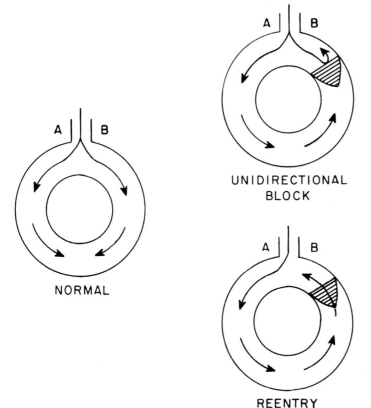

UNIDIRECTIONAL
BLOCK

NORMAL

REENTRY

FIG. 4–2. The mechanism by which unidirectorial block can precipitate reentrant arrhythmias. The hatched lines on pathway B represent a region of unidirectional block, through which a wave traveling only in one direction can be propagated.

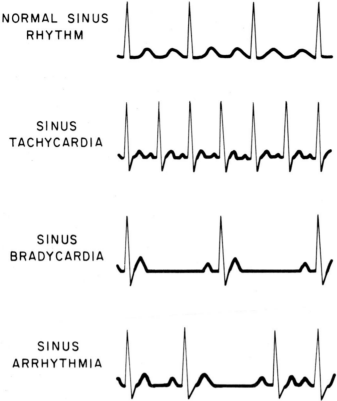

NORMAL SINUS
RHYTHM

SINUS
TACHYCARDIA

SINUS
BRADYCARDIA

SINUS
ARRHYTHMIA

FIG. 4–3. Normal sinus rhythm at a rate of 60 beats per minute, sinus tachycardia at a rate of 120 per minute, sinus bradycardia at a rate of 40 per minute, and sinus arrhythmia at an irregular rate.

anism is likely to be sinus in origin. Variations in the sinus rate are common because of the sensitivity of the sinus to neural input and circulating catecholamines. *Sinus tachycardia* (Fig. 4–3) occurs with strenuous exercise or strong emotion. A chronic *sinus bradycardia* may be present in the athlete. Most normal people experience some variability from beat to beat, called *sinus arrhythmia*, owing to the respiratory effects of atrial filling, with the heart rate reflexly increasing during inspiration.

Sinus tachycardia can, however, be caused by underlying disease and can reflect (1) a response to serious stress, as in hypoxemia or fever; (2) an attempt to maintain cardiac output in the face of hemorrhage, dehydration, or inadequate myocardial pumping (congestive heart failure); or (3) irritation of the sinus node (pericarditis or atrial infarction). It can also be the only clue to otherwise apathetic hyperthyroidism.

Sinus bradycardia may reflect increasing vagal discharge from reflexes triggered during nausea, or it may reflect an inferior myocardial infarction. Additionally, sinus bradycardia may be associated with hypothyroidism.

The loss of normal sinus arrhythmia may be associated with dysfunction of normal autonomic reflexes, and is seen as part of the dysautonomia of diabetes mellitus.

Ordinarily, therapy for sinus bradycardia and sinus tachycardia consists solely of treatment of underlying diseases. However, severe and symptomatic sinus bradycardia may at times require cardiac pacing.

ATRIAL ARRHYTHMIAS

If normal P waves are not identifiable, the EKG should be scanned for abnormal P waves. Bizarre and variable P waves suggest that various ectopic atrial foci are taking their turn driving the heart. This type of arrhythmia is known as a *wandering atrial pacemaker* (Fig. 4–4), which in itself is not clinically significant. If the rate accelerates to more than 100 beats per minute, it is known as *multifocal atrial tachycardia*, not uncommonly seen in patients with chronic lung disease or pulmonary embolism.

The next step is to determine whether the pacemaker is located in the atria, the A-V node, or the ventricles. If the QRS complex is narrow and normal in appearance, activation within the ventricles must have progressed over the normal pathways, and the pacemaker must be in the A-V node or above. Inverted P waves, which may proceed or follow the QRS complex, may represent retrograde conduction from the ventricles. In this instance, there is a P wave associated with each QRS complex, but the primary pacemaker lies below the atria.

Arrhythmias that arise within or above the A-V node are called *supraventricular arrhyth-* mias. There are three common supraventricular arrhythmias: *atrial fibrillation, paroxysmal atrial tachycardia,* and *atrial flutter.*

Atrial fibrillation (Fig. 4–5) is a common disorder in which multiple atrial foci "fire" independently, bombarding the A-V node with more than 300 discharges every minute. The ventricular response is irregular and depends on the refractoriness of the A-V node. Rates may vary anywhere from 30 to 300 beats per minute. The hemodynamic effects of atrial fibrillation result from the loss of atrial "kick" and from heart rates that are too slow or too fast to maintain cardiac output. Atrial fibrillation is easily recognized on the EKG. The undulating baseline reflects the shivering, noncontracting atrium. The electrocardiogram is devoid of formed P waves, and the QRS complexes are spaced irregularly. Atrial fibrillation occurs in many varieties of cardiac and noncardiac disease. It may reflect atrial stretch (a factor in mitral stenosis) or ischemia (myocardial infarction), and can accompany hyperthyroidism or pulmonary embolism. Atrial fibrillation may occur in paroxysms, but it is often a stable rhythm and can last many years.

In *atrial flutter*, the atria contain a small re-entrant pathway circulating at about 300 times per minute and giving rise to regular atrial flutter waves (Fig. 4–6). The number of waves that gets through to the ventricles again depends upon the refractoriness of the A-V node, and may vary from beat to beat. The ventricular response is usually regular or regularly irregular. Atrial flutter is seen in the

FIG. 4–4. A wandering atrial pacemaker. Note the irregularities in the shape of the P wave as well as the irregular rhythm.

WANDERING
ATRIAL
PACEMAKER

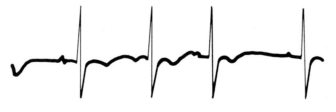

atrial fib = irreg.
flutter = reg or reg irreg.

ATRIAL
FIBRILLATION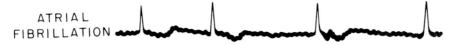

FIG. 4–5. Note the absence of formed P waves and the irregular rhythm.

same diseases in which atrial fibrillation is seen. Atrial flutter is an unstable rhythm and frequently reverts to normal sinus rhythm or changes to atrial fibrillation.

Paroxysmal atrial tachycardia (PAT) is also a re-entrant circuit. Its rate is slower than atrial flutter, ranging between 140 and 220 beats per minute. P waves are usually not visible. The most important physiologic distinction between PAT and atrial flutter is that the reentrant circuit in PAT includes the A-V node. PAT can accompany myocardial injury, but in healthy hearts it frequently is an intermittent phenomenon. In some people it can be triggered by caffeine, nicotine, or the catecholamines used in antiasthmatic medications. PAT may also be a problem in the Wolff-Parkinson-White syndrome in which an accessory muscle bundle bypasses the A-V node producing an anatomic reentry loop.

Carotid Sinus Massage. Recognizing the irregularity of atrial fibrillation is fairly easy. It is more difficult to categorize a regular supraventricular tachycardia that is going at a rate of 150 beats per minute. The possibilities include sinus tachycardia, paroxysmal atrial tachycardia, and atrial flutter in which only one of every two atrial beats gets through to the ventricle (2:1 block). Carotid sinus massage provides a means to distinguish among these possibilities.

The carotid sinus lies at the bifurcation of the internal and external carotids, just under the angle of the jaw near the thyroid cartilage (Fig. 4–7). It contains the carotid baroreceptor. Increasing blood pressure stretches the baro-

receptor and triggers a reflex decrease in the heart rate. The baroreceptor cannot distinguish between internal and external pressure, and can be "fooled" into triggering a vagal reflex by gentle external massage. The patient must be lying flat and should be monitored continuously. The procedure is not without risk, and several precautions should be observed:

1. Never press both carotids simultaneously, or blood flow to the cortex may be totally occluded.

2. Always listen first over the carotid artery to ensure that there are no bruits. Dislodging an arteriosclerotic plaque may result in a cerebrovascular accident.

3. Have resuscitation equipment nearby. Some carotid baroreceptors are so sensitive that massage may precipitate cardiac arrest.

4. Never press the carotid artery for more than a few seconds.

With gentle pressure to the carotid artery, sinus tachycardia will slow gradually and reaccelerate upon release, making the P waves more easily visible. In atrial flutter the ventricular response will slow in a regular fashion (that is, 2:1, 3:1, and so on) as the A-V node becomes more refractory under vagal influ-

FIG. 4–6. Note the saw-tooth "flutter" waves that are conducted to the ventricle with degrees of block varying from 2:1 to 4:1.

ATRIAL
FLUTTER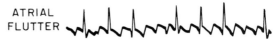

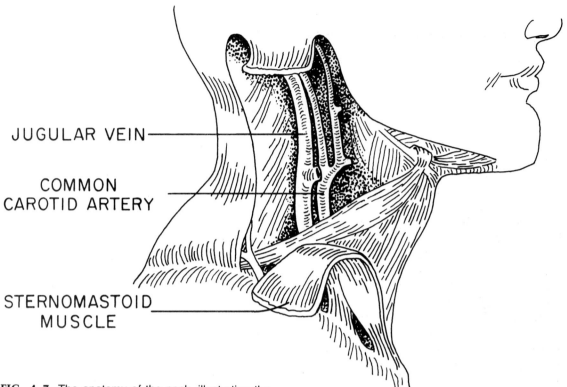

JUGULAR VEIN

COMMON
CAROTID ARTERY

STERNOMASTOID
MUSCLE

FIG. 4–7. The anatomy of the neck, illustrating the relationship of the jugular vein, the common carotid artery, and the sternomastoid muscle. The bifurcation of the common carotid artery is shown; this is the point at which gentle pressure should be applied during carotid sinus massage.

ence. Flutter waves may become visible. PAT may revert abruptly to normal sinus rhythm with carotid sinus pressure because the reentrant circuit involves the A-V node.

Treatment of Atrial Arrhythmias

The urgency of intervention depends on the degree of hemodynamic compromise, the patient's symptoms, and the cause of the arrhythmia. For example, a patient with mitral stenosis who is chronically in atrial fibrillation with a ventricular response of 70 to 80 beats per minute and who is comfortable, requires no immediate therapy to convert the rhythm to normal sinus rhythm. Similarly, emergency therapy is not required in the young patient with paroxysmal atrial tachycardia who is disturbed only by palpitations or an uneasy feeling of breathlessness. On the other hand, immediate cardioversion is necessary in the patient whose atrial arrhythmia has precipitated hypotension, pulmonary edema, angina, or central nervous system dysfunction.

The most rapid means of cardioversion is electrical. The patient is given a short-acting anesthetic, and equipment for intubation is kept available in case of arrest. The paddles are placed on the chest and back, and a DC shock is applied between them. The amount of power that is required varies with the arrhythmia. Atrial flutter, for example, is very sensitive to low voltages, whereas PAT and rapid atrial fibrillation may require more than 100 watt-seconds for conversion to sinus rhythm. Electrical cardioversion is usually a safe procedure, although it may on rare occasions induce cardiac arrest. Digitalis intoxication has been reported to heighten the risk of asystole and ventricular fibrillation.

If the patient's condition is stable, less urgent therapy is appropriate:

1. *Atrial fibrillation* has two undesirable side-effects: (a) it causes hemodynamic deterioration at very slow or very rapid heart rates, and (b) clots can collect in the fibrillating atrium that may subsequently embolize. If the heart rate is too rapid, digitalis and propranolol can slow the ventricular response by effects on the atria and A-V node. Cardioversion to normal sinus rhythm is desirable, but cannot always be achieved. Reversion to a normal rhythm can be attempted electrically or with drugs, usually quinidine. Quinidine, however, has one important side-effect in atrial fibrillation: it is *vagolytic*, enhancing conduction through the A-V node. Thus, in a patient with a modest ventricular response to atrial fibrillation, quinidine may suddenly cause an acceleration of the ventricular response to 200 to 300 beats per minute before the drug is able to convert the atrial rhythm. Most patients should therefore be pretreated with digoxin to block the A-V node before quinidine cardioversion is attempted.

The need for anticoagulation in atrial fibrillation is still debated. Patients with both mitral stenosis and atrial fibrillation carry an extraordinarily high risk of embolism and should be anticoagulated. In some centers, most patients with chronic atrial fibrillation are anticoagulated. This is a sensible approach, but evidence supporting the use of anticoagulation is convincing only for patients with mitral stenosis underlying the atrial fibrillation. If possible, patients should also be anticoagulated before attempts at elective cardioversion, since reversion to normal sinus rhythm is sometimes accompanied by embolization.

2. *Atrial flutter* is an inherently unstable rhythm. As is the case with atrial fibrillation, the ventricular response can be modulated with digoxin or propranolol. Under coverage of these drugs and following therapy of possible noncardiac precipitants, atrial flutter may spontaneously convert to normal sinus rhythm or to atrial fibrillation. Electrical cardioversion is quite simple, however, and requires low voltage.

3. In patients with *paroxysmal atrial tachycardia*, methods other than carotid sinus massage can be tried to increase vagal tone, thus breaking the re-entrant loop through the A-V node and returning the rhythm to normal sinus. These include the Valsalva maneuver, immersing the face in water (diving reflex), or causing the patient to gag. Drug therapy may eventually be required. Either digitalis or propranolol can be given intravenously to break PAT. Occasionally, the use of other drugs may become necessary: (1) Anticholinesterases can directly increase vagal tone, and (2) phenylephrine raises blood pressure, thus stimulating the carotid sinus reflex. Long-term therapy after a burst of PAT is rarely indicated, but avoidance of nicotine and caffeine is advisable.

Verapramil blocks the slow inward current that underlies the prolonged action potential of cardiac cells. It may soon come to be the drug of choice for the treatment of supraventricular tachycardias, including paroxysmal supraventricular tachycardia, atrial flutter, and atrial fibrillation. In many cases, intravenous administration will result in conversion to normal sinus rhythm. In others, it will slow the rate of ventricular response to atrial flutter or fibrillation. It also acts as a coronary vasodilator and is under investigation for use in patients with coronary artery disease. Its

a. fib - digoxin followed by quinidine
a flutter - low volt shock, digoxin a propranolol } Verapamil
PAT - digitalis a propranolol.

severe side-effects include a worsening of heart failure, bradycardia, transient asystole, and hypotension. It should therefore be avoided in patients with sick sinus syndrome or severe congestive heart failure and in patients taking β-adrenergic blocking drugs.

VENTRICULAR ARRHYTHMIAS

The presence of a wide or bizarre QRS complex means either that the origin of the arrhythmia is ventricular, or that the origin is supraventricular and the impulse is being conducted aberrantly. The latter sequence of events can be caused by diffuse heart disease, or it can occur when the heart rate becomes too rapid to permit normal completion of the repolarization sequence. A feature that suggests that the rhythm is supraventricular with aberrant conduction is the presence of a P wave preceding each QRS complex. Occasionally, an ectopic atrial P wave can be found on the EKG. If this is followed by a bizarre QRS complex identical to the one in the arrhythmia, it suggests that the origin of the arrhythmia is supraventricular.

It is important to distinguish ventricular from supraventricular arrhythmias. The physical examination can be helpful. In ventricular arrhythmias, atrial contraction no longer has a constant relation to ventricular contraction. As the ventricle contracts, the atrioventricular valves will sometimes be completely open and sometimes partially or completely closed. The excursion of the closing A-V valves will therefore vary in intensity, being softer with smaller excursions and louder with broader excursions. Occasionally, the atria contract against closed A-V valves, and this will produce "cannon" A waves in the jugular veins.

Ventricular origin is suggested by *fusion beats*—QRS complexes appearing as a cross between the bizarre and the normal QRS—

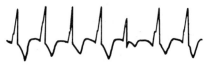

VENTRICULAR TACHYCARDIA

FIG. 4–8. Note the wide, bizarre-shaped complexes and the presence of one fusion beat.

that indicate simultaneous activation from both above and within the ventricle.

As a final definitive maneuver, a recording pacemaker can be placed near the His bundle. His bundle recordings can show whether the activation is proceeding in the normal direction, that is, from atrium to His bundle to ventricle.

When tachycardia originates as an ectopic focus or a re-entry loop within the ventricle, it is called *ventricular tachycardia* (Fig. 4–8). The rate is usually 150 to 250 beats per minute. Ventricular tachycardia can be a medical emergency, presaging cardiac arrest. As the rate increases, the arrhythmia becomes more unstable. Ventricular tachycardia is almost always associated with intrinsic cardiac disease. Persistent ventricular tachycardia may be stable enough to allow attempts at cardioversion with intravenous lidocaine, but electrical cardioversion is often necessary. Short runs of ventricular tachycardia are not uncommon immediately after a myocardial infarction (see Chap. 3).

Ventricular fibrillation is a terminal rhythm of a dying heart. There is no concerted cardiac pumping, and the EKG reveals only an undulating baseline. Ventricular fibrillation is an indication for cardiopulmonary resuscitation (see Chap. 1) and immediate electrical defibrillation.

Drug Therapy for Ventricular Arrhythmias

The most frequently used medications for ventricular arrhythmias are quinidine, pro-

(add Quinid ← Vtach afib) IV lidoc.
+ procainam) or cardiover̄

cainamide, and lidocaine. These drugs affect both specialized conducting tissue and actively pumping myocardial cells. By altering the rate of ion fluxes across individual cells, these drugs can supress some ectopic foci and affect the rate of conduction of the action potential through the heart, thus disturbing and breaking re-entrant circuits.

Side-effects are common. Each of these drugs interferes with conduction down the His bundle, leading to a wider QRS complex and, potentially, to complete heart block. Each can also cause depression of contractility; lidocaine is less of a myocardial depressant than quinidine or procainamide.

* *Quinidine* can be administered orally or parenterally. The oral route significantly reduces the risk of adverse cardiovascular side-effects. The drug is eliminated almost entirely by hepatic metabolism and can accumulate to toxic levels in patients with liver disease. Serum quinidine levels can help guide the patient's dosage; if these are not available, careful monitoring of prolongation of the QRS and QT intervals can help prevent overdosage. Toxic side-effects are common, necessitating discontinuation of the drug in 30% of patients. These side-effects are usually gastrointestinal, including especially diarrhea and nausea. On rare occasions, quinidine has been implicated as the cause of sudden death from ventricular fibrillation. Allergic reactions, such as fever or thrombocytopenia, also occur infrequently. Patients taking digoxin when quinidine therapy is initiated should have serum digoxin levels monitored, because quinidine increases the serum digoxin concentration. A recently introduced drug, *disopyramide*, has similar therapeutic effects. It is purported to have fewer gastrointestinal side-effects, but it has more prominent anticholinergic side-effects, especially urinary retention. Its elimination is primarily renal.

* The half-life of *procainamide* depends on renal and hepatic function, and the dosage must be adjusted accordingly. Side-effects are very common. Most patients eventually develop antinuclear antibodies during long-term therapy, and one-third develop a lupus-like syndrome with skin rash, arthralgias, pleuritis, or pericarditis. The short half-life of about three hours necessitates taking procainamide at inconveniently brief intervals.

* *Lidocaine* is a potent anti-arrhythmic agent, but at present oral congeners are available only experimentally, so that the drug must be administered parenterally. Its metabolism is primarily hepatic. Toxic reactions are usually manifested in the central nervous system, and include depression, confusion, and seizures.

* *Bretylium* may be successful in converting ventricular fibrillation that is resistant to lidocaine and multiple attempts at DC cardioversion. Bretylium depresses the release of norepinephrine from sympathetic neurons, producing a chemical sympathectomy. Thus, it causes the predictable side-effect of orthostatic hypotension, which is usually responsive to infusions of volume.

Who should receive these medications? The patient suffering hemodynamic or ischemic consequences of an arrhythmia requires electrical cardioversion. Subsequent chemical prophylaxis, at least temporarily, is prudent. Drug therapy is also sensible for patients with ventricular arrhythmias who fall into one of the following categories:

1. A patient undergoing a myocardial infarction is at high risk for ventricular tachycardia and should receive lidocaine as prophylaxis. If a ventricular tachycardia supervenes during lidocaine therapy, procainamide or quinidine may be added.

2. After an episode of sudden death presumed to be arrhythmic in origin, initiation of therapy with chronic quinidine or procainamide seems judicious, despite the absence of unequivocal data supporting this empirical approach. An experimental protocol currently

under study in several centers involves the use of a pacemaker to stimulate ventricular tachycardia, in the hope of triggering the arrhythmia responsible for sudden death. This technique permits evaluation of the effectiveness of various drugs and dosages in treating the induced arrhythmia.

3. A patient who, two to three weeks after myocardial infarction, continues to have frequent ventricular ectopic beats is at an increased risk for sudden death. It is not known whether antiarrhythmic prophylaxis can prevent such deaths, but most physicians treat such patients with quinidine. Procainamide, with its severe side-effects and short intervals between doses, is a second line drug for use in these patients.

4. A patient who manifests frequent ventricular ectopy without evidence of infarction presents a therapeutic dilemma. These patients range from those with ectopy as a manifestation of significant underlying heart disease to those with ectopy as an incidental and unimportant problem. Some are at high risk for ventricular fibrillation and some are not. Some can benefit from antiarrhythmic drugs, and some simply suffer their side-effects. Many clinicians choose to treat only patients with ectopy who have evidence of significant underlying ischemic or cardiomyopathic heart disease. Others also treat patients who manifest salvos of ventricular tachycardia or runs of two or three consecutive ectopic beats, or whose EKG gives evidence of multifocal ventricular origin.

Sometimes drug therapy cannot prevent recurrent ventricular tachycardia. In some of these patients, endocardial mapping will indicate a small irritable focus from which the arrhythmia originates, and surgical removal of that region of myocardium may abolish the arrhythmia. A promising new approach takes advantage of the observation that some arrhythmias can be "overdriven" by bursts of electrical stimulation delivered by a ventric-

ular pacemaker. These pacemakers can be activated externally by radio frequency and programmed for appropriate stimulation parameters. Patients can thus successfully terminate their arrhythmias outside of the hospital.

BRADYARRHYTHMIAS AND HEART BLOCK

A slow heart rate may be due to sinus bradycardia, sinus node arrest, or blockage within the normal conduction pathway, allowing pacemakers outside of the sinus node to drive the heart. Heart block means that conduction has stopped. It can occur anywhere along the conduction pathway. Heart block can be a normal physiologic response, such as, for example, the inability of the A-V node to accommodate and transmit all atrial impulses during atrial fibrillation. Heart block can also result from ischemic damage or fibrosis along the conduction pathway.

Heart block occurs in three varieties: (1) In first degree A-V block, the PR interval is prolonged to greater than 0.20 seconds, implying unusually long delays in the A-V node. (2) In second degree A-V block, some atrial beats do not penetrate the A-V node, and some of the P waves are therefore not followed by QRS complexes. Second degree A-V block comes in two varieties: Type I or Wenckebach block reflects disease within the A-V node. It is reflected by progressive lengthening of the PR interval until, finally, a P wave fails to conduct, a QRS complex is dropped, and the cycle resumes. Type II block derives from disease below the A-V node and is manifested by a QRS complex being dropped without changes in the preceding interval. (3) In third degree A-V block, no P waves reach the ventricle, and the ventricle contracts with its own escape pacemaker unrelated to atrial activity.

First degree A-V block and Wenckebach type second degree block pose <u>no immediate concern</u> to the physician. Both can occur during digitalis therapy, with increased vagal tone in a healthy individual, or uncommonly with inflammation of the A-V node (as may occur in patients with rheumatic fever). They may also occur transiently during an inferior myocardial infarction, reflecting involvement of the A-V node, and usually do not require therapy.

<u>Type II second degree block and third degree A-V block</u> usually reflect <u>disease below the A-V node</u>, and are <u>more worrisome</u>. They are most commonly caused by damage to the conduction system by idiopathic sclerosis (Lenegre's disease) and fibrocalcific degeneration of the myocardium (Lev's disease). They may also be caused by an extensive anterior myocardial infarction or diffuse disease of the myocardium. In chronic conduction system disease, sudden syncopal attacks (Stokes-Adams attacks) occur without warning, caused by momentary ventricular standstill. Perma-nent pacemakers can prevent further syncopal attacks, and are indicated for these patients.

BIBLIOGRAPHY

Bigger JT, Dresdale RJ, Heissenbuttel RH et al: Ventricular arrhythmias in ischemic heart disease: Mechanism, prevalence, significance and management. Prog Cardiovasc Dis 19:255–300, 1977

Connolly ME, Kersting F, Dollery CT: The clinical pharmacology of beta-adrenoreceptor-blocking drugs. Prog Cardiovas Dis 19:203–234, 1976

Goldreyer BN: Mechanisms of supraventricular tachycardias. Annu Rev Med 26:219–228, 1975

Treatment of cardiac arrhythmias. Medical letter 20:113–120, 1978

Heissenbuttel R, Bigger J: Bretylium tosylate: A new available antiarrhythmic drug for ventricular arrhythmias. Ann Intern Med 91:229–238, 1979

Warner H: Therapy of common arrhythmias. Med Clin North Am 58:995–1017, 1974

Zipes D, Troup PJ: New antiarrhythmic agents: Amiodarone, aprindine, disopyramide, ethmozin, mexiletine, tocainide, verapamil. Am J Cardiol 41:1005–1024, 1978

5 Valvular Heart Disease

The most important consideration in caring for patients with valvular heart disease is the timing of surgery. Not every patient requires surgery, but if an appropriate opportunity for surgical correction is missed, irreversible heart failure may supervene and surgery will then carry an unacceptably high mortality. Medical therapy involves antibiotic prophylaxis given at appropriate times (for example, during dental work) to prevent infection of the scarred valves, as well as treatment of the heart failure and arrhythmias that complicate valvular heart disease.

The normal heart valve is a diaphanous, wispy sheet of connective tissue. The mitral valve is composed of two such leaflets, the tricuspid, aortic, and pulmonic valves of three. Mechanisms of buttressing vary from valve to valve. For example, the leaflets of the aortic valve are attached only at their base to a ring of fibroelastic tissue. The mitral valve, in contrast, has a complex system of supports composed of chordae tendineae, strands of fibrous tissue running from the tips of the leaflets to papillary muscles projecting from the endocardial surface of the ventricle.

Valvular disease can take two forms:

A valve becomes *incompetent* when leaflets are torn or distorted by scar, so that they can no longer appose; when they lose support, as occurs with rupture of the chordae tendineae; or when the valve ring is loosened by dissecting blood or pus.

A valve becomes *stenotic* with narrowing of the orifice by scar or by a congenital anatomic defect.

HEMODYNAMIC CONSEQUENCES AND NATURAL HISTORY OF VALVULAR DISEASE

Mitral stenosis

Rheumatic heart disease accounts for nearly all cases of mitral stenosis. The lesion runs a leisurely course, and initial symptoms are often delayed until 15 to 20 years after the insult.

With narrowing of the mitral orifice, pressures in the left atrium rise in order to maintain the flow of blood from the left atrium to the left ventricle. The left atrium enlarges and pulmonary venous and pulmonary capillary pressures rise, sometimes with consequent pulmonary edema.

Early in the course of mitral stenosis, shortness of breath is only noted during strenuous exercise, when the venous return increases. In addition, the tachycardia accompanying exercise reduces the length of time available for the left atrium to empty (*i.e.*, reduces the length of diastole). Later, symptoms occur even at rest, and are exacerbated by lying flat. An average of seven years separates the onset of symptomatology from complete incapacity. At that time, the two cusps have become adherent at their lateral borders, reducing the orifice to less than 1 cm² (normally 4 to 6 cm²). The valve often becomes surrounded by calcium deposits. When left atrial pressures rise to about 25 torr, dyspnea, and orthopnea may result from the pulmonary edema. Pulmonary pressures may eventually become high enough to cause right heart failure. When the right heart fails, there may appear to be a temporary grace period in the patient's course. Episodes of pulmonary edema cease, since the right heart is no longer capable of overloading the left side. Tricuspid regurgitation may appear. When this point is reached, damage to the heart and lungs may be too extensive and irreversible for surgery to be of any benefit.

Approximately 30% of patients with mitral stenosis, for unknown reasons, follow a different course in the initial stages of their illness. In these patients, the pulmonary vasculature constricts early in the disease with consequent cor pulmonale and right heart failure, and with less pulmonary edema.

The symptoms and complications of mitral stenosis are several:

1. Dyspnea and orthopnea and attacks of frank pulmonary edema are often induced by exercise, pregnancy, or uncontrolled atrial fibrillation. These occur especially frequently in younger patients in whom neither reactive pulmonary arterial vasoconstriction nor right heart failure has occurred, both of which would protect the left heart.

2. Hemoptysis (see Chap. 20).

3. Systemic and pulmonary embolization are very common, especially in patients with atrial fibrillation.

4. Atrial fibrillation is presumably precipitated by disturbances in left atrial electrophysiology, but does not appear to correlate with the severity of the stenosis. It is important not only because of the hemodynamic embarrassment it may cause, but because it contributes to the predisposition to embolization.

The typical course of mitral valvular disease can be summarized as follows: The initial rheumatic attack occurs between the ages of 8 and 12. Subsequently, the valve begins to stenose, but there are no symptoms until about age 30, at which time the patient begins to experience dyspnea on exertion. In the absence of adequate therapy, the disease progresses, often culminating in death by age 40. The course may be interrupted by bouts of pulmonary edema, especially in patients who become pregnant or who experience other precipitants such as bronchitis or atrial fibrillation. Atrial fibrillation at first occurs sporadically, and then persists chronically, and contributes to episodes of pulmonary or systemic embolization. Early death may be caused by pulmonary edema or emboli; otherwise, the patient endures progressive increments in left atrial and pulmonary arterial pressures, and eventually the symptoms of right heart failure become apparent (see Chap. 8).

Mitral Regurgitation

Several pathologic processes can give rise to mitral regurgitation in addition to rheumatic mitral valve disease: (1) Papillary muscle dysfunction results from infarction at the base of the muscle or from distortion of the ventricular anatomy in the dilated hearts of patients with congestive heart failure. This can prevent adequate coaptation of the valve; (2) endocarditis can destroy the valve; (3) unusually, massive calcification of the mitral annulus, of unknown etiology, may distort the anatomy enough to cause mitral regurgitation; (4) mitral valve prolapse, a common and usually benign syndrome, only rarely deteriorates with resulting fulminant insufficiency. It is described more fully below.

In mitral regurgitation, the left ventricle ejects blood back into the left atrium during systole. The left ventricle and left atrium dilate to accommodate both the forward stroke volume and the regurgitant volume. The left ventricle adapts well to the increased volume burden, increasing its compliance so that the end diastolic pressure does not rise until late in the course of the illness. Consequently, the patient with chronic mitral regurgitation tolerates the long-standing left atrial and left ventricular distention with few complaints until quite late in the disease. The dilated left atrium holds the large regurgitant volume with only moderate increases in pressure so that the incidence of pulmonary edema, hemoptysis, and systemic embolization is low compared with that in mitral stenosis. Eventually, however, left ventricular failure does ensue. Exhaustion and exercise intolerance—due to low cardiac output—not infrequently predominate over symptoms of pulmonary congestion.

Acute mitral regurgitation in which the patient does not have the benefit of the hemodynamic compensations of chronic mitral regurgitation is, in contrast, catastrophic, frequently accompanied by shock and acute pulmonary edema. Surgical intervention may be necessary and lifesaving. Acute mitral regurgitation can be caused by papillary muscle rupture (as opposed to dysfunction), which may accompany myocardial infarction; by rupture of one or several chordae which can occur in patients with chronic rheumatic mitral disease, with or without superimposed endocarditis; sometimes in patients without any obvious cause; and occasionally related to the syndrome of mitral valve prolapse.

Aortic Stenosis

There are two major causes of aortic stenosis: rheumatic fever and the congenitally bicuspid valve. When rheumatic fever is the cause, the aortic valve is never involved alone, but is affected in combination with the mitral valve and sometimes the tricuspid valve. Isolated aortic stenosis is usually due to a congenitally bicuspid valve; the valve usually functions normally at birth and throughout development, but later becomes scarred and produces symptoms by the fourth or fifth decade. The common degenerative changes of the normal aortic valve, seen in people over 70 years of age, frequently cause a systolic murmur, but rarely progress far enough to produce significant stenosis.

During normal systole, when the aortic valve is open, the pressures in the left ventricle and the aorta are equal. In a patient with aortic stenosis, a pressure gradient develops across the valve. The patient remains asymptomatic during the early stages of the lesion, unless there is concurrent coronary artery disease. When the lesion becomes "critical," necessitating surgical intervention, the peak systolic gradient across the stenotic valve exceeds 50 torr (i.e., the pressure in the ventricle is 50 torr greater than the pressure in the aorta). The ventricle hypertrophies, the myocardial demand for oxygen increases, and the end diastolic pressure rises because of the loss of left ventricular compliance.

When any one of a triad of symptoms appears—angina pectoris, symptoms of left ventricular failure, or syncope—the patient's life expectancy without surgery is less than five years, and 15% to 20% of patients will die of sudden death.

1. Angina portends an average life expectancy of five years, and presumably reflects the

inability of the coronary blood flow to meet the increased requirements of a hypertrophied myocardium. In about 50% of patients with aortic stenosis and angina, the angina occurs without significant arteriosclerosis of the coronary arteries. The characteristics and precipitants of the pain are similar to those of the angina that accompanies coronary artery disease, and it responds to nitroglycerin.

2. Syncope predicts an average survival of only three years. Some patients do not experience true syncope, but describe only exertional "light headedness"; their prognosis is equally grim. Syncope often accompanies exertion. Its origin is unknown, possibly arrhythmic, possibly an inappropriate hemodynamic reflex similar to the Bezold-Jarisch reflex, in which stretching of the ventricle causes peripheral vasodilatation and bradycardia. Acute left ventricular decompensation accompanying the increased stress of exercise may also be at fault.

3. The most ominous symptoms are those associated with left ventricular failure—dyspnea on exertion and orthopnea. They portend an average survival of less than two years.

Aortic Regurgitation

Isolated aortic regurgitation is caused by many of the same diseases that cause aortic stenosis. About one-third of cases are rheumatic in etiology. Some of the remainder are due to syphilitic aortitis, various disorders of the connective tissue including ankylosing spondylitis, and myxomatous degeneration. Distortion of the root of the aortic valve, as occurs in Marfan's syndrome or with hypertension, may also produce progressive incompetence.

The major hemodynamic consequence of aortic regurgitation is volume overload of the left ventricle. At first the ventricle compensates by dilatation. Furthermore, there is a reflex peripheral vasodilatation that makes it easier for the ventricle to empty. The ventricle handles the increased volume load for some time without serious consequences, but symptoms of left ventricular failure eventually appear and angina may develop.

Acute aortic regurgitation, seen with endocarditis or following trauma, is a catastrophe. The rapid rise in ventricular end diastolic pressure precipitates pulmonary edema, and the ventricle may not be able to maintain adequate forward cardiac output.

EVALUATION OF VALVULAR HEART DISEASE

The initial evaluation of valvular heart disease involves four essential areas:

1. History. The history should be probed for evidence of rheumatic fever, heart failure, endocarditis, angina, or syncope.

2. Physical examination. The heart should be carefully auscultated for subtle murmurs, quiet clicks, and soft gallop sounds, and the precordium should be palpated for suggestions of atrial or ventricular hypertrophy and enlargement. The neck veins should be inspected to estimate right atrial pressures and to detect abnormalities of wave form that may suggest, for example, tricuspid regurgitation. Gentle palpation of the carotid arteries permits a preliminary evaluation of the nature and degree of aortic valvular stenosis or regurgitation. Evidence of both right and left heart failure should be diligently sought.

3. Chest x-ray. The chest x-ray should be viewed with special consideration given to detecting evidence of chamber enlargement, valve calcification, and pulmonary edema.

4. Electrocardiogram. The EKG should be evaluated for evidence of chamber hypertrophy and arrhythmias.

The Normal Cardiac Cycle. Figure 5–1 illustrates the left ventricular and aortic pressures during systole, with the timing of the

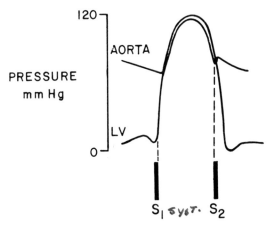

FIG. 5–1. Hemodynamic pressure tracings from the aorta and left ventricle, showing their relationships to each other and to the normal heart sounds.

normal heart sounds beneath. Although the following description focuses only on the events occuring on the left side of the heart, clearly an analogous cycle occurs on the right side.

At the onset of left ventricular systole, the left ventricle contracts, and pressures in that chamber rise above those in the left atrium, closing the mitral valve. This produces the first heart sound, S_1. As soon as the left ventricular pressure exceeds the pressure in the aorta, the aortic valve opens. The left ventricle and the aorta therefore have equal pressures during the emptying of the left ventricle.

As the left ventricle finishes its contraction, the ventricular pressure begins to fall, and as soon as it drops below the aortic pressure, the aortic valve closes, producing the second heart sound, S_2. Auscultation reveals two components to the S_2; the first is the sound of aortic valve closure (A_2) and the second is the sound of pulmonic valve closure (P_2). During inspiration, A_2 and P_2 move slightly apart (S_2 is said to be split), reflecting increased venous return

$$A_2 \longrightarrow P_2$$

to the right ventricle and thus delayed closing of the pulmonic valve.

When the declining left ventricular pressure drops below the pressure in the left atrium, the mitral valve opens, and the left ventricle and left atrium have equal pressures.

Heart Murmurs. Disease of the heart valves rarely presents without an accompanying murmur. A murmur is caused by turbulent blood flow across a valve, the result either of distorted anatomy or an increased volume of flow. The character, location, intensity, and direction of radiation of a murmur can be clues to the location and severity of the lesion. Figure 5–2 shows the timing of the most common cardiac murmurs.

During systole, the aortic and pulmonic valves are open and the mitral and tricuspid valves are closed. Systolic murmurs are therefore due either to stenosis of the aortic or pulmonic valves or to incompetence of the mitral or tricuspid valves.

During diastole, the aortic and pulmonic valves are closed, the mitral and tricuspid valves are open. Diastolic murmurs therefore suggest incompetence of the aortic or pulmonic valves or stenosis of the mitral or tricuspid valves.

The radiation of murmurs is usually along the direction of the jet underlying them; thus, for example, the murmer of mitral regurgitation radiates toward the axilla, and the murmur of aortic stenosis toward the neck.

Mitral Stenosis

The diastolic murmur of mitral stenosis has several characteristic features:

1. The first heart sound is accentuated. The elevated left atrial pressure keeps the valve wide open at the onset of ventricular contraction so that it snaps shut over a wider excursion than is normal. A loud snapping S_1 may

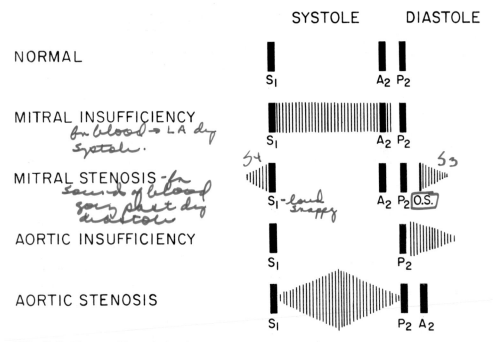

Handwritten annotations:
MITRAL INSUFFICIENCY — *for blood → LA dg Systole.*
MITRAL STENOSIS — *Sound of blood going past dg diastole*
S4
S3

FIG. 5–2. The position of the heart sounds and murmurs in several valvular lesions.

be the only auscultatory clue to early mitral stenosis.

2. The opening snap of the stenosed mitral valve occurs early in diastole and produces a short, high-pitched sound following S_2. The opening snap must be distinguished from a widely split S_2, which usually exhibits respiratory variation, and from a loud S_3. The latter is rarely heard in pure mitral stenosis and occurs later in diastole than the opening snap; it has a much lower pitch, and is heard better with the bell of the stethoscope. The interval between the S_2 and the opening snap reflects the abnormal pressure gradient across the valve. As the stenosis worsens, the atrial pressure rises and causes the valve to open progressively earlier in diastole. The opening snap thus moves closer to S_2.

3. A mid-diastolic rumble is produced by turbulent flow across the valve. It is low-pitched and often distinctly localized to the cardiac apex. The murmur is best detected using the bell of the stethoscope while having the patient lie in the left lateral decubitus position, placing the cardiac apex close to the anterior chest wall.

4. In many patients, a presystolic accentuation of the murmur immediately precedes the S_1. This sound is produced by the augmentation of flow upon left atrial contraction and is usually lost when atrial fibrillation develops.

In addition to the auscultatory examination, other physical findings can help in the evaluation of mitral stenosis. The classic "mitral facies," characterized by a malar flush and cyanosis of the lips, is not commonly seen. In pure mitral stenosis, an elevated jugular venous pressure signifies right ventricular hypertrophy or failure, a consequence of secondary pulmonary hypertension. Because the left ventricular diastolic pressure is normal, the apical impulse would be expected to have a normal contour and normal timing. A parasternal heave therefore suggests pulmonary hypertension and right ventricular hypertrophy.

A chest x-ray (Fig. 5–3) can show a large left atrium (straightening of the left heart border, widening of the carinal angle, displacement of a barium-filled esophagus on lateral view) and reveal evidence of pulmonary edema and, late in the disease, right ventricular enlargement.

In the absence of atrial fibrillation, large biphasic P waves suggest left atrial enlargement on the electrocardiogram. An M-mode echocardiogram can suggest the presence of mitral stenosis by revealing diminished velocity of closure of the anterior leaflet in diastole (a decreased E-F slope), and parallel anterior movement of both leaflets in diastole instead of their normal divergent opening. The echocardiogram cannot, however, predict the severity of the stenosis.

Mitral Regurgitation

A systolic murmur is produced at the mitral area when the valve is incompetent. The murmur of mitral regurgitation is holosystolic, heard at the cardiac apex, and typically radiates posteriorly into the axilla. Occasionally, the murmur radiates to the base and can there be confused with the murmur of aortic stenosis. The murmur is typically accompanied by a soft or absent S₁ and a loud third heart sound (S₃). The S₃ may be followed by a short diastolic rumble reflecting excess flow across the valve. The compensatory chamber enlargement can often be felt on palpation as a gentle rocking motion.

The *prolapsing mitral valve* produces a distinctive systolic murmur accompanied by one or more midsystolic clicks, usually due to redundant mitral leaflet tissue. This is a common syndrome, and occurs in as many as

10% of the healthy young female population. It is important to distinguish this lesion from more serious cardiac lesions. Specific maneuvers during auscultation produce characteristic changes: decreasing the ventricular volume (by having the patient stand or perform a Valsalva maneuver) causes the clicks and murmur to occur earlier; increasing the ventricular volume (by having the patient squat) causes the clicks and murmur to occur later, and they may even disappear. These patients should be given appropriate antibiotic prophylaxis for subacute bacterial endocarditis. Rarely, complications may ensue; these include endocarditis, acute fulminant mitral regurgitation, ventricular and atrial arrhythmias, and sudden death. Usually the syndrome is asymptomatic. However, it should be considered in any young patient who presents with an arrhythmia or unexplained syncope.

Aortic Stenosis

The murmur of aortic stenosis is a rough, low-pitched sound best heard at the base of the heart, and radiating to the neck and along the carotids. As shown in Figure 5–2, it begins shortly after S₁ and peaks in midsystole; the murmur is thus said to be diamond-shaped. The impulse of the enlarged left ventricle is somewhat displaced and is discrete and sustained. In significant stenosis, a systolic thrill may be palpable at the base. The carotids feel weak and the impulse delayed (*pulsus tardus et parvus*).

An S₄ gallop suggests that the atrium is emptying into a noncompliant ventricle. An S₃ gallop is a sign of left ventricular failure and is not due to aortic stenosis *per se*. If the valve retains some freedom of motion, an ejection sound may also be heard. The intensity of the ejection sound diminishes as calcification sets in. As the disease progresses, aortic closure may be progressively delayed, producing a single S₂ when the aortic sound

FIG. 5–3. Thirty-one-year-old woman with mitral stenosis. Chest radiograph, posteroanterior view. Note the slight evidence of left atrial enlargement, marked by enlargement of the left atrial appendage below the pulmonary artery on the left heart border, and the double density just to the right of the spine. There is some redistribution of pulmonary blood flow compatible with elevations of pressures in the pulmonary vasculature.

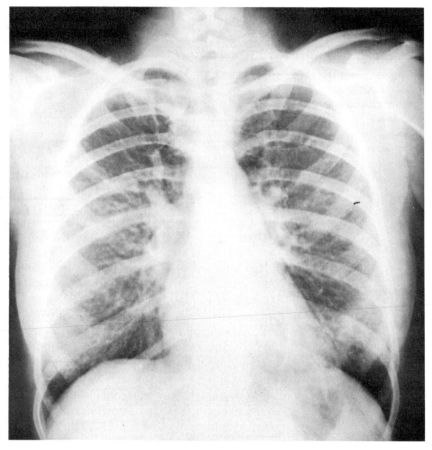

A

merges with the pulmonic sound. When the aortic sound is delayed beyond the pulmonic sound it is referred to as paradoxic splitting. Systolic pressures are usually not abnormally low.

The qualities of the murmur do not correlate well with the severity of the aortic stenosis. In fact, with very severe aortic stenosis, the ventricle may pump so inadequately that no murmur is generated. A better guide to the severity of the lesion can be obtained from the quality of the carotid upstroke, the presence of a systolic thrill, and the delay of A_2.

The obstruction to left ventricular outflow produces concentric thickening of the ventricular wall, and the x-ray picture often appears normal. A careful eye may sometimes pick up a suggestion of fullness of the left ventricular contour on the PA film. The left atrium may also be enlarged from having to pump into a noncompliant ventricle, but it may also be enlarged because of associated mitral valve disease.

Fluoroscopy may reveal calcification in the region of the aortic valve. Calcification is invariably present in the adult with severe aortic stenosis, and its absence strongly suggests that the degree of aortic stenosis is not significant. Recently, the echocardiogram has

FIG. 5–3. (cont.) Lateral view which better demonstrates the left atrial enlargement as shown by indentation of the barium-filled esophagus. The right ventricle is enlarged.

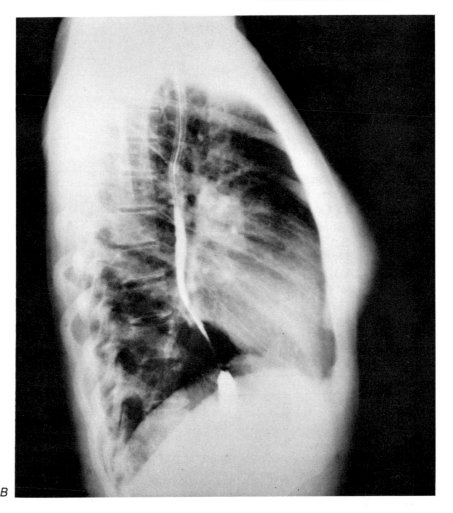

B

been used successfully to predict the severity of aortic stenosis.

The characteristic findings of left ventricular hypertrophy and strain are found in the EKG: increased QRS voltage, ST segment depression, and T wave inversion in standard leads I and aVL, and in the left precordial leads. An increase in P wave voltage suggests left atrial hypertrophy. Left bundle branch block or intraventricular conduction defects are not uncommon.

Asymmetric Septal Hypertrophy. True valvular aortic stenosis must be distinguished from asymmetric septal hypertrophy (ASH, also referred to as idiopathic hypertrophic subaortic stenosis, IHSS). In ASH, dramatic hypertrophy of the left ventricle is accompanied by pronounced asymmetric hypertrophy of the interventricular septum. During contraction, the hypertrophied septum approximates the anterior mitral valve leaflet and obstructs forward flow. Obstruction of the aortic outflow tract is not fixed, but varies throughout the cardiac cycle. The carotid pulse has a bisferiens contour, in which a rapid upstroke is followed by a rapid descent (due to the obstruction) and then a second slow rise in pressure.

Any maneuver that diminishes ventricular size will enhance the obstruction and the murmur. Thus, the Valsalva maneuver, exercise, upright posture, and amyl nitrate all intensify the murmur of ASH. Additionally, any hemodynamic intervention that increases contractility enhances the murmur. For example, under normal conditions, when an extrasystolic beat occurs, the ensuing ventricular contraction is stronger and the intensity of the pulse is enhanced (postextrasystolic potentiation). In ASH, the increased contractility of the postextrasystolic beat leads to decreased flow through the outflow tract, and the pulse pressure of the postextrasystolic beat is significantly diminished.

Any maneuver that expands the ventricle will reduce the obstruction and the murmur. Passive leg raising, supine posture, and pharmacologic constriction of the arteries all diminish the murmur of ASH.

Aortic Regurgitation

The murmur of aortic regurgitation is a decrescendo diastolic murmur occurring shortly after S$_2$. In rheumatic valvular disease, it is best heard at the left sternal border. With disease of the aortic root, as in syphilis, auscultation is often better at the right border. Another diastolic murmur may be mixed in with the murmur of aortic regurgitation. This diastolic murmur is called the *Austin Flint murmur*. The timing and quality of this murmur resemble mitral stenosis. The Austin Flint murmur probably derives from the regurgitant stream striking the anterior leaflet of the mitral valve and causing it to vibrate. It does not signify disease of the mitral valve.

During long-standing aortic regurgitation, the body adapts to the lesion by reflexly vasodilating the peripheral arterioles. This may help to minimize the regurgitant flow. The resultant wide-open circulation causes many of the characteristic signs of aortic regurgitation: (1) a widened pulse pressure, with a dramatically reduced diastolic pressure; (2) a distinctive pulse that rapidly rises and rapidly collapses; (3) pistol shot sounds over the large arteries, which reflect the rapid flow of blood; and (4) pronounced capillary pulsations that are especially obvious in the nail beds. The bounding pulses cause the uvula, the whole head, or even the whole body to bounce. None of these signs can be directly related to the severity of the underlying disease.

The chest film in aortic regurgitation reveals a boot-shaped elongation of the left ventricle. The electrocardiogram may suggest left ventricular hypertrophy. The echocardiogram reveals indirect evidence of aortic regurgitation: the regurgitant stream produces a high frequency stuttering of the anterior leaflet of the mitral valve, and causes premature closure of the mitral valve.

THERAPY FOR VALVULAR HEART DISEASE

Mitral Stenosis —anticoag/ diuretics

All patients with mitral stenosis complicated by atrial fibrillation should be anticoagulated to prevent embolism. Some clinicians advocate anticoagulating almost all patients with mitral stenosis. Diuretics should be employed as necessary for relief of dyspnea and the symptoms of right heart failure. These patients, like all patients with rheumatic heart disease, require antibiotic prophylaxis against subacute bacterial endocarditis. Digitalis has no role in the treatment of mitral stenosis, except for controlling the ventricular rate in atrial fibrillation.

Once symptoms begin and before pulmonary hypertension supervenes, catheterization should be performed. The size of the mitral orifice can be calculated from pressure measurements. If the orifice is less than approximately 1.5 cm^2, surgery should be performed. In a young patient with a noncalcified valve and without mitral regurgitation, the valve can be split surgically allowing the patient an additional period of time before a prosthetic valve is needed. In other patients, the valve should be replaced. Operative mortality is about 5% to 10%, but is significantly worse if right ventricular failure has developed. Many surgeons use tissue valves rather than prosthetic valves to avoid the need for long-term anticoagulation in some patients.

Mitral Regurgitation *dig. diuretics*

Surgery is often the only option for the patient with acute mitral regurgitation. Without operative intervention, the patient may die from refractory pulmonary edema and shock. In patients with chronic mitral regurgitation, operation may occasionally be avoided. Early symptoms can be treated with digitalis and diuretics and afterload reduction. Catheterization with dye injection is needed to evaluate the degree of mitral regurgitation and the extent to which the regurgitation derives from disease of the valve and/or from myocardial and papillary muscle dysfunction. As with all the other valvular diseases, evaluation for surgery should be considered before flagrant left or right heart failure supervenes.

Aortic Stenosis *dig. diur., ⊖ salt NTG*

For the patient with aortic stenosis, the complications of surgery and a life with a pros-

thetic valve are significant. It is, therefore, wise to delay catheterization and operation until the onset of symptoms, but before there is significant evidence of left ventricular failure. The major exception to this rule is the young patient in whom significant aortic stenosis is often asymptomatic. Such patients may die suddenly if surgery is delayed. Catheterization is done to determine the pressure gradient across the valve and the degree of accompanying coronary artery disease (coronary bypass grafting is often necessary) and to ensure that the obstruction is at the valvular and not the subvalvular (or rarely, supravalvular) level.

Medical management consists of the use of digitalis, diuretics, and salt restriction for congestive heart failure, and nitroglycerin for angina. Once significant aortic stenosis is suspected and confirmed, valve replacement should be expedited. Operative mortality is as low as 5% for patients in good condition and as high as 30% for those with heart failure. The operation can be performed with excellent results even in the elderly. Patients have a significantly better long-term survival with an operation than without.

ASH is handled differently from aortic stenosis. *ASH* Patient education is important in order to avoid unnecessary Valsalva maneuvers (e.g., playing a tuba) and fluid depletion. The dynamic obstruction, which depends on contraction of the hypertrophied system, can be diminished by β-adrenergic blockade, which diminishes myocardial contractility. Verapamil has been as effective as propranolol in some studies. Digitalis should generally be avoided, because the drug's positive inotropic effect can worsen the obstruction. However, if atrial fibrillation occurs, the loss of an atrial kick can be catastrophic, and adequate rate control with digitalis may be lifesaving. Occasionally, patients cannot be medically managed and must undergo surgical excision of the hypertrophied muscle.

Aortic Regurgitation

The timing of surgery is critical in patients with aortic regurgitation, since there is a point of no return for the decompensated ventricle. Several clinical clues have been found to be helpful and suggestive of imminent deterioration if surgery is postponed. These include (1) moderate left ventricular enlargement on PA chest x-ray film, (2) electrocardiographic changes suggestive of left ventricular hypertrophy and strain, and (3) a difference in diastolic and systolic blood pressures of more than 100 torr. Once symptoms of congestive failure appear, surgery should not be postponed beyond the stage at which minimal diuresis suffices. In acute aortic regurgitation rapid surgical valve replacement may be life-saving.

RHEUMATIC FEVER

Acute rheumatic fever is generally a disease of childhood and adolescence. It develops after pharyngeal infections with group A streptococci and presumably reflects an immunologic disorder triggered by the infection.

The immediate symptoms are fever, carditis, and a migratory polyarthritis. Less common manifestations include (1) *chorea*, a neurologic disturbance characterized by sudden and uncontrollable jerky movements and emotional lability; (2) *erythema marginatum*, an evanescent serpiginous rash; and (3) *subcutaneous nodules* found over the extensor surfaces of bony prominences. These manifestations can appear at different times during the illness. During the evaluation of valvular heart disease, it is important to question the patient thoroughly about any such childhood illnesses.

The carditis affects the pericardium, myocardium, and endocardium (electrocardiographic changes are common). In some patients, the carditis may follow a fulminant course, leading to death from acute valvular insufficiency, heart failure, or arrhythmias. More often, however, the carditis is silent during the acute phase, and if extracardiac manifestations do not develop, the patient will first come to medical attention later in life for valvular disease, without any recollection of acute rheumatic fever.

Rheumatic fever is a recurrent illness, and patients who suffer carditis in the first attack are more likely to suffer it during subsequent attacks. Following an attack of acute rheumatic fever, therefore, it is mandatory to initiate prophylaxis against group A streptococci; this consists of monthly injections of benzathine penicillin. The penicillin may be discontinued after age 18, unless the risk of exposure to streptococcal infections is high. Antibiotics should also be administered before invasive dental or surgical procedures in any patient with evidence of valvular heart disease.

BIBLIOGRAPHY

Glancy, DL, Epstein S: Differential diagnosis of type and severity of obstruction to left ventricular outflow. Prog Cardiovasc Dis 14:153–191, 1971

Fowler NO, van der Bel-Kahn JM: Indications for surgical replacement of the mitral valve with particular reference to common and uncommon causes of mitral regurgitation. Am J Cardiol 44:148–157, 1979

Goodnight S: Antiplatelet therapy for mitral stenosis? Circ 62:466–468, 1980

Koster FE: Diagnosis and management of complications of prosthetic heart valves. Am J Cardiol 35:872–885, 1975

Roberts WC, Perloff JK: Mitral valvular disease: A clinicopathologic survey of the conditions causing the mitral valve to function abnormally. Ann Intern Med 77:939–975, 1972

Spagnuolo M, Kloth H, Taranta A et al: Natural history of rheumatic aortic regurgitation: Criteria predictive of death, congestive heart failure, and angina in young patients. Circulation 44:368–380, 1971

Wood P: Diseases of the Heart and Circulation. Philadelphia, JB Lippincott, 1968

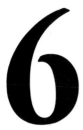

6

Cardiomyopathy

Cardiomyopathy means disease of the heart muscle. Through common usage, the term has been restricted to exclude valvular, congenital, and coronary heart disease. Three broad categories of cardiomyopathy are recognized:

Congestive (dilated) cardiomyopathy. Congestive cardiomyopathy is the most common form of cardiomyopathy. A chest x-ray reveals a large heart with evidence of biventricular heart failure.

Restrictive (nondilated, nonhypertrophic) cardiomyopathy. In the United States, restrictive cardiomyopathy is almost always due to amyloidosis. A chest x-ray shows a heart of nearly normal size, but the patient has evidence of heart failure. Stiff ventricles, which restrict filling, are responsible for the symptoms of heart failure.

Hypertrophic (nondilated) cardiomyopathy. Although hypertrophic cardiomyopathy is uncommon, it has recently been much discussed. Asymmetrical hypertrophy of the myocardium produces a characteristic clinical picture in which signs of obstruction to aortic outflow accompany evidence of restriction to filling.

CONGESTIVE CARDIOMYOPATHY

The problems of the patient with congestive cardiomyopathy include congestive heart failure, arrhythmias, and pulmonary emboli. The typical patient suffers a relentless progression of right and left heart failure, evolving over weeks and sometimes years. The precise date of onset of the illness is often poorly recalled. The history is remarkable for the steadily progressive nature of the deterioration. This history is unlike that of the patient with repeated heart attacks, who frequently recalls periods of stability punctuated by episodes of acute decompensation (presumably, new myocardial infarctions), during which symptoms acutely and significantly worsen.

Congestive cardiomyopathy is generally idiopathic in origin, but in some patients it can be associated with alcoholism, infections, and the peripartum period.

Idiopathic Congestive Cardiomyopathy
Signs of R + L Heart Failure

In patients with congestive cardiomyopathy, the heart is grossly enlarged. Mural thrombi are present, and mild hypertrophy and scattered fibrosis are seen histologically. It is not known why the myocardial cells lose their ability to pump. As systolic function deteriorates, the ejection fraction falls and the heart dilates as it attempts to compensate (Chapter 7). The patient, therefore, usually arrives in the emergency room because of congestive heart failure. Other less common presenting symptoms are the result of arrhythmias and systemic (e.g., renal) and pulmonary emboli. High left atrial pressures result in interstitial pulmonary edema, with dyspnea, orthopnea, and sometimes frank alveolar pulmonary edema. High right atrial pressures, evidenced by bulging neck veins, contribute to peripheral edema and ascites. The patient is generally fatigued from the poor cardiac output and his skin is cold and clammy from the consequent vasoconstriction. The blood pressure is normal or low and the pulse weak. Sinus tachycardia, atrial fibrillation, and atrial and ventricular ectopy are common. The apex beat is displaced laterally, reflecting an enlarged left ventricle. The enlarged right ventricle may be felt heaving just to the left of the sternum. The murmurs of mitral regurgitation or tricuspid regurgitation are not infrequently heard, and are related to direct involvement of the papillary muscles and to their malalignment in the enlarged ventricles. Both S_3 and S_4 gallops are almost always heard. The electrocardiogram is rarely normal, but the changes are nonspecific. These include low voltage, nonspecific ST and T wave abnormalities, an abnormal axis, and sometimes a suggestion of left ventricular hypertrophy, as well as atrial and ventricular ectopy. Bundle branch block may be present. Q waves may falsely suggest an old infarction. The chest x-ray reveals enlargement of all the chambers, and often interstitial or alveolar pulmonary edema.

Differential Diagnosis. An aggressive approach to diagnosis should be taken before accepting the diagnosis of congestive cardiomyopathy and rejecting the possibility of other, potentially treatable forms of congestive heart failure. These other disorders have their own hallmarks:

1. *Ischemic coronary artery disease* may be marked by angina or myocardial infarction, or it may be clinically silent. Most cases of congestive heart failure in elderly patients are secondary to repeated myocardial infarctions, and thus the term *cardiomyopathy of coronary artery disease* has been coined. At present, it makes no therapeutic difference whether the patient's disease is classified as cardiomyopathy of coronary artery disease or idiopathic cardiomyopathy.

2. *Ventricular aneurysms* are regions of akinesia (total lack of motion of part of the ventricular wall) or dyskinesia (paradoxic systolic expansion of part of the wall). Aneurysms usually develop in regions of infarcted myocardium. They rarely rupture, but if large enough, they disrupt left ventricular output and result in congestive heart failure. If the remaining myocardium is adequate, resection of an aneurysm may significantly ameliorate symptoms of heart failure. Gated blood pool scans provide a noninvasive way of outlining the defect, but angiography remains the only reliable diagnostic test.

3. *A pericardial effusion* (see Chap. 9) may be evident as an enlarged heart on the chest x-ray. Clinically, however, the patient does not have heart failure: the lungs are free of pulmonary edema. Unless tamponade results in severe impairment to cardiac filling, there will be no evidence of diminished cardiac output or elevation of systemic venous pressures. Pericardial effusions may be seen on echocardiography in patients with cardiomyopathy as part of the generalized pattern of fluid retention.

4. *Aortic stenosis* may be silent, especially late in the disease when left ventricular function has deteriorated and little blood flows

through the valve. Cardiac fluoroscopy should be undertaken in all patients with unexplained congestive heart failure in order to detect aortic valve calcification. Critical aortic stenosis almost never occurs in the adult without calcification of the valve. Valve replacement can be curative even in the critically ill elderly patient.

5. *Right heart failure* from cor pulmonale presents with systemic venous congestion and right-sided cardiomegaly, and is only rarely difficult to diagnose. An echocardiogram reveals a normal-sized left ventricle.

6. *Mitral regurgitant* murmurs are not uncommon in cardiomyopathy. The valve structure may be distorted by ventricular dilatation, and, in addition, the myopathic process can affect the papillary muscles. If the murmur is not noted prior to the onset of congestive failure, exclusion of primary mitral valvular disease is difficult. One strong indicator of primary mitral valve disease is the finding of well-maintained ventricular contractility on gated blood pool scan, echocardiogram, or angiogram.

Alcoholic Congestive Cardiomyopathy

Two syndromes of heart failure are related to alcohol abuse—alcoholic cardiomyopathy and beriberi heart disease.

The more common is alcoholic cardiomyopathy, a dilated cardiomyopathy with no distinctive pathology to differentiate it from idiopathic cardiomyopathy and with the identical clinical and physiologic progression. Alcohol ingestion acutely diminishes left ventricular function, and many alcoholics have mild left ventricular dysfunction. The development of the full-blown cardiomyopathy, however, requires five to ten years of heavy, regular drinking. If drinking continues after the development of cardiomyopathy, death is predictable within two to three years. In the majority of patients, abstinence results in stabilization or a return to normal. Interestingly, the alcoholic patient with cardiomyopathy rarely has cirrhosis.

Beriberi heart disease is part of the systemic illness of thiamine deficiency. It is not restricted to alcoholics, and has been diagnosed in teenagers with restricted, "junk food" diets. Although the patient has a large heart and pulmonary and systemic edema, the disease differs greatly from idiopathic and alcoholic cardiomyopathy, and is mentioned here only because of its association with alcohol abuse. The patient has a hyperdynamic circulation (evidenced by a bounding pulse, an enormous cardiac output of up to 17 liters per minute, and warm skin because of arterial vasodilatation); there is an accompanying peripheral neuritis. Edema clears rapidly after thiamine is given, and heart size returns to normal within a few weeks of its administration.

Toxins other than ethanol may be responsible for some cases of congestive cardiomyopathy. For example, cobalt, once used as a beer foam stabilizer, was related to an epidemic of fulminant congestive cardiomyopathy in Quebec in the 1960's, and doxorubicin and daunorubicin, two antineoplastic agents, may cause irreversible heart failure, especially when combined with radiation to the heart.

Congestive Cardiomyopathy Associated with Infection

In the United States, acute myocarditis is generally caused by Coxsackie B virus infections. It is manifested by fever, arrhythmias, chest pain, and *transient* congestive heart failure, which resolves without important sequelae. Nonspecific ST and T wave abnormalities may persist in the electrocardiogram. Treatment consists of salt restriction, administration of diuretics for heart failure, and rest. Digitalis should be used with caution, since these patients have a tendency to digitalis toxic arrhythmias.

Outside the United States, infectious causes of cardiomyopathy are more common. Several million South Americans, for example, have chronic Chagas' heart disease with insidious congestive heart failure, arrhythmias, and right bundle branch block. The source of the illness is infection by the endemic parasite *Trypanasoma cruzi.*

Congestive Cardiomyopathy During the Puerperium

New congestive heart failure appearing in the puerperium is a rare cause of congestive cardiomyopathy in the United States. However, it is the most common cardiac disease in some parts of Africa. The disease often remits spontaneously, but (at least in the United States) future pregnancies carry a high risk of recurrence.

Many other systemic illnesses, notably hemochromatosis, sarcoidosis, and the muscular dystrophies, occasionally manifest biventricular failure and arrhythmias. With the recent advent of transvenous biopsy of the right ventricle, it should become possible to determine how often such illnesses underlie cases currently treated as idiopathic cardiomyopathy. It will be helpful to make this determination, since the congestive heart failure of hemochromatosis may respond to iron removal by weekly phlebotomy, and that of sarcoidosis to corticosteroids.

Therapy. In cases of congestive cardiomyopathy in which a particular cause can be identified, specific intervention is possible. The patient with alcoholic cardiomyopathy should be repeatedly encouraged to abstain from alcohol, and the patient with peripartum cardiomyopathy should be discouraged from future pregnancies.

In the absence of contraindications, warfarin should be used to anticoagulate all patients with congestive cardiomyopathy in order to reduce the risk of emboli. Diuretics are employed and titrated for maximum symptomatic improvement. Furosemide is often used in combination with a potassium-sparing diuretic, such as spironolactone. The difficulty with the use of diuretics is that the cardiac output decreases with the diminishing blood volume and venous return. This may become apparent as clinical evidence of dehydration (dry mucous membranes, loss of skin turgor) and a rising BUN. Isordil dinitrate and hydralazine, two unloading agents (Chapter 7), may also be helpful in ameliorating symptoms that derive from poor cardiac output and venous congestion.

Digitalis is not always useful, but may be tried empirically. If there is no obvious clinical improvement, there is no reason to continue the drug.

In the younger patient without significant multiorgan disease, cardiac transplantation offers a final therapeutic option. (With proper patient motivation and institutional commitment, Stanford University Medical Center has achieved a 43% two-year survival.)

RESTRICTIVE CARDIOMYOPATHY

Like the congestive cardiomyopathies, the restrictive cardiomyopathies can present with evidence of right or left atrial hypertension (*i.e.*, venous congestion or pulmonary edema, respectively), and with electrocardiographic abnormalities. In contrast to the congestive cardiomyopathies, however, the heart is usually only slightly dilated. An infiltrate around or within the myocardial cells produces the "stiff" heart characteristic of this syndrome. The hemodynamic alterations resemble those of constrictive pericarditis: The systolic (pumping) function of the heart is fairly well maintained, but diastolic pressures are high. Ventricular pressures may be elevated from the onset of diastole or may start low and rapidly increase to a plateau (similar to the "dip and plateau" of pericardial constriction Chap. 9).

In the United States, amyloid infiltration is responsible for nearly all cases of restrictive cardiomyopathy. Symptoms derive from pulmonary or systemic venous congestion. Infiltration of the myocardium causes electrocardiographic abnormalities of low voltage, axis deviation, bundle branch block, and atrial and ventricular ectopy.

It is important to distinguish restrictive cardiomyopathy from constrictive pericarditis, since pericardial resection is a cure for the latter. Although noninvasive tests may be helpful in diagnosis (e.g., pericardial calcification suggests pericardial disease), even cardiac angiography may not be definitive, and final diagnosis may require a percutaneous transvenous ventricular biopsy or open thoracotomy.

The heart failure of amyloidosis progresses over a course of months to years, and spontaneous resolution has not been observed. Patients with amyloid heart disease are unusually susceptible to digitalis toxic arrhythmias and derive no demonstrable benefit from that drug.

In some equatorial countries, a type of restrictive cardiomyopathy called endomyocardial fibrosis is responsible for up to one-fourth of deaths from heart disease. The disease is thought to result from an immunologic disorder involving the endocardium. Patches of fibrosis replace normal endocardium and sometimes obliterate the ventricular chambers. The only effective therapy appears to be surgical débridement.

HYPERTROPHIC CARDIOMYOPATHY

Hypertrophy of the myocardium is a predictable and normal response of heart muscle cells to work, especially when subject to large pressure loads. However, a spectrum of hypertrophic myocardial diseases has been identified in which hypertrophy, especially of the septum of the heart, occurs without identifiable stress. These disorders are referred to as asymmetric septal hypertrophy (ASH) (See Chap. 5). The septum may be rendered adynamic from the bizarre and disorganized muscle bundles that characterize (but are not pathognomonic of) the disease. There is a strong familial tendency with an autosomal dominant mode of inheritance. However, many of the patients in these families display ASH on echocardiography, but have no symptoms.

The problems encountered by patients with ASH are caused by a stiffened ventricle that restricts diastolic filling, and, less often, from actual obstruction of ventricular output. Obstruction, when it occurs, is caused by the abutment of the anterior leaflet of the mitral valve on the hypertrophied septum, thus obliterating the outflow tract of the left ventricle. The relative roles of diastolic restriction and systolic obstruction in the symptomatology of this syndrome (i.e., angina, exertional syncope, dyspnea and sudden death) are still debated. Sudden death does not appear to be related to the degree of obstruction. When the systolic murmur of obstruction is present, its characteristics reflect the dynamic nature of the stenosis. Thus, maneuvers that shrink the ventricular cavity (volume depletion, nitrates, the Valsalva maneuver) or enhance myocardial contractility (isoproterenol or digitalis) augment the obstruction and the murmur. Those that dilate the ventricle (volume repletion) or lessen the vigor of myocardial contractility (propranolol) diminish the obstruction. Relief of angina and syncope may be achieved in many of these patients with β-adrenergic blockade. If symptoms prove refractory, surgical excision of part of the hypertrophied septum may be necessary and is often helpful. Unfortunately, neither propranolol nor surgery prevents the high incidence of sudden death.

BIBLIOGRAPHY

Dash H, Johnson R, Dinsmore RE et al: Cardio-myopathic syndrome due to coronary artery disease. Br Heart J 39:733–739, 1977

Goodwin JF: Clarification of the cardiomyopathies. Mod Concepts Cardiovasc Dis 41:41–46, 1972

Henry WL, Clark CE, Roberts WC et al: Differences in distribution of myocardial abnormalities in pa-tients with obstructive and nonobstructive asym-metric septal hypertrophy (ASH). Circulation 50:447–455, 1974

Kawal C, Wakabayashi A, Matsumara T, Yui Y: Reappearance of beriberi heart disease in Japan. Am J Med 69:383–386, 1980

Oakley CM: Clinical recognition of the cardio-myopathies. Cir Res 34, 35 (suppl II): 11-152—11-167, 1974

Segal JP, Stapleton JF, McClellan JR et al: Idiopathic cardiomyopathy: Clinical features, prognosis and therapy. Curr Prob Cardiol 3, No. 6:1–48, 1978

Shah PM: Hypertrophic cardiomyopathy. Ann Rev Med 28:235–250, 1977

7

Congestive Heart Failure

When the ventricles of the heart are no longer able to fulfill their role as pumps, the patient is said to be in heart failure. Since the function of the ventricles is to empty the venous reservoir into the arterial circulation, heart failure leads to overfilling of the venous system and underperfusion of the arterial system.

Either or both ventricles can fail. If the right ventricle fails, the systemic veins become congested (reflected in an increased jugular venous pressure) and the elevated back pressure causes peripheral edema, ascites, and an enlarged, tender liver. If the left ventricle fails, the pulmonary venous and pulmonary capillary pressures rise. Fluid leaks into the pulmonary interstitium and alveoli, producing pulmonary edema. Unless there is accompanying right ventricular failure, systemic venous congestion is not part of the picture of left ventricular failure. With failure of either ventricle, easy fatigability and renal failure may become prominent as cardiac output diminishes.

MECHANISMS OF HEART FAILURE

When the right ventricle fails it is usually a result of increased pulmonary arterial pressures which derive from lung disease or left ventricular failure. Congenital heart disease or acquired lesions of the tricuspid or pulmonary valve may also cause right ventricular failure.

Left ventricular failure can result either from "overwork" of the ventricle from massive or multiple myocardial infarctions, or from intrinsic disease of the heart muscle. The left ventricle performs work as it ejects a volume of blood under pressure, and the extent of work is determined by the blood pressure and the stroke volume. Overwork can therefore derive either from a pressure overload (hypertension, aortic stenosis) or a volume overload (mitral regurgitation, thyrotoxicosis). In terms of energy expenditure, pressure work is more costly than flow work.

The more a myocardial cell is stretched in diastole, the more it contracts during the next systole. Thus, extending this concept to the whole heart, the greater the end-diastolic volume the more vigorous the ensuing systolic contraction (Fig. 7–1). When the heart fails, it operates on a lower curve and pumps out less blood at any given end-diastolic volume. In order to maintain stroke volume, the failing heart must therefore operate at a higher end-

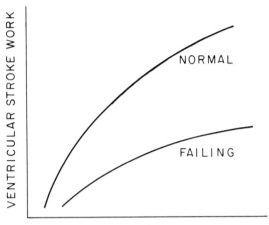

FIG. 7–1. The Starling curves of a normal and failing myocardium, showing that the failing ventricle generates less work than does the normal ventricle at any given ventricular end diastolic volume.

diastolic volume. A failing heart is therefore an enlarged heart.

The failing left ventricle has several clinical characteristics: (1) The elevated left ventricular end-diastolic pressures are transmitted back to the pulmonary capillaries, producing pulmonary edema and dyspnea; (2) poor cardiac output can cause fatigue, renal failure, and sometimes a change in mental status; and (3) the kidneys retain sodium and water, expanding the plasma volume and exacerbating the pulmonary congestion. This stimulus to retain sodium and water originates at least in part from reflexes triggered by atrial stretch.

CLINICAL PROGRESSION

The patient with early congestive heart failure is often not aware of his predicament, and the first evidence of failure may be the discovery of a large heart on a chest x-ray (Fig. 7–2). Suspicion may also be aroused by discovering electrocardiographic evidence of infarction or signs of valvular disease.

As cardiac function worsens, fatigue and dyspnea become apparent. The patient may unconsciously have begun to limit his physical activity. Physical examination may now reveal a resting tachycardia and peripheral vasoconstriction, the latter an attempt to maintain blood pressure. An abnormal diastolic filling sound, the S_3, can be heard.

The patient eventually begins to experience dyspnea at rest. The failing ventricle is unable to handle the increased venous return associated with a recumbent position, and the patient requires more pillows at night to elevate his head and avoid shortness of breath. The patient may suddenly awake severely short of breath and rush to open a window in order to "get more air." This phenomenon is referred to as *paroxysmal nocturnal dyspnea*. As left ventricular function further deteriorates, the patient notes dyspnea even when sitting still.

When a patient's pulmonary capillary pressures rise high enough to cause fluid to leak into the interstitium and alveoli of the lung, he is said to have *pulmonary edema*. The severity of the symptoms depends not only on the pressures in the pulmonary circuit, but also on the acuteness of decompensation. Patients who have chronically elevated pulmonary venous pressures (e.g., patients with mitral stenosis) tolerate high pulmonary pressures with less distress (and probably less fluid leakage) than patients who are acutely decompensating from a first myocardial infarction. The protection afforded by chronic pressure elevations may derive from chronic changes in the interstitium.

The progression from mild respiratory discomfort to fulminant pulmonary edema may evolve over years (in patients with chronic valvular disease or hypertension) or minutes (in patients with massive myocardial infarctions or acute aortic or mitral regurgitation).

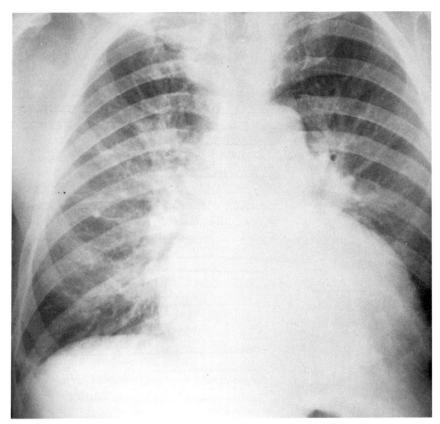

FIG. 7–2. Chest radiograph showing left ventricular failure.

Frequently, a patient remains stable at one level of clinical compromise until the heart is stressed by new ischemia or a large salt and volume load.

EVALUATION AND THERAPY

It is important to determine the underlying etiology of the heart failure as well as the immediate precipitant that led to the worsening of symptoms and brought the patient to the hospital.

The major diseases underlying heart failure are disease of the heart muscle (such as my-ocardial infarction or cardiomyopathy), rheumatic valvular or congenital heart disease, hyperthyroidism, and hypertension. Following successful resolution of the acute decompensation, these must be appropriately treated.

Common acute stresses on the myocardium include (1) an acute volume or salt load (a bag of potato chips or a pizza), (2) ischemia or new infarction, (3) arrhythmias, (4) hypoxemia (from lung disease or a pulmonary embolus), and (5) stresses to which the body responds with an increased cardiac output, such as fever, anemia, or thyrotoxicosis. The patient's ability to handle each of these stresses depends upon the severity of the underlying illness.

Appropriate therapy depends upon the stage of illness. Therapy for the earliest outpatient stages of heart failure consists of dietary salt restriction to lower blood volume, weight loss for the obese patient, and treatment of remediable precipitants. Later, pharmacologic intervention becomes necessary.

Three classes of drugs—digitalis, diuretics, and unloading agents—comprise the core of the medical armamentarium for treating congestive heart failure. Most physicians prefer to initiate therapy with gentle diuretics (such as hydrochlorthiazide) and later substitute more potent ones (such as furosemide). Some begin with, or add, digitalis, an agent that increases myocardial contractility (although not all patients respond to this drug). Nitrates, agents that dilate peripheral arteries and veins, "unload" the heart and may serve to lessen discomfort.

Digitalis

Digitalis is the name of a group of steroid compounds extracted from plants. Since Withering's observation in 1785 that extracts of the foxglove plant help patients with "ascites, anasarca and hydrops pectoris," digitalis has remained an integral part of the therapy of congestive heart failure.

On the molecular level, digitalis inhibits the sodium-potassium ATPase, an enzyme responsible for the membrane transport of sodium and potassium. Therapeutically, digitalis is used to improve cardiac contractility. It is extremely effective in experimental animals, but helps only some patients with heart failure. It is not known how it improves contractility (some propose it does so because of an increase in intracellular calcium) or why it is not uniformly successful. A second, more consistently beneficial, use for digitalis is in the treatment of arrhythmias (see Chap. 4).

Digitalis has a very low therapeutic index.

Several radioimmunoassays for determining digitalis levels are available, including one for the most widely used type of digitalis preparation—digoxin. There is no way to predict what serum level will be of benefit to a given patient. Since digoxin is excreted through the kidneys, serum digoxin levels do not have to be repeatedly checked once a stable dose has been achieved unless there is deterioration of renal function. If the creatinine clearance falls, the digoxin dose must be reduced.

Serum potassium levels must be carefully monitored, since hypokalemia predisposes to digitalis toxicity. Because many patients receive both digitalis and diuretics, hypokalemia is a common problem.

Toxic levels of digitalis produce central nervous system effects, including anorexia, nausea, vomiting, and abnormal vision (with blurring and a yellow cast to colors). Cardiac toxicity is more worrisome, and results from (1) heart block due to increased vagal tone and (2) increased automaticity from the direct enhancement of nonsinus pacemakers. Any arrhythmia can be caused by digitalis toxicity. The most common include ventricular ectopy, junctional tachycardias, and paroxysmal atrial tachycardia with block. Massive (suicidal) overdoses not only cause arrhythmias, but can also cause hyperkalemia from poisoning of the sodium-potassium ATPase.

Discontinuing the drug, ensuring adequate oxygenation, and repleting potassium are usually adequate to treat most mild manifestations of toxicity. Phenytoin or lidocaine effectively suppresses digitalis-induced ectopy. Atropine and temporary pacemakers may become necessary if heart block develops. Direct countercurrent shock may itself precipitate lethal arrhythmias in the face of digitalis toxicity. Fragments of antibodies to digitalis have recently been introduced to reverse massive overdosage, but this technique is still experimental.

Diuretics

Diuretics are agents that stimulate urine flow by enhancing sodium and water excretion. Most diuretics act directly by poisoning the enzyme systems within the kidney that are responsible for reabsorbing chloride or sodium.

Thiazides inhibit sodium and chloride reabsorption primarily in the distal segment. Water accompanies the increased excretion of sodium chloride. Side-effects include (1) hypokalemia, from the distal secretion of potassium, (2) hyperuricemia, and (3) hyperglycemia. The serum potassium must be checked regularly and replaced either with food high in potassium (such as bananas) or with supplements of potassium chloride.

Furosemide is more potent than the thiazides. It reduces intravascular sodium chloride and water by inhibiting chloride reabsorption—and hence reabsorption of the accompanying sodium ions—in the ascending loop of Henle. Hyponatremia, hypokalemia, and hypochloremia may result with subsequent metabolic alkalosis. Potassium should therefore be replaced in the form of the chloride salt, rather than as potassium gluconate.

Spironolactone is a competitive inhibitor of aldosterone. It therefore interferes with the reabsorption of sodium and the secretion of potassium. Therefore, in contrast to the thiazides and furosemide, spironolactone can cause hyperkalemia. *Triamterene* also causes potassium retention while enhancing sodium excretion. It acts on a different tubular site than spironolactone.

Unloading Agents

It has been shown experimentally that isolated papillary muscles stretched with a weight in a water bath contract more rapidly when the load is decreased—hence the term "unloading." Vasodilating drugs unload a failing ventricle by affecting the arterial impedance, the systemic venous compliance, and the left ventricular volume. Different vasodilators affect these variables to different degrees. Thus, patients with heart failure, manifested primarily as poor perfusion, benefit from different drugs than do those suffering from pulmonary congestion. *Hydralazine*, for example, is chiefly an arteriolar vasodilator. By reducing the arterial impedance, hydralazine allows the failing heart to increase its output. Thus, patients with evidence of poor perfusion (fatigue or an increasing blood urea nitrogen, BUN) benefit most from this drug. On the other hand, venodilators, such as the *nitrates*, cause pooling of blood in the capacitance veins, reducing cardiac filling pressures and ameliorating pulmonary edema.

PULMONARY EDEMA

The balance of hydrostatic and oncotic pressures normally does not allow a significant net flux of fluid from the pulmonary capillaries into the pulmonary interstitium and alveoli. If, however, the hydrostatic pressure inside the capillary increases (*e.g.*, in patients with left ventricular failure), fluid can be forced out of the vasculature. Leakage rarely occurs unless the pulmonary capillary wedge pressure exceeds 18 torr.

In the early stages of pulmonary edema, fluid leaks into the interstitium. Because the alveolar surface is clear, this stage is marked less by hypoxemia than by dyspnea and tachypnea, which accompany the stiffening of the lung. If pressures remain elevated, fluid eventually moves into the alveolar air spaces. In the most severe cases, the pulmonary edema fluid froths into the trachea.

Leakage of fluid into the lung is not always a result of hemodynamic compromise, but

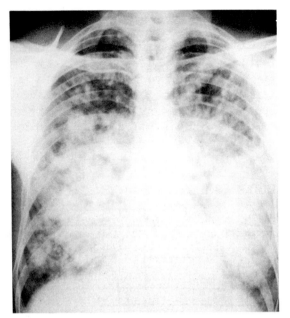
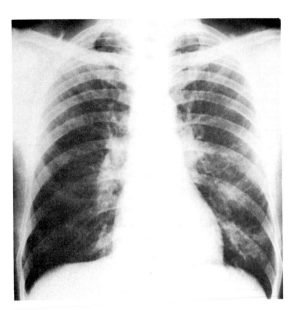

FIG. 7–3. Chest radiograph showing the classic "butterfly pattern" of pulmonary edema (*left*) and its resolution (*right*). The patient was a 29-year-old man whose uremic pulmonary edema cleared after dialysis.

can be the result of injury to the endothelium or epithelium. When this occurs, the fluid that leaks has a high protein content. Circulating or inhaled toxins are frequently invoked as the etiology for this type of pulmonary edema.

Evaluation and Treatment

The clinical status of the patient is the most important determinant of how aggressively one should treat the patient with pulmonary edema. If the patient is comfortable, a cautious approach can be taken despite a chest x-ray showing severe congestion. Conversely, aggressive measures may be necessary in the acutely dyspneic patient even if the chest x-ray reveals only minimal interstitial fluid.

Anxiety and discomfort cause a predictable hypertension and sinus tachycardia, but these require no therapy. Signs which are cause for concern include a sluggish sensorium, evidence of respiratory fatigue, and the presence of frothing, pink-tinged, pulmonary edema fluid. The height of the jugular veins does not correspond to any measure of left ventricular function. An S_3 and rales are present.

Electrocardiographic evaluation for arrhythmias or myocardial infarction should be performed immediately, and any arrhythmia (except sinus tachycardia) should be appropriately treated. A chest x-ray should be obtained, even though it is often a poor guide to the patient's clinical status. Radiologic findings (Fig. 7–3) lag behind the pathology in both the onset and resolution of pulmonary edema. Obtaining arterial blood gases is not a first priority, and an arterial puncture often serves only to distress the patient even more.

The object of therapy is to improve oxygenation and redistribute fluid away from the lungs, either into the capacitance veins or out the kidneys. The patient automatically assumes the most comfortable position unless thwarted by the physician. He should be seated upright with legs dangling in order to reduce the venous return. No discomfort is more frightening than dyspnea, and constant reassurance is critical at this and at every stage of therapy. One hundred percent oxygen therapy by face mask should be started at once, and an intravenous line should be inserted. Unless critically hypoxemic, patients with pulmonary edema rarely require intubation.

In the acutely dyspneic patient, the drug of choice is intravenous *morphine sulfate*. Recent work suggests that morphine acts centrally on the cardiovascular centers of the brain stem to produce venodilation. The resultant relief of dyspnea can be dramatic. Diuretics should follow. Some diuretics have slight immediate dilating effects on the veins, but their most important action, that of diuresis, is delayed. In desperate situations, a phlebotomy of about 500 ml of blood can be lifesaving. This maneuver is especially helpful in patients with renal failure, who are unable to respond adequately to diuretics. Some still employ tourniquets on four limbs to reduce venous return from the extremities, but this approach rarely benefits the patient. Oxygen, morphine, diuretics, and phlebotomy should be the staples of therapy.

BIBLIOGRAPHY

Biddle TL, Yu P: Effect of furosemide on hemodynamics and lung water in acute pulmonary edema secondary to myocardial infarction. Am J Cardiol 43:86–90, 1979

Cohn JN, Franciosa JA: Selection of vasodilator, inotropic or combined therapy for the management of heart failure. Am J Med 65:181–188, 1978

Fishman AP: Heart Failure. New York, McGraw-Hill, 1978

Marcus FI: Current status of therapy with Digoxin. Curr Probl Cardiol 3, No. 5:1–44, 1978

8

Cor Pulmonale

Cor pulmonale is the term applied to right ventricular enlargement secondary to pulmonary hypertension. A dramatic example can be found in rats that have ingested seeds of the West Indian shrub *Crotalaria*. Arteriolitis and medial hypertrophy result in pulmonary arterial pressures that soar beyond the pumping capacity of the right ventricle. The right ventricle dilates in its effort to maintain stroke volume and ultimately fails.

Cor pulmonale in man is a less exotic, generally chronic disease, evolving over months or years. One important exception is found in the patient who experiences a massive pulmonary embolus, and in whom right heart failure progresses swiftly, culminating in death—a condition referred to as *acute cor pulmonale*.

The primary diagnostic and therapeutic problem in cor pulmonale is to identify and treat the cause of pulmonary hypertension. There are only two sources of pulmonary hypertension: obliterative anatomic disease of the pulmonary vasculature, and physiologic pulmonary arterial vasoconstriction. Congenital heart disease and dysfunction of the left side of the heart can also raise pressures within the pulmonary circuit, but these are excluded from the definition of cor pulmonale.

Obliteration of the Pulmonary Vasculature. The obliteration of the pulmonary vasculature can produce pulmonary hypertension only when the loss of vasculature is extensive. The highly distensible pulmonary tree can accommodate even the removal of an entire lung with only a modest increase in blood pressure. Similarly, the widespread vascular loss associated with emphysema is usually tolerated well by the patient. Thus, it is the rare patient in whom pulmonary hypertension results from the loss of vasculature.

Blockage may be caused by multiple pulmonary emboli (Chap. 17), thrombi, as in sickle cell anemia (see Chap. 45), or parasites, as in schistosomiasis. Sometimes, no inciting agent can be discovered. Such cases, in which there is no evidence of chronic lung disease, heart disease, or emboli, are called *primary pulmonary hypertension* (Fig. 8–1). Those most commonly affected are females between the ages of 20 and 40. Pathologically, they evidence a triad of concentric intimal fibrosis, necrotizing arteritis, and plexiform lesions of the small pulmonary arteries (probably reflecting a healing phase of the necrotizing arteritis). The etiology is unknown; however, an association has been noted with Raynaud's syndrome and connective tissue disease. It is also

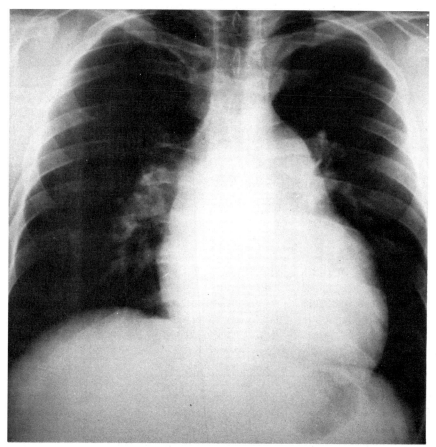

FIG. 8–1. Chest radiograph of a patient with primary pulmonary hypertension. Note the large heart, prominent hilar vessels, and marked decrease in peripheral pulmonary vascular markings.

possible that some cases are caused by substances in the diet. In Switzerland, for instance, an epidemic of pulmonary hypertension followed the introduction of the appetite-depressant aminorex, and resolved following the banning of the drug. The clinical manifestations of the early stages of primary pulmonary hypertension are subtle. Definitive diagnosis requires cardiac catheterization and, frequently, a lung biopsy. Right ventricular pressures rise and eventually approach systemic pressures. There is no curative therapy, and the disease is almost always fatal.

Pulmonary Arterial Vasoconstriction. Pulmonary hypertension is much more frequently the result of pulmonary arterial vasoconstriction. Unlike other vascular beds, the pulmonary arteries constrict upon exposure to hypoxemia and acidosis. Hypoxia of any kind raises pulmonary arterial pressures; upon correction of the hypoxia, pressures return to normal. If hypoxia persists chronically, the media of the vessels hypertrophies and pulmonary arterial pressures become irreversibly elevated. The perpetuation of pulmonary hypertension derives partly from the loss of vasculature owing to the underlying lung disease and partly from the hypertrophied media itself, which appears to be hyperresponsive to hypoxemia and contributes directly to the loss of vascular distensibility.

Chronic hypoxemia implies that ventilation is inadequate to oxygenate the blood. It may be due to diffuse lung disease, an inadequate ventilatory drive, or deformed or ineffective chest bellows. In the United States, *chronic obstructive lung disease* underlies most cases of cor pulmonale. Respiratory acidosis combines with chronic hypoxemia to elevate resting mean pulmonary arterial pressures to 30 torr (normal 15–20). With exercise or fever, or during an acute hypoxemic episode accompanying an exacerbation of the lung disease, pressures may transiently rise even further, frequently exceeding 50 torr. The degree of pulmonary hypertension correlates fairly well with both the FEV_1 and the severity of hypoxemia. The so-called "pink puffer" with pure emphysema (Chap. 13) rarely suffers cor pulmonale until his blood gases begin to deteriorate.

In patients with normal lungs, chronic hypoxemia can result from: (1) congenital or acquired blunting of the ventilatory drive, (2) distortion of the chest wall (kyphoscoliosis) or inadequacy of the respiratory musculature (poliomyelitis or myasthenia gravis), or (3) upper airway obstruction. Some people experience marked upper airway obstruction during sleep, with resultant periods of apnea and hypoventilation. This condition has been dubbed the *sleep-apnea syndrome* and has been associated with, among other things, enlarged tonsils and obesity. In some patients with "central" alveolar hypoventilation, hypotonia of the oropharyngeal muscles during sleep is responsible for most of the clinical symptoms. It is therapeutically important to recognize when one of these syndromes is responsible for cor pulmonale. Just like pa-

tients with chronic obstructive pulmonary disease, these people may suffer respiratory arrest if oxygen is administered in an uncontrolled fashion. Additionally, specific therapeutic options are becoming available for their treatment.

CLINICAL COURSE

Cor pulmonale has two stages. First, the right ventricle hypertrophies and enlarges as it struggles to keep up with the load of pulmonary hypertension. Later, the ventricle fails and dilates, cardiac output becomes inadequate even under mildly stressful conditions, and systemic veins become congested. Signs of early cor pulmonale are rarely dramatic—a loud P_2, signaling pulmonary hypertension, and a right ventricular sternal or epigastric heave, suggesting right ventricular hypertrophy. A right ventricular S_3 gallop, venous congestion, peripheral edema, and ascites mark the onset of a later stage of cor pulmonale, that of right ventricular failure with accompanying sodium and water retention. The presence at this stage of jugular venous "V" waves and a pulsatile liver may suggest tricuspid regurgitation.

The electrocardiogram may confirm the diagnosis, especially in a patient with a normal-shaped chest. The most reliable changes are large R waves or inverted T waves in the right precordial leads. Less diagnostic but still suggestive are "peaked" P waves ("P" pulmonale), right axis deviation of greater than 110 degrees, and right bundle branch block. Patients who have suffered acute decompensation of chronic obstructive lung disease may manifest acute reversal of these electrocardiographic changes with correction of their hypoxemia. Unfortunately, the patient with chronic obstructive pulmonary disease usually has an enlarged or distorted chest cage, rotated heart, and flat diaphragms, making the electrocardiogram less useful as a diagnostic tool. Only one-third of patients with chronic obstructive pulmonary disease who prove to have an enlarged right ventricle at autopsy display the characteristic electrocardiographic changes during life. Overexpanded lungs similarly reduce the utility of the chest x-ray as a measure of right ventricular enlargement. However, the appearance of enlarged pulmonary arteries and pruned peripheral vessels supports the diagnosis of pulmonary hypertension.

THERAPY

Generally, in patients with underlying lung disease, only correction of that disease with restoration of adequate arterial oxygenation can reverse cor pulmonale. When right ventricular failure complicates cor pulmonale, diuretics are the essential addition to the standard regimen of controlled oxygenation and the treatment of infection. Since the lungs share in the fluid retention associated with right ventricular failure, diuresis improves gas exchange in addition to relieving the discomfort of edema and ascites. Desperation may prompt one to attempt more aggressive therapy, but this is usually without any clear benefit. Digoxin, for example, is of little value. Although digoxin may enhance right ventricular output, most patients with chronic lung disease have a normal cardiac output anyway, and the drug only raises pulmonary arterial pressures further. In addition, concomitant hypoxemia and acidosis heighten susceptibil-

ity to the arrhythmias associated with digitalis toxicity. Some selected patients with primary pulmonary hypertension have been found to exhibit a satisfactory response to vasodilators, such as diazoxide or hydralazine.

Patients with normal lungs who hypoventilate present similar therapeutic problems and will occasionally afford unique options for the reversal of hypoxemia. Patients with intermittent upper airway obstruction may benefit from a tracheostomy. Those who are overweight often improve with weight loss. Patients with a blunted ventilatory drive from myxedema return to normal ventilatory status within weeks of starting thyroxine therapy. Central respiratory stimulants, such as progesterone, have enjoyed modest success, but none has received adequate long-term trials to permit a proper assessment of benefits and risks.

BIBLIOGRAPHY

Edwards WD, Edwards JE: Clinical primary pulmonary hypertension: Three pathologic types. Circulation 56:884–888, 1977

Fishman AP: Chronic cor pulmonale. Am Rev Resp Dis 114:775–794, 1976

Fishman AP: Hypoxia on the pulmonary circulation: How and when it acts. Circ Res 38:221–231, 1976

Rubin LJ, Peter RH: Oral hydralazine therapy for primary pulmonary hypertension. N Engl J Med 302:69–73, 1980

Wood P: The Eisenmenger syndrome. Br Med J 2:701–709, 2:755–762, 1958

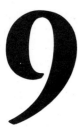

Pericardial Disease

With the exception of the back of the left atrium, the entire heart is enveloped by the pericardium. The visceral pericardium is a diaphanous membrane that is separated from the fibrous parietal pericardium by 25 to 35 ml of fluid contained in the pericardial space. The functions of the pericardium have been difficult to determine because even total absence of the pericardium does not result in any obvious clinical manifestations. The pericardium comes to the physician's attention only when it is the site of inflammation or effusion. Pericardial disease occurs in three forms:

Acute pericarditis is the most common and most benign form of pericardial disease. Fluid accumulates in the pericardial space, and pain derives from inflammation of the pericardium.

Pericardial tamponade is life-threatening. Large amounts of fluid fill the pericardial space and stretch the pericardium so taut that it interferes with ventricular filling.

Constrictive pericarditis is a state of chronic inflammation. The inflamed pericardium becomes adherent to the myocardium, reducing myocardial compliance and causing an elevation of systemic venous pressures.

ETIOLOGY

The inflammation of pericarditis can be caused by any infectious agent, uremia, blunt chest trauma, myocardial infarction, or neoplastic disease, or it may be part of the diffuse serosal inflammation associated with connective tissue diseases.

Most often the etiology is viral and the disease benign and self-limited. Purulent (bacterial) pericarditis is rare, but it has a mortality rate of 50%. It can arise by contiguous spread from the lungs, the mediastinum, or the heart (especially after cardiac operations), or may result from a systemic bacteremia. Tuberculous pericarditis has become an uncommon disease in developed countries; evidence of pulmonary tuberculosis may be absent, and the diagnosis is often made upon postmortem examination.

Forty to fifty percent of patients with uremia develop evidence of pericarditis. Pericarditis in these patients has been proposed to be caused by a circulating toxin. It usually responds well to dialysis, but may require pericardiocentesis or, rarely, pericardiectomy. The pericarditis of uremia may uncommonly progress to tamponade, but constrictive pericarditis is almost unknown.

Primary tumors of the pericardium are rare, and neoplastic involvement usually represents metastatic spread from lung carcinoma, breast carcinoma, malignant melanoma or lymphoma. Evidence of cardiac metastases usually becomes apparent only late in the course of the cancer. Clinical evidence of carcinomatous pericardial disease usually implies extensive invasion not only of the pericardium, but of neighboring intrathoracic structures as well.

ACUTE PERICARDITIS

The hallmarks of pericarditis are chest pain, a friction rub, and electrocardiographic changes. The pain is characteristically sharp and stabbing and is felt in the chest or across the top of the shoulders. The intensity of the pain is affected by respiration and position.

The scratchy auscultatory sounds called pericardial friction rubs are caused by inflammation of the visceral and parietal pericardial surfaces. Friction rubs frequently have three components, corresponding to atrial contraction, ventricular systole, and ventricular diastole. Rubs are usually ephemeral, but they can persist despite the accumulation of large amounts of pericardial fluid. They are best heard during forced expiration with the patient leaning forward.

The electrocardiographic changes indicate epicardial injury, and include components similar to those of myocardial infarction—ST segment elevation and T wave inversion. However, unlike the EKG of myocardial infarction, the ST segment is concave upward, and the T wave does not become inverted until the ST segments have returned to baseline. Most important, these repolarization abnormalities are not restricted to just a few leads, and they do not exhibit the reciprocal changes associated with the localized injury of a myocardial infarction. Supraventricular arrhythmias are common, especially paroxysmal atrial fibrillation. Atrial and ventricular premature beats are also frequently seen.

Acute viral pericarditis usually improves over a day or two, but may run a fluctuating course. There is no specific therapy; bed rest and analgesia are the only remedies. Aspirin often suffices, but indomethicin or even a brief course of high-dose corticosteriods may be necessary for the relief of pain. It remains debatable whether or not to hospitalize patients with acute viral pericarditis. In general, it is advisable to hospitalize patients over 40 years old in whom signs and symptoms of pericarditis may instead derive from a myocardial infarction. In addition, any patient should be hospitalized if there is suspicion of bacterial pericarditis (as evidenced by the stigmata of sepsis or the suggestion of pneumonia on physical examination and chest radiograph), if there has been preceding chest trauma, if there is a complicating systemic illness, and, of course, if there is any hemodynamic compromise (evidence of tamponade). Younger patients with viral pericarditis may be allowed to recover at home if they have a companion to keep an eye on them. They should return in a day or two for re-evaluation. Several tests should be obtained before the patient leaves the hospital, including an electrocardiogram and blood samples for culture, ANA, and viral antibodies (convalescent titers should be determined later). A chest radiograph is taken to evaluate heart size and to rule out pneumonia. Almost every patient will get an echocardiogram, but because the echo beam visualizes only a small sector of the heart it may be a less useful guide than the chest radiograph. All patients should have a skin test for tuberculosis (PPD).

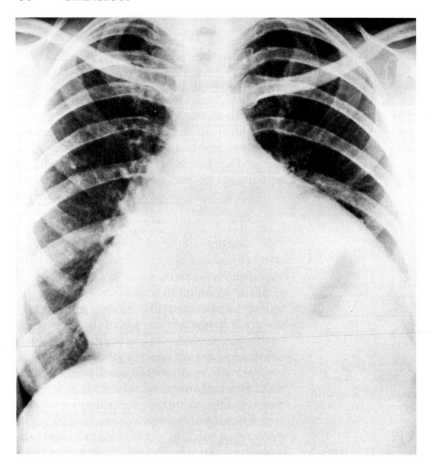

FIG. 9–1. Chest radiograph showing a large pericardial effusion.

PERICARDIAL TAMPONADE

Almost all cases of pericarditis are accompanied by an effusion (Fig. 9–1). When fluid accumulates rapidly, the pericardium may be unable to stretch adequately or rapidly enough to accommodate it. The heart is then compressed and ventricular filling is inhibited. If the pericardium is noncompliant, hemodynamic compromise may occur with small pericardial volumes; if it is compliant, or if fluid accumulates slowly, tamponade may not occur until the pericardial space is filled with hundreds of milliliters of fluid. Cardiac output at first may be maintained by tachycardia.

Eventually, however, this compensatory mechanism fails, and the blood pressure drops.

The tamponaded heart is typically quiet to auscultation. Hemodynamic evidence of tamponade includes elevated venous pressures, tachycardia, low arterial blood pressure, and pulsus paradoxus (*i.e.*, a drop in systolic blood pressure of more than 10 torr with inspiration). A smaller inspiratory fall in blood pressure is normal. The exaggerated fall in patients with tamponade is caused by at least two mechanisms:

1. Upon inspiration, pressures in the thoracic cavity diminish and venous return increases. The right ventricle enlarges and im-

pinges on the left ventricle. Ordinarily, this causes only a slight decrease in the ejection volume of the left ventricle. Patients with tamponade, however, have a tight pericardium and an exaggerated inspiratory increase in venous return due to elevated venous pressures, and there is not enough room for the left ventricle to fill normally at the same time that the right ventricle is filling. Thus, the left ventricular ejection fraction is significantly diminished.

2. The decrease in intrathoracic pressure caused by inspiration is transmitted to the myocardium, but not to the extrathoracic arteries. This effectively raises the arterial afterload on the heart and makes it more difficult for the myocardium to empty. Thus, patients with asthma who have an exaggerated inspiratory effort and patients with very poor myocardial performance will also have pulsus paradoxus. During severe tamponade, the blood pressure may actually decrease to zero during inspiration.

If the patient is temporarily stabilized, confirmation of the diagnosis of tamponade can be obtained by cardiac catheterization. More often, however, the immediate situation is critical and urgent therapy is mandatory. The patient's cardiac output should be enhanced by infusions of large volumes of fluid. A needle is then inserted in the pericardial space, and the effusion is aspirated. This procedure is done with a long needle attached to an electrocardiographic lead. The EKG records an "injury current" (ST segment changes) if the myocardium is punctured. The needle is inserted just to the left of the xiphoid and under the ribs, and angled cephalad and toward the spine. This approach avoids the anterior descending coronary artery, internal mammary artery, and left pleura. Removal of even 25 ml of fluid can be lifesaving. Because coronary laceration or myocardial puncture can accompany this procedure, it should not be repeated frequently. Surgical pericardiectomy

may then become the only effective intervention.

CONSTRICTIVE PERICARDITIS

A chronically inflamed pericardium eventually scars, calcifies, and adheres to the myocardium, interfering with venous return. The resulting clinical picture resembles that of right heart failure. The neck veins are elevated and swell with inspiration, since the right atrium is unable to accommodate the increased venous return of inspiration. This inspiratory rise in jugular venous pressure is referred to as Kussmaul's sign. Hemodynamic measurements within the chambers reveal characteristic changes as the ventricles fill rapidly from the high venous pressures but soon reach their maximum expansion with very high end diastolic pressures.

Because the rigid shell of the pericardium prevents the respiratory increase in diastolic filling, respiratory variations in blood pressure and pulsus paradoxus are not part of the overall picture. An early diastolic "knock" may be heard, but pericardial rubs are rare. The chest x-ray often reveals a small heart and clear lungs, and, in about 50% of patients, pericardial calcification. Atrial fibrillation, low voltages, and nonspecific T wave changes are common. Confirmation of the diagnosis by cardiac catheterization is mandatory.

Clinically, constrictive pericarditis progresses insidiously, often without obvious cardiac symptomatology. Chest pain is infrequent, since the active inflammatory stage has resolved. Ascites or peripheral edema may develop, reflecting elevated venous pressures. In fact, patients with ascites or cirrhosis deriving from constrictive pericarditis may be mistakenly treated as though they have primary liver disease. Fatigue suggests decreased cardiac output. Dyspnea is common, but its origin is obscure: pulmonary congestion is not a part of constrictive pericarditis, and the left heart is protected from overload by the restriction of venous return. Elevated venous pressures may interfere with lymphatic drainage from the gut; the consequent loss of gastrointestinal protein is referred to as *protein-losing enteropathy*. The nephrotic syndrome may develop, although its cause is unknown. Both the nephrotic syndrome and protein-losing enteropathy of chronic pericarditis may abate upon surgical stripping of the pericardium.

The initiating episode is often never identified, and the etiology of chronic constrictive pericarditis frequently remains unknown. The pathology is generally nonspecific, with only calcification and fibrosis. Diagnosis of constrictive pericarditis is nevertheless important, because surgical stripping of the pericardium will frequently relieve the patient's symptoms.

BIBLIOGRAPHY

Fowler NO Physiology of cardiac tamponade and pulsus paradoxus. Mod Concepts Cardiovasc Dis 47, No. 11, 12:109–113, 1978

Fowler NO, Manitsas GT: Infectious pericarditis. Prog Cardiovasc Dis 16:323–336, 1973

Harvey WP: Auscultatory findings in disease of the pericardium. Am J Cardiol 7:15–20, 1961

Hirschmann JV: Pericardial constriction. Am Heart J 96:110–122, 1978

Rooney JJ, Crocco JA, Lyons HA: Tuberculous pericarditis. Ann Intern Med 72:73–81, 1970

10 Hypertension

Hypertension, both systolic and diastolic, is a risk factor for a multitude of potentially life-threatening illnesses. Although usually asymptomatic, hypertension is associated with an increased risk of angina, myocardial infarction, congestive heart failure, renal failure, and hemorrhagic and thrombotic strokes. Although hypertension can affect anyone at any age, black males in particular appear to be at an increased risk.

Normal blood pressure is usually defined as 120/80 torr. Individuals with blood pressure exceeding 160/95 torr are generally considered to have hypertension.

Successful treatment of hypertension decreases the incidence and rate of recurrence of stroke, diminishes left ventricular hypertrophy (determined by chest x-ray and EKG), increases survival in patients with renal insufficiency, and reduces the chances that the patient's hypertension will progress to malignant hypertension. With each increment in blood pressure, the risk of end-organ disease increases, and thus even partial blood pressure reduction is beneficial. At present, however, there is little evidence that the incidence of sudden death and myocardial infarction diminishes when hypertension is controlled.

ETIOLOGY

Primary Hypertension

The etiology of more than 95% of hypertensive disease remains unknown. It appears to be multifactorial, involving a complex interplay between the hemodynamic effects of the central nervous system, the peripheral adrenergic system and circulating catecholamines, and the volume regulatory effects of the renin-angiotensin-aldosterone system. Hemodynamic measurements have shown that the blood pressure can be elevated by increases in the peripheral vascular resistance or cardiac output.

Secondary Hypertension

Occasionally, a specific disorder of one of the control systems previously mentioned may cause hypertension. Patients with these disorders are said to have secondary hypertension. Although such disorders account for less than 5% of all hypertensive disease, they are often curable and are thus of great diagnostic importance. Before accepting the diagnosis of primary hypertension, all causes of secondary hypertension must be excluded.

Patients at risk for secondary hypertension include: (1) young (less than 25 years of age) and elderly (more than 65 years of age) patients with newly diagnosed hypertension, (2) patients with very severe or accelerated forms of hypertension, and (3) patients with hypertension that does not readily respond to conventional medical therapy.

The Renin-Angiotensin System. In the pioneering experiments of Goldblatt in 1934, constriction of a single renal artery was found to produce chronic hypertension. It is now known that renal hypoperfusion leads to augmented release of the enzyme, renin. Renin activity within the circulation leads to the activation of the peptide, angiotensin II. Angiotensin has two actions: it is a potent vasoconstrictor, and it stimulates the adrenal cortex to release aldosterone, a mineralocorticoid hormone that mediates sodium retention.

The most common cause of renovascular hypertension is discrete atherosclerotic narrowing of the renal artery, usually occurring in the elderly. The lesion is often surgically correctable. Other causes of renovascular hypertension include fibromuscular disease of the renal arterial wall (seen in young women), localized aneurysms, and various space-occupying lesions of the kidney, such as cysts and tumors, which produce unilateral renin release through local distortion of the intraparenchymal renal vasculature. Renin-secreting tumors of the kidney have also been described.

In a patient with renovascular hypertension, a rapid sequence intravenous urogram may reveal shortening of the affected kidney. In addition, the appearance of the dye is delayed in the diseased kidney, and, when finally present, the dye persists late into the study. Renal arteriography can provide the definitive diagnosis by delineating the site and extent of the vascular stenosis.

Not every stenosis, however, produces renovascular hypertension, and surgical correction of all identifiable lesions would lead to a disappointingly low rate of cure. In order to select only the proper candidates for surgical cure, the functional consequences of a stenotic lesion must be defined by renal venous catheterization. With unilateral disease, the renin activities in blood samples obtained from the veins of the affected kidney should be at least twice that of the unaffected kidney, indicating augmented renin release from the diseased kidney and suppression of renin release from the other. If this criterion is fulfilled in a hypertensive patient with arteriographic evidence of unilateral renovascular disease, the chance for a surgical cure is high. The recent availability of agents that block the conversion of angiotensin I to angiotensin II should enhance the diagnostic accuracy of these tests and may in the future offer a therapeutic alternative to surgery.

Adrenal Gland. Hypertension caused by diseases of the adrenal gland can usually be treated successfully with surgery.

Adrenal Cortex. Primary aldosteronism is a hypertensive disorder caused by an excess of the mineralocorticoid hormone, aldosterone. It should be suspected in any patient who presents with hypertension and hypokalemia (in the absence of diuretic therapy). The hypertension is usually mild. Primary aldosteronism is most commonly caused by hyperplasia of the zona glomerulosa; benign adenomas of the adrenal cortex can also secrete excess amounts of aldosterone. Salt and water retention with consequent volume expansion are responsible for the elevated blood pressure. Peripheral edema is rare. The diagnosis can be established by finding elevated aldosterone levels (with normal levels of cortisol and ACTH). The hallmark of the disease is the suppression of plasma renin activity produced by the sustained, autonomous volume expansion.

Patients with *Cushing's syndrome* can also develop hypertension (Chap. 29). Although cortisol has only weak mineralocorticoid activity, it can lead to sodium retention when present in excess. The precise etiology of the hypertension, however, is not understood.

Adrenal Medulla. The adrenal medulla has a prominent effect on the blood pressure through the production and release of the catecholamines, epinephrine and norepinephrine. When a tumor of the chromaffin cells of the adrenal medulla is present, the uncontrolled production of these catecholamines can produce a hypertensive syndrome (see Chapter 29).

Cardiovascular System. The only known correctable cardiovascular abnormality responsible for hypertension is *coarctation of the aorta*, a congenital anomaly characterized by an infolding of the aortic wall that constricts the aortic lumen. Coarctation produces delayed and markedly diminished pulses in the lower extremities, and sustained hypertension. The pathogenesis of the hypertension is far from clear. Although renal ischemia would seem to be a logical explanation, this does not seem to be true, since plasma renin activity is usually normal.

Many patients with uncomplicated coarctation (without other accompanying anomalies) are asymptomatic, although some may complain of headaches or exertional claudication. The key finding on physical examination is a difference in the systolic pressure between the arms and legs. In older children and adults, the musculature of the lower extremities may be underdeveloped. The physical examination is also noteworthy for a systolic murmur that originates from the coarctation. The murmur is best heard in the back between the scapulae. If the collateral circulation is well developed, pulsatile flow may be palpated in the intercostal spaces.

The chest x-ray is frequently diagnostic, exhibiting the classic "three sign" along the left heart border, produced by the aortic constriction and the silhouettes of the prestenotic and poststenotic vascular dilatations. In the presence of well-developed collateral flow, erosion of the inferior bony margin produces pathognomonic "rib notching."

Surgical correction of the luminal obstruction is curative in the majority of patients, although hypertension may persist or reappear in the later decades. Life-long prophylaxis for infectious endocarditis is mandatory.

END-ORGAN COMPLICATIONS OF HYPERTENSION

Cardiovascular Complications

Hypertension is a major risk factor in the development of atherosclerotic coronary vascular disease, with consequent angina pectoris and myocardial infarction. The sustained increase in the mean arterial pressure can also lead to left ventricular hypertrophy. The concentric hypertrophy of the left ventricular wall that results from chronic hypertension may be reflected in the electrocardiogram, although the EKG is an insensitive and by no means quantitative guide to the degree of hypertrophy. EKG findings may include (1) prominent R waves in leads primarily measuring activity of the left ventricular wall (greater than 2.5 mV in leads V_5 or V_6, or greater than 2.0 mV in leads I or aVL), (2) deep S waves in leads V_1 or V_2, and (3) inverted T waves with downsloping ST segments in lateral chest leads (referred to as "strain"), (4) left atrial enlargement, (5) and intraventricular conduction delays.

Evidence of left ventricular hypertrophy is frequently detected on the physical examination and on the electrocardiogram of untreated patients. Palpation of the chest can reveal an unusually pronounced and prolonged apical impulse. Eventually, left ventricular dilatation and congestive heart failure may develop.

Dissection of the aorta is a serious complication of long-standing hypertension. The forward pulsatile flow of blood produces an intimal tear in the aorta and permits blood to dissect between the intima and media for variable distances along the length of the aorta. The intima is particularly susceptible to hemodynamic stress at the two sites where the aorta is nonmobile: in the ascending aorta above the aortic valvular ring, and immediately distal to the left subclavian artery. Predisposing conditions for aortic dissection include hypertension and diseases that weaken the aortic media (*e.g.*, Marfan's syndrome).

Aortic dissection is characterized clinically by the acute onset of severe tearing pain in the anterior chest that radiates to the interscapular region. Patients are often extremely agitated and anxious. A chest x-ray usually demonstrates widening of the superior mediastinum. The diagnosis should be confirmed by contrast arteriography, which will demonstrate a false lumen or narrowing of the true lumen.

The consequences of aortic dissection are profound and potentially fatal, depending upon the location of the intimal tear. In *Type I aortic dissection*, the intimal tear occurs in the ascending aorta. The dissection may extend distally for variable lengths, and can proceed all the way to the aortic bifurcation. In 50% of patients, the dissection also proceeds proximally, producing acute aortic regurgitation or hemopericardium. Disastrous sequelae may occur when this second, or false, lumen occludes the ostia of the major arterial branches, including the coronary, carotid, renal, and mesenteric vasculature. The clinical presentation may therefore include my-

ocardial infarction, arrhythmias, stroke, mesenteric infarction, acute renal failure, or cardiac tamponade. Type I aortic dissection occurs primarily in patients under 65 years of age and is the most lethal form of the disease.

Type II dissection also involves the ascending aorta, but the dissection does not extend to the origin of the great vessels. Marfan's syndrome and other connective tissue disorders are the major predisposing factors. Hypertension does not play an important role.

Patients with *Type III dissections* are almost all elderly patients with atherosclerosis and hypertension. The tear occurs in the descending aorta so that sequelae result from hypoperfusion of the vascular tree distal to the left subclavian artery.

Therapy of aortic dissection depends upon the site of the intimal tear. Proximal dissection must be treated surgically with resection of the involved portion of the aorta. The prognosis with medical therapy alone is dismal. Death results from compromise of critical vessels or rupture of the aorta into the pericardium.

Patients with distal dissection respond more favorably to medical treatment. Therapy is directed toward rapidly reducing the blood pressure with nitroprusside or ganglionic blocking drugs (*e.g.*, trimethaphan). Reducing the rate of rise of the systolic pressure with each heart beat is thought to be beneficial, and may be accomplished with drugs that block the β receptor. Surgery is usually reserved for patients in unrelenting pain or with radiographic evidence of progression.

Renal Complications

Aging produces progressive intimal thickening of the intrarenal arteries and hyalinization of the glomeruli. This process may be accelerated by hypertension. It is called *nephrosclerosis*, and results in small, shrunken kidneys and azotemia.

Central Nervous System Complications

Hypertension can have devastating effects upon the intracerebral vasculature. Transient ischemic attacks, thrombotic strokes, rupture of intracranial aneurysms, and hypertensive intracerebral hemorrhages all can complicate the course of moderate to severe hypertension. An even more common form of end-organ damage in the nervous system is the retinopathy of hypertension, which produces fundoscopically detectable vascular changes (arteriovenous nicking is one of the earliest changes), hemorrhages, and exudates in a graded fashion.

AN APPROACH TO THE DIAGNOSIS AND THERAPY OF HYPERTENSION

A significant reduction in morbidity and mortality can result from a concerted effort to diagnose and treat arterial hypertension. Even patients with mild hypertension—those with a diastolic pressure between 95 and 100 torr—and patients with only systolic hypertension should be treated.

Because of the great prevalence of the disease and the cost of implementing a complete laboratory evaluation, there is much disagreement about what constitutes an adequate hypertensive assessment. From the foregoing discussion, certain elements of the evaluation appear to be essential (see list which follows). The serum electrolytes, particularly the potassium level, serve as an adequate screen for many of the causes of secondary hypertension. The extent of end-organ damage should be assessed with a plain chest x-ray, electrocardiogram, urinalysis, and serum creatinine.

If the history or physical examination suggests the possibility of secondary hypertension, one or more of the specific screening modalities may be employed: a rapid sequence intravenous urogram; plasma renin or aldosterone assay; 24-hour urine collection for

The Diagnostic Approach to Hypertension

Routine
Serum electrolytes
Serum creatinine
Plain chest x-ray
Electrocardiogram
Urinalysis
Desirable
Fasting blood sugar
Serum lipids
Screening for secondary causes, where indicated
Rapid sequence IV urogram
Plasma renin activity
Plasma aldosterone
24-hour urine catecholamines, metanephrine, vanillylmandelic acid, 1 mg overnight dexamethasone suppression test

catecholamines, vanillylmandelic acid, and metanephrine; and plasma cortisol determination after overnight dexamethasone suppression (see Chap. 29). Positive findings from any of these screening tests should be pursued in the appropriate manner. If no cause of secondary hypertension can be ascertained, the patient can be presumed to have primary hypertension.

The therapy of hypertension should be adjusted for the patient's age and the severity of the pressure elevation. Precipitous lowering of the blood pressure in patients whose vessels are occluded by atherosclerosis may precipitate stroke or myocardial infarction.

In many patients, the initial intervention should be to restrict salt intake. In obese patients, weight loss alone can greatly ameliorate hypertension. Increased physical activity (walking or jogging) can also be effective in lowering the blood pressure.

If the blood pressure cannot be brought

down to normal levels using the above modalities, drug therapy is required. The goal in treating hypertension is to bring the blood pressure within the normal range, or as close to it as possible (see Flow Sheet, p. 77).

The *oral diuretics* are most frequently chosen as the initial approach to blood pressure control. These drugs often lower the blood pressure to desired limits when used alone, and can be incorporated into a multidrug regimen to minimize the sodium retention that complicates the use of most other antihypertensive drugs.

The diuretics fall into three categories: thiazides, loop diuretics, and aldosterone antagonists.

1. The *thiazides* act on the cortical diluting segment to prevent sodium reabsorption. Their use is complicated by hypokalemia, and potassium replacement may be required. All thiazides share the potential side-effects of hyperglycemia and hyperuricemia; the latter may unmask latent gouty arthritis.

2. *Furosemide* is a thiazide derivative that affects the ascending limb of the loop of Henle. It is a much more potent natriuretic agent than the thiazides, and can therefore cause more profound electrolyte disturbances. For this reason, furosemide has little role in antihypertensive therapy in patients in whom the thiazides can be used.

3. *Spironolactone* is an aldosterone antagonist that blocks the effects of aldosterone on the distal tubule. It is a weak diuretic. Spironolactone is potassium-sparing and can produce hyperkalemia, epigastric distress, and breast tenderness or gynecomastia. *Triamterene* is another commonly used potassium-sparing diuretic.

If diuretic therapy does not yield adequate control, the addition of a second agent is indicated, either a direct vasodilator, a central nervous system agent, or a β-adrenergic blocker.

Hydralazine is typical of the drugs that produce vasodilatation through direct relaxation of the arteriolar smooth muscle. It is a short-acting drug and is rapidly inactivated by the liver when given orally. With any route of administration, the rapid reduction of blood pressure can produce profound reflex tachycardia.

Propranolol is a β-adrenergic receptor antagonist. Its antihypertensive effect may be achieved through blockade of sympathetically mediated renin release and through action at regulatory sites within the central nervous system and within the heart itself. It should be used only with great caution in patients who have evidence of left ventricular failure or reactive bronchoconstriction.

Methyldopa is the prototype of a centrally acting antihypertensive. In addition to its action on the central nervous system, it suppresses renin release and produces only minimal orthostatic hypotension. An undesired sedative effect is commonly seen. Other side-effects include a reversible elevation of hepatic serum transaminases, hyperprolactinemia with lactation, and a Coombs' positive hemolytic anemia.

Clonidine exerts its antihypertensive effect through its effects on central nervous system alpha receptors. The hypotensive response to clonidine is characterized by a reduction in the cardiac output at rest. Because the reflex control of vascular resistance is not impaired, orthostatic hypotension is a rare complication. However, a withdrawal syndrome with signs of sympathetic excess, including tachycardia, hypertension, and arrhythmias, may appear within 36 hours after abrupt cessation of clonidine therapy.

Reserpine is a long-acting, centrally acting sympatholytic drug. It is usually used in concert with a diuretic or other antihypertensive agent. Like clonidine, reserpine preserves the peripheral vascular reflexes, so that postural hypotension is rarely a problem. The use of reserpine is limited by its many troublesome

Therapy of Hypertension: A Flow Sheet

Non-pharmacologic Therapy
        weight loss
        increased physical activity
        moderate salt restriction
        relaxation and avoidance of stress

Group I   *Thiazide diuretic* (± a potassium sparing diuretic or KCI replacement therapy, especially in the elderly)

if hypertension persists, add:

Group II *Propranolol* (or other β-blocking drug)
        or
        Methyl-dopa (occasionally, *propranolol plus* one of the other Group II drugs must be added to the diuretic to achieve blood pressure control)
        or
        Clonidine
        or
        Reserpine
        or
        Hydrala-zine

if hypertension still persists, try:

Group III *Prazosin*
        or
        Guanethidine

side-effects, which include bradycardia, cutaneous flushing, excess salivation, nasal congestion, stomach cramps, and depression. The drug is contraindicated for patients with known affective disorders or peptic ulcer disease.

Prazosin is a new antihypertensive medication that blocks alpha-adrenergic receptors. It is especially useful in combination with a diuretic or a β-blocking drug in patients with severe hypertension. Patients may experience severe orthostatic hypotension and even syncope after taking the first dose.

Patients who do not adequately respond to some combination of these agents should receive a trial of *guanethidine, a sympathetic blocking agent*. The drug is a powerful antihypertensive, but unfortunately it exhibits several undesired effects, including severe orthostatic hypotension, diarrhea, weakness, and impotence. These effects are usually severe enough to limit its application, but in certain patients blood pressure control can only be achieved with this drug.

It has been conclusively demonstrated that the control of hypertension significantly decreases morbidity and mortality. Unfortunately, it is often difficult to convince the patient of the necessity of lifelong therapy for a disease that is usually asymptomatic. Whatever the mode of therapy in hypertensive disease, patient education and reinforcement are essential to a successful outcome. Weight reduction and dietary restriction of sodium should be stressed repeatedly, and the patient's blood pressure must be monitored frequently until sustained control is achieved at the desired level. Pharmacotherapy will probably be required indefinitely, even when the blood pressure is reduced to desired limits.

MALIGNANT HYPERTENSION

Malignant (or accelerated) hypertension is a potentially fatal complication of hypertension. The blood pressure that will precipitate a hypertensive emergency varies with each patient and is dependent upon the etiology and duration of the preceding hypertension. Thus, although a diastolic blood pressure of greater than 140 torr is conveniently used to define patients at risk for a hypertensive crisis, the absolute level is less important than the associated physical findings. In addition to the dangerous elevation of blood pressure, the syndrome of malignant hypertension includes advanced retinal changes, papilledema, progressive oliguric renal failure, and hypertensive encephalopathy. The clinical presentation of hypertensive encephalopathy may include headache, seizures, coma, or agitation.

The pathogenesis of malignant hypertension is unclear. It is associated with intimal hyperplasia of small renal arteries that produces a characteristic fibrinoid necrosis. This, in turn, leads to high circulating levels of renin, which undoubtedly contribute to the dramatic increase in blood pressure.

To prevent a potentially lethal outcome and to preserve renal function, aggressive measures must be undertaken to lower the blood pressure in a rapid and controlled manner. It must be emphasized that this rapid approach to blood pressure reduction should be reserved for patients who exhibit papilledema, oliguria, or encephalopathy. Therapy must be initiated in the emergency room and continued in the intensive care unit.

Initial blood pressure reduction is frequently achieved with a bolus injection of *diazoxide*; it begins to work within several minutes. This potent vasodilator can precipitate hypotension and coronary ischemia, and may cause hyperglycemia. It is not a suitable medication for continued therapy. *Hydralazine* can also provide immediate blood pressure reduction.

If intra-arterial pressure monitoring is available, *nitroprusside* allows minute-by-minute titration of the blood pressure. For refractory patients, a ganglionic blocking agent such as trimethaphan can be used.

Methyldopa has a delayed onset of action (approximately several hours) when given orally or intravenously, and is therefore not of immediate benefit.

Once the patient's blood pressure is stabilized at a lower level, a change to oral antihypertensive agents is feasible. These include diuretics, propranolol, or methyldopa.

All of the rapidly acting antihypertensive agents have profound effects and side-effects, and must be used with extreme care. It is occasionally advisable to monitor the arterial pressure continuously with an intra-arterial catheter. In most patients, the goal should be an initial reduction of the diastolic pressure to approximately 100 torr, followed by a gradual reduction to the desired end point.

BIBLIOGRAPHY

Dunn MJ, Tannen RL: Low renin hypertension. Kidney Int 5:317–325, 1974

Foster JH, Maxwell MH, Franklin SS et al: Renovascular occlusive disease. Results of operative treatment. JAMA 231:1043–1048, 1975

Fries ED: The clinical spectrum of essential hypertension. Arch Intern Med 133:982–987, 1974

Gifford RW Jr, Tarazi RC: Resistant hypertension: Diagnosis and management. Ann Intern Med 88:661–665, 1978

Gifford RW Jr, Westbrook E: Hypertensive encephalopathy: Mechanisms, clinical features and treatment. Progr Cardiovasc Dis 17:155–175, 1974

Graham RM, Pettinger WA: Drug therapy: Prazosin. NEJM 300:232–236, 1979

Hypertension detection and follow-up program cooperative group: Five-year findings of the hypertension detection and follow-up program. JAMA 242:2562–2571, 1979

Koch Weser J: Diazoxide. N Engl J Med 294:1271–1273, 1976

O'Malley K, O'Brien E: Management of hypertension in the elderly. N Engl J Med 302:1397–1401, 1980

Palmer RF, Lasseter KC: Sodium nitroprusside. N Engl J Med 292:294–297, 1975

Shand DG: Propranolol. N Engl J Med 293:280–285, 1975

Slater EE, DeSanctis RW: The clinical recognition of dissecting aortic aneurysm. Am J Med 60:625–633, 1976

Pulmonary Disease

11

Pulmonary Function Tests

Pulmonary function tests are used to assess the nature and severity of lung disease as well as to quantify the progression of disease and its response to therapy. In recent years, in the hope of identifying nascent pulmonary disease at an early and reversible stage, the scope of pulmonary function tests has expanded to include the assessment of pulmonary function in persons who are free from respiratory symptoms, but who have been exposed to suspected toxins, most commonly those from cigarette smoking.

The most widely available pulmonary function tests are spirometry and arterial blood gas determinations. In the near future, tests of small airway function and ventilatory drive will probably become routine at most centers.

VITAL CAPACITY AND FORCED EXPIRATORY VOLUME

The vital capacity (VC) is the maximum volume a person can exhale, and is equal to the volume of air in the lungs at full inspiration (total lung capacity, TLC) minus the volume of air that is left after full exhalation (residual volume, RV). Diseases that obstruct the airways, such as chronic obstructive pulmonary

disease and asthma, make emptying difficult and incomplete and thereby increase the residual volume and decrease the vital capacity (Fig. 11–1). The total lung capacity may actually increase, but never to a greater degree than does the residual volume. Restrictive lung diseases, such as scleroderma, stiffen the lungs and decrease the total lung capacity, residual volume, and vital capacity.

Measuring the volume forcefully exhaled in one second, starting at total lung capacity, gives the measurement known as the FEV_1 (forced expiratory volume in one second). The FEV_1 is normally greater than 75% of the vital capacity. It decreases with obstructive—but not with restrictive—processes.

If the spirometer is connected to an oscilloscope, simultaneous measurements of flow and volume can be recorded and graphed. The standard maneuver is to have the patient forcefully exhale and inhale his vital capacity while the instantaneous flow is plotted against the lung volume on the oscilloscope. This series of measurements is called a *flow-volume loop*.

The shape of the loop varies characteristically with different disorders. The exhalation limb of the loop for several different types of lung diseases is shown in Fig. 11–2. Reduction

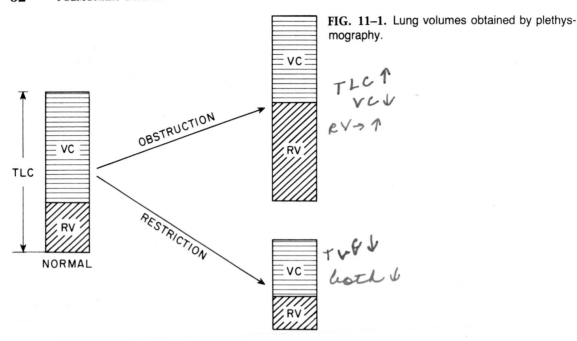

FIG. 11–1. Lung volumes obtained by plethysmography.

TLC ↑
VC ↓
RV → ↑

T↓ ↓
both ↓

of flow suggests obstructive lung disease. Since obstructive processes often affect the small airways first, exacerbating their tendency to collapse at small lung volumes, such processes can manifest themselves at their earliest stages by reducing flow at low lung volumes (50% or 25% of the vital capacity). For this reason, pulmonary function test printouts often include the midexpiratory flow at 50% of vital capacity ($MEF_{50\%VC}$). Restrictive lung diseases, on the other hand, present a narrower loop, since the total lung volume shrinks, but the overall shape remains essentially normal. The most important use of the flow-volume loop is in the diagnosis of a large airway obstruction, such as in tracheal stenosis. Such diseases flatten the curve by obstructing the flow of air early in expiration (Fig. 11–2) in contrast to patients with small airway disease.

SMALL AIRWAY DISEASE

Because of their vast number and large total volume, small airways contribute little resistance to airflow. Thus, for example, widespread disease of the 2- to 3-mm bronchi that occurs in smokers remains silent on both spirometry and on the flow-volume curve until the disease is almost incapacitating. Tests have therefore been developed that can highlight small airway disease early in its course.

The density dependence test makes use of the different physics of airflow in large as opposed to small airways. Flow in the large airways, normally turbulent, improves with breathing low-density helium mixtures. Flow in the small airways is more laminar, and does not improve upon breathing helium. Some 80 to 90% of the airway resistance in

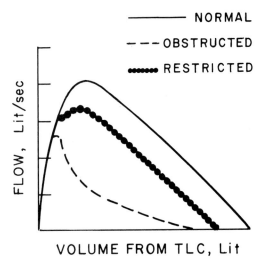

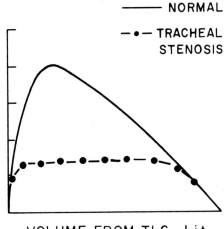

FIG. 11–2. The flow-volume curves showing the pattern of early diminution in flow seen in obstructive lung disease and the uniform plateau diagnostic of stenosis in the trachea.

healthy individuals involves the large airways, and flow therefore improves markedly with helium breathing. Smokers, on the other hand, in whom resistance to airflow includes a disproportionate contribution from the small airways, do not show any improvement. They lose this normal density dependence even before the shape of the standard flow-volume curve is affected.

The *closing volume test* takes advantage of two factors:

1. Small airways located at the base of the lungs are subject to more positive pleural pressure because of the weight of the lung, and tend to collapse during expiration. These airways normally collapse only at end expiration (RV), but may collapse earlier in expiration if the supporting structure of the lung is lost (emphysema) or the airway patency is obstructed (bronchitis).

2. With inspiration, alveoli at the base of the lung undergo twice the volume change as alveoli located at the apex. A breath of oxygen therefore selectively dilutes air in the basal alveoli.

The closing volume test is performed by having the patient inhale oxygen, and then measuring the concentration of nitrogen in the next exhaled breath. The exhaled air contains a low concentration of nitrogen (diluted by the oxygen) until the basal alveoli close. Without their contribution, the nitrogen concentration rises. This break in the curve is referred to as the *closing volume.* In the airway disease caused by smoking, the small bronchi lose their support and collapse earlier, and the closing volume rises.

BLOOD GASES

Oxygen. The partial pressure of oxygen in the blood (Pa_{O_2}) is approximately 100 torr in normal youngsters, and approaches 80 torr in the elderly. A low Pa_{O_2} can result either from inhaling air with a low oxygen concentration (*e.g.,* at high altitudes) or from lung disease. Only two disease processes can cause hypoxemia: hypoventilation and diffusion abnormalities.

Hypoventilation means that ventilation is inadequate to oxygenate the blood and to remove carbon dioxide. *Focal alveolar hypoventilation* is seen in obstructive lung diseases, where some, but not all, airways are narrowed and their alveoli underventilated. This situation produces a ventilation/perfusion (V/Q) abnormality: Blood passes through a region of inadequate ventilation and returns unoxygenated to the heart. The effect is that of an anatomic right-to-left shunt. The unoxygenated blood mixes with the blood that has passed through adequately oxygenated regions, and the final saturation of the blood returning to the heart is below normal. In *global alveolar hypoventilation*, all alveoli share equally in the impaired ventilation. Global alveolar hypoventilation can result either from an abnormal ventilatory drive (*e.g.,* Pickwickian syndrome or hypothyroidism) or from a distorted or weak chest wall (*e.g.,* kyphoscoliosis or myasthenia gravis).

Diffusion abnormalities result from destruction of alveolar-capillary membranes, either from emphysema or interstitial inflammation. The extent of compromise can be determined by measuring the amount of carbon monoxide absorbed from a single breath of gas containing carbon monoxide. Hypoxemia that is due to a diffusion abnormality often becomes marked only with exercise. It is still not known how much of the measured diffusion abnormality reflects actual thickening and obstruction at the alveolar-capillary interface and how much reflects a ventilation/perfusion mismatch.

Carbon Dioxide. Carbon dioxide retention occurs in all forms of global alveolar hypoventilation, and can also occur in severe cases of focal alveolar hypoventilation. It does not occur with diffusion abnormalities, because CO_2 diffuses rapidly across the alveolar membranes even in these patients.

REGULATION OF VENTILATION

A low Pa_{O_2} stimulates ventilation by means of arterial chemoreceptors. A high Pa_{CO_2} stimulates ventilation by means of a central nervous system chemoreceptor. The ventilatory response to abnormal blood gases varies from individual to individual and from population to population. The Sherpa inhabitants of the Himalayas are chronically exposed to a low Pa_{O_2} and increase their ventilation only minimally with progressive hypoxemia. Many patients with chronic bronchitis manifest a blunted response to carbon dioxide, and rely almost totally on the hypoxic drive to breathe. The ventilatory drive can be measured by administering gases of variable mixtures of oxygen and carbon dioxide and measuring the ventilatory response.

A technique that more accurately reflects the instantaneous drive to breathe has recently been developed. This test measures the inspiratory force generated when the airway is suddenly occluded while the person is breathing varying mixtures of oxygen and carbon dioxide.

BIBLIOGRAPHY

Bass H: The flow volume loop: Normal standards and abnormalities in chronic obstructive pulmonary disease. Chest 63:171–176, 1973

Cherniack NS: The clinical assessment of the chemical regulation of ventilation. Chest 70:274–281, 1976

Hodgkin JE: Evaluation before thoracotomy. West J Med 122:104–109, 1975

Rodarte JR, Hyatt RE, Rehder K et al: New tests for the detection of obstructive pulmonary disease. Chest 72:762–768, 1977

12

**Respiratory
Failure**

Few situations provoke more anxiety than the acutely dyspneic patient. Typically, the patient is sitting forward, his blue hands gripping any fixture to support the labor of his accessory muscles of respiration. Despite vigorous tachypnea, the patient is exchanging little air and is often unable to spare a breath even to give a history.

The immediate therapeutic question seems to be straightforward: Should the patient be intubated? The answer, however, frequently requires knowledge of the patient's clinical history that is unattainable during the acute event. One must then weigh the many potential complications of mechanical ventilation against the risks of hypoxia, hypercarbia, and respiratory acidosis.

Evaluation of the patient's clinical status, interpretation of arterial blood gas tensions, and institution of therapy should all be tempered by whether or not the patient has been suffering from chronic lung disease before the acute decompensation. Patients chronically exposed to low tissue oxygen tension, either because they live at a high altitude or because they have chronic lung disease, develop compensatory mechanisms to enhance oxygen delivery (such as changes in the oxygen dissociation curve and increases in red blood cell

number). They tolerate a given level of hypoxemia better than a patient who is acutely suffering respiratory decompensation for the first time. Similarly, the patient who chronically retains CO_2 because of obstructive lung disease can be expected to have an elevated Pa_{CO_2} as well as a compensatory increase in serum HCO_3^-. A previously healthy patient, however, should have a low arterial CO_2, since he will be hyperventilating in an attempt to maintain his arterial P_{O_2}. When this patient begins to retain CO_2 it suggests that the respiratory muscles have fatigued and respiratory arrest is imminent. A further consideration is that patients with prior CO_2 retention experience blunting of their CO_2-dependent drive to breathe. They rely upon a low arterial P_{O_2} as their only ventilatory stimulus. If high levels of oxygen are delivered in inspired air this drive is removed and they stop breathing. On the other hand, it is appropriate, and may be lifesaving, to administer 100% oxygen to patients without a history of carbon dioxide retention.

Patients may have normal lungs but still suffer from alveolar hypoventilation if their lung bellows do not, or cannot, move enough air. This may be due to disorders of neurons that control breathing or to distortion or weakness of the thoracic musculature. Since all alveoli share in the hypoventilation in these patients, they are said to have "global" or "general" alveolar hypoventilation.

HYPOXIA

People vary in their sensitivity to hypoxia. Oxygen demands vary with fever, activity, nutrition, thyroid function, and hepatic disease.

Hypoxia derives largely from two pulmonary disorders:

1. **Right-to-left shunts** within the lung. In healthy persons, 2.5% of the cardiac output is shunted within the lung and is not oxygenated. In some patients with severe pulmonary disease, this figure can rise to as high as 50%.

2. **Alveolar hypoventilation** may be divided pathophysiologically into two varieties, "global" and "regional."

If patients have normal lungs, hypoventilation may be associated with hypothyroidism, muscle weakness, dysautonomia, medullary disease (e.g., poliomyelitis), drugs, or severe metabolic alkalosis. Some patients suffer global hypoventilation because of intermittent upper airway obstruction, a problem referred to as the "sleep-apnea syndrome." Patients with this condition hypoventilate during the night because of the upper airway obstruction, and are therefore always sleepy during the day. Eventually, via undefined pathways, nocturnal hypoventilation causes a blunting of their ventilatory drive. The Pickwickian syndrome, a term used to describe obese patients with hypersomnolence and polycythemia, is related to the sleep-apnea syndrome.

Chronic obstructive pulmonary disease causes hypoxemia because of "regional" hypoventilation (Chap. 13). Some alveoli are poorly ventilated because of obstructive lesions in the airways, bronchoconstriction, atelectasis, and loss of the supporting structures of the bronchial walls.

Central nervous system function is a fairly good clinical indicator of severe hypoxia. As the Pa_{O_2} decreases, mental proficiency and concentration decline. Headache, anorexia, insomnia, and delerium supervene, and eventually culminate in respiratory arrest when hypoxemia becomes severe enough to cause central respiratory depression. Recovery from an acute hypoxic insult can be protracted. A Pa_{O_2} of less than 20 is incompatible with life. Patients suffering chronic hypoxemia, either from lung disease or from living at a high altitude, tolerate low arterial oxygen levels with fewer ill effects.

Hypoxic damage to other organ systems may also be significant. Diminished renal glomerular filtration with sodium and water retention contributes to the edema that often accompanies acute pulmonary failure. A general decrease in muscle tone can be demonstrated. The liver enzymes SGOT and LDH may increase and there may be pathologic evidence of centrilobular necrosis. Gastric motility is diminished and gastric acid secretion heightened, and there appears to be an increased incidence of gastrointestinal bleeding. Hypoxic depression of myocardial contractility can be masked by the circulatory adjustments of tachycardia and vasoconstriction. If hypoxemia is severe, a myocardial infarction may result.

HYPERCARBIA AND RESPIRATORY ACIDOSIS

A Pa_{CO_2} of greater than 45 implies that the ventilatory apparatus can no longer keep up with the metabolic production of carbon dioxide. Pa_{CO_2} levels of 80 to 90 are narcotic and cause respiratory depression. Even before this end state is reached, however, the acidosis that results from carbon dioxide accumulation is a serious threat to the patient (Chap. 21).

The direct toxic manifestations of an increased Pa_{CO_2} are primarily neurologic. As the Pa_{CO_2} exceeds 80, the patient experiences a decrease in cognitive function. Headache, hypersomnolence, and asterixis and tremor appear. These are sometimes accompanied by diaphoresis and conjunctival suffusion. Eventually, coma supervenes.

Cardiac arrhythmias are a regular accompaniment of respiratory failure. The precise contribution of hypoxemia, hypercarbia, and acidosis to the genesis of these arrhythmias often cannot be resolved. The presence of arrhythmias contributes to the decision whether to intubate a patient. The most common arrhythmias are supraventricular, especially paroxysmal atrial tachycardia or multifocal atrial tachycardia; ventricular ectopy and ventricular tachycardia also appear frequently and carry a poor prognosis. Ventricular fibrillation is not uncommon in acute respiratory failure.

THERAPY

Intubation

Intubation is mandatory in any patient with a Pa_{O_2} of less than 20 or a Pa_{CO_2} of more than 80 to 90; otherwise, no absolute levels of Pa_{O_2} or Pa_{CO_2} should be accepted as dictating intubation. Rather, it becomes critical to determine whether the patient has a history of chronic lung disease and how fulminant the deterioration has been.

Patients with chronic lung disease develop compensatory mechanisms to ensure adequate oxygen delivery (such as shifts of the oxygen dissociation curve) and to buffer chronic respiratory acidosis, and thus they can tolerate levels of hypoxemia and hypercarbia that can be life-threatening in a previously healthy patient. They may be perfectly comfortable with a baseline Pa_{O_2} of 60 and a Pa_{CO_2} of 50. For these patients, chronic carbon dioxide retention is part of their physiologic readjustment to chronic lung disease and reflects their blunted carbon dioxide drive to breathe. These patients respond chiefly to the hypoxic drive to breathe, and aggressive oxygen therapy may suppress ventilation and lead to respiratory arrest.

For patients with previously normal lungs, the carbon dioxide-induced drive to breathe is still intact, and a Pa_{CO_2} of 50 suggests that fatigue has set in. Rapid deterioration is predictable if intubation is not expedited.

The lucidity of the patient's sensorium is perhaps the most useful measure of the need for intubation in acute respiratory failure. The patient in acute distress will be obstreperous, agitated, and confused. Respiratory muscle fatigue may be manifested as discoordination of the diaphragm and intercostal muscles. Contraction of the intercostal and accessory muscles alone causes the diaphragm to be drawn upward with consequent inward movement of the abdomen during inspiration.

As the arterial blood gases worsen and respirations quicken, two questions should be answered:

1. How long will it be before either muscular fatigue or carbon dioxide narcosis causes respiratory arrest or before hypoxemia, acidosis, and hypercarbia precipitate arrhythmias?

2. What components of the patient's distress are acutely reversible?

A tight-fitting mask and continuous positive pressure breathing may be useful initially, but eventually the progression of hypoxemia and hypercarbia may demand intubation.

The advantages of intubation include (1) the ability to ensure maximum delivery of oxygen. This can be accomplished without immediate worry about blunting ventilation because the respirator ensures that breathing continues;

(2) the application of positive end-expiratory pressure to keep the lungs inflated throughout the respiratory cycle and thereby prevent atelectasis; (3) suctioning of secretions in a patient with an ineffective cough; and (4) the ability to relieve the patient of dyspnea, thereby giving him a feeling of well-being and security.

Complications. The endotracheal tube breaches the normal laryngeal and mucosal barriers to infection. Colonization by unusual organisms almost always occurs, and these may produce pneumonia. Secretions can accumulate because of the loss of effective cough mechanisms. Frequent suctioning is therefore important in managing these patients. Pneumothorax and pneumomediastinum, though rare, may occur, especially in patients with obstructive airway disease. Permanent tracheal stenosis and tracheomalacia may plague the patient after intubation, although these problems are less common now that tracheal tubes with soft balloons are available. The patient's mobility is limited, postural drainage is time-consuming, and the tendency to thromboembolism and venous stasis disease is heightened. Other problems include malfunction of the ventilator, kinking or plugging of the endotracheal tube, intubation of only the right main stem bronchus, and unintentional hyperventilation. For some patients, intubation may cause severe psychological trauma.

Positive pressure breathing interferes with venous return, especially in the volume-depleted patient, and can drastically reduce the cardiac output. Massive gastric dilatation, presumably from leakage of air back to the mouth and then swallowed into the stomach, can—in extreme cases—cause gastric rupture. Several kilograms of free water can be retained, caused partly by the additional 500 ml of water that enter the patient each day by means of the heated nebulizer, but also by the increased transatrial pressure and resultant reflex release of antidiuretic hormone.

The need for mechanical ventilation in a patient with chronic lung disease predicts a poor outcome, with a 30% in-hospital mortality, the cause of which is usually nonpulmonary. The prognosis in a patient with previously healthy lungs is slightly more hopeful. There is a 20% mortality in the intensive care unit, and those who survive often experience no significant residual pulmonary dysfunction.

Weaning the Patient. When infection is under adequate control by means of antibiotics, pulmonary edema resolved, metabolic alkalosis reversed, and the trend to improved pulmonary function clearly established, mechanical ventilation may no longer be necessary. In addition to the Pa_{O_2} and Pa_{CO_2}, several other criteria can be helpful in determining the adequacy of ventilation. Intubation is still required when:

1. The vital capacity is less than 15 ml/kg (normal, 65 to 75 ml/kg),

2. The gradient of P_{O_2} between the alveoli and the arterial blood while the patient is breathing 100% oxygen is greater than 450 torr (normal 25 to 65 torr), or

3. The inspiratory force is less than 25 cm H_2O (normal, 75 to 100 cm H_2O).

Many patients, especially those with previously abnormal lungs or those who have undergone long intubations, become dependent upon their ventilators. Their reliance on ventilatory supports derives from muscle weakness caused by poor nutrition, inactivity and diaphragmatic discoordination.

Often within 30 minutes after the cessation of mechanical ventilation, radiographic evidence of atelectasis develops, dyspnea returns, and hypoxemia and carbon dioxide retention begin again. It may then be necessary to wean the patient from his ventilator over many days by using "intermittent mandatory ventilation," in which the ventilator delivers a guaranteed number of breaths per minute. As the patient's respiratory drive and coordination are restored, the number of mandatory breaths can be progressively reduced. The addition of positive pressure at end expiration helps to prevent airway closure and atelectasis.

Other Therapeutic Interventions

Whether or not the patient is intubated, other therapeutic modalities must begin immediately. (The use of bronchodilators is described in Chap. 15.)

Positioning the Patient. Only trial and error can determine the most comfortable and most efficient posture for gas exchange for the dyspneic patient. No single position should be maintained without interruption or else secretions will accumulate and edema collect in dependent tissues. Most patients, especially the markedly obese and patients recovering from abdominal operations, feel more comfortable and have a higher Pa_{O_2} sitting than lying down. The patient with one diseased lung may benefit if placed in the lateral decubitus position with the diseased lung uppermost. This posture appears to increase blood flow to the healthy lung.

Oxygen Therapy. The dangers of oxygen therapy include suppression of the drive to breathe and the direct toxicity of oxygen. The patient with previously normal lungs relies on the carbon dioxide drive to breathe, and—except for the possible threat of oxygen toxicity—there is no reason to limit oxygen delivery. On the other hand, the patient with chronic alveolar hypoventilation has a blunted and ineffective ventilatory response to increasing Pa_{CO_2}, and relies on the hypoxic drive to breathe. In this patient, oxygen must be delivered carefully, slowly increasing the FiO_2

(the oxygen concentration of inspired air) and repeating arterial blood gases 20 minutes after each increment in oxygen delivery. If significant carbon dioxide retention begins to occur, the FiO_2 must immediately be lowered. The supplemental oxygen should not be turned off completely, however, since this may cause a precipitous drop in Pa_{O_2}.

In patients with abnormal lungs, the Pa_{O_2} can usually be increased from 25 torr (barely enough to support a healthy person) to 40 torr, with progressive increments of only 4% to 7% in FiO_2. Slight carbon dioxide retention will probably occur, but usually only on the order of 10 torr. Small changes in Pa_{O_2} markedly improve oxygen delivery to the tissues in the hypoxemic range generally encountered (Pa_{O_2} of 25 to 50), and only rarely should attempts be made to surpass a Pa_{O_2} of 60. The addition of more oxygen usually does little to improve oxygenation (because of the presence of large shunts), and, if it does, it then engenders the problems of carbon dioxide retention and narcosis. The Venturi masks that can be set for an FiO_2 of 24% or 28% have proved to be most convenient for safe graded oxygen delivery in the nonintubated patient.

The threat of oxygen toxicity must be considered in patients with and without severe underlying lung disease. High oxygen concentrations damage the lungs at both the alveolar and cellular levels. An oxygen-filled alveolus is prone to *absorption collapse* as oxygen is rapidly absorbed down a high concentration gradient (from alveolus to capillary), leaving the air space without gas. Direct cytotoxicity may be mediated by a reaction product of oxygen, called superoxide. Superoxide is normally rendered harmless by the enzyme superoxide dismutase, but this protection can be overwhelmed by high oxygen concentrations. Oxygen may also interfere with mucociliary function. High oxygen concentrations eventually damage the epithelium and endothelium and result in the accumulation of alveolar and interstitial edema. Although individual sensitivities to oxygen vary, it appears that an FiO_2 of less than 40% can be given safely for weeks. Any FiO_2, even 100%, is safe for 24 hours, but for longer periods of time an FiO_2 exceeding 60% is hazardous.

Positive End Expiratory Pressure (PEEP). The required FiO_2 can be reduced by positive end expiratory pressure (during mechanical ventilation) or continuous positive pressure (during spontaneous breathing), in which the expiratory port is submerged under 5 to 20 cm of water. Positive pressure prevents collapse of the airways at end expiration. It has proved to be especially helpful in treating patients with pulmonary edema and with the acute respiratory distress syndrome of the adult (see later in chapter). Patients with obstructive disease do not benefit from PEEP, and are predisposed to develop tension pneumothoraces. In all patients, PEEP can decrease cardiac output by interfering with venous return. Volume infusions may then be required to maintain the cardiac output.

↓ CO
↓ VR

Carbon Dioxide. The Pa_{CO_2} can be rapidly lowered and easily regulated by changing the tidal volume and the rate of mechanical ventilation. There is little evidence corroborating the early concern that precipitous changes in carbon dioxide tension precipitate hypotension and seizures. However, there is no reason to reduce the Pa_{CO_2} below the patient's baseline, since this would precipitate respiratory alkalosis. Bicarbonate should play no role in the treatment of respiratory acidosis unless the patient is so acidotic that circulatory collapse and the accumulation of lactic acid pose real dangers.

Diuresis and Digoxin. Diuresis often dramatically improves oxygenation because some of these patients are suffering in part from left ventricular failure. The chest x-ray, usually an excellent guide to treating pulmonary edema, is often of little use in patients with chronic lung disease. In these patients, pulmonary edema appears as regional patchy infiltrates rather than as the classic diffuse haze seen in patients with otherwise normal lungs. During acute respiratory decompensation, diuretics should be administered in order to improve oxygenation, not to rid the patient of peripheral edema. Patients with cor pulmonale may therefore derive only little benefit from diuresis, and may even suffer hypotensive episodes if fluid loss proceeds too rapidly. Neck veins and peripheral edema are not an appropriate guide to filling pressure of the left ventricle. It is precisely these patients, in whom the degree of left ventricular failure is uncertain, who will benefit therapeutically from direct measurement of the pulmonary capillary wedge pressures using a Swan-Ganz catheter. Some patients with severe lung disease and right ventricular failure do seem to develop left ventricular failure without clear-cut disease of the left ventricle itself. It is not understood why the left ventricle often fails along with the right ventricle in severe lung disease. Possible causes include hypoxemia, concomitant coronary artery disease, and the adverse mechanical effects of the failing right ventricle. In any case, digoxin should be avoided in the acute phase of respiratory failure when metabolic derangements predispose to digoxin toxicity. The drug should be used, however, as necessary to control appropriate arrhythmias. The common arrhythmia of respiratory distress, multifocal atrial tachycardia, is usually refractory to digoxin.

Hypoventilation. Reversible causes of hypoventilation should be remedied. Hypothyroidism is associated with a depressed hypoxic ventilatory drive, and ventilation improves over weeks with thyroid replacement. Metabolic alkalosis, secondary to the chloride and potassium depletion of diuretics, is a ventilatory depressant. It must be vigorously treated with potassium chloride or hydro-chloric acid (if severe). Acetazolamide administration may acidify the blood by inhibiting carbonic anhydrase and producing a proximal tubular acidosis. If liver function is adequate, some favor chloride replacement with ammonium chloride. The use of respiratory stimulants is not accepted. Analeptics, such as doxapam, are fraught with side-effects and should only be a last, desperate resource.

ADULT RESPIRATORY DISTRESS SYNDROME

One of the unforeseen offshoots of the war in Southeast Asia was an increased awareness and understanding of the "shock lung syndrome," sometimes graphically referred to as DaNang lung. This syndrome was epitomized by the soldier who had suffered nonthoracic injuries and had become hypotensive. Rushed to the base hospital, he would be quickly and successfully resuscitated with saline, blood, and oxygen. He would be resting comfortably only to decompensate suddenly with respiratory distress, tachypnea, and cyanosis. A chest x-ray would reveal progressive, patchy edema and atelectasis (Fig. 12–1). As the lungs stiffened and filled with fluid, oxygenation would swiftly deteriorate and death would occur within 24 to 48 hours.

It subsequently became apparent that this clinical pattern represented the final pathway of many metabolic and physical injuries of the lung. An identical picture could be seen not only after hemorrhagic shock, but also in patients with pancreatitis, fat emboli, septic shock, massive aspiration pneumonia, drug ingestions, and viral penumonia, and in the postoperative course, especially after cardiopulmonary bypass. There was often a period of grace between the insult and the development of respiratory failure. The syndrome was named the adult respiratory distress syndrome (ARDS). Undoubtedly, with further research, each of these disorders will be found to bear its own distinctive markers, clinically, pathologically, and therapeutically.

The nature of the common insult is not yet understood. Possibilities include direct hypoxic damage, selective loss of surfactant production, and the effects of proteolytic enzymes released locally or carried by the blood.

Descriptive studies have failed to find the expected uniformity of pathologic damage. Perhaps the most elegant study has looked at the pulmonary damage associated with septicemia. Initially, there is fragmentation of the type 1 alveolar epithelial cells. Edema and hemorrhagic inflammatory infiltrates are found in the alveoli and interstitium, and the lung becomes boggy with congestive atelectasis. Later, surfactant-secreting type 2 cells begin to proliferate and the interstitium is overwhelmed with new collagen fibers and cells. A loss of capillarity becomes evident. The physiologic changes mirror the pathologic destruction: The filled alveoli underlie the progressive right-to-left shunting and consequent refractory hypoxemia, and the boggy and fiber-filled interstitium makes the lung noncompliant and necessitates tremendous inflation pressures.

The hypoxemia of ARDS is caused by venous-to-arterial shunting. An FiO_2 of 100% cannot abolish the hypoxemia, because the shunted blood never sees a ventilated alveolus and will continue to depress the arterial oxygen concentration.

The extent of shunting is usually measured while the patient is receiving 100% oxygen. As shown in Figure 12–2, the oxygen dissociation curve is almost flat at a high Pa_{O_2}, and thus even small depressions in oxygen content caused by shunting bring about large falls in the Pa_{O_2}. The degree of shunting is expressed in the P_{O_2} gradient between alveolus and artery $(PA_{O_2} - Pa_{O_2})$, where, on 100% oxygen,

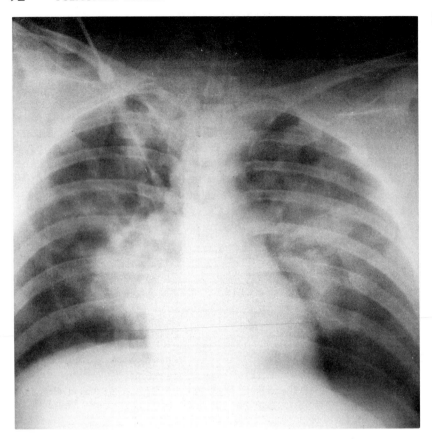

FIG. 12–1. Chest radiograph showing "Shock lung."

$PA_{O_2} = P_{barometric} - PA_{H_2O} - PA_{CO_2} = 760 - 47 - 40 = 673)$.

As respiratory distress worsens, the alveolar-arterial oxygen difference rises from 25 torr to more than 500 torr, and the shunt rises from 5% to greater than 50% of the total pulmonary blood flow.

Therapy. Therapy for ARDS is extremely frustrating. Pressure-cycled ventilators are ineffective. Instead, volume-cycled ventilators are used with prolonged inspiration and positive end-expiratory pressures in the hope of expanding atelectatic regions. Potentially toxic levels of inspired oxygen are often required to maintain adequate arterial oxygenation.

Other therapeutic questions remain unanswered, largely because the mélange of syndromes incorporated under the rubric "ARDS" obscures possible helpful distinctions. For example, diuresis and albumin infusions can help relieve pulmonary edema in some patients, but albumin is only effective when an intact capillary membrane is present to permit an oncotic gradient to be established between the circulation and the interstitum. Therefore, diuresis and albumin infusions cannot be uniformly recommended since they cannot benefit those regions of the lung that are already destroyed. If fat emboli are contributing to the damage, albumin may be beneficial because of its fatty acid binding capability.

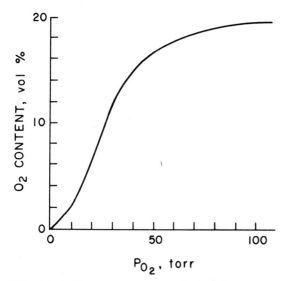

FIG. 12–2. The normal oxygen dissociation curve.

Short courses of high dose (1 to 2 grams) methylprednisolone have been used with encouraging results. As the course of steroids becomes more prolonged, septic complications may ensue.

BIBLIOGRAPHY

Asmundsson T, Kilburn KH: Survival after acute respiratory failure. Ann Intern Med 80:54–57, 1974

Bachofen A, Weibel ER: Alterations of the gas exchange apparatus in adult respiratory insufficiency associated with septicemia. Am Rev Respir Dis 116:589–615, 1977

Campbell EJM: The management of acute respiratory failure in chronic bronchitis and emphysema. Am Rev Respir Dis 96:626–639, 1961

Fishman AP: Shock lung: A distinctive nonentity. Circulation 47:921–923, 1973

Murray JF: Mechanisms of acute respiratory failure. Am Rev Respir Dis 115:1071–1078, 1977

Pierce AK, Robertson J: Pulmonary complications of general surgery. Annu Rev Med 28:211–221, 1977

Pontoppidan H, Geffin B, Lowenstein E: Acute respiratory failure in the adult. N Engl J Med 287:690–698, 743–752, 799–806, 1972

Pontoppidan H, Wilson R, Rie M et al: Respiratory intensive care. Anesthesiology 47:96–116, 1977

Rastegar A, Thier SO: Physiologic consequences and bodily adaptations to hyper- and hypocapnia. Chest 62 (Suppl):28S–34S, 1972

Zwillich CW, Pierson DJ, Creagh CE et al: Complications of assisted ventilation. Am J Med 57:161–170, 1974

13

Chronic Obstructive Pulmonary Disease

Patients with chronic obstructive pulmonary disease (COPD) are traditionally separated into two categories: those with chronic bronchitis and those with emphysema. Both diseases cause airway obstruction—bronchitis from inflammation, inspissated mucus and bronchospasm, and emphysema from the loss of buttressing tissue around the airways. In addition, both are accompanied by dyspnea and hypoxemia. The clinical progression and pathophysiology of the two diseases, however, are very distinctive.

The division of COPD into these two categories is not entirely satisfactory for two reasons: First, a person only rarely falls neatly into a single category. Bronchitis and emphysema frequently coexist in the same patient, although why this is so is unclear. It is possible that one disorder predisposes to the other, or, more simply, that they derive from similar insults (i.e., smoking). Some have even suggested a linked genetic predisposition. Second, whereas chronic bronchitis is a *clinical* diagnosis, made by documenting cough and sputum production for at least three months a year for two consecutive years, emphysema is a *pathologic* diagnosis, made by demonstrating enlarged airspaces and the loss of alveolar tissue.

The clinical course of COPD is extremely varied. Nevertheless, patients generally display two patterns of symptoms superimposed on each other: (1) A progressive worsening of underlying lung function. This is manifested primarily by progressive dyspnea, fatigue, and exercise intolerance. (2) Intermittent exacerbations. This most often results from upper respiratory or lung infections. In addition, these patients have little respiratory reserve, and any stress such as mild congestive heart failure or a pulmonary embolus may result in rapid clinical deterioration.

Patients with COPD usually come to the hospital only during an exacerbation of their illness. The question of intubation frequently arises in patients with severe respiratory decompensation (see Chap. 12). In this chapter, however, we will be primarily concerned with the nature of the underlying disease and the care of patients who require less drastic intervention. The spectrum of patients under consideration ranges from those whose only evidence of decompensation is increased sputum production, to those severely dyspneic and febrile from a purulent bronchitis, to those whose efforts to expectorate their tenacious sputum are thwarted by bronchospasm.

The patient with COPD suffers essentially from two sets of problems:

1. Wheezing and dyspnea reflect both reversible brochospasm and irreversible bronchial obstruction.

2. Hypoxemia and hypercarbia result from chronic alveolar hypoventilation. Chronically, the major detrimental effect of hypoxemia and hypercarbia is pulmonary hypertension with consequent cor pulmonale. (The metabolic effects are discussed in Chap. 21.)

Therapeutic intervention is aimed at relieving respiratory distress and acutely and chronically improving arterial oxygenation.

Once chronic lung disease becomes clinically symptomatic, the prognosis is poor with a 5-year mortality of 50%, predominantly from lung disease. The progression of the disease is relentless and can be monitored by the increasing severity of the underlying ventilatory impairment (for example, FEV_1), and the presence of carbon dioxide retention. The first episode of respiratory failure heralds even more rapid decompensation, with two of every three patients dying within the next two years.

CHRONIC BRONCHITIS

Patients with chronic bronchitis range from those without clearcut clinical evidence of airway obstruction to those so crippled by the disease that the slightest physical exertion— even just buttoning a shirt—can bring on severe dyspnea. Any discussion of the natural history of the disease must be tempered by an awareness of this wide spectrum of clinical involvement.

The two entities most often implicated in the development of chronic bronchitis are smoking and recurrent infections.

Smoking. In 1963, a study in Chilliwack, British Columbia, revealed that chronic bronchitis and obstructive lung disease were four times more common in male smokers than in male nonsmokers. With the advent of new tests of small airway disease, significant obstruction has been found in many asymptomatic smokers. Pathologists have also begun to remark on the consistency of early inflammatory changes in the bronchi of young smokers. Fortunately, early damage and symptomatology can be reversed with the cessation of smoking.

Numerous toxins in cigarette smoke interfere with respiratory and bacteriocidal lung function and have adverse systemic effects. These include (1) acrolein, a constituent of cigarette smoke (and an excellent tissue fixative), which interferes with macrophage and ciliary function; (2) nitrogen dioxide, which damages epithelium; (3) hydrogen cyanide, which poisons respiratory enzymes and has been suggested as the cause of tobacco amblyopia; (4) carbon monoxide, which impairs the oxygen carrying capacity of the blood (carboxyhemoglobin can attain blood levels of 5% to 10% in smokers); (5) polycyclic hydrocarbons, whose possible carcinogenicity has been receiving increasing attention.

Air pollution has also been implicated in the development of chronic lung disease. A temperature inversion in a polluted city can be lethal to a patient with COPD. Epidemiologic evidence suggests that air pollution can also adversely affect the lungs of children. Even healthy children manifest reduced airway conductance during days of heavy pollution.

Infection. Bouts of infection often punctuate the slowly progressive debility of chronic bronchitis. The resulting clinical deterioration, which often precipitates a hospital visit, is marked by increasing sputum production and purulence. The tracheobronchial tree, sterile in healthy people, is chronically colonized by bacteria in patients with chronic bronchitis. Ineffective ciliary motion, altered mucus, and perhaps less effective macrophage function all contribute to the successful invasion and growth of bacteria in the bronchitic lung. Two potential pathogens are commonly grown from the tracheal secretions of patients with chronic bronchitis, *Hemophilus influenza* and the pneumococcus. It is not clear whether these organisms are pathogenic in these patients, since the bacterial flora does not change drastically during exacerbations. On the other hand, more than one-third of exacerbations coincide with evidence of mycoplasma pneumonia or viral infection. Epidemiologic evidence suggests a potential role for repeated childhood respiratory infections in the predisposition to adult chronic lung disease.

Pathophysiology

The lungs of patients dying of bronchitis display an increased number of bronchial goblet cells, enlarged mucus glands, squamous metaplasia of the epithelium, mucosal edema, and lumens filled with mucous and inflammatory cells. The increased sputum production characteristic of chronic bronchitis results from secretions in the upper airway. The airway obstruction is the result of fibrotic narrowing and mucus plugging of the many smaller (2 to 3 mm) airways. Destructive emphysema often accompanies the bronchitis.

The hypoxemia of a patient with bronchial obstruction derives from the shunting of venous blood past unventilated alveoli. This blood mixes with blood that has been adequately oxygenated in other healthier regions of the lung so that the oxygen content of the blood that finally returns to the left side of the heart is reduced.

The reasons for the retention of carbon dioxide (alveolar hypoventilation) are less clear. Part of the explanation is that when the work of breathing is increased by rising airway resistance, the ventilatory response to CO_2 is blunted. There is also evidence of diminished sensitivity of central respiratory neurons to CO_2 in these patients, and, in addition, there is a component of respiratory muscle fatigue.

The effects of hypoxia on the pulmonary vasculature play a crucial role in the progression of the disease. Hypoxia causes pulmonary vasoconstriction, and thus produces pulmonary hypertension, which eventually leads to cor pulmonale and right heart failure. At this stage, the jugular veins protrude, the liver enlarges (passive congestion), the ankles swell (edema), and ascites collects.

A stocky habitus and bull neck often coincide with the clinical picture of the patient severely ill with chronic bronchitis and chronic alveolar hypoventilation. This paradigm is referred to as the *blue bloater*.

EMPHYSEMA

The patient with emphysema loses both air spaces and blood vessels, and thus displays less ventilatory-perfusion mismatch than does the patient with chronic bronchitis. Early in the course of the disease, therefore, the patient may be able to maintain levels of oxygenation adequate to prevent pulmonary hypertension and right heart failure. Rosy-cheeked, free from edema, and often of more asthenic build than the blue bloater, the emphysematous patient has been referred to as the *pink puffer*. Although bouts of bronchitis or pneumonia may precipitate transient hypoxemia and cor pulmonale, these patients are distinguished from blue bloaters by the absence of severe hypoxemia and chronic cor pulmonale until late in the disease.

The lungs of the patient with emphysema are made compliant by the loss of tissue. Ventilation is therefore less arduous, and, perhaps because of this, carbon dioxide retention is only a late complication of emphysema. In addition, patients with emphysema may have a more sensitive ventilatory response to carbon dioxide than do patients with chronic bronchitis, and therefore they retain less carbon dioxide with the same degree of obstruction.

The emphysematous patient complains of dyspnea rather than excessive sputum production. The physical examination reflects the loss of elastic recoil of the lungs. The diaphragms are flat and the chest wall is enlarged to accommodate the expanded lungs. On chest x-ray, the heart looks small in comparison to the "hyperinflated" lungs (Fig. 13–1).

Only rarely does a smoker manifest more emphysema than bronchitis. The purest variety of emphysema is a result of an inherited deficiency of the enzyme α_1-antitrypsin. α_1-antitrypsin is a glycoprotein in human serum that inhibits trypsin and other proteases. At least 20 different α_1-antitrypsin phenotypes have been distinguished. Genetic studies reveal that the glycoprotein derives from a single locus with co-dominant alleles; each person can therefore make at most two types of α_1-antitrypsin (one from each parent's chromosomes). Each type of α_1-antitrypsin has been electrophoretically isolated and labeled, for example, M or Z. In persons with the common normal phenotype, MM, both chromosomes provide α_1-antitrypsin of variety M. Some phenotypes, such as ZZ, lead to less than normal amounts of α_1-antitrypsin activity. ZZ homozygotes have very low levels and have a great tendency to develop emphysema at a young age. The resultant emphysema affects the alveolar walls more than the terminal bronchioles and is termed *panlobular*. The chest x-ray shows widespread emphysematous damage, especially to the lung bases. Smoking accelerates the lung deterioration.

EVALUATION AND THERAPY

It is important to recognize the limitations of available therapy for chronic obstructive pulmonary disease. No treatment currently exists for the irreversible lung destruction of emphysema, and although many of the symptoms of chronic bronchitis can be alleviated, no form of therapy has been shown to alter its inevitable downhill course. Objective measurements of pulmonary function are also not infallible guides to treatment since some modes of therapy may reduce the patient's discomfort without objective remission.

The decision whether to intubate the patient, and the utility of the history and physical examination in defining the degree of urgency, are discussed in Chapter 12. It is important to emphasize the need to search for and identify the specific precipitant of the patient's worsening condition. Often this is an acute upper airway infection, and, less often, a pneumonia.

The patient's respiratory distress is not necessarily a result of worsening intrinsic lung disease. Heart failure can masquerade as worsening COPD, and questions relating to cardiac arrhythmias and salt load are therefore appropriate. The possibility of a pulmonary embolus must also be considered. Emboli are not uncommon in these patients, who lead inactive lives and whose legs are frequently swollen with edema. The patient's condition may also have been exacerbated by the inappropriate administration of high concentrations of oxygen during the ambulance ride.

The examination of the patient should include a careful assessment of the degree of ventilatory impairment (estimated by the respiratory rate, the length of the expiratory phase, and the need for accessory muscles in inspiration) and an evaluation for the presence of cor pulmonale. Diaphragmatic fatigue may

FIG. 13–1. Chest radiograph of a 58-year-old man with emphysema. (*A*) Posteroanterior view.

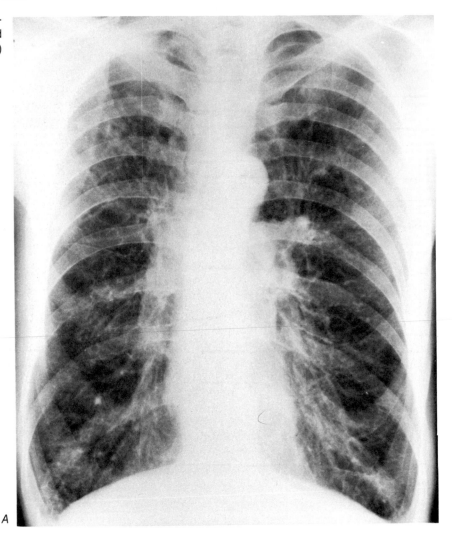

A

be reflected by inward movement of the abdomen during inspiration.

Therapy should begin as soon as possible. A severe episode of respiratory decompensation usually requires low flow oxygen and agents to relieve bronchospasm. Bronchodilators, such as theophylline derivatives and adrenergic agents, help relieve the bronchospastic component so common in COPD, and deserve a trial in virtually all patients (see

Chap. 15). In some patients, other modes of therapy may also deserve an empirical trial, including corticosteroids, antibiotics, and chest physical therapy.

Oxygen

The aim of oxygen therapy should be to maintain arterial oxygenation sufficient to support tissue oxygenation without suppressing the drive to breathe. This can usually be

FIG. 13–1. (cont.). (B) Lateral view.

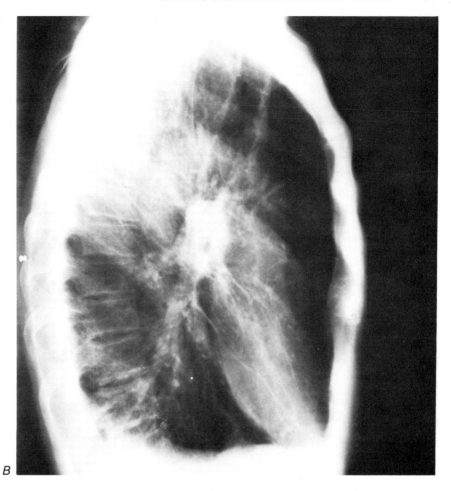

B

achieved with a Pa_{O_2} between 40 and 60 torr. A Pa_{O_2} of 60 is approximately the threshold for the hypoxic drive to breathe, and if exceeded, the patient will rely more upon his carbon dioxide-stimulated drive to breathe. However, as discussed previously, patients with COPD have a blunted carbon dioxide drive; even when breathing room air they tend to exhibit hypercapnia and respiratory acidosis. A Pa_{O_2} of 60 must therefore not be exceeded, or hypoventilation will become even worse.

Reasonable oxygen levels can be achieved by delivering oxygen by calibrated low flow, slowly increasing the FiO_2 from 24% to 28%, and so on. Acutely, low flow oxygen can improve the Pa_{O_2}, reduce pulmonary hypertension, and restore mental acuity. Chronically, low flow oxygen therapy can increase exercise tolerance, ameliorate the symptoms of cor pulmonale, and diminish compensatory erythrocytosis.

Corticosteroids

Because steroids have been useful in treating the bronchospasm of asthma, they have also been widely employed in the treatment of COPD. Clinical experience dictates that they should not be used automatically, since they are frequently without benefit, and their long-term use is fraught with complications. Some patients, however, respond dramatically. The complications of systemic corticosteroids—adrenal suppression, osteoporosis, fluid retention, hyperglycemia, and an increased susceptibility to infection—can be avoided in patients who can be maintained on the inhaled form of steroids.

Antibiotics

If a pneumonia or upper airway tract infection is present, every attempt should be made to identify the organism. Appropriate antibiotic therapy should then be instituted. Even in patients without a pneumonia, however, *Hemophilus influenza* and the pneumococcus can frequently be grown from the tracheal secretions of patients with chronic bronchitis. It is likely that these organisms are opportunistic, grafted onto an epithelium injured by a virus or an inhaled toxin, and not responsible for the injury initiating the respiratory decompensation. Nevertheless, some of the symptomatology may originate from bacterial infection, since antibiotics shorten the course and reduce the discomfort of severe and moderate exacerbations. It is therefore common to give a short course (*i.e.*, 7–10 days) of a broad spectrum antibiotic (such as tetracycline) for such episodes. The clinical response to antibiotic therapy does not correlate with the organism found in sputum cultures. If fever and purulent sputum are still present two days after the initiation of therapy, repeat cultures should be taken to uncover unusual pathogens.

Physical Therapy

Postural drainage with chest percussion has demonstrable benefit for patients with bronchiectasis and cystic fibrosis, but remains of unproven value in COPD. Some patients, perhaps those with a bronchiectatic component, may benefit. The use of physical therapy must therefore remain empirical.

Several techniques are currently used to enforce slow, deep breathing, and in this way increase the tidal volume. Therapists teach patients to use their abdominal muscles during expiration, to position their body to relax the accessory muscles, and to exhale through pursed lips. If these techniques help the patient, they should be used. Controlled trials have demonstrated no consistent benefit. On the other hand, exercise conditioning, with supplemental oxygen, if necessary, has been shown to increase exercise tolerance.

BIBLIOGRAPHY

Anderson DO, Ferris BG, Zickmantel R: The Chilliwack Respiratory Survey, 1963, part IV: The effect of tobacco smoking on the prevalence of respiratory disease. Can Med Assoc J 92:1066–1076, 1965

Burrows B: Physiologic variants of chronic obstructive lung disease. Chest 58(suppl 2):415–416, 1970

Derenne J-Ph, Macklem PT, Roussos H; The respiratory muscles: Mechanics, control, and pathophysiology. Part III. Am Rev Resp Dis 118:581–601, 1978

Diener CF, Burrows B: Further observations on the course and prognosis of chronic obstructive lung disease. Am Rev Respir Dis 111:719–724, 1975

Hugh-Jones P, Whimster W: The etiology and management of disabling emphysema. Am Rev Respir Dis 117:343–378, 1978

Lertzman MM, Cherniack RM: Rehabilitation of patients with chronic obstructive pulmonary disease. Am Rev Respir Dis 114:1145–1165, 1976

Tager I, Speizer FE: Role of infection in chronic bronchitis. N Engl J Med 292:563–571, 1975

14

Lung Cancer and
Pulmonary Nodules

In the United States, nearly 100,000 patients die each year of lung cancer. To reduce this number, the internist must accept two mandates: to promote vigorously the cessation of smoking and to attempt to detect carcinoma in its earliest stages. The only hope of curing cancer of the lung is to find a surgically resectable lesion, since, with the exception of oat cell carcinoma, remissions can only very rarely be obtained by chemotherapy. Early suspicion of the disease is therefore crucial, especially in patients who are considered to be at high risk. Those who are at high risk include both men and women over the age of 45 years with a long history of heavy smoking.

There are essentially four pathologic varieties of lung cancer, each with its own distinctive histologic and clinical hallmarks:

1. Squamous cell carcinoma comprises about 30% of all lung tumors, and presumably derives from metaplastic squamous cells lining the bronchi. The tumor grows rapidly, invading and often obstructing bronchi, and leading to cavitation. Typical presenting symptoms are cough and hemoptysis. The sputum cytology is usually positive.

2. Small cell (predominantly oat cell) tumors comprise about 25% of lung tumors. These probably derive from cells located within bronchial glands. Small cell tumors have usually metastasized by the time of diagnosis.

3. Adenocarcinomas arise peripherally and are sometimes found in association with old scars of pulmonary infarcts or infection. A subgroup of bronchiolo-alveolar tumors derives from epithelial cells and spreads along the existing alveolar network.

4. Large cell carcinoma is the name applied to the remaining cancers of the lung, and includes anaplastic and giant cell tumors.

Evidence of lung carcinoma can be obtained in three ways:

1. By recognizing symptoms caused by the tumor. Symptoms can be due to the local spread of the tumor, to the distant effects of metastases, or, as part of certain ill-defined neurohormonal syndromes, to so-called paraneoplastic effects.

2. As an incidental finding on chest x-ray.

3. By screening high-risk populations.

SYMPTOMATIC PRESENTATION

Pulmonary Symptoms

The pulmonary symptoms of lung cancer are nonspecific.

101

Cough is the most common symptom, present in 75% of patients. It usually reflects the presence of a tumor of the main bronchus or lobar bronchi that is causing irritation or obstruction. A chronic, nonproductive cough is likely to come from an irritating, nonobstructive lesion of the main bronchus.

Sputum production, on the other hand, is more often associated with obstructive lesions, such as may occur with tumors located around the lobar bronchi. Blood-tinged sputum or hemoptysis occurs in more than 30% of patients, and should always raise the suspicion of cancer.

Dyspnea is present in more than 50% of affected patients, and is frequently the initial symptom. A variety of mechanisms can cause dyspena in patients with lung cancer, including: (1) airway obstruction, (2) pleural effusions, and (3) stretching of intrapulmonary J receptors (stretch receptors located within the pulmonary interstitium).

The symptoms mentioned thus far also occur in patients with chronic obstructive pulmonary disease, the same population of male smokers at high risk for lung cancer. These patients require regular, periodic x-ray examinations and cytologic analysis of sputum, especially if any symptoms begin to worsen.

If *pneumonia* develops in patients at risk for lung cancer, sputum should be sent for cytologic as well as bacteriologic analysis. Pneumonia frequently develops in a lobe whose airway has been obstructed by a tumor. The bacteriology is the same as ordinary infectious pneumonias, but the onset of clinical illness may be more gradual and the rate of resolution slower. Recurrence of pneumonias in the same area suggests an obstructing lesion. Because air flow is blocked by obstructing lesions, increased breath sounds and fremitus (the classic findings of pneumonia) are often not heard.

There are several *thoracic syndromes* that are associated with lung cancer:

1. Pleural exudates (see Chap. 18).
2. Superior vena cava syndrome. Occlusion of the superior vena cava is usually due to external compression. Lung cancer is the most common cause, and centrally located right-sided tumors are responsible in the majority of cases. The symptoms can be abrupt in onset, and include edema, suffusion, and cyanosis of the face and arms, and often marked orthopnea. Cerebral hypoperfusion can produce prominent neurologic symptoms, including headache, dizziness, behavioral changes, and even coma. The severity of symptoms is related to the completeness of the obstruction and the rate of occlusion, because slowly progressive obstruction allows time for collaterals to form. Diagnosis of the superior vena cava syndrome is made by angiography. Treatment must be rapid in severe cases, and consists of diuretics and irradiation. Steroids and single dose chemotherapy have also been used with success.

3. Involvement of the recurrent laryngeal nerve. The sudden development of hoarseness suggests that lung cancer has involved the recurrent laryngeal nerve (Fig. 14–1). In one large series, hoarseness was the presenting symptom in 20% of patients with lung cancer. Indirect laryngoscopy can confirm the diagnosis by demonstration of unilateral vocal chord paralysis. If the result of the chest x-ray examination is negative, mediastinal tomograms may reveal the tumor.

4. Pancoast tumor. A Pancoast tumor is a subpleural tumor located in the superior sulcus. Pain is the most common initial symptom, and is the result of the tumor impinging on the rich neural network (the brachial plexus) in this area. Shoulder pain is particularly common. When the nerve roots C8 and T1 are involved, pain is experienced in the forearm along the ulnar distribution. At this

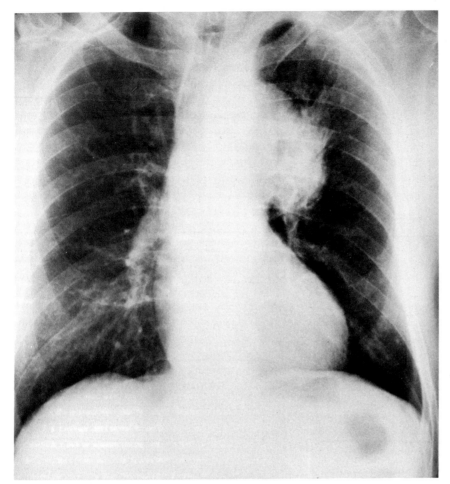

FIG. 14–1. Chest radiograph of a patient with carcinoma of the lung. The patient presented with hoarseness due to entrapment of the recurrent laryngeal nerve.

stage in the patient's evaluation, the diagnosis is often missed. Even if a chest x-ray is obtained, it may fail to reveal the tumor, since it is usually small and submerged within the other shadows at the apex. Apical lordotic radiographs are needed to provide the clearest view of the area. Ipsilateral muscle weakness frequently follows the pain. The patient may also develop an ipsilateral Horner's syndrome, which includes ptosis, miosis, and enophthalmus caused by disturbance of the sympathetic chain. Since the peripheral location of Pancoast tumors makes cytologic diagnosis by sputum cytology or bronchoscopy unlikely, a needle biopsy is necessary.

Metastatic Effects

The symptoms of lung cancer metastases depend on the organ involved and the size of the secondary tumor. The most common sites of metastases are the brain, the liver, and bone. Many are asymptomatic and go unsuspected until found at postmortem examination. Two-thirds of brain metastases are asymptomatic during life. In fact, the finding of a tumor anywhere in the body therefore dictates that careful radiographs of the lung should be taken to determine whether lung cancer is the primary source. Oat cell carcinomas metastasize early and widely. When diagnosed in the lung, they should be assumed to have already spread. Oat cell metastases have a predilection for the endocrine glands, as well as the more typical sites of lung cancer metastases.

Paraneoplastic Effects

Neuromuscular symptoms affect up to 10% of patients with lung cancer, and may appear years before the primary tumor becomes evident. It is when these symptoms are the patient's first complaint that the possibility of an occult lung cancer should be considered.

The most common syndrome of patients with lung cancer is mild weakness of the proximal musculature, sometimes accompanied by diminished deep tendon reflexes but without sensory findings. The electromyogram (EMG) reveals a denervation pattern. Another neurologic syndrome involves a sensorimotor peripheral neuropathy whose most prominent symptom is a sensory ataxia. Cerebrospinal fluid (CSF) analysis reveals increased protein without a pleocytosis. Many of these patients have a progressively deteriorating neurologic course. Chest x-rays should be taken of every patient who develops either of these syndromes.

The *Eaton-Lambert syndrome* is a disorder of the neuromuscular junction that causes weakness of the pelvic girdle and thigh muscles. This syndrome is found in association with many tumors, including thymomas and lymphomas, and is seen with oat cell carcinoma of the lung. Despite its superficial resemblance to myasthenia gravis, the Eaton-Lambert syndrome can be distinguished because it spares the ocular muscles and muscle strength improves with repeated contractions (unlike the progressive weakening of myasthenia). The EMG shows facilitation of the action potential with repeated stimuli. The Eaton-Lambert syndrome may respond to guanidine hydrochloride, but not to acetylcholinesterase inhibitors.

Two connective-tissue syndromes are frequently associated with lung cancer: clubbing and hypertrophic pulmonary osteoarthropathy (HPO). *Clubbing* is enlargement of the distal portions of the fingers and toes due to hypertrophy and soft-tissue inflammation. It is associated with many other diseases and is in no way diagnostic of lung cancer.

Hypertrophic pulmonary osteoarthropathy can be found in approximately 3% of patients with lung cancer, most often in those with tumors that involve the pleura, and least often in those with oat cell carcinoma. Patients complain of pain and swelling of the joints, but there is actually little joint involvement, although mildly inflammatory effusions occasionally are present. Rather, the disease is a proliferative periostitis with a propensity for the distal long bones of the legs and arms. There is swelling and pain over the involved bones, which are often very tender. The inflammatory reaction can be so marked that it may give the impression of deep venous thrombosis or cellulitis. X-rays of the long bones may reveal a marked periosteal reaction, and bone scans may show a pattern of increased uptake. Prompt relief is sometimes afforded by surgical thoracic sectioning of the vagus. Anti-inflammatory agents are rarely effective.

A variety of endocrine disorders can arise

in the setting of lung cancer. These are felt to be due to ectopic production of hormones or hormone-like substances by the tumor.

Hypercalcemia is the most common syndrome associated with lung cancer, and is seen most frequently with squamous cell carcinoma. X-rays of the lungs should always be taken in a patient with unexplained hypercalcemia. Hypercalcemia in these patients may be due to secretion of parathyroid hormone-like peptides.

Oat cell carcinoma is associated with the syndrome of inappropriate ADH secretion, but this disorder has so many causes that it is not a specific marker for lung cancer. On the other hand, ectopic ACTH production leading to Cushing's syndrome is very often caused by oat cell carcinoma. Muscle wasting is prominent, but otherwise these patients may lack the typical appearance of a patient with Cushing's syndrome (see Chap. 29).

DIAGNOSIS

In previously well patients who develop hemoptysis, dyspnea, hoarseness, or a new or changing cough, or in whom an obstructive lesion is suspected, the first diagnostic procedures include a chest x-ray and three sputum cytologies. The chest x-ray is positive in 90% of patients with symptomatic lung cancer. The result of the sputum cytology establishes the diagnosis in 75% of patients, and can be positive even when the lesion is not visible on x-ray.

If either the chest x-ray or sputum cytologies is positive, the patient should be bronchoscoped. (The only exceptions are patients in whom oat cell carcinoma has been diagnosed and patients with demonstrated advanced metastatic disease.) Bronchoscopy can confirm the diagnosis and localize the lesion.

If both the chest x-ray and sputum cytolo-

gies are negative, bronchoscopy should be reserved for patients experiencing hemoptysis or entrapment of the recurrent laryngeal nerve, and patients who are at high risk for lung cancer (*e.g.*, heavy smokers). Patients in whom milder symptoms persist may also eventually require bronchoscopy. The benefits *versus* the risks of bronchoscopy in a patient with a negative chest x-ray and worsening cough, dyspnea, or a "suspicious" pneumonia are unknown.

The Solitary Pulmonary Nodule

Lung cancer is not always symptomatic, and the first evidence of cancer may be the incidental finding of a solitary pulmonary nodule on chest x-ray (Fig. 14–2). The detection of a small rounded lesion in the lung poses a diagnostic dilemma: Is the lesion malignant, or not? More than 75% of nodules discovered in this way are benign, and one would therefore like to determine whether the lesion is malignant in order to avoid the necessity of resecting all lesions.

Among the benign lesions one must consider in the differential diagnosis, the most common are the granulomas. Among these, the most frequently encountered are tuberculomas, histoplasmomas and coccidioidomas. The latter two are generally confined to endemic areas. Positive skin tests cannot by themselves confirm the diagnosis, since an individual may simply have been exposed to the organism at some time in the past, but sputum stains can be valuable. Other benign lesions include hamartomas (benign connective-tissue tumors), circumscribed pneumonias, and, rarely, bronchogenic cysts.

Many x-ray criteria have been proposed as aids in determining the malignancy of a solitary pulmonary nodule. The two most reliable criteria are growth rate and calcification. If a lesion has been present for two or more

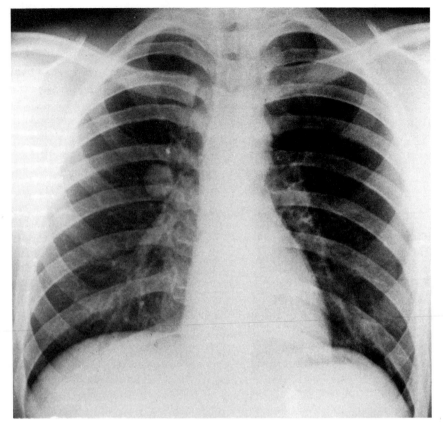

FIG. 14–2. Chest radiograph of a solitary nodule in the right lung of a 16-year-old boy with soft-tissue sarcoma.

years without any detectable change in size, it is almost certainly benign. Extremely rapid growth suggests an inflammatory rather than a malignant lesion. Diffuse calcification is common in benign lesions and is extremely rare in malignant ones. About 30% of granulomas and hamartomas present with calcification.

Unless the x-ray picture is clear-cut or unless responsible organisms can be found in the sputum, the potential malignancy of a solitary pulmonary nodule cannot be determined through noninvasive means. Before proceeding with surgery, however, many clinicians advocate the use of either percutaneous biopsy, which can produce a diagnosis in up to 90% of patients, or fiberoptic bronchoscopy with transbronchial biopsy and brush biopsy.

When the decision to go to surgery has been made, mediastinoscopy should be considered. This procedure requires general anesthesia and is usually combined with a thoracotomy. Approximately one-third of patients whose lesions had initially appeared resectable will be discovered to have mediastinal metastases that make resection untenable.

Resection of the lesion results in definitive diagnosis, and many patients ultimately undergo surgery. A solitary nodule should be resected unless (1) it can be proved to be benign beyond any reasonable doubt, (2) the patient is in such a debilitated state that surgery poses too great a risk, or (3) there is evidence of metastatic spread. Thoracotomy is a low-risk procedure in young patients (mortality less than 1%), but in elderly patients with coronary atherosclerosis or obstructive lung disease, the mortality increases to 5% to 10%. The risk must be weighed against the evidence of improved 5-year survival time with resection of malignant lesions. Several studies reveal a 50% or more 5-year survival with resection, compared with an 8% 5-year survival for all patients with lung cancer.

The nonsurgical options for therapy of lung cancer are discouraging. A variety of multi-agent chemotherapeutic regimens are in use, but none of these offers a cure. The best results with chemotherapy have been obtained with oat cell carcinoma. More than 70% of patients achieve a remission that may last more than 12 months. However, with the exception of patients with oat cell carcinoma, chemotherapy for nonresectable lung cancer should be approached cautiously, because it may only exacerbate the patient's suffering. Radiation therapy is an important palliative tool, especially in patients with the superior vena cava syndrome. Radiation may also be used for treating brain metastases and localized bone pain.

BIBLIOGRAPHY

Feinstein AR, Gelfman NA, Yesner R: The diverse effects of histopathology on manifestations and outcome of lung cancer. Chest 6:225–229, 1974

Greco FA, Oldham RK: Small cell lung cancer. N Engl J Med 301:355–358, 1979

Hyde L, Hyde LI: Clinical manifestations of lung cancer. Chest 65:299–306, 1974

Lillington GA: The solitary pulmonary nodule—1974. Am Rev Respir Dis 110:699–707, 1974

Richardson RH, Zavala DC, Mukerjee PK et al: The use of fiberoptic bronchoscopy and brush biopsy in the diagnosis of suspected pulmonary malignancy. Am Rev Respir Dis 109:63–66, 1974

15

Asthma

Asthma is rarely lethal. Its major impact lies instead in its great prevalence and in its ability to cripple patients both functionally and emotionally. Two to three percent of the adult population in the United States have asthma, about half of whom experience the onset in adult life.

PATHOPHYSIOLOGY

The underlying disorder in asthma is hyperreactivity of the bronchial musculature of both the large and small airways to various stimuli. This is manifested by intermittent attacks of wheezing, dyspnea, and cough.

This bronchospastic component is superimposed upon a number of chronic pathologic changes. These include hypertrophy and hyperplasia of the mucus glands and goblet cells, thickening of basement membranes, and filling of bronchial lumens with desquamated epithelial cells, eosinophils, and inspissated mucus. The bronchi of patients with status asthmaticus (*i.e.*, life-threatening attacks refractory to therapy with hydration and bronchodilators) are always plugged with this adherent exudate. Significant permanent destruction is rare.

Evidence of the pathologic changes taking place in the pulmonary tissue can be detected in the sputum coughed up during an acute attack. The sputum may be filled with (1) distal airway casts composed of respiratory epithelial cells (Curschmann's spirals); (2) compact clusters of columnar epithelial cells (Creola bodies), and (3) Charcot-Leyden crystals and eosinophils.

Precipitants of Asthma Attacks

All asthmatics exhibit a proclivity to bronchoconstriction in response to diverse stimuli. These stimuli may include airway irritants such as dust, charcoal, or sulfur dioxide; pharmacologic agents such as histamine, methacholine, or prostaglandin $F_2\alpha$; and biologic antigens such as ragweed pollen and tree bark.

Many asthmatics suffer airway obstruction during *exercise*, which often peaks after the exercise is stopped. Apparently, running causes bronchospasm more often than does swimming. Many asthmatics can "run through" their attack. Hyperventilation, hypoxemia, and acidosis do not appear to be responsible for exercise-induced asthma. Inhalation of cold air exacerbates it. The precise cause is not known. Premedication with bron-

$\downarrow CO_2$

chodilators or disodium chromoglycate may reduce the incidence and severity of exercise-induced asthma, and hypnosis has been used with some effectiveness.

In many asthmatics, the primary precipitant appears to be *emotional stress*.

Upper respiratory tract infections lower the threshold for bronchospasm, perhaps by sloughing epithelium over irritant receptors, and is a common precipitant of acute attacks.

A subset of patients is susceptible to bronchospasm that is provoked by *aspirin* and other anti-inflammatory agents, such as indomethacin. Aspirin sensitivity is often associated with the syndrome of nasal polyposis and sinusitis. A single aspirin tablet can precipitate fulminant bronchospasm, rhinitis, urticaria, pruritis, and hypotension.

Another group of patients is sensitive to *environmental pollutants*. Some previously asymptomatic persons first experience asthma symptoms when they move to areas of heavy pollution. This is especially common among military personnel, and such names as Tokyo-Yokohama asthma have been used to describe their particular susceptibility. Many workers first discover their tendencies to asthma at their site of employment. Thus, there is woodworker's, baker's, and meat-wrapper's asthma, to name a few.

In England, asthma is frequently a manifestation of *allergic bronchopulmonary aspergillosis*. Patients with this condition are sensitive to *Aspergillus fumigatus*. The disease is characterized by wheezing, eosinophilia, fleeting pulmonary infiltrates, and eventual bronchial destruction with proximal bronchiectasis.

Mechanisms of Bronchial Hyperreactivity

Two pathways link the asthma precipitants discussed above with the resultant bronchial smooth muscle contraction:

1. The local pathway. Sensitized mast cells release histamine and SRS-A (slow reacting substance of anaphylaxis), both potent bronchoconstrictors.

2. The reflex pathway. Reflexes are triggered by submucous irritant receptors, and the efferent information is carried by the vagus nerve to stimulate the bronchial smooth muscle.

The local pathway is an example of type I immune hypersensitivity and is mediated by IgE, an immunoglobulin that binds to the surfaces of mast cells. IgE molecules are antigen specific and bind particular allergens. When an allergen bridges two surface-bound IgE molecules, the mast cell degranulates, releasing histamine and SRS-A, as well as other molecules, including eosinophilic chemotactic factor of anaphylaxis (ECF-A) leukotrienes and prostaglandins. Mast cell release is dependent on intracellular levels of cyclic 3′, 5′-adenosine monophosphate (cyclic AMP). High levels of cyclic AMP appear to inhibit secretion.

Two asthmatic populations can be identified:

1. Those in whom local immunologic factors predominate are said to have *allergic asthma*. Allergic asthma usually has its onset in childhood and is associated with a family history of atopy that may include seasonal asthma, hives, or eczema. People with allergic asthma often have high serum levels of IgE and manifest positive responses to skin tests and to provocative exposures to specific antigens.

2. Those in whom neural triggers presumably predominate are said to have *nonallergic asthma*. This more often begins in adulthood. Frequently there is no family history of atopy, skin tests are negative, and serum IgE levels are normal. This population may have hypersensitive vagal receptors.

The distinction between these populations, however, is highly artificial, since the two varieties frequently coexist.

CLINICAL PRESENTATION AND LABORATORY FINDINGS

The typical hospital visit follows days of fluctuating symptoms. The severity of an acute asthma attack can be difficult to assess. The clinical hallmarks of the asthmatic state—wheezing, coughing, and dyspnea—do not correlate in any predictable fashion with lung function. There are, however, two signs that, when present, suggest severe pulmonary compromise: (1) the presence of pulsus paradoxus and (2) the use of accessory muscles (e.g., the sternocleidomastoids) to aid in inspiration. The latter can be detected by looking for retractions in the neck and between the ribs. Either of these signs suggests an FEV_1 of less than 25% of normal.

Pulmonary function tests show changes in all mechanical aspects of lung function: a diminution of flow rates, evidence of bronchoconstriction and airway obstruction, and elevations of the residual volume and total lung capacity (see Chap. 11). The vital capacity is reduced because the residual volume is so markedly elevated.

Even when both the physician and the patient agree that the acute attack has subsided, pulmonary function tests reveal residual defects of small airway function. The FEV_1 remains only 50% of normal, and the residual volume 200% of normal. The FEV_1 is the first value to return to normal following an acute attack. Abnormalities in the airflow rates, residual volume, and arterial blood gases may persist for days.

Arterial blood gases during an acute attack routinely reveal hypoxemia, hypocarbia, and respiratory alkalemia. Only when the obstruction becomes so severe that the FEV_1 falls to less than 20% of normal does the Pa_{CO_2} reach 40, signifying impending respiratory failure. Very few acute episodes will be severe enough to produce respiratory acidosis and carbon dioxide retention, and these are often related to the use of sedatives. The signs of impending catastrophe are not subtle, and include altered mental status, obvious exhaustion, and the disappearance of wheezing (suggesting progressive airway occlusion); a pneumothorax may underlie an acute decompensation.

The usual asthmatic attack is brief, treated by the patient with inhaled bronchodilators, and does not require hospital admission. However, when the patient with asthma arrives in the emergency room complaining of a severe attack the threshold for admission should be low. A course of intensive in-hospital therapy can abbreviate an attack that, if only partially treated at home, would wax and wane over many days due to incomplete resolution of mucous plugging of the airways and residual bronchoconstriction. Furthermore, once the obstruction progresses to plugging of the airways, the patient will become refractory to bronchodilators. This state—status asthmaticus—may be lethal. It often requires intubation.

If the clinical assessment suggests severe bronchospasm, therapy should be initiated immediately. A CBC and differential should be obtained before therapy because the therapeutic agents, such as catecholamines and corticosteroids, raise the white blood cell count by themselves. Leukocytosis suggests infection, and an eosinophil count of more than 350/mm³ correlates with disease activity and can be used to adjust the steroid dosage. Some patients with asthma, however, do not have eosinophilia even during attacks.

Differential Diagnosis

If the diagnosis of asthma is not obvious or if the etiology of the asthma is uncertain, the chest x-ray and electrocardiogram can be helpful. The chest x-ray is invaluable for documenting pneumonia or pneumothorax. An electrocardiogram is likely to show the peaked P waves of P-pulmonale or right axis deviation.

The EKG is otherwise nonspecific, unless a silent myocardial infarction with pulmonary edema is being confused with acute asthma.

Critical mitral stenosis or left ventricular dysfunction with pulmonary edema can be indistinguishable from asthma at the bedside. Heart sounds, murmurs, and gallops can be obscured by wheezes. Less frequently, recurrent pulmonary emboli may present with wheezing. An angiogram may then be necessary to make the diagnosis. Upper airway obstruction can be differentiated from asthma by the presence of stridor and harsh tracheal sounds.

Bronchopulmonary aspergillosis can be diagnosed by immediate hypersensitive skin reactions to aspergillus antigen, identification of precipitating antibodies to aspergillus, elevated serum IgE levels, repeated cultures of aspergillus from the sputum, and the findings of characteristic destruction and bronchiectasis of the central airways.

If violaceous facial flushing, hypotension, tachycardia, and diarrhea accompany bronchospasm, a serotonin-secreting carcinoid should be suspected, and urine should be obtained for a 5-hydroxyindole acetic acid (5-HIAA) determination.

THERAPY

Therapeutic intervention for a patient experiencing an asthma attack involves (1) improving gas exchange, (2) mobilizing secretions, and (3) alleviating bronchospasm with drugs.

Oxygenation

Adequate oxygenation can generally be maintained with supplemental oxygen. An FiO_2 of 28% is usually sufficient. Repeated arterial blood gases are not necessary unless the patient is in severe distress. Hypoxemia and hypocarbia are the rule. Although they may persist even past discharge, they are of no particular prognostic value. As discussed above, however, an elevated or even normal Pa_{CO_2} during an asthmatic attack signals impending respiratory arrest. Immediate intubation should be considered.

Mobilization of Secretions

Mobilization of secretions can be accomplished with adequate fluid replacement. There is no evidence that overhydration is helpful, and, especially in the older patients, care must be taken to avoid pulmonary edema. Ultrasonic nebulizers can help individual patients, but some aerosols actually cause bronchoconstriction. Use of nebulizers more than every three to four hours or without accompanying nebulized bronchodilators can be counterproductive. As airways open, previously inspissated secretions appear, and deep coughing and postural drainage become helpful. Expectorants and mucolytic agents have no demonstrable value.

Pharmacologic Intervention

Unless the asthma patient is to be intubated, sedatives should be avoided because of the danger of hypoventilation. Infection should be treated. Even if no organism can be identified in the sputum and even if the x-ray is clear, many advocate a brief course of a broad-spectrum antibiotic, such as tetracycline, on the assumption that a bronchitis may be present.

The primary goal of therapy is to relieve bronchospasm. This can be accomplished by action at two loci: (1) the mast cell population must be stabilized, and (2) the bronchial smooth muscle cells must be relaxed. Both these objectives can be achieved through pharmacologic effects on intracellular cyclic AMP, which, in high concentrations, inhibits mast cell release and causes bronchial smooth muscle relaxation.

Three classes of pharmacologic agents are currently employed: β-adrenergic agents, theophylline, and corticosteroids.

β-adrenergic agents are sympathomimetic drugs that selectively bind to β-receptors on heart cells (β₁ receptors) and on mast cells and bronchial smooth muscle cells (β₂ receptors). Receptor-binding leads to stimulation of adenylate cyclase, the enzyme controlling cyclic AMP synthesis.

Epinephrine (or its derivative, ephedrine) has long been the mainstay of asthma therapy. Although it relieves bronchoconstriction via β₂ receptors, epinephrine also binds to β₁ receptors and thus accelerates the heart rate. In young patients unlikely to be harmed by tachycardia, a subcutaneous injection of epinephrine (which may be repeated every 20 to 30 minutes) should be the initial therapy. If there is no response after 2 to 3 injections, further injections will probably not be helpful.

Recently, more selective β₂ agents have become available. Their major side-effect is muscle tremor. If subcutaneous epinephrine fails or seems inadvisable because of cardiac complications, these β₂ agents offer an attractive alternative. Oral terbutaline can be a helpful addition. (Given subcutaneously, it is little more selective than epinephrine.) Metaproterenol aerosol is useful as a prophylaxis against asthma attacks, and a few puffs can be helpful during acute bronchospasm.

Some continue to advocate isoproterenol (a nonselective β agent) aerosol. However, there are two major drawbacks to the use of isoproterenol: (1) excessive usage has been associated with an increase in the death rate from asthma, presumably because of its cardiac effects; and (2) isoproterenol may desensitize the bronchial β-receptors, thus impairing sympathetically mediated bronchodilation. In addition, presumably by altering lung perfusion characteristics, isoproterenol has sometimes been found to decrease the Pa$_{O_2}$ in spite of the fact that it improves airway function. This problem can be remedied with supplemental oxygen.

Theophylline (usually given in its ethylenediamine form, aminophylline) inhibits the degradation of cyclic AMP. If the drug is not already part of the outpatient regimen, an intravenous loading dose is required. The loading dose can then be followed by a constant intravenous infusion. Theophylline metabolism is unpredictable, so that serum levels should be measured and the patient carefully observed for side-effects. These include both minor effects (e.g., nausea, abdominal discomfort, and anorexia) and major effects (e.g., supraventricular arrhythmias, tachycardia, and seizures). Titration is easiest when the drug is given intravenously. Rectal suppositories should be avoided because of their erratic absorption.

If neither the β-adrenergic agents nor theophylline has worked, glucocorticoids can provide dramatic relief. Their effect, however, is not measurable for three hours and does not peak until 12 hours after the initial dose. Their mechanism of action may involve limiting local inflammation by decreasing leukocyte accumulation and function.

The steroid-dependent asthmatic who cannot be weaned to low dose or alternate day programs is at risk for infection, osteoporosis, purpura, hypotension, diabetes, and adrenal cortical suppression. Although inhaled steroids (beclamethasone) may chronically spare these side-effects, they are ineffective during an acute episode. Any patient experiencing an asthma attack who has been on high dose steroids within the previous 9 to 12 months requires supplemental glucocorticoids. The adrenal function remains suppressed for up to one year, and an acute asthma attack constitutes an enormous stress. If feasible, steroids should be tapered off over the 10 days following the acute episode. Rapid removal is ill-advised because of the prolonged and slowly reversible residua of asthma.

A variety of other agents have been tried in the treatment of asthma. *Cromolyn sodium*, an inhaled powdered derivative of a substance called khellin, does not help in acute asthma, although prophylactic use prevents wheezing induced by antigens or exercise. It appears to act by stabilizing mast cell membranes. Unfortunately, it is an expensive drug and is often ineffective in the adult population.

In an as yet poorly defined subset of asthmatics, inhaled *anticholinergic drugs* have been demonstrated to prevent or ameliorate wheezing. Atropine

Intubation and assisted ventilation are required in only a very few patients with status asthmaticus. Even in these patients, mucus plugs clear within a day or two, and sensitivity to catecholamines returns.

BIBLIOGRAPHY

Austen KF, Orange RP: Bronchial asthma: the possible role of the chemical mediators of immediate hypersensitivity in the pathogenesis of subacute chronic disease. Am Rev Respir Dis 112:423–436, 1975

McFadden ER Jr, Ingram RH Jr: Exercise-induced asthma. N Engl J Med 301:763–769, 1979

Rebuck AS, Read J: Assessment and management of severe asthma. Am J Med 51:788–798, 1971

Rosenberg M, Patterson R, Mintzer R et al: Clinical and immunologic criteria for the diagnosis of allergic bronchopulmonary aspergillosis. Ann Intern Med 86:405–414, 1977

Saunders NA, McFadden ER: Asthma: An update. Disease-a-Month 24, No. 11:1–49, 1978

Van Dellen RG: Theophylline. Mayo Clin Proc 54:733–745, 1979

16

Pleuritic Chest Pain and Pneumothorax

Only the parietal pleura has pain fibers (supplied by the intercostal nerves), and irritation of these nerve endings may be responsible for the pain of pleural disease. The pain is almost always unilateral and well localized. It is rapid in onset, sharp, and exacerbated by deep breathing and coughing. The pain is often severe enough to prompt the patient to seek immediate medical attention.

Despite the distinctive characteristics of pleuritic chest pain, it can be difficult to distinguish from pericardial and chest wall pain.

Pericardial pain can also be sharp and aggravated by respiration. Unlike the patient with pleuritic pain, however, the patient with pericardial pain can sometimes be relieved by changes in position, such as sitting up and bending forward. In addition, the pain is frequently substernal in pericardial but not in pleural disease. Inflammation of the pericardium and the pleura can occur concurrently.

Chest wall pain commonly occurs secondary to trauma. It can also result from an inflammatory process, usually costochondritis. This entity, also called *Tietze's disease*, occurs most often in young adults. The patient presents with anterior chest pain that is ex-

acerbated by coughing, movement, and occasionally by deep inspiration. Unilateral swelling and tenderness of one costochondral junction (frequently the second) may be found. Although costochondritis is a self-limited process, it may persist for months. It is best treated with aspirin or other anti-inflammatory agents. Severe cough can produce a musculoskeletal pain that is located at the insertion of the abdominal muscles at the inferior costal margin, and the pain can sometimes be elicited by contraction of the abdominal musculature.

Various signs and symptoms are associated with pleuritic chest pain, and these generally depend upon the underlying cause of the pain. Two findings, however, are common to almost all: (1) the patient will be splinting the affected side; and (2) because the tidal volume can be quite low, the patient will increase his respiratory rate to maintain minute ventilation.

CAUSES OF PLEURITIC CHEST PAIN

Any disease of the pleura can produce pleuritic chest pain. These diseases are most conveniently divided into infectious and noninfectious etiologies.

114

Acute Infectious Causes

Although many acute infectious diseases of the lung present with pleuritic chest pain, it is rarely the only symptom. Frequently present are fever, chills, and a cough that is either nonproductive or productive of purulent sputum. The chest x-ray findings can simplify the differential diagnosis by placing the condition within one of three basic groups: (1) pain associated with parenchymal infiltrates, (2) pain associated with isolated effusions, and (3) pain associated with a clear chest x-ray.

1. A *parenchymal infiltrate* abutting on the pleura suggests that a pneumonia underlies the pleuritic pain. Pleuritic chest pain is present in over 50% of patients with bacterial pneumonias, but less often in patients with viral, mycoplasmal, and rickettsial pneumonias.

2. A smaller group of patients presents with x-ray findings of *pleural effusions without any evidence of parenchymal disease.* These patients also have fever and malaise, but frequently have no cough or one that is only mild and nonproductive. The major disease entities that fall into this group are postprimary tuberculosis and empyema.

Tuberculosis. The most common setting for pleural disease in tuberculosis is the early postprimary period, when there is no evidence of parenchymal disease. Symptoms of acute infection often accompany pleuritic pain, especially in young persons. Although the skin test is most often positive, a definitive diagnosis of tuberculosis may be difficult at this stage. There is usually a pleural effusion, but this is positive for acid-fast bacteria in only a minority of cases. The highest diagnostic yield comes from culturing Cope needle biopsy specimens of the pleura, but even these findings

are negative in up to 33% of patients. When the tubercle bacilli are not found, treatment must frequently be empiric.

Empyema. The presence of pleuritic pain, a pleural effusion, and the signs and symptoms of an acute infection must raise the possibility of an infected pleural space even without x-ray evidence of parenchymal involvement. Empyema may spread from a subdiaphragmatic infection, such as an abscess, from a pneumonia that has resolved from partial treatment, or from seeding of the pleural space in the setting of a bacteremia. Diagnosis and therapy depend upon thoracentesis and surgical drainage.

3. *Epidemic pleurodynia* is an acute infectious disease of children and young adults that may cause pleuritic chest pain *without producing any positive x-ray findings.* A prodrome of headaches, myalgias, and malaise often precedes the onset of pain. In the older patient, typical pleuritic chest pain is likely to be present. Young children complain of abdominal pain more often than of chest pain. Fever is almost invariably present, and some patients have a nonproductive cough. The disease usually runs its course within a week. Coxsackie B virus is the most common etiologic agent. The disease entity occurs in community epidemics that cluster in the summer and fall months. The diagnosis is made by the proper clinical presentation in the appropriate epidemiologic setting.

Acute Noninfectious Causes

Pulmonary Embolus. In several large series, the incidence of pleuritic chest pain in patients with pulmonary emboli ranges from 10% to 70%. Pleuritic chest pain is rarely the only symptom of an embolus.

In diagnosing the cause of pleuritic chest pain, the distinction between a pulmonary

FIG. 16–1. Chest radiograph showing a tension pneumothorax on the left (*A*) that had reexpanded with the exception of a small residual pneumothorax at the apex of the left lung (*B*).

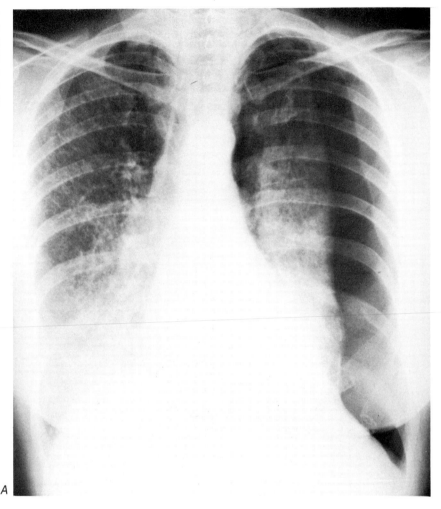

A

embolus and an acute infectious process can be difficult. Fever can occur with a pulmonary embolus, though it rarely rises above 100° to 102°F, and rigors are unusual. The white blood cell count may be elevated (as in any stressful situation), and a cough may be present, although it is either nonpurulent or bloody. In general, the white cell count, fever, and cough are less impressive in a pulmonary embolus than in bacterial pneumonia. (A complete discussion of pulmonary embolus can be found in Chapter 17.)

Other causes of pleuritic chest pain include diseases that can cause inflammation of the pleura. These include diffuse inflammatory disorders such as systemic lupus erythematosis and rheumatoid arthritis.

Spontaneous Pneumothorax. Pneumothorax, the presence of air in the pleural space, can arise spontaneously or secondarily as a result of trauma to the chest. The vast majority of spontaneous pneumothoraces occur in healthy individuals, usually men in their 20s

FIG. 16–1. (cont.).

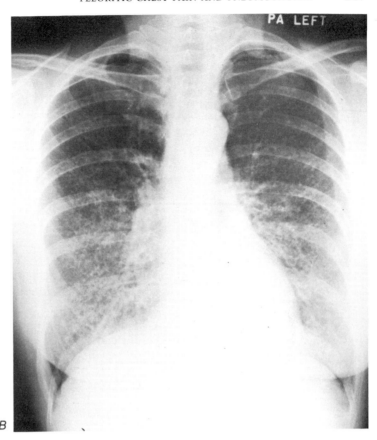

B

and 30s with a tall, asthenic habitus. About 80% occur when the individual is at rest, and are believed to result from the spontaneous rupture of apical alveoli. Air then dissects along the septa to form small blebs that subsequently rupture. Most spontaneous pneumothoraces occur in healthy persons, but a great many pulmonary diseases have been associated with spontaneous pneumothorax, including tuberculosis, chronic obstructive pulmonary disease, pulmonary fibrosis, asthma, carcinoma, and sarcoidosis.

The cardinal symptom of spontaneous pneumothorax is the sudden onset of pleuritic chest pain. Most patients also experience some dyspnea. The lung collapses under its own elastic recoil, and is suddenly underventilated despite continued perfusion. The resulting ventilation/perfusion abnormality leads to hypoxemia. The patient becomes acutely tachypneic and dyspneic. Over the next 24 hours, reflex vasoconstriction in the involved lung shifts the flow of blood to the healthy lung, thereby ameliorating the hypoxemia. By this time the patient no longer feels dyspneic, even though the size of the pneumothorax may be unchanged.

The size of a pneumothorax is defined as the percentage of the hemithorax occupied by pleural air, and determines the clinical signs that are present. When the pneumothorax exceeds 50%, one may be able to detect decreased breath sounds and hyperresonance. Larger pneumothoraces may produce marked aberrations of lung function, and the patient may become extremely dyspneic and cyanotic. The underlying pulmonary function of the patient determines just how large a pneumothorax can be tolerated before respiratory embarrassment occurs. Even a very small pneumothorax in a patient with poor lung function can push him toward respiratory failure.

The chest x-ray is the best tool for the diagnosis of a pneumothorax. The visceral pleural edge is visible as a line outlined against the partially collapsed lung (Fig. 16–1). In small pneumothoraces, the pleural edge can be difficult to see, so an x-ray should be taken at full expiration to maximize the collapse of the lung. This maneuver increases the radiodensity of the lungs and thus, by contrast, may reveal an otherwise inapparent collection of air. Pneumothoraces are almost always unilateral, but bilateral collections of air can be seen in a small percentage of cases.

The majority of spontaneous pneumothoraces are self-limited events. The leak in the visceral pleura presumably seals itself, the accumulation of air ceases, and the free air is gradually resorbed. One study determined that the rate of resorption is about 1% to 2% of the pleural air per day. The treatment of small pneumothoraces can therefore involve nothing more than reassurance and patience. However, with larger pneumothoraces, two factors determine whether surgical intervention is necessary: (1) the extent of the cardiopulmonary compromise and (2) the length of time one is willing to wait for pulmonary function to return to normal. Generally, pneumothoraces of less than 15% are left alone, but it is impossible to define a precise cutoff.

If intervention is required, there are two possible approaches available to the physician. The air can be aspirated either through a large bore needle placed into the anterior second or third intercostal space, or through an indwelling thoracotomy tube. The needle is easy to use and brings rapid results, but there is always the danger of a pleural tear as the lung expands. A purported advantage of the tube is that it may stimulate pleural inflammation and scarring, thereby protecting against recurrences.

Recurrences are a problem, and occur in about 25% of patients. The more recurrences a person has, the more likely he is to experience them in the future. In one study, the incidence of recurrence after three previous episodes approached 85%. They may or may not be on the same side as the initial event; when they do occur on the same side, the possibility of an underlying structural lesion must be considered. Recurrent pneumothoraces in one hemithorax should lead one to consider obliterating that pleural space by instilling sclerosing agents or physical abrasives.

Tension Pneumothorax. Rarely, a tear that leads to a spontaneous pneumothorax fails to seal spontaneously, and air enters the pleural space. As air accumulates, through a flap-valve-type mechanism that allows air to enter but not to leave the pleural space, it compresses the lung. This is called a tension pneumothorax. Continual positive pressure in the pleural space compromises ventilation by collapsing the lung. The pressure of the pleural air also impinges on the mediastinal structures, obstructing venous return, and thereby reducing cardiac output and producing hypotension.

A tension pneumothorax is an acute emergency. The patient experiences dyspnea, chest pain, cyanosis, and hypotension. Physical examination reveals a large pneumothorax with the trachea and the mediastinum shifted to the unaffected side.

The diagnosis can be established by placing a needle into the second intercostal space.

The needle is connected to a saline-filled syringe from which the plunger has been removed. If air bubbles out of the needle during the full respiratory cycle, the diagnosis of pneumothorax is confirmed. (If a pneumothorax is not present, the water provides a seal.) A large thoracotomy tube is placed to evacuate the pleural space.

Secondary Pneumothorax. Most secondary pneumothoraces (*e.g.*, pneumothoraces occurring in the setting of trauma) are seen on surgical services. However, they occur in two other settings that the clinician must be aware of.

Secondary pneumothorax may be seen after the insertion of a subclavian line or after placing a transthoracic pacemaker. To ensure that a traumatic pneumothorax has not been precipitated, an x-ray should be taken after an attempt at a subclavian puncture.

A second cause is barotrauma-related pneumothoraces, not uncommonly encountered in patients on respirators. Patients with emphysema or other bullous lung diseases are particularly susceptible. The incidence of pneumothoraces increases when positive end-expiratory pressure (PEEP) is used, especially at high pressures. Any patient on a respiratory device who develops worsening blood gases or hypotension (especially when associated with a significant rise in peak inspiratory pressure) must be suspected of having a pneumothorax, and a chest x-ray should be obtained. Raising the level of PEEP because of deteriorating gases merely exacerbates the problem. Many of these patients develop subcutaneous emphysema, in which air dissects under the skin making it crepitate. Subcutaneous emphysema is usually painless and requires no specific therapy.

BIBLIOGRAPHY

Killen DA, Goggel WG: Spontaneous Pneumothorax. Boston, Little, Brown, 1968

Kumar A, Falke KJ, Geffin B et al: Continuous positive pressure ventilation in acute respiratory failure: effects on hemodynamics and lung function. N Engl J Med 283:1430–1436, 1970

Sacks PV, Kanarek D: Treatment of acute pleuritic pain. Am Rev Respir Dis 108:666–669, 1973

17

Pulmonary Thromboembolism

When a piece of a thrombus in a deep vein of the leg breaks loose and lodges in the lungs, it is referred to as a pulmonary thromboembolism. It is a common problem both in and out of the hospital, and is estimated to cause approximately 50,000 deaths each year in the United States.

Many of those who die succumb suddenly to a massive embolus before medical intervention is possible. In the remaining patients, adequate anticoagulation can reduce mortality to less than 5%.

Even a healthy youngster can have a pulmonary embolus, but the majority of emboli are dealt with silently and expeditiously by endogenous thrombolytic mechanisms. For emboli to become symptomatic, they must compromise the expansive pulmonary circulation, either through size or number.

Four clinical syndromes of pulmonary embolism can be distinguished: (1) massive pulmonary emboli with acute cor pulmonale; (2) subacute recurrent small pulmonary emboli with chronic cor pulmonale; (3) acute pulmonary emboli with infarction; and (4) pulmonary emboli without either cor pulmonale or infarction. It will become apparent from the following sections that there is some overlap among these categories.

1. *Massive Pulmonary Emboli.* This term is applied when the pulmonary vasculature is occluded to the extent that it interferes with right ventricular output. The patient experiencing massive emboli faces a life-threatening catastrophe. Although massive emboli comprise only 10% of thromboembolic events, they account for at least 50% of deaths from pulmonary emboli.

A massive pulmonary embolic event is usually defined by the resultant obstruction of two lobar pulmonary arteries. However, this strict criterion neglects the importance of the patient's underlying clinical state. For example, the elderly patient whose pulmonary vasculature is already compromised by emphysema will tolerate a clot much more poorly than a young, healthy individual.

Only a minority of patients with massive pulmonary emboli survive long enough to be hospitalized. Those who reach the hospital arrive frightened, cold, clammy, tachypneic, and often diaphoretic and hypotensive. The neck veins are distended. Auscultation of the chest may reveal a right-sided S_3, and sometimes a systolic murmur can be heard over the involved vessel. The EKG may show evidence of right ventricular strain, right bundle branch block, P pulmonale, or right axis deviation. More frequently, there are only nonspecific changes in the ST segment, T wave, and QRS complex compatible with infarction or axis deviation. The chest x-ray may reveal a loss of vascular markings in the region of the lungs supplied by the involved vessel. Radionuclide scanning and angiography can confirm the diagnosis (see later in chapter).

2. *Subacute Recurrent Small Pulmonary Emboli.* This is an uncommon pattern of thromboembolism in which repeated thromboemboli reach the lung silently. The patient complains only of continuous and slowly progressive dyspnea, and sometimes of an ill-defined precordial discomfort. The dyspnea becomes especially marked with exercise. The chest x-ray is clear and the arterial blood gases are unremarkable except for evidence of hyperventilation (decreased Pa_{CO_2}). At this stage, the diagnosis is often missed, and the patient's complaints dismissed as psychogenic. Eventually the recurrent small emboli and the associated reactive intimal fibrosis occlude enough pulmonary vasculature to raise pulmonary arterial pressures to systemic levels, and the syndrome of cor pulmonale becomes obvious. The patient becomes severely dyspneic and edematous. Therapy with anticoagulation is generally futile at this stage, and usually the patient dies. The distinction between the syndrome of recurrent pulmonary emboli and the syndrome of primary pulmonary hypertension is often made only at autopsy.

3. *Acute Pulmonary Emboli with Infarction.* Only about 10% of emboli cause clear-cut infarction. Clinical manifestations of tissue necrosis include pleuritic pain, a pleural friction rub, a pleural effusion, and, occasionally, hemoptysis. Tachypnea and breathlessness are noted in all patients, but can be overshadowed by pleuritic chest pain and hemoptysis.

A chest x-ray may reveal a radiopaque density that abuts on the pleura and protrudes toward the heart (Hampton's hump). Following the embolic event, infarction takes hours to develop and becomes evident only on the second day of hospitalization. An accompanying fever and leukocytosis may suggest the diagnosis of pneumonia.

4. *Pulmonary Emboli without Cor Pulmonale or Infarction.* Most pulmonary emboli do not cause immediate death, cor pulmonale, or infarction. Patients present only with dyspnea, tachypnea, tachycardia, and often a sense of apprehension. Unless there is clear-cut evidence or a high index of suspicion of co-existent deep venous thrombophlebitis, the diagnosis is often missed. This is unfortunate, because postmortem examination suggests that many patients with undiagnosed and untreated emboli eventually die of recurrent pulmonary emboli.

Resolution

Pulmonary emboli resolve in three stages: (1) by fragmentation, physical lysis, and peripheral dispersion of the clot, which occurs immediately; (2) by action of the fibrinolytic system, which occurs over hours to days; and (3) by organization and eventual recanalization, continuing over days to weeks.

The rate at which the vessel is reopened depends on the nature of the clot and on the local condition of the lung. Clots that are organized before embolization—the result of long-term venous disease—resolve more slowly than fresh clots. Lungs previously damaged by disease clear emboli more slowly than healthy lungs.

Resolution begins immediately, and within a day or two angiography reveals clearing of approximately 20% of the involved vasculature. Only rarely is dissolution of the clot complete before the fourth day. It usually takes four to six weeks for a repeat angiogram or lung scan to return to normal, and in some cases remnants of the clot remain permanently. The normalization of pulmonary hypertension corresponds with clearing of the angiogram.

Mechanisms of Clinical Symptomatology

Dyspnea and tachypnea may derive from distortion of the interstitium around small lodged emboli, causing irritation of the local J receptors. Stimulation of these receptors in animals has been shown to produce tachypnea.

Hypoxemia is extremely common, even with relatively small pulmonary emboli, but the reason for its high incidence remains unclear. At least two mechanisms that may contribute to hypoxemia have been described: (1) alveoli collapse in the neighborhood of occluded vessels, possibly due to the loss of surfactant; and (2) factors released from platelets and mast cells cause local bronchoconstriction. The blood flowing past underventilated alveoli is not adequately oxygenated, and consequently contributes to hypoxemia.

The mechanical effects of vessel occlusion by the clot fail to account totally for the occurrence of pulmonary hypertension. Associated pulmonary arterial vasospasm may also be important, mediated by local release of vasoactive substances and by neural reflexes.

DIAGNOSIS

The major reason pulmonary emboli are missed is that the diagnosis is not considered. This is particularly true in patients with emboli unassociated with cor pulmonale or infarction. Few clinicians fail to consider the diagnosis of pulmonary emboli in the tachypneic patient with pleuritic chest pain and hemoptysis or with dramatic evidence of disease of the deep venous system (see discussion later in chapter); however, most emboli are not accompanied by infarction, and venous disease is frequently silent. The diagnosis of pulmonary thromboembolism should therefore be considered in any patient who is susceptible to venous stasis (at bed rest or preoperatively) and who experiences any acute cardiopulmonary decompensation, including dyspnea, new tachypnea, hypoxemia, arrhythmias, and evidence of decreased cardiac output.

Short of angiography, diagnostic confirmation of an embolic event is extremely difficult. Most patients with pulmonary emboli are hypoxemic, but 15% have a Pa_{O_2} greater than 85 torr. In the absence of cor pulmonale, the electrocardiogram reveals only tachycardia and nonspecific ST and T wave abnormalities. Serum enzyme patterns that were previously thought to suggest embolism (i.e., increased LDH, increased bilirubin, and normal SGOT) have not proven to be reliable.

In the absence of pulmonary infarction, the chest x-ray provides only nonspecific hints. Disappearance of vascularity suggests blockage of an artery by an embolus. Focal atelectasis and edema often occur in the region of occlusion, and appear as transient opacities. There may also be elevation of one hemidiaphragm.

Lung Perfusion and Ventilation Scans

A lung perfusion scan is performed by injecting microspheres or macroaggregates of radioactively labeled albumin into the circulation. These particles are slightly larger than the pulmonary capillaries and get caught in the pulmonary vascular bed. Any region receiving less than the normal amount of blood supply is conspicuous by the absence of radioactivity. When a perfusion scan is normal, it rules out a pulmonary embolus. Abnormal scans, however, are unreliable, reflecting any lung process that infringes on the vasculature. Many patients with a positive perfusion scan will, on subsequent angiogram, reveal no abnormalities. Among the diseases that can produce perfusion defects are several parenchymal lung diseases, such as emphysema, tumors, and pneumonia.

Enhanced diagnostic specificity can be achieved by performing a ventilation scan. The patient inhales a radioactive gas that is unable to reach areas in which the bronchi are not patent. By demonstrating continued ventilation to a region with absent perfusion, the clinician can feel more confident of the diagnosis of a pulmonary embolus. On the other hand, a matched ventilation/perfusion defect, in which corresponding areas of both scans are abnormal, is generally accepted as evidence against the possibility of a pulmonary embolus. However, because pulmonary emboli can cause local bronchoconstriction, even such matched defects are an unreliable means of ruling out a pulmonary embolus. The ventilation scan is also not sensitive enough to pick up many intrinsic diseases of the lung that may be simultaneously affecting the perfusion scan. In summary, radionuclide scanning is inadequate to establish the diagnosis of a pulmonary embolus, and should be used only to rule out an embolic event.

Angiography

Angiography is the definitive procedure for the diagnosis of pulmonary embolism (Fig. 17–1). Because of the hazards of anticoagulation, angiographic confirmation of a pulmonary embolus is desirable. The drawbacks of angiography include the invasiveness of the procedure, its discomfort, the dangers of dye allergy and volume load in an elderly patient with tendency to heart failure, difficulties of interpretation, and variable readings among different observers. If angiography is not available, clinical suspicion and the perfusion scan must be relied upon.

DEEP VEIN THROMBOSIS

Nearly all significant pulmonary emboli derive from the deep veins located between the knees and the hips. It is therefore not unreasonable to state that virtually all deaths from pulmonary emboli reflect the failure to recognize and treat deep vein thrombosis. Only very infrequently does an embolus tear off a mural thrombus in the right atrium or ventricle in patients with right heart failure. Venous clots can certainly form elsewhere (e.g., in varicose veins, in inflamed prostatic veins, and as a result of superficial thrombophlebitis near intravenous sites), but these clots either do not embolize or are small enough to allow rapid clearance. The only other significantly worrisome source is the pelvic veins, which occasionally shower infected emboli in association with a septic abortion.

A host of situations predisposes to deep vein thrombosis, including circulatory stasis and damage to the endothelial surface. Prolonged bed rest, especially during the postoperative period, congestive heart failure, or fracture of a lower extremity, often precedes deep vein thrombosis and pulmonary emboli. Diseases associated with deep vein thrombosis include malignancy (especially of the pancreas, lungs, and stomach), diabetes, obesity, and peripheral arterial disease. The mechanisms of linkage between these diseases and deep vein thrombosis remain uncertain. Whether the oral contraceptive pill predisposes to deep vein thrombosis is still uncertain.

Low dose subcutaneous heparin, in doses too small to even prolong the PT or PTT, prevents deep vein thrombosis and subsequent pulmonary emboli. The only complication of

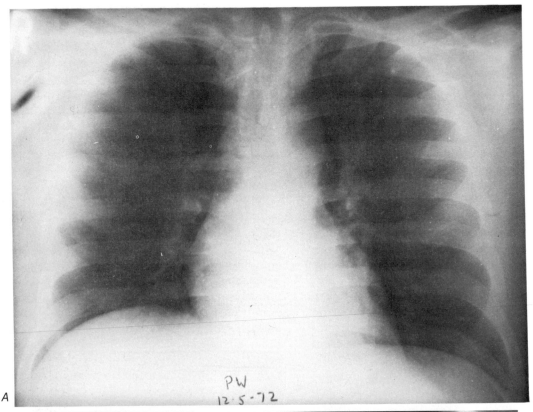

A

PW
12·5·72

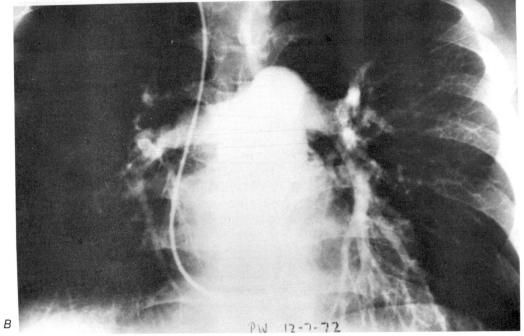

B

PW 12-7-72

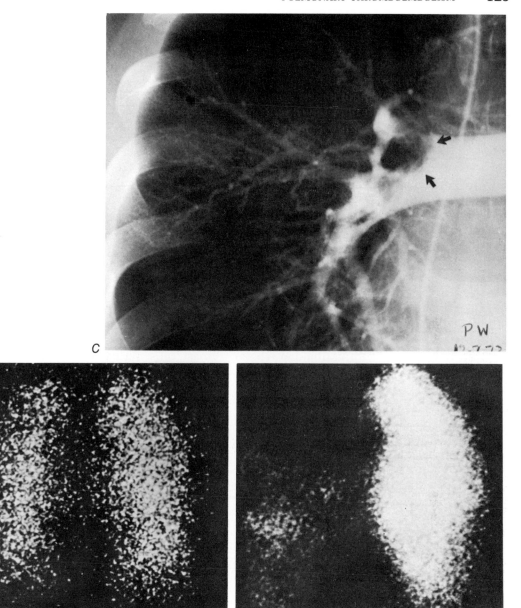

C

PW

D,E PE

FIG. 17–1. (A), Chest radiograph, (B and C), angiogram, and (D and E), lung scan on a patient with a massive pulmonary embolus in the right lung. (A) The chest radiograph is not at all diagnostic. (B) The angiogram suggests obstruction of the vessels to the right lung. However, the embolus is not clearly seen until close-up views (C) are taken. (D) The ventilation scan is normal. (E) The perfusion scan, however, is dramatic and shows a marked defect in the right lung. The patient was a 31-year-old man who had suffered shortness of breath for 3 weeks before diagnosis of pulmonary emboli to the right upper lobe and right lower lobe was made.

low dose therapy is an increased risk of wound hematomas. Subcutaneous heparin should be administered to all patients over 40 years of age who are undergoing abdominothoracic surgery or who are chronically debilitated and bedridden with congestive heart failure, stroke, or malignancy. It should also be given to high risk patients with obesity, diabetes, or previous deep vein thrombosis or pulmonary emboli, who will be at rest for a prolonged time. Subcutaneous heparin should begin before an operation because deep venous thromboses can form during the procedure. Subcutaneous heparin appears to be ineffective, however, in operations that release large amounts of tissue thromboplastin. The latter include extensive bone surgery (especially on the hip) and abdominal prostatectomy. Subcutaneous heparin should also be avoided during neurosurgery, because it may increase bleeding into the brain.

Both the physical examination and laboratory techniques used to confirm the presence of deep venous thromboses rely on two phenomena: (1) obstruction of venous return with concomitant edema and reduced flow and (2) local inflammation with erythema, tenderness, and a palpable venous cord. Clinical examination reveals at most 50% of deep venous thromboses and falsely suggests the diagnosis 30% of the time. If the initiation of anticoagulation depends on the diagnosis of deep vein thrombosis, confirmation by venography is mandatory. The side-effects of this procedure are local irritation and the risk of dye anaphylaxis. If anticoagulation is to be started regardless of the presence or absence of deep vein thrombosis, as in patients with a known pulmonary embolus, a less invasive—and less accurate—procedure may suffice. Impedance plethysmography, for example, makes use of changes in the electrical impedance of the legs to reflect changes in blood volume, and can thus be used to diagnose thrombotic interruption of flow in large

proximal leg veins. ^{125}I-fibrinogen can be incorporated into an actively forming thrombus, but it is not accurate in diagnosing thrombi in the proximal veins and will be negative in patients whose thrombus has already formed. This study carries a risk of hepatitis and is primarily used as a research tool.

THERAPY

Anticoagulation is aimed chiefly at preventing recurrences of pulmonary emboli. Because of the chronic nature of the underlying venous disease, many patients with one episode soon suffer repeated thromboembolic events, and may eventually succumb to them. Anticoagulation dramatically reduces this risk.

Heparin

Heparin is a mucopolysaccharide found in mast cells. Its intrinsic physiologic function is still uncertain, but its ability to inhibit the clotting of blood has been known since its discovery by a medical student in 1916. Heparin combines with the platelet cofactor, antithrombin III, to inhibit specific proteins of the coagulation cascade, thereby prolonging the activated partial thromboplastin time (PTT). The half-life of heparin, and hence the duration of its anticoagulant activity, varies greatly among patients.

In 10% to 20% of patients, treatment is complicated by bleeding around intravenous sites, in the retroperitoneum, in the gastrointestinal tract, or in wounds. A constant infusion of heparin seems to predispose to bleeding less often than intermittent bolus administration. Protamine, a heparin antagonist, should be available in case of emergency. Fortunately, other side-effects of heparin, including thrombocytopenia, hypersensitivity reactions, and osteoporosis with prolonged use, are rare.

Because of the danger of recurrent emboli,

the risk of not heparinizing a patient can be great. Early initiation of heparin therapy can reduce the mortality from a recurrence of pulmonary embolism to 3% from a predicted 30% without anticoagulation. Only a few conditions should therefore be considered contraindications to using the drug. These include the presence of a significant hemorrhage or hemophilia and the danger of intracranial, intrathecal, or intraocular bleeding from trauma, surgery, subacute bacterial endocarditis, or intracranial metastases. Patients with a known history of peptic ulcer disease can be heparinized, but must be watched very closely.

Warfarin

Warfarin is the most frequently used oral anticoagulant. It slows clotting by depleting clotting factors II, VII, IX, and X. These factors all depend on vitamin K for their synthesis. Warfarin blocks vitamin K-dependent synthesis, probably by interfering with the conversion of precursor proteins into the actual clotting factors. The prothrombin time reflects the activity of the extrinsic pathway, which involves factor VII, and is a sensitive index to the adequacy of anticoagulation. The major drawback to using this drug is its interaction with many other drugs. Some drugs diminish the response to warfarin by inducing degradative hepatic enzymes (barbiturates), or by decreasing absorption (cholestyramine). Other drugs enhance warfarin's effect by inhibiting metabolism (disulfiram) or by displacing warfarin from albumin binding (phenylbutazone). Aspirin interferes with platelet function, and aspirin and anticoagulants used in combination predispose to hemorrhage.

Fibrinolytic Agents

The new fibrinolytic agents, such as urokinase, lyse the clot, and accelerate the resolution of pulmonary emboli. The addition of fibrinolytic therapy, however, increases the frequency of hemorrhagic complications without significantly decreasing mortality, and should not be a part of standard therapy. It remains to be seen whether a role for such agents will be found in life-threatening massive pulmonary emboli.

Therapeutic Protocol

Heparin is the drug of first choice because of the immediacy of its action, its potency, and its ready reversibility by protamine. It may be given either by intermittent intravenous boluses or by continuous infusion. A continuous infusion is preferred, and the dose is regulated to maintain the PTT at 1.5 to 2.5 times normal. Chronic oral anticoagulation with warfarin should be begun before heparin is stopped. The two drugs should be given together for three to five days until there is adequate depletion of the vitamin K-dependent clotting factors. Outpatient administration of warfarin is continued for about four months.

If embolism continues from the legs despite adequate anticoagulation or if anticoagulation is contraindicated, surgery may be required. The inferior vena cava can be clipped with a serrated device or—in patients too sick for anesthesia—an umbrella of tongs can be passed down the jugular vein to lodge in the inferior vena cava. Despite rapid development of venous collateralization, recurrent emboli are rare following inferior vena cava clipping. The umbrella has the disadvantage of occasionally migrating from its place of insertion.

In the setting of massive pulmonary embolism with persistent shock and hypoxemia, the only recourse may be an attempt at embolectomy, a procedure that requires the patient to be put on cardiopulmonary bypass. The benefit of embolectomy remains questionable. The mortality exceeds 50%, and some patients die from alveolar hemorrhage after successful removal of the embolus.

AIR, TALC, AND FAT EMBOLI

Air can enter the venous system accidentally through an open CVP line or during hemodialysis. The estimated lethal bubble size is 200 ml. When the foaming bubble lodges in the right ventricular outflow tract or pulmonary artery, it can obstruct the cardiac output. Physical examination reveals tachypnea, hypotension, diffuse wheezes, and a mill wheel murmur from air churning in the pulmonic valve. The patient should be placed in a left lateral decubitus position to float the foam out of the right ventricular inflow and outflow tracts. If possible, hyperbaric 100% oxygen should be employed.

Narcotic addicts may inadvertently inject enough talc to produce numerous microemboli. Pulmonary hypertension may then result from a granulomatous reaction to these microemboli.

An otherwise uneventful recovery from long bone trauma may be interrupted by evidence of fat embolization. Twenty-four hours after the injury, a low grade fever, tachypnea, and tachycardia appear. Evidence of systemic embolization may include confusion, agitation, and a petechial rash of the torso and conjunctivae. Pulmonary involvement is manifested by dyspnea and cyanosis. Rarely, shock and coma may supervene, and the patient dies of adult respiratory distress syndrome. The diagnosis can be confirmed by finding fat globules in the urine and by an elevation of serum lipase. Treatment is unsatisfactory at present. Some clinicians suggest using albumin to bind free fatty acids. Systemic corticosteroids may be used to reduce inflammation.

BIBLIOGRAPHY

Barritt DW, Jordan SC: Anticoagulant drugs in the treatment of pulmonary embolism. A controlled trial. Lancet 1:1309–1312, 1960

Dalen JE, Haffajee CI, Alpert JS et al: Pulmonary embolism, pulmonary hemorrhage, and pulmonary infarction. N Engl J Med 296:1431–1435, 1977

Kakkar VV: Deep vein thrombosis. Circulation 51:8–19, 1975

Moser KM: Pulmonary embolism. Am Rev Respir Dis 115:829–852, 1977

O'Reilly RA: Vitamin K and the oral anticoagulant drugs. Ann Rev Med 27:245–261, 1976

Stein PD, Dalen JE, McIntyre KM et al: The electrocardiogram in acute pulmonary embolism. Prog Cardiovasc Dis 17:247–257, 1975

18

Pleural Effusions

The pleural space is filled with a thin film of pleural fluid maintained between the visceral and parietal pleura. The pleural fluid serves two essential functions: (1) It acts as an adhesive between the chest wall and the lung, preventing the lung from collapsing under the force of its own elastic recoil; and (2) it serves as a lubricant between the lung and the chest wall during respiratory movement. The pleural fluid is continually being formed and removed. It enters the pleural space from capillaries located at the parietal pleura, and is resorbed by the lymphatics and capillaries of the visceral pleura. The exact mechanics of the forces governing the production of pleural fluid are unknown, but the traditional Starling forces are most probably involved.

INITIAL EVALUATION

A pleural effusion is defined as any abnormal accumulation of fluid in the pleural space. The clinical manifestations vary from patient to patient. Many are asymptomatic. *Dyspnea* is common in patients with large, rapidly accumulating effusions or with preexisting pulmonary disease that has already compromised pulmonary function. *Cough* and *chest discomfort* are also common complaints. The chest pain is frequently pleuritic in nature.

The interposition of fluid between lung and chest wall gives rise to the physical findings, which include diminished breath sounds and dullness to percussion. Dullness to percussion is also found with parenchymal consolidation, but in such patients breath sounds are increased. Rales may be heard over the lung tissue adjacent to the effusion, denoting areas of compressive atelectasis.

The most sensitive diagnostic tool is the chest x-ray (Fig. 18–1). With small effusions of 200 to 500 ml, x-ray findings are generally limited to blunting of the costophrenic angles, best seen by looking at the posterior angle on the lateral film. Larger effusions produce more dramatic changes, including elevation of the lung, a mediastinal shift, and a large radiopacity at the lung base that tapers along the lateral chest wall in the shape of a meniscus. The chest radiograph can give definitive evidence of an effusion if the fluid can be shown to "layer out" on decubitus views.

TRANSUDATES AND EXUDATES

Effusions are divided into two categories:

FIG. 18–1. Chest radiograph showing a tuberculous pleural effusion on the left.

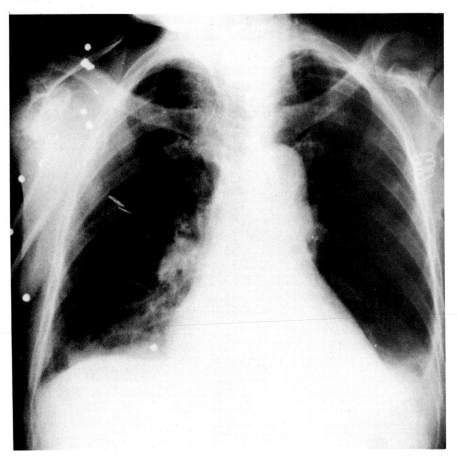

1. A *transudate* is an ultrafiltrate of plasma and is characteristically low in protein. A transudate can develop when the systemic or pulmonary capillary pressures increase, or when the colloid osmotic pressures decrease. The most common cause of pleural transudates is congestive heart failure. The mechanism of formation may be related to elevations in the venous hydrostatic pressure. Transudates are also seen in cirrhosis and the nephrotic syndrome.

2. *Exudates* are rich in protein and can be produced by any inflammatory or infiltrative process that involves the lung. The common denominator in many of these situations is increasing capillary permeability. Inflammatory involvement of the capillary walls permits leakage of a protein-rich exudate into the pleural space. Obstruction of lymphatic outflow will also lead to exudate formation. Exudative effusions can result from carcinoma, infection, infarction, pulmonary emboli, pancreatitis, Dressler's syndrome, rheumatoid arthritis, systemic lupus erythematosis, and other less common disorders. Carcinoma and infections are the leading causes of exudative pleural effusions.

Malignancy

Carcinoma is the leading cause of pleural exudates in the adult. Lung cancer is most

FIG. 18–1. (cont.). The effusion is seen especially well on the lateral view.

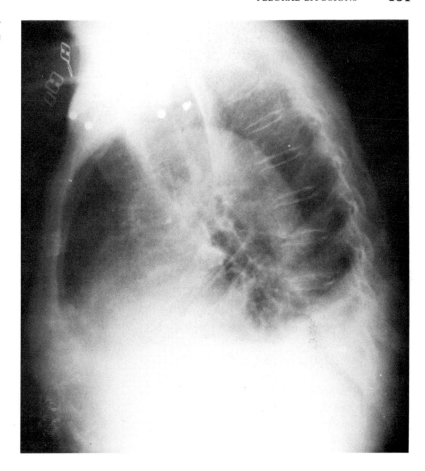

often responsible, and adenocarcinoma in particular is a common culprit, presumably because it tends to be a peripheral lesion. Cancers of the breast, ovary, and stomach commonly metastasize to the lung and cause effusions. Not all malignant effusions are exudates.

Seventy-five percent of these patients have symptoms that derive from their pleural involvement. In 40% or more of such patients, symptoms related to the effusion may be the first indication of disease. The chest x-ray reveals bilateral effusions in up to one-third of patients with malignant effusions, and most patients have effusions that exceed 500 ml. The majority of chest x-rays reveal parenchymal disease as well, either an infiltrative lesion or one or more discrete tumor masses. The presence of a malignant effusion generally signifies widely metastatic disease.

Infection

Pleural exudates associated with infection do not always contain infectious organisms, and are often only inflammatory reactions to a parenchymal pneumonia. Tuberculosis commonly causes effusions, and a pleural exudate is frequently seen in early tuberculosis. Pneumococcal pneumonia produces effusions in about 10% of cases, Klebsiella in 30 to 40%, *Staphylococcus aureus* in 50%, and *Streptococcus pyogenes* in up to 80%. Anaerobic pulmonary infections produce pleural effusions in about 35% of cases. Up to 20% of cases of mycoplasmal pneumonia have small transient effusions, which may be bilateral. In viral pneumonias, effusions occur in 10 to 20% of cases.

DIAGNOSIS

Because the diagnostic possibilities differ greatly depending upon whether an exudate or an transudate is present, it is important to make this distinction in every patient with an unexplained pleural effusion. This can be done only with a diagnostic thoracentesis. *All unexplained effusions should be tapped.* In addition, if the fluid is interfering with respiratory function, a therapeutic tap should be performed even if the diagnosis has been established. On the other hand, a newly diagnosed pleural effusion that appears to be associated with heart failure can usually be watched to see whether it resolves with treatment of the underlying cardiac disease. If the effusion fails to resolve, a diagnostic thoracentesis is advisable.

There is an abundance of studies questioning or espousing the virtues of examining almost every conceivable component of pleural fluid. Currently, lactic dehydrogenase (LDH) and protein measurements are used in making the important distinctions between exudates and transudates. The exact criteria most commonly used in establishing the presence of an exudate are:

1. the ratio of total protein in the effusion to total serum protein is greater than 0.5
2. the LDH in the effusion exceeds 200 I.U.
3. the ratio of the LDH in the effusion to the serum LDH is greater than 0.6.

If all three criteria are used, diagnostic accuracy exceeds 95%. The diagnostic accuracy of the LDH ratio increases as the ratio itself increases. It is very unusual to find a transudate with an LDH ratio greater than 1. The presence of LDH in exudates is due to its release by active phagocytes and possibly by malignant cells.

Other criteria have also been employed, but have not proved to be as useful. Specific gravity correlates grossly with protein content, but is not as accurate as the protein ratio. White blood cell counts in the pleural fluid exceeding 10,000 rarely occur in transudates, but also occur in only a minority of exudates. The red blood cell count is rarely helpful, and even minor trauma during the tap can alter its value considerably. However, grossly bloody pleural effusions are generally associated with malignancy, pulmonary emboli, or trauma. The finding of very low levels of pleural fluid glucose has been claimed to be associated with several causes of exudates, such as empyema, tuberculosis, and rheumatoid arthritis, but this test has not proven to be very useful in reaching a specific diagnosis.

The same diagnostic thoracentesis used to differentiate a transudate from an exudate can be used to help establish the specific etiology of the effusion. To prevent the necessity for a repeat thoracentesis, some of the fluid obtained from the original tap should therefore be saved for culture, stains for bacteria (including AFB), a complete blood count and differential, and cytology.

Malignant Effusions

The diagnosis of a malignant effusion relies on two procedures. *Cytological examination* of the fluid demonstrates malignant cells in 50 to 60% of patients with malignant effusions. *Closed pleural biopsy* is also positive in 50 to 60% of patients. Together, these procedures have a diagnostic yield of 85 to 90%. Improved diagnostic yields are achieved by examining large amounts of fluid and doing repeated taps. Because there must be fluid present in order to do a closed biopsy, the original diagnostic tap should not drain the pleural space dry. Recurrence of malignant effusions is common and, if they interfere with ventilation, can be treated by instilling sclerosing agents (such as tetracycline) into the pleural space.

Pleural Effusions Associated with Infections

There are three types of effusions associated with pulmonary infections: empyema, loculated sterile effusions, and simple sterile effusions.

Empyema, or infection of the pleural space, is almost always found in association with pneumonic infection. It is rarely caused by seeding of the pleural space in the course of a bacteremia or by extension from a subdiaphragmatic abscess. Anaerobic empyema developing during the course of an aspiration pneumonia is probably the most common form of pleural space infection. Among aerobic bacterial pneumonias, staphylococcus and streptococcus are common causes of empyema. The treatment of empyema is surgical drainage plus high dose antibiotics to treat bacteremia and prevent seeding of other tissues.

Simple sterile effusions generally resorb spontaneously but *loculated sterile effusions* may be a persistent source of respiratory embarrassment, and frequently require chest tube drainage for resolution.

Empyema is diagnosed by a positive culture. Gram-stain is helpful if positive, but is frequently unrevealing. Prior treatment with antibiotics may obscure culture results. High white blood cell counts with a predominance of polymorphonuclear leukocytes, as well as a low pleural fluid glucose, support the diagnosis of empyema, but neither finding is diagnostic. Determination of the pleural fluid pH can sometimes be of value in distinguishing the different types of parapneumonic effusions. Several studies have shown that if the pleural fluid pH is less than 7.2, the effusion will be either an empyema or a loculated effusion, and therefore will likely require chest tube drainage. The use of this criterion is only valid in parapneumonic effusions.

Other Causes of Pleural Effusions

Additional studies may be useful in determining the specific etiology of a nonmalignant and noninfectious pleural exudate. About 10% of cases of pancreatitis are associated with pleural effusions, and these are associated with high levels of pleural fluid amylase. Unfortunately, about 10% of cases of malignant effusions also have high amylase levels. Complement levels are reported to be decreased in effusions associated with rheumatoid arthritis or systemic lupus erythematosis (LE). The finding of LE cells in an effusion is pathognomonic for lupus. Ultimately, the identification of the cause of exudative effusions in situations such as pulmonary emboli, pancreatitis, Dressler's syndrome, and connective-tissue diseases rests more with the total clinical picture than with any esoteric finding in the pleural fluid.

BIBLIOGRAPHY

Black LF: The pleural space and pleural fluid. Mayo Clin Proc 47:493–506, 1972

Leff A, Hopewell PC, Costello J: Pleural effusion from malignancy. Ann Intern Med 88:532–537, 1978

Light RW, Macgregor MI, Luchsinger PC et al: Pleural effusions: The diagnostic separation of transudates and exudates. Ann Intern Med 77:507–513, 1972

Rabin CB, Blackman NS: Bilateral pleural effusion: Its significance in association with a heart of normal size. Mt Sinai J Med 24:45, 1977

19

Aspiration Syndromes

Aspiration occurs in individuals who have lost the normal coordinated mechanism that permits air to enter the trachea while preventing the passage of liquid and solid material.

Pulmonary aspiration, especially in the hospital population, is a common event. Under the rubric "aspiration pneumonia" lies a variety of distinct clinical syndromes. These range from sudden respiratory arrest to the indolent course of a necrotic pneumonitis that may evolve over weeks or months. The characteristics of each syndrome depend upon:

1. whether the aspirate is composed primarily of particulate or liquid gastric contents,
2. the acidity and volume of the aspirate,
3. the lipid content of the aspirate,
4. whether infectious organisms are present.

Acidity

It has been possible to correlate the acidity of gastric aspirates with mortality. When the pH is below 1.8, the mortality rate approaches 100%. As the pH rises, the mortality rate falls rapidly.

The destructive effects of acidic aspirates (pH less than 3.5) are accomplished quickly; the damage is done within minutes. The initial lesion is a chemical burn that destroys cells all the way from the bronchi to the alveoli. Surfactant is lost and atelectasis follows within minutes. Over the next few hours there is a considerable exudation of fluid into the alveoli with hemorrhaging and consolidation. All these processes combine to produce significant hypoxia. In addition, the volume of the exudate may be sufficient to bring about hypovolemia and hypotension.

Aspiration of gastric contents when the pH is greater than 3.5 produces a more varied pathology. The precise picture depends upon the chemical nature of the aspirate and whether food particles are present. The extent of parenchymal damage is less than with acidic aspirates, but atelectasis and alveolar edema do develop, again giving rise to hypoxia. In both nonacidic and acidic aspirates, the extent of the pulmonary compromise increases with the volume of the aspirated material.

Lipid Content

The chemical nature of the aspirate may significantly affect the clinical presentation. One syndrome in particular is worth noting in this regard: _Lipoid pneumonia_ is a chronic aspiration syndrome that results from the aspiration of fat. It is encountered most often in the elderly. Mineral oil, used as a base for many nose drops or taken orally as a laxative, is the most common offender. Aspirated mineral oil is ingested by alveolar macrophages, but is poorly metabolized. Oil droplets can be seen in the interstitial tissues surrounded by a mononuclear inflammatory reaction. The alveolar interstitium thickens and fibrosis develops.

The diagnosis of lipoid pneumonia can be difficult. The patient is frequently asymptomatic, and when symptoms are present, they are usually nonspecific, with only a nonproductive cough and dyspnea. A chest x-ray shows evidence of an alveolar infiltrate that ultimately progresses to localized fibrosis; the discovery of a scarred density on x-ray may misleadingly raise the spectre of bronchogenic cancer. A history of exposure to mineral oil is certainly helpful in making the diagnosis, and the finding of lipid-laden macrophages in the sputum or in bronchoscopic washings should suggest lipoid pneumonia. However, lipid-laden macrophages cannot always be detected, and more definitive procedures, such as a lung biopsy for a tissue diagnosis, may be required.

Infection

Perhaps the most important consideration in aspiration syndromes is the role of infection. There are two ways in which bacterial infection can become a factor: (1) through superinfection of a lung already damaged by sterile aspiration, and (2) through direct aspiration of infected material.

Superinfection. The lung's defenses against bacterial infection can be severely compromised by aspiration damage. Several studies have shown that 50% or more of patients develop a pulmonary infection following fluid aspiration. Such infections are not immediately apparent, and may only become noticeable in time.

The clinical recognition of the development of superinfection in the setting of pulmonary aspiration can be very difficult. The patient may develop fever, a cough with purulent sputum, and leukocytosis, and there may be x-ray findings of consolidation. These signs and symptoms, however, can also be present in aspiration uncomplicated by infection. Suspicion of superinfection should be very high if the symptoms persist or become more severe. It is important to examine properly obtained samples of sputum regularly for organisms. The infecting bacteria are commonly aerobes, and include staphylococcus, streptococcus, pneumococcus, and gram-negative organisms.

Aspiration Infection. Direct aspiration of infected material may produce a syndrome considerably different from destructive aspiration followed by superinfection. Unlike the latter, there may be little pulmonary damage by the aspiration event itself; the aspiration event may even go entirely unnoticed. Presumably, a small occult focus of infection develops from the heavily contaminated aspirate. The source of the aspiration is the oropharynx. Although people all have bacteria in their mouths and upper airways, in the majority of cases of aspiration infections, poor dental hygiene provides a predisposing setting.

The clinical findings of aspiration infection can be quite varied. Most often the patient presents with the symptoms of indolent infection—malaise, fever, and cough. Aspiration infections acquired outside the hospital commonly have longer symptomatic periods than in-hospital infections, averaging one to six weeks, although symptoms may persist for months. Any of several x-ray patterns can be observed: empyema, pulmonary abscess (Fig.

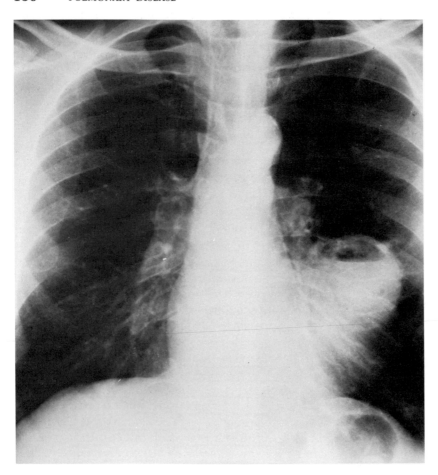

FIG. 19–1. Chest radiograph of a lung abscess.

19–1), necrotizing pneumonia, or pneumonitis. Empyema rarely occurs alone and is usually associated with one of the other parenchymal lesions.

Ninety percent of aspiration infections occurring in the community involve anaerobic organisms. This is not surprising since the majority of the normal inhabitants of the oropharynx are anaerobes. About 50% of these infections involve mixtures of anaerobic and aerobic organisms.

In-hospital aspiration infections involve gram-negative aerobes in up to 70% of cases. This also is not unexpected, since the oro-pharynx of the hospitalized patient is rapidly colonized with gram-negative aerobes. One organism associated with aspiration infection that is not a normal inhabitant of the oropharynx is *Bacteroides fragilis*, a gram-negative anaerobe present in 10% to 25% of cases. *Bacteroides fragilis* is usually resistant to penicillin, whereas most other anaerobes are highly sensitive to the drug.

Suspicion of an occult aspiration should be greatly enhanced by the discovery of anaerobes in the sputum, since aspiration is by far the most common cause of anaerobic pleuropulmonary infections. Less common settings include seeding from a distant site of anaerobic infection, and the presence of structural lesions of the lung. Foul-smelling sputum has been touted as indicating the presence of anaerobes, but it occurs in only about 50% of cases of anaerobic infection. In addition, sputum production may not begin until one or two weeks following infection.

Because the oropharynx normally is heavily colonized with anaerobes, sputum samples must be obtained from transtracheal aspirates or empyema fluid. Anaerobic cultures should always be made. Gram-staining will frequently reveal a mixed flora of slender pleomorphic gram-negative rods representing organisms such as bacteroides and fusobacterium, and tiny gram-positive cocci suggesting anaerobic streptococcus. Blood cultures are usually negative.

The course of anaerobic aspiration infections is often long and indolent, although acute fulminant infections do occur. Even after the institution of proper antibiotic therapy, fever and signs of a pneumonic process may persist for weeks.

COMMON SETTINGS FOR ASPIRATION

Healthy persons frequently aspirate oral contents during sleep, but the volume of the aspirate is small and intact respiratory defense mechanisms protect the lung from the establishment of infection.

Clinically significant aspiration occurs most frequently in patients with depressed mental status, including coma, stupor, seizures, postictal state, drunkenness, and anesthesia. Anatomic and physiologic aberrations, notably esophageal diverticuli and dysphagia secondary to neuromuscular dysfunction, can provide fertile settings for aspiration. Nasogastric tubes destroy the integrity of the esophageal sphincters, permitting aspiration of gastric contents. Tracheostomies predispose to aspiration, but the risk can be minimized by using a large volume, low pressure cuff. Finally, vomiting and subsequent aspiration are not infrequent during cardiopulmonary resuscitation.

DIAGNOSIS

When the aspiration event is observed, the diagnosis is obvious. Unfortunately, the majority of aspirations are either unwitnessed or silent. The diagnosis of aspiration then depends on accumulating several indirect pieces of evidence. Certainly, the existence of any predisposing factor is helpful. The presence of necrotizing pneumonia, lung abscess, or any proven anaerobic pulmonary infection should raise one's index of suspicion.

The location of the infiltrate on x-ray can be extremely valuable in diagnosing aspiration. Aspiration occurs most frequently with the patient on his back, and the aspirate therefore settles into the dependent areas of the lung; these include the superior segments of the lower lobes, the posterior segment of the right upper lobe, and the superior segment of the left upper lobe. Aspiration infiltrates are often bilateral.

Large particles can obstruct major bronchi with the resultant acute onset of dyspnea and cyanosis, focal loss of breath sounds, and eventually the loss of lung volume. Thus, evaluation of airway patency is critical for any patient who goes into acute respiratory distress. Nasotracheal and posterior pharyngeal suction should be applied to remove any obstruction that may be the source of the distress. If foodstuffs or recognizable gastric contents are returned with suction, the diagnosis of aspiration is virtually a certainty.

TREATMENT

Both mechanical and pharmacologic therapeutic modalities are used in the treatment of aspiration syndromes.

Endotracheal suctioning, especially when the aspiration event is witnessed, is an important maneuver that should be tried at once to remove any accessible aspirated material, as well as to stimulate the patient to cough up deeper material. If the clinical picture strongly suggests a large particulate obstruction, bronchoscopy should be carried out to remove the offending matter. Bronchial lavage was once recommended, but the current feeling is that it probably has little place in the treatment of aspiration. If respiratory failure supervenes, ventilatory support will be necessary just as in other causes of pulmonary failure; no specific maneuvers are applicable to aspiration.

The pharmacologic approach to aspiration has traditionally centered around the use of steroids and antibiotics. Despite a number of controversial studies, there is no firm evidence that steroid administration favorably affects the course of a patient with pulmonary aspiration. There are several studies suggesting that steroid administration may increase the incidence of gram-negative pneumonia in patients who have aspirated gastric contents.

Despite the mixed nature of many aspiration infections, clinical experience indicates that treatment of the anaerobes alone is generally sufficient. Since the majority of anaerobes are susceptible to penicillin, this is the drug of choice. *Bacteroides fragilis*, however, is often insensitive to penicillin. Fortunately, this organism is usually present as part of a mixed anaerobic flora, and the use of penicillin is usually adequate.

Treatment of in-hospital aspirations can usually be dictated by culture results, but finding enteric-looking gram-negative rods on a sputum gram-stain suggests that penicillin may not be enough. Most of these aerobic gram-negative rods are enteric organisms or pseudomonas. Treatment often requires broader spectrum drugs or aminoglycosides.

The difficulty in treating pulmonary aspiration is rarely in choosing the right drug, but rather in determining whether a patient has developed an infection in the setting of an aspiration syndrome. It is often necessary to wait and monitor the patient for a period of time. However, because infection is so common in pulmonary aspiration, it is reasonable to ask why one should not presumptively treat all aspirations for infection. Many clinicians do just that, using penicillin to cover the possibility of anaerobic infection. Although this method of treatment may be reasonable, there are no prospective studies examining the benefits *versus* the harms of such an approach. Potential harms lie in giving a patient a drug he may not need and in the possibility of selecting for resistant organisms.

Cases of aspiration associated with an anaerobic empyema or abscess may not heal with antibiotic therapy alone. In such cases, antibiotic treatment should be continued, but should be supplemented by drainage procedures such as an indwelling chest tube or bronchoscopy.

BIBLIOGRAPHY

Bartlett JG, Gorbach SL: The triple threat of aspiration pneumonia. Chest 68:560–566, 1975

Bartlett JG, Gorbach SL, Finegold SM: The bacteriology of aspiration pneumonia. Am J Med 56:202–207, 1974

Cameron JL, Fuidema GD: Aspiration pneumonia: Magnitude and frequency of the problem. JAMA 219:1194–1196, 1972

Wynne JW, Modell JH: Respiratory aspiration of stomach contents. Ann Intern Med 87:466–474, 1977

20

Hemoptysis, the coughing up of blood, is difficult to ignore. This is fortunate, because even if the patient coughs up only enough blood to stain the sputum, there is usually underlying disease. If hemoptysis is massive (more than 200 ml/day) and allowed to go untreated, the patient usually dies from asphyxiation.

ASSESSMENT

The first concern in the treatment of patients with hemoptysis should be to determine whether the blood is truly coming from the lungs. A careful history and physical examination should enable one to distinguish bleeding from the tracheobronchial tree from a nosebleed (epistaxis) or bleeding from a throat lesion. Even a cursory examination will usually suffice to distinguish hemoptysis from hematemesis, but confusion may arise if the patient has first vomited and then aspirated the blood. Blood that has been in the stomach will be acidic and will contain remnants of food, whereas blood coming from the lungs will be alkaline and will contain alveolar macrophages laden with hemosiderin.

Small amounts of blood (blood-tinged sputum) most often, but not invariably, come from lung infections, especially bronchitis. Approximately 20% of patients coughing up *moderate* amounts of blood prove to have carcinoma of the lung. Most others will be found to have mitral stenosis or lung infections. In about 15% of patients, no etiology will be found; in general, the prognosis for these patients is good.

Massive hemoptysis is usually infectious in origin, due to tuberculosis, bronchiectasis, or a lung abscess.

CAUSES OF HEMOPTYSIS

Cancer

Unless an infectious etiology is certain in patients with hemoptysis, bronchoscopy must be performed to rule out cancer. Even an abscess, unless incontrovertibly related to an episode of aspiration, must be directly visualized, since it may be due to a necrotic cancer or a bronchus obstructed by cancer. Bronchoscopy can be useful in localizing and characterizing a carcinoma that is heralded only by hemoptysis, even when the chest x-ray remains clear and sputum cytologies are negative.

Lung Abscess 30–50

Thirty to fifty percent of patients with lung abscess have hemoptysis at some time in the course of their illness. Following massive and fatal hemoptysis from a lung abscess, a postmortem examination may reveal a pulmonary artery opening directly into the abscess cavity.

Bronchiectasis

Permanently dilated bronchi can result either from congenital deformations or from necrotizing pneumonias. Dilated and poorly epithelialized inelastic bronchi invite repeated infection. Bleeding is a result of the chronic inflammatory process ulcerating into the fragile anastomotic vascular network that is usually present. Hemoptysis is usually accompanied by cough and voluminous sputum production. A chest x-ray is occasionally diagnostic. More often, confirmation of the diagnosis depends upon bronchography, in which the bronchi are outlined with radiopaque dye. Bronchography is quite uncomfortable for the patient, and should be reserved for use only in anticipation of surgery.

Tuberculosis

Hemoptysis may occur during the active inflammatory stage of tuberculosis. Acid-fast bacilli can often be found in the sputum. The blood comes from endobronchial or cavitary ulcerations of either the pulmonary veins (red blood) or the pulmonary arteries (dark blood). Hemoptysis can also be caused by the residua of tuberculosis. These include aspergillus infections of cavities, postinflammatory bronchiectasis, and migration of calcified lymph nodes (broncholithiasis) through bronchial walls. Fatal pulmonary hemorrhage can result from aneurysms of intracavity pulmonary arteries (Rasmussen's aneurysms). If it weren't for the tendency of pericavity vessels to thrombose, hemorrhage might even be more common in tuberculosis.

Mitral Stenosis 40%

Forty percent of patients with mitral stenosis experience hemoptysis. Massive hemorrhage is rare; when it occurs, it invariably does so early in the disease, often predating dyspnea. The source of this hemorrhage is the bronchial veins. In mitral stenosis, these vessels form a plentiful, vulnerable submucosal anastomotic collateral system shunting blood between the high pressure pulmonary veins and the low pressure systemic veins. Early in the course of mitral stenosis, this anastomotic network carries a large volume of blood, and is easily disrupted by coughing or by acute elevations in left atrial pressure. Later in the disease, as cardiac output diminishes and systemic venous pressures increase, massive hemorrhage is less likely, but pink-stained pulmonary edema froth may accompany the episodic dyspnea. At this point, hemoptysis associated with pulmonary emboli becomes more likely.

Other Disorders

There are several rare disorders in which hemoptysis is a major clinical component.

Goodpasture's syndrome is an immunologic disease affecting the lungs and kidneys. It is caused by circulating antibodies directed against cross-reacting components of the renal glomeruli and pulmonary alveoli. Hemoptysis is often the first sign of disease, and almost always occurs at some point in the course of the illness. Hemoptysis can be alleviated by bilateral nephrectomy, plasmaphoresis, and the use of cytotoxic agents.

Several varieties of *pulmonary vasculitis* are associated with hemoptysis. Wegener's granulomatosis is associated with granulomas throughout the lung and upper respiratory

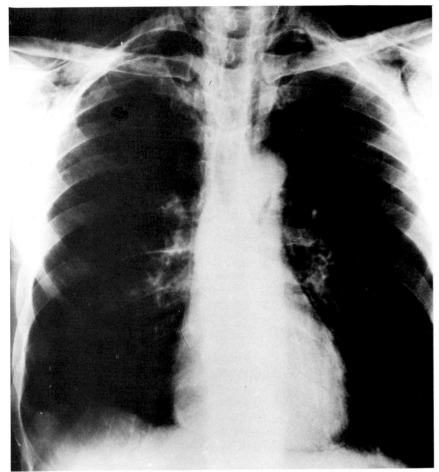

FIG. 20–1. Chest radiograph showing mediastinal emphysema and subcutaneous emphysema following bronchoscopy.

tract. Connective tissue diseases, including systemic lupus erythematosis, can evoke a pulmonary vasculitis and, rarely, hemoptysis.

Pulmonary hypertension, whether it is idiopathic, the result of high altitude exposure, or a sequela of congenital systemic-to-pulmonary shunts, can lead to hemoptysis.

Other disorders that can cause hemoptysis but do not require bronchoscopy include pulmonary embolism, coagulation disorders, lung trauma due to puncture by a broken rib or projectile, avulsion of the tracheobronchial tree by blunt trauma, and irritation and necrosis of the mucosal lining by inhaled fumes or smoke.

EVALUATION AND THERAPY

The bleeding site may be auscultated as localized rales, rhonchi or wheezes, or may be seen on a chest x-ray. The physical findings can be misleading, however, since rales and wheezes may reflect a focal pneumonitis from aspirated blood rather than the primary focus.

Some patients report that they can sense the location of the hemorrhage.

Bronchoscopy allows direct visualization of the tracheobronchial tree and has revolutionized pulmonary medicine, especially in the evaluation of tumors, abscesses, obstruction, and hemoptysis of unknown etiology.

The flexible fiberoptic bronchoscope consists of a bundle of optical fibers. The image passes to the viewer unchanged regardless of the degree of the angle of bend of the fibers. The patient is given a local anesthestic and a tranquilizer, and the bronchoscope is directed through the nose, through the vocal cords, and into the trachea and orifices of each of the main and segmental bronchi. A site of bleeding or obstruction can be seen, secretions can be obtained for culture or cytology, and the lesions can be brushed or biopsied.

For massive hemoptysis, the rigid bronchoscope is preferred. It is a hollow tube and permits better control for direct visualization and packing of a site of hemorrhage.

Although bronchoscopy is an uncomfortable procedure, the significant dangers are few. The tube causes partial airway obstruction that may result in decreases in arterial oxygenation. Rarely, an attempt at biopsy may produce a pneumothorax, mediastinal emphysema (Fig. 20–1), or significant hemorrhage.

If the blood loss does not exceed 200 ml for 24 hours, therapy for hemoptysis consists of treating the underlying disease. Massive pulmonary hemorrhage, however, can be rapidly fatal without immediate surgical intervention. When a bleeding site is identified, the patient should be placed so that the bleeding site is as low as possible in the hope of protecting the airways of the other lung. If the degree of respiratory compromise is severe, the healthy lung can be intubated for protection.

The surgeon next assesses operability. If nonsurgical temporizing measures are attempted, an 80% mortality can be expected in these patients. Mortality with surgical intervention is about 20%. If necessary to halt the bleeding, even lesions of active tuberculosis or an untreated lung abscess can be removed without an unacceptable risk of infectious complications. The major contraindications to surgery include advanced bilateral pulmonary disease, an inability to localize the lesion, widespread metastatic carcinoma, and severe pulmonary functional impairment.

BIBLIOGRAPHY

Crocco JA, Rooney JJ, Fankushen DS et al: Massive hemoptysis. Arch Intern Med 121:495–498, 1968

Schwartz R, Myerson RM, Lawrence LT et al: Mitral stenosis, massive pulmonary hemorrhage, and emergency valve replacement. N Engl J Med 275:755–758, 1966

Smiddy JF, Elliott RC: The evaluation of hemoptysis with fiberoptic bronchoscopy. Chest 64:158–162, 1973

Renal Disease

21

Fluids, Electrolytes, and pH Homeostasis

WATER, SODIUM, AND POTASSIUM

The total body fluid occupies two compartments: an extracellular compartment, containing the plasma volume and the interstitial fluids, and an intracellular compartment.

Water freely crosses cell membranes and distributes throughout both the extracellular and intracellular compartments.

Sodium chloride, on the other hand, is restricted primarily to the extracellular space. It is kept outside of cells by membrane-bound pumps and counterbalances the osmotic force generated by intracellular proteins. When sodium chloride is ingested, it remains in the extracellular space and therefore draws water out of the cells until the osmotic equilibrium is restored. Thus, the ingestion of salt tends to expand the extracellular volume. For this reason, salty solutions, such as normal saline (0.9% sodium chloride), are given to patients whose plasma volume is low.

Although changes in the plasma volume and serum sodium concentration are in many ways interdependent, for most purposes it is profitable to view them as separate entities.

Plasma Volume

The plasma volume is primarily a function of the total *amount* of sodium in the body. If the amount of sodium that is ingested exceeds the amount that is excreted (positive sodium balance), the plasma volume rises, because the excess sodium retains water in the extracellular space. As a result, the glomerular filtration rate increases, and the excess sodium and water are excreted by the kidney to restore the normal plasma volume. However, a patient with compromised cardiac function may experience an attack of acute pulmonary edema before the kidneys can excrete the excess sodium load.

If the net sodium balance is negative (excretion exceeds ingestion), the plasma volume falls. If the fall is precipitous or severe, the patient manifests signs of hypovolemia: orthostatic hypotension, dry mucous membranes, a resting tachycardia, absent axillary sweat, poor skin turgor, and a low jugular venous pressure. These manifestations reflect the body's attempt to minimize further salt loss and maintain adequate blood pressure in the face of a decreased plasma volume.

145

The plasma volume is most directly sensed by volume-sensing receptors in the atria of the heart and controlled by means of the renin-angiotensin-aldosterone axis.

Serum Sodium Concentration

The *concentration* of sodium reflects primarily the body's state of water balance, and is a measure of how much the sodium has been diluted by water. Because water freely distributes across plasma membranes, the concentration of sodium, as well as the concentration of all other salts, decreases with water overload and increases with water depletion. The serum sodium concentration is thus an accurate gauge of the serum osmolality, and for practical purposes the two are often used interchangeably. Hyperosmolar states are therefore often hypernatremic states. An important exception is hyperglycemia, when hyperosmolality results from a dramatically increased glucose concentration.

In most instances, regulation of the serum sodium concentration is achieved by pathways that regulate the serum osmolality by adjusting the body's water balance. These pathways originate in the osmoreceptors of the brain. The osmoreceptors are stimulated by a 2% rise in the serum osmolality, and trigger both the release of antidiuretic hormone (ADH) and the thirst mechanism.

In summation, hypovolemia and hypervolemia are primarily sodium problems; hyponatremia and hypernatremia are primarily water problems. Clinical evaluation utilizes this distinction, although it must be stressed that these concepts are true only to a first approximation.

HYPONATREMIA

The kidney can excrete almost any water-load presented to it, and it is therefore extremely difficult to become hyponatremic by drinking dilute fluids unless there is an underlying disorder of the kidneys or of the ADH-secretory mechanism. Most patients tolerate hyponatremia well. Symptoms usually arise only when the sodium concentration falls precipitously below 125 mEq/liter. The symptoms of precipitous hyponatremia are predominantly neurologic. They progress from mild confusion and anorexia to nausea, vomiting, and eventually to convulsions, coma, and death.

Hyponatremia implies only that there is too much water relative to the amount of solute in the body. Hyponatremia can therefore occur with excess total body water (overhydration), normal total body water (euhydration), or even low total body water (dehydration).

Hyponatremia with Overhydration

Edematous States. Congestive heart failure, the nephrotic syndrome, and cirrhosis are all associated with hyponatremia. The reasons for these associations are not clear. Some have suggested that the "effective" intravascular volume may be decreased, leading to a stimulation of ADH secretion.

Syndrome of Inappropriate ADH (SIADH). Several disorders can result in the circulation of too much ADH or ADH-like substances with consequent hyponatremia (see Chap. 26). Some *tumors,* especially oat cell carcinomas of the lung, secrete biologically active ADH-like material. *Disorders of the central nervous system,* including meningitis and encephalitis, may directly affect the osmoreceptors that regulate ADH secretion. *Pulmonary infections* are occasionally reported to cause a decreased serum sodium concentration by an unknown mechanism. Numerous *drugs,* especially clofibrate and the oral hypoglycemic chlorpropamide, either enhance the secretion of ADH or potentiate the kidneys' response to the hormone.

Hyponatremia with Euhydration

The prolonged use of *diuretics* may cause hyponatremia without any evidence of dehydration. It has been postulated that in this circumstance the kidneys are directly responsible for retaining excess free water.

Some individuals may have a "reset osmostat," in which the osmoreceptor has reestablished its point of equilibrium at a serum osmolality below 280 mOsm. These patients have normal pituitary, adrenal, ADH, and renal function, and their responses to water loading and water restriction are normal. Compensatory mechanisms always return the osmolarity to the same, although lowered, set point.

Hyponatremia with Dehydration

Patients who have hyponatremia with dehydration present with clinical evidence of diminished intravascular volume. Sodium loss may occur by way of the kidneys or by a nonrenal route.

Renal loss may result from the use of diuretics, from adrenal insufficiency, or, rarely, from a salt-losing renal disease.

If the urine of a patient with hyponatremia with dehydration contains less than 10 mEq of sodium per liter, a nonrenal source is likely. With severe volume depletion, the regulation of volume becomes more critical than the regulation of osmolality, and ADH secretion increases. Thus, in a patient experiencing severe volume depletion from repeated vomiting, diarrhea, or excessive sweating, hyponatremia may result if these sodium-containing fluid losses are replaced solely with water.

Therapy of Hyponatremia

Hyponatremia is often discovered only incidentally, and usually requires no specific therapeutic intervention. Water restriction generally suffices. Severe symptomatic hyponatremia can be reversed with an infusion of hypertonic saline, but the serum sodium should only be returned to approximately 125 mEq/liter.

It is important to recognize that a low serum sodium concentration can be an artifact of measurement. In patients with hyperlipidemia or extreme hyperproteinemia, sodium is excluded from a water-free space in the plasma sample, and a lower value will be reported per milliliter of plasma even though the concentration of sodium per milliliter of plasma water is normal.

HYPERNATREMIA

Hypernatremia develops when the water loss exceeds the sodium loss. Water may be lost (1) by way of the kidneys, because of inadequate ADH secretion (see Chap. 26 for a discussion of diabetes insipidus) or a poor renal response to ADH (nephrogenic diabetes insipidus), (2) by way of the skin (burns, sweat), or (3) by way of the lungs. Even when water wasting is massive, as in some patients with diabetes insipidus, normal thirst mechanisms can prevent hypernatremia unless the patient is obtunded, comatose, or institutionalized without access to water. Patients with a high risk for developing hypernatremia therefore include those with strokes or those who have recently had neurosurgical procedures, that is, those who acquire diabetes insipidus from an intracranial event and whose cognitive functions are compromised. Hypernatremia is treated by slowly replacing the lost water.

POTASSIUM

Potassium is preferentially restricted to the intracellular space by the same membrane pumps that exclude sodium. The extracellular concentration of potassium is carefully maintained at only 3.5 to 5.0 mEq/liter. For many cells, the gradient of potassium across the membrane provides the basis for the resting membrane potential. For excitable and secretory cells (and perhaps for all other cells), potassium currents determine the repolarization phase of action potentials and are linked to metabolic events within the cytosol that control repetitive neuronal activity and secretion.

Total body potassium is regulated by the kidney. The major determinants of the concentration of potassium in the extracellular space are (1) the pH and (2) the level of total body potassium stores.

During acidosis, H⁺ ions enter the cells in exchange for potassium, thereby raising the extracellular potassium concentration. During alkalosis, potassium enters the cells and the extracellular potassium falls. Since membrane potentials depend upon the ratio of intracellular to extracellular potassium, small changes in the extracellular concentration can greatly affect excitable tissues.

The total amount of potassium in the body is regulated by renal secretion, which in turn is under three controlling influences: (1) *Aldosterone* increases potassium secretion. (2) *Delivery of sodium* to the distal tubule determines the extent of sodium reabsorption. Increased sodium delivery (*e.g.,* in patients on diuretic therapy) causes the inside of the tubule to become more electronegative, enhancing potassium secretion as the ion moves down its electrical gradient. (3) The *potassium and H⁺ ion concentrations* within the renal tubular cell also contributes to the regulation of potassium secretion. Alkalosis increases the intracellular concentration of potassium and thus provides more potassium for secretion. At the same time, there are fewer intracellular H⁺ ions competing with the potassium for the same or similar pumps.

Maximal renal potassium secretion will occur in states associated with high aldosterone, a high delivery of sodium to the distal tubule, and alkalosis. This combination is not uncommon in patients on diuretics, and it is the reason that hypokalemia is so prevalent in those patients.

Hypokalemia

Hypokalemia, like hyponatremia, is generally well-tolerated. The affects of hypokalemia are usually subtle and often include only skeletal muscle weakness. If hypokalemia is profound or occurs rapidly, the patient may experience nausea, impaired gastrointestinal motility, impaired urinary concentrating ability, arrhythmias, and carbohydrate intolerance.

The patient on digitalis must have his serum potassium checked regularly, since hypokalemia increases the risk of digitalis toxicity. The reason for this interaction is not clear, but may be related to (1) changes in the binding of digitalis by cells, (2) the interaction of potassium and digitalis with ion currents, or (3) the nature of the underlying cardiac disease.

Potassium may be lost through the kidneys or the gastrointestinal tract, or it may shift into cells:

1. There are several clinical situations associated with increased renal potassium loss. (a) The use of diuretics is the most common cause of potassium loss. All common diuretics, except those designed to interfere with potassium secretion (triamterene and spironolactone), cause significant potassium loss. (b) The osmotic diuresis that occurs, for example, in diabetic ketoacidosis, can produce hypokalemia. (c) States of hyperaldosteronism increase the renal secretion of potassium. (d) Renal tubular acidosis can also produce hypokalemia (discussion follows).

2. Gastrointestinal causes of hypokalemia include prolonged vomiting, diarrhea, and fis-

tulous drainage. Alkalosis associated with prolonged vomiting results in poor renal potassium conservation, and contributes significantly to the hypokalemia.

3. Intracellular shifts of potassium have been described in an unusual familial disorder known as hypokalemic periodic paralysis. Attacks of weakness or even complete paralysis are accompanied by the transient movement of potassium into cells with resultant hypokalemia. It is unlikely that hypokalemia alone is responsible for the exceptional weakness.

The therapy for hypokalemia can generally proceed slowly, employing oral or intravenous supplementation with potassium chloride. Only when the serum potassium is below 2 mEq/liter in a patient with paralysis or electrocardiographic changes (flattened or inverted T waves with prominent U waves) should potassium infusions ever be carried out at a rate greater than 10 mEq/hour.

Hyperkalemia

Significant hyperkalemia (potassium concentrations greater than 6.5 mEq/liter) may cause ventricular fibrillation and cardiac standstill. The progression of hyperkalemia can sometimes be followed on the electrocardiogram, although the electrocardiographic changes are neither invariable nor specific (Fig. 21–1). Initially, the T wave becomes tall and peaked. Next, the PR interval becomes prolonged and the P wave diminishes in size. Eventually, the QRS complex widens, the P wave disappears, and the QRS complex and T wave merge to form a "sine wave." These electrocardiographic changes portend cardiac arrest.

The causes of hyperkalemia are (1) inadequate renal excretion of potassium and (2) the movement of potassium out of cells.

Inadequate renal excretion can derive from renal failure, from the absence of aldosterone, or from diuretics that inhibit potassium se-

cretion. In patients with anuric renal failure, the potassium concentration will rise about 0.5 mEq/liter per day. In any patient with compromised renal function, the administration of large potassium loads can cause iatrogenic hyperkalemia.

Acute hyperkalemia can result from massive cell death. The source of the potassium is usually muscle. Potassium is released from necrotic muscle after massive crush injuries or following acute arterial emboli. Less often, the red blood cell is the source of potassium, either as a result of hemolysis or internal hemorrhage. In patients with thrombocytosis or leukemic leukocytosis, apparent hyperkalemia may be an artifact of cell lysis within the blood sample (see Chap. 49).

The therapy for hyperkalemia must be adjusted to the severity of the electrolyte disturbance. In the most severe cases, when the potassium concentration is greater than 8 mEq/liter or when there are electrocardiographic changes in the QRS complex or P wave, the cardiac toxicity must be countered by an infusion of calcium gluconate. The

FIG. 21–1. An electrocardiogram showing severe hyperkalemia.

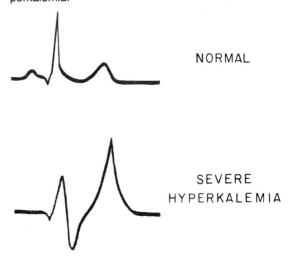

NORMAL

SEVERE
HYPERKALEMIA

therapeutic effect should be immediate. The excess potassium must then be moved back into the cells by alkalinization with sodium bicarbonate. Glucose, in combination with small doses of insulin, is also given to enhance the movement of potassium into the cells. The effects on potassium concentration should be noticeable in less than an hour. Finally, potassium-trapping resins (Kayexalate) can be given orally or rectally to remove potassium from the body. These resins exchange sodium for potassium and may therefore cause volume overload by providing a large sodium load. The resins are constipating, so a nonreabsorbable solute, sorbitol, is given simultaneously to induce diarrhea. The resins take several hours to achieve their maximal effect on the potassium concentration. In more refractory cases, dialysis may become necessary.

In less acute cases, with slightly lower potassium levels, the resin alone will suffice. In most cases of moderate hyperkalemia, however, especially when potassium levels are below 6.5, no immediate therapy is necessary and the underlying condition can be treated first.

PRINCIPLES OF SALT AND WATER THERAPY

Many patients who enter the hospital are too ill to ingest their daily fluid and electrolyte requirements, and therefore require intravenous maintenance therapy. Basal requirements can be estimated by allowing for (1) a loss of about 1000 ml of water per day—500 ml through the kidneys and another 500 ml as insensible losses from the lungs and skin—(2) a loss of 20 mEq/day of potassium, an obligate loss from the kidneys, and (3) a need for about 150 to 200 grams/day of carbohydrate to prevent protein catabolism. The renal excretion of sodium is quite flexible, and in

most patients with normal renal function can be reduced almost to zero with sodium restriction. These requirements can be met with appropriate combinations of saline and glucose solutions with the addition of potassium chloride. In some patients, fluid and electrolyte losses may exceed basal requirements. Thus, for example, insensible losses increase with fever and hyperventilation. Losses attributed to vomiting or diarrhea can be replaced either directly by measuring the ionic content and volume of the vomitus or diarrhea or indirectly by using standard estimates (see Table 21–1).

Fluid therapy should always be thoroughly monitored. Intake and output can be quantitated by taking daily measurements of body weight. This is especially critical in patients suffering from renal failure. Patients at bed rest lose approximately 0.3 kg of lean body mass per day, so that losses in excess of this may represent inadequate fluid replacement or severe catabolism.

REGULATION OF pH: ACIDOSIS AND ALKALOSIS

Virtually all cellular functions are dependent upon careful regulation of the pH. Enzyme function, membrane and action potentials, muscle contraction, and fertilization of o-ocytes all directly or indirectly depend upon the H^+ ion activity. At the intracellular level, the ability of the mitochondrion to generate ATP by oxidative phosphorylation is a function of the pH gradient across the mitochondrial membrane.

Most biologic reactions function most efficiently at an extracellular pH of about 7.4. To maintain this pH, the body relies on a series of buffer systems and on removal of excess acid or alkali by excretion through the kidneys and lungs.

Table 21–1

| | Na$^+$ | K$^+$ | mEq/L | | |
			H$^+$	Cl$^-$	HCO$_3^-$
gastric secretion	40	10	90	140	—
diarrheal fluid	50	35	—	40	45

Modified from Freitag JJ, Miller LW: Manual of Medical Therapeutics, 23rd ed. Boston, Little, Brown & Co, 1980

Buffers. The body possesses both intracellular and extracellular buffers. Each buffer has an unique affinity for the H$^+$ ion, and so will be more or less protonated at any given pH. All the body buffers are in equilibrium at any given time. Thus, if the ratio of protonated buffer to nonprotonated buffer is known for any one of the buffer systems, it is then possible to predict both the pH and the ratio for any other buffer system. This fact was appreciated by L. J. Henderson, who formulated the only equation needed to understand acid-base balance, the Henderson-Hasselbalch equation:

$$pH = pK_B + \log \frac{(B)}{(B \cdot H^+)}$$

in which (B) is the concentration of nonprotonated buffer, (B·H$^+$) is the concentration of protonated buffer, and pK is a constant that is characteristic of each buffer, describing its affinity for the H$^+$ ion.

Because a change in any one of these variables in one buffer system (B) necessitates a change in the other buffers (e.g., C), the following equation is true:

$$pH = pK_B + \log \frac{(B)}{(B \cdot H^+)}$$
$$= pK_C + \log \frac{(C)}{(C \cdot H^+)}$$

Thus, the ratio of any one of the buffer pairs can be used to predict the pH. In practice, the ratio employed most frequently is that of the *bicarbonate-carbonic acid buffer system:*

$$CO_2 + H_2O \rightleftharpoons H_2CO_3 \rightleftharpoons HCO_3 + H^+$$

The pK of this buffer system is 6.1, and the resultant Henderson-Hasselbalch equation is:

$$pH = 6.1 + \log \frac{(HCO_3^-)}{(H_2CO_3)}$$

Excretion. Any acid or alkaline load, whether introduced exogenously or produced endogenously, is buffered immediately. However, in order to restore these buffer systems, the load must be excreted. This is accomplished by means of the lungs, which release carbon dioxide, and the kidneys, which secrete acids and generate new bicarbonate. The responses of the lungs and kidneys are much slower than the immediate effects of chemical buffering (discussion later).

Acidosis and Alkalosis

Acidosis means that the body is exposed to an acid load, and *alkalosis* means exposure to an alkaline load. *Acidemia* refers specifically to the arterial pH, indicating that it is less than 7.36. *Alkalemia* means that the arterial pH is greater than 7.44. A patient can have acidosis without acidemia when two concurrent acid-base disorders coexist, for example, when the effects of acidosis and alkalosis on the total H$^+$ ion concentration cancel each other, so that the arterial pH remains normal. If there is no second counterbalancing pH disturbance, however, acidosis will result in at least a slight acidemia: the body's buffering and excretory homeostatic mechanisms cannot completely restore the pH to normal.

Cells and Serum

Immediate buffering of an acid or alkaline load is dependent upon the extracellular bicarbonate system and intracellular phosphate and protein. Such loads are buffered equally in the intracellular and extracellular spaces. The body's total buffer stores are only about 12 mEq to 15 mEq/kg body weight. In severe acidosis, the release of calcium salts into the circulation from bone may provide some additional buffering potential.

Lungs

The daily metabolism of fats and carbohydrates produces dissolved CO_2 that is easily hydrated by the enzyme carbonic anhydrase, producing about 13,000 mEq of carbonic acid per day. CO_2 and H_2CO_3 are in equilibrium $(CO_2 + H_2O \rightleftharpoons H_2CO_3)$, and when the lungs excrete CO_2 they drive the reaction to the left, effectively diminishing the concentration of carbonic acid.

Kidneys

A second chronic source of acid is the nonvolatile (non-CO_2) acids that result from fat and carbohydrate metabolism (H_2SO_4, H_3PO_4, and uric acid). This metabolism produces about 70 mEq of acid per day. The kidney handles this load in two ways: (1) it excretes acids by secreting H^+ ions into the tubular lumen, where they meet appropriate anions (*i.e.*, phosphate) and leave the body; and (2) it excretes H^+ ions in the form of NH_4^+, and thus generates new bicarbonate to replace any losses. The kidney cells produce ammonia from organic amines, such as glutamine. The ammonia diffuses back into the lumen where it traps the H^+ ion as NH_4^+, which is not able to diffuse back into the cell. The ability of the kidney to increase urinary ammonium secretion underlies its ability to handle a chronic acid load. Furthermore, the kidney reclaims, largely in the proximal tubule, any filtered bicarbonate.

Nomograms

Nomograms, such as that shown in Figure 21–2, predict how well the pH can be readjusted by the body's homeostatic mechanisms. The nomograms have been developed by studying the responses of populations with acute and chronic metabolic and respiratory disorders. The direction of compensation can be predicted by the form of the Henderson-Hasselbalch equation below:

$$pH = pK + \log \frac{(HCO_3^-)}{\text{constant} \times Pa_{CO_2}}$$

The pK is that of carbonic acid, 6.1. This equation substitutes the Pa_{CO_2}, which is readily measured, for carbonic acid, which is not. This simplication is feasible because CO_2 and H_2CO_3 are in equilibrium, related by the constant (0.031 mmol/liter/torr Pa_{CO_2}) which is the solubility factor for carbon dioxide dissolved in blood. The equation reveals that maintenance of a normal pH requires that the *ratio* of HCO_3^- to Pa_{CO_2} remains unchanged.

With acidosis resulting from the ingestion of acid or the development of renal failure (metabolic acidosis), the HCO_3^- is lowered and the ratio can be maintained by a reduction in the Pa_{CO_2}. This is achieved through hyperventilation, in which the lungs effectively blow off excess CO_2.

The response to acidosis resulting from respiratory failure (respiratory acidosis), with alveolar hypoventilation and an increasing Pa_{CO_2}, is renal synthesis of new bicarbonate. The greater the respiratory acidosis, the higher the compensatory rise in the serum HCO_3^-. Overcompensation, however, is never

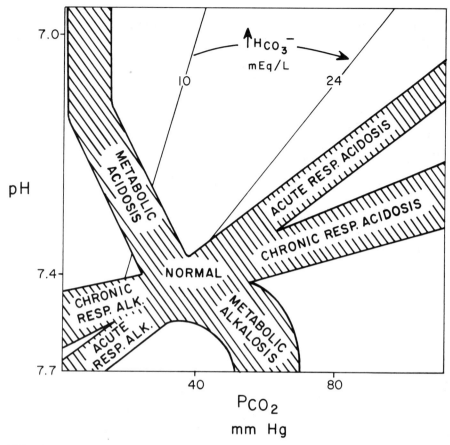

FIG. 21–2. The acid-base nomogram derived from studies of populations with the various disorders of acid–base balance described in the text.

achieved. In fact, in any chronic pH disturbance, the pH always remains slightly biased in the direction of the primary disorder.

RESPIRATORY ACIDOSIS

A Pa_{CO_2} of greater than 45 (alveolar hypoventilation) implies that the ventilatory apparatus can no longer keep up with the metabolic production of carbon dioxide. This results in an acidosis. The buffering of carbonic acid is accomplished in two phases.

1. Acutely, all changes in the Pa_{CO_2} are buffered by cellular proteins. As the Pa_{CO_2} rises, the concentration of carbonic acid rises. The carbonic acid dissociates to H^+ and HCO_3^-. The H^+ ion enters cells in exchange for sodium and potassium, and is buffered by cellular proteins. This leaves a bicarbonate ion in the extracellular space. Fifty percent of the compensatory rise in serum bicarbonate in acute respiratory acidosis arises by this mechanism. Most of the remainder of the HCO_3^- is produced within red blood cells. Carbon dioxide enters the red blood cell,

where it is hydrated to form carbonic acid. This dissociates to H^+ ion and bicarbonate. Hemoglobin buffers the H^+ ion, and the bicarbonate is transported out of the cell in exchange for chloride. These reactions are completed within about ten minutes. These cellular systems only partially buffer an acute carbonic acid load, and there is still a large change in the H^+ ion concentration for each increment in the Pa_{CO_2} (0.7 nM H^+ ion/liter for each torr rise in the Pa_{CO_2}).

2. During chronic respiratory acidosis there is an increase in the H^+ ion excretion in the form of urinary ammonium. Thus, in chronic respiratory acidosis, the pH changes less for the same change in Pa_{CO_2} than it does in acute respiratory acidosis (0.3 nM H^+ ion/liter for each torr rise in the Pa_{CO_2}). The kidney does not overcompensate for the lungs' problems, and the pH does not completely return to 7.40.

Patients with chronic hypercarbia (*e.g.*, due to chronic obstructive pulmonary disease) are better able to prevent marked H^+ ion concentration changes during acute episodes of ventilatory decompensation because they have chronically elevated HCO_3^- levels. The greater the initial bicarbonate, the greater must be the change in the Pa_{CO_2} to produce any given change in pH.

RESPIRATORY ALKALOSIS

Alveolar hyperventilation of any etiology can *acutely* lower the Pa_{CO_2} of arterial blood to less than 36 torr. The patient is typically lightheaded and complains of paresthesias, numbness, and tingling, especially around the mouth and in the fingers. If the respiratory alkalosis becomes severe, the patient may become unconscious. Hyperventilation is usually the result of anxiety. Other stimuli that can cause alveolar hyperventilation include pain, salicylates, intracranial hemorrhage, fever, and sepsis.

Chronic alveolar hyperventilation is asymptomatic, perhaps partly because renal compensation returns the arterial pH toward normal. The stimulus to chronically hyperventilate may come from the "stiff" lungs of diffuse interstitial lung disease, from the hypoxemia of high altitude or cyanotic congenital heart disease, or from high progesterone during pregnancy.

Only the acute hyperventilation of anxiety requires therapy specifically directed to raising the Pa_{CO_2}—rebreathing into a paper bag. This allows the patient to inhale an atmosphere enriched in CO_2. This simple maneuver is combined with reassurance to the patient that his symptoms derive from a benign and reversible problem.

METABOLIC ACIDOSIS

In metabolic acidosis, the bicarbonate concentration is lowered. There are many causes of metabolic acidosis, and one of the essentials for diagnosis is calculation of the "anion gap."

Anion Gap. The sum of the predominant extracellular anions (chloride and bicarbonate) is normally less than the concentration of the predominant extracellular cation (sodium). This difference [$Na^+ - (Cl^- + HCO_3^-)$], expressed in mEq/liter, is referred to as the anion gap. The normal anion gap is less than 12 to 14 mEq/liter, and represents phosphate, sulfate, protein, and other endogenously produced or exogenously administered anions. Metabolic acidosis can present with either a widened or a normal anion gap.

Acidosis with a Widened Anion Gap. There are only a limited number of disorders that cause a metabolic acidosis with a widened anion gap. In these disorders, the offending substance is an acid that dissociates into a H^+ ion (producing the acidosis) and an accompanying anion (producing the widened anion gap). These disorders include toxic ingestions (salicylates, paraldehyde, methanol, or ethylene glycol) or states of acid retention (uremia, diabetic ketoacidosis, or lactic acidosis). Each of the ingestions has accompanying clinical clues. Salicylates may directly stimulate the respiratory center causing a respiratory alkalosis; paraldehyde, a hypnotic drug partially excreted through the lungs, has an unmistakable odor; methanol, an alcohol substitute, causes blindness and optic disk hyperemia; ethylene glycol, a component of antifreeze, is metabolized to oxalate, and calcium oxalate crystals may be found in the urine.

Uremia causes acidosis with a widened anion gap only late in its course.

The acidosis of diabetic ketoacidosis occurs secondary to production of acetoacetic and β-hydroxybutyric acids. The bedside detection of ketonuria and ketonemia relies upon the colorimetric reaction of nitroprusside with acetoacetate. Because these tablets do not measure beta-hydroxybutyrate, the severity of the acidosis may be significantly underestimated when beta-hydroxybutyrate is the predominant ketone body.

Lactic acidosis occurs (1) with tissue hypoxia, in states of shock or respiratory failure, or (2) in several poorly understood states that presumably affect cellular metabolism and interfere with the normal aerobic pathways. Frequently, the acidemia of diabetic ketoacidosis also has a component of lactic acidosis, and the hypoglycemic agent phenformin has caused lactic acidosis.

Acidosis with a Normal Anion Gap. Metabolic acidosis with a normal anion gap results from the loss of bicarbonate by way of either the kidney or the gastrointestinal tract. The loss of bicarbonate is balanced by an elevation of chloride in the serum, and patients are said to have a *hyperchloremic acidosis.* Because the chloride rises as the bicarbonate declines, the anion gap does not change.

A depletion of bicarbonate can result from the loss of bicarbonate-rich fluid in patients with diarrhea or pancreatic fistulae. In patients with a ureterosigmoidostomy, the ureter is reimplanted into the sigmoid colon where the urinary contents, exposed for a prolonged period to the colon, exchange urinary chloride for serum bicarbonate, with subsequent excretion of an alkaline urine.

Bicarbonate depletion may also occur in patients with *renal tubular acidosis.* The kidney normally controls the extracellular bicarbonate concentration by (1) reabsorbing filtered bicarbonate, 90% of which is accomplished by the proximal tubule, and (2) generating new bicarbonate. The latter is accomplished by means of the dissociation of H_2CO_3 into H^+ and HCO_3^-. The secreted H^+ ion is trapped within the lumen as ammonium (NH_4^+) or complexed with other buffers, primarily phosphate. The HCO_3^- is reabsorbed into the blood. The production of ammonia by the kidney is flexible, and it can be stimulated over several days to handle an increasing acid load.

When an otherwise normal kidney cannot adequately excrete H^+ ions, the disorder is termed renal tubular acidosis. There are two major subtypes:

1. In *proximal renal tubular acidosis,* the ability of the proximal tubule to reabsorb HCO_3^- is compromised, HCO_3^- is lost, and acidemia develops as the limited capacity of the distal tubule to reabsorb the flood of HCO_3^- is overwhelmed. Eventually, the serum HCO_3^- concentration declines to the point at which the proximal tubule is able to reabsorb most of the reduced HCO_3^- load. The remainder is reclaimed in the distal tubule, and the urine can then be acidified to a pH of less than 5.3. Proximal renal tubular acidosis can be caused by toxic injury to the renal tubular

cells, for example, by heavy metals or by Bence Jones proteins in patients with multiple myeloma, but more often it occurs as part of a generalized disorder of proximal tubular functions.

2. In *distal renal tubular acidosis*, the proximal reabsorption of bicarbonate is adequate, but the ability of the distal tubule to secrete H^+ ions is compromised. The urine pH remains above 5.3 even if the patient is given a load of acid. Hypercalciuria and renal stone formation frequently accompany the defect in urinary acidification.

An Approach to Acidosis

The measurement of arterial pH does not by itself clarify the nature of the process leading to a disturbance of the acid–base balance, but tells only the net result of all simultaneous disorders of and compensations for H^+ ion imbalance. It is clinically important to ascertain whether the primary disturbance is respiratory or metabolic and whether it is acute or chronic. These determinations can be clear-cut if the patient's history and blood gases are compatible with an isolated respiratory or metabolic disturbance, but more confusing if there is a mixed metabolic–respiratory problem.

Thus, for example, consider two patients, both with a respiratory acidosis marked by CO_2 retention and an arterial P_{CO_2} of 70 torr: one has chronic respiratory acidosis from obstructive lung disease and the other has acute respiratory acidosis because of hypoventilation from a heroin overdose. The patient with chronic lung disease will have some prior degree of renal compensation, and his serum HCO_3^- will be chronically elevated, for example, to 35 mEq/liter. This partially offsets the acidosis, so that the arterial pH is 7.31. In contrast, the serum HCO_3^- of the patient with acute respiratory acidosis from heroin overdosage will be only 27 mEq/liter, since the kidneys have not had time to generate new HCO_3^-. His arterial pH will be 7.19.

Consultation of the nomograms confirms that the first patient's blood gases are compatible with chronic respiratory acidosis with some metabolic compensation, and that the second patient has an acute respiratory acidosis. However, if the serum HCO_3^- of the patient with a heroin overdose was only 15 mEq/liter, and his pH consequently 6.94, it would fall outside of the range of acute respiratory acidosis and suggest the presence of a second simultaneous metabolic acidosis. This could be confirmed by an increased anion gap and might be explained, if the patient were hypotensive, by a concomitant lactic acidosis.

In general, a metabolic acidosis in which the pH is greater than 7.2 is tolerated well enough, allowing primary therapy to be directed at the underlying disorder. However, a much lower pH may interfere with normal cardiac and vascular functions and will become self-perpetuating if not treated adequately with the administration of bicarbonate. Although there is no accurate way to predict the absolute bicarbonate requirements of a patient with metabolic acidosis, the base deficit is usually equal to about one-half the body weight (in kilograms) multiplied by the difference between the normal bicarbonate concentration and the measured bicarbonate. No more than one-half the calculated base deficit should be administered at one time, especially if delivered by a central venous line, because (1) a large alkaline load can be toxic to the heart, and (2) as the patient improves and begins to correct his acidosis, the alkaline load may push the patient into alkalemia.

METABOLIC ALKALOSIS

The kidney is responsible for nearly all cases of metabolic alkalosis. Only very rarely does alkali ingestion or injection underlie this pH imbalance. The kidney causes alkalosis by the secretion of H^+ ions.

The most common cause of metabolic alkalosis is a combination of *volume depletion and chloride depletion*, resulting either from the use of diuretics or from vomiting. The kidney attempts to maintain the plasma volume by reabsorbing sodium. It does so in an electroneutral fashion, either by reabsorbing a chloride ion with a sodium ion, or by secreting hydrogen or potassium ions in exchange for sodium. In the face of chloride depletion, however, the tubule must rely more upon H^+ ion secretion. This produces and maintains an alkalosis (volume regulation thus seems to take precedence over pH homeostasis). This condition has been referred to as "contraction alkalosis." The ability of the lungs to compensate for a metabolic alkalosis with hypoventilation is limited by the hypoxemia that would result, and the lungs therefore play only a small ameliorative role. Administration of sodium chloride cures the alkalosis.

Two less common causes of metabolic alkalosis are *hypokalemia* and *adrenal cortical overactivity*. Depletion of intracellular potassium results in increased H^+ ion secretion by the renal tubular cells. Mineralocorticoids directly stimulate H^+ ion (and potassium) secretion. Alkalosis in these patients does not respond to sodium chloride administration, but rather to treatment of the adrenal disease or to repletion of potassium chloride.

Metabolic alkalosis by itself does not produce any obvious symptoms. If hypocalcemia is also present, tetany may result because alkalosis decreases the proportion of calcium that exists in the ionized form.

Only rarely is metabolic alkalosis so severe and so refractory to conventional volume and potassium chloride replacement that acid administration is required. When necessary, however, hydrochloric acid may be administered by a central venous catheter. It must be diluted in large volumes of intravenous solutions before administration. Arginine hydrochloride can be given in a more concentrated form, but the arginine exchanges with intracellular potassium and may precipitate hyperkalemia in patients with renal insufficiency, especially if there is concomitant hepatic failure which prevents the metabolism of arginine.

BIBLIOGRAPHY

Bear R, Gribik M: Assessing acid–base imbalances through laboratory parameters. Hosp Practice Nov, 157–165, 1974

Cox M, Sterns RH, Singer I: The defense against hyperkalemia: The roles of insulin and aldosterone. N Engl J Med 299:525–532, 1978

Emmett M, Nairns R: Clinical use of the anion gap. Medicine 56:38–100, 1977

Garella S, Dana C, Chazan J: Severity of metabolic acidosis as a determinant of bicarbonate requirements. N Engl J Med 289:121–126, 1973

Leaf A: The clinical and physiologic significance of the serum sodium concentration. N Engl J Med 267:24–30, 77–83, 1962

Moses AM, Miller M: Drug-induced dilutional hyponatremia. N Engl J Med 291:1234–1239, 1974

Rastegar A, Thier SU: Physiologic consequences and bodily adaptations to hyper- and hypocapnia. Chest 62:28S–34S, 1972

Ross EJ, Christie SBM: Hypernatremia. Medicine 48:441–473, 1969

Seldin D, Rector F: The generation and maintenance of metabolic alkalosis. Kidney Int 1:306–321, 1972

22

Acute Renal Failure

The sudden loss of renal function is termed acute renal failure. The most common cause is renal hypoperfusion, in which the kidneys fail as a result of ischemia. Other causes of acute renal failure include certain forms of intrinsic renal disease, such as rapidly progressive glomerulonephritis, which may evolve quickly enough to present as acute failure. A host of nephrotoxic agents, including heavy metals, aminoglycoside antibiotics, substances released during rhabdomyolysis, and others, can also produce acute renal failure. Finally, acute bilateral ureteral obstruction can be responsible. If both kidneys are functioning and healthy, this requires the unlikely occurrence of simultaneous blockage of both ureters or a single obstruction distal to the bladder. In men, who are the usual victims of postrenal obstruction, the latter is most frequently due to disease of the prostate gland.

ACUTE TUBULAR NECROSIS

Acute renal failure not due to obstruction or intrinsic renal disease is called acute tubular necrosis (ATN). It is most commonly caused by renal ischemia, and less often by toxins. Renal ischemia can result from bleeding, shock from any cause, anaphylaxis, or can occur during surgery (especially operations that involve the abdominal aorta), cardiopulmonary resuscitation, obstetric emergencies, and so forth.

The term acute tubular necrosis is actually somewhat of a misnomer, since the syndrome can occur without any histologic abnormalities. Commonly, however, there is some degree of tubular necrosis that may be extensive or mild, patchy or diffuse. There may be casts of material in the lumens of tubules and variable degrees of interstitial inflammation. Despite extensive research into the pathophysiology of ATN, no clear-cut, unifying picture has emerged.

Although patients may present with dramatic and even total failure of all aspects of renal function, the majority of those who survive recover full renal function. The challenge to the hospital staff, therefore, is to keep the patient alive through the days to weeks of renal failure during which there is a high mortality rate. The mortality rate varies greatly depending upon the etiology and the overall clinical status of the patient. In general, patients with severe underlying disease have a mortality rate of 50% to 70%, whereas ATN secondary to an obstetrical disaster, such as uterine hemorrhage or a septic abortion, carries a much lower death rate.

Diagnosis

When ATN occurs during the hospital course of a medical or surgical patient, the diagnosis is usually easy to make. The patient's previous renal function is generally known and the acuteness of renal deterioration is therefore readily documented. Furthermore, the ability to demonstrate the presence of a culpable toxin or vascular event to explain the sudden onset of renal failure greatly aids in making a correct diagnosis. In all patients, whether acute renal shutdown occurs in the hospital or out, postrenal obstruction must be suspected and ruled out by appropriate anatomical studies (see Chap. 24).

Laboratory. Basic laboratory tests in ATN typically show the following results:

1. The serum blood urea nitrogen (BUN) and creatinine levels are elevated.

2. The urinary sodium is elevated, usually exceeding 50 mEq/liter (the urinary sodium may be unreliable as a guide to the presence of ATN when the patient has been using diuretics).

3. The urinary sediment generally reveals renal epithelial cells and pigmented cellular casts (casts are molds of tubules formed by the accumulation of cells or proteinaceous material).

The BUN and creatinine rise progressively during the course of the patient's illness, so that the exact levels at any given time depend on how long the patient has been in acute renal failure. Furthermore, the extent to which the BUN and creatinine are elevated, both absolutely and in relation to each other, varies considerably. The catabolic state of the patient also influences the levels of both these parameters; hypercatabolic states such as fever or sepsis will increase these values.

Perhaps 25% of all patients with ATN will experience some amount of gastrointestinal bleeding during their course. The catabolism of blood proteins by bacteria within the intestine produces urea, and thus will raise the BUN disproportionately to the creatinine. On the other hand, major tissue trauma with rhabdomyolysis leads to large increases of serum creatinine derived from muscle creatine stores.

Additional findings in the urinary sediment can aid in the specific etiologic diagnosis. For example, urate crystalluria suggests the possibility of acute urate nephropathy, and myoglobinuria suggests myoglobin-induced acute renal failure. The casts of ATN are distinctly different from those of acute renal failure of other etiologies. Thus, red blood cell casts are found in glomerulonephritis, and leukocyte casts and clumps in active pylonephritis. Less specific are hyaline casts, which are composed of proteinaceous material consisting largely of a normal tubular mucoprotein (called the Tamm-Horsfall protein). Hyaline casts are found in some normal persons and, in greater numbers, in patients with almost any renal disease. Granular casts are speckled hyaline casts, and can also be seen with all types of renal disease.

Acute versus Chronic Renal Failure. A common and difficult problem is posed by the patient arriving in the emergency room in whom laboratory examination reveals renal failure (*i.e.*, an elevated BUN and creatinine), but for whom no medical history is available regarding any previous renal disease. Once obstruction is ruled out, the primary question is whether the renal failure is acute or a consequence of end-stage chronic renal disease. The entire uremic syndrome (see Chap. 23), with the exception of the bony changes of renal osteodystrophy and the uremic peripheral neuropathies, can also be seen in acute renal failure.

The history may indicate a cause for acute failure. Since the most common cause of acute renal failure is renal ischemia, an episode or reason for hypoperfusion and hypovolemia should be sought. The use of diuretics and the findings on physical examination of obvious dehydration suggest a setting compatible with ATN.

The size of the kidneys on abdominal x-ray may be of help. The kidneys are of normal size in acute renal failure, whereas in most cases of end-stage chronic renal failure they are small. Exceptions to the latter include amyloidosis, diabetic renal disease, and rapidly progressive glomerulonephritis.

Prerenal Azotemia. Many patients present with a picture of hypovolemia and elevated BUN and creatinine levels that is consistent with ATN, but who actually have a syndrome known as *prerenal azotemia*. In these patients, decreased perfusion pressure to the kidney resulting from diminished cardiac output (e.g., as a result of cardiac disease or hypovolemia) results in a series of complex physiologic reflexes that represent, in part, a homeostatic attempt to maintain volume. Salt and water reabsorption in the tubules rises. Because the tubular flow rate decreases, there is an increased back diffusion from the tubules of filtered urea, and the BUN also rises. In general, the glomerular filtration rate is maintained, so that the serum creatinine does not rise, at least in the early or mild stages of hypoperfusion. With severe hypoperfusion, however, the serum creatinine does rise, reflecting some decrease in the filtration rate.

In clear-cut cases, laboratory values should distinguish prerenal azotemia from ATN. These laboratory differences directly reflect the different pathogenetic mechanisms. In general, the BUN rises "out of proportion" to the creatinine in prerenal azotemia, and the ratio of BUN to creatinine in the serum generally rises to greater than 15–20 to 1. The urinary sodium should be extremely low in prerenal azotemia, because of the reabsorption of sodium from the tubules. It must be em-phasized that oral diuretics can confuse the use of the urinary sodium as a diagnostic tool, and are also common contributors to prerenal azotemia. Therapy for prerenal azotemia is simple and effective: volume replacement.

Course and Complications

There are two clinical phases in the syndrome of acute tubular necrosis: renal failure and recovery.

Renal Failure. The period of renal failure usually lasts one to two weeks, but may persist for months. During this phase, the patient must receive intensive support if he is to survive.

Although patients have traditionally been thought to have oliguria during the phase of renal failure (producing less than 800 ml of urine per day), approximately 50% of patients with acute tubular necrosis do not have oliguria. Nephrotoxic agents are likely to cause nonoliguric acute tubular necrosis, but there is no way to predict who will have oliguria and who will not. Patients with nonoliguric acute tubular necrosis generally experience milder symptoms, because they retain some ability to excrete solutes. They still develop uremia and the other problems of renal failure, because the amount of solute they excrete does not keep up with the accumulation of uremic substances within the body.

The major complications of the period of renal failure are (1) fluid and electrolyte imbalances, (2) infections, and (3) uremia.

1. Volume overload and water intoxication pose serious dangers. Once the patient is in the hospital, the most common cause of circulatory overload and hyponatremia is iatrogenic.

2. Potassium, hydrogen ions, and phosphate are produced endogenously and accumulate during renal failure. The serum potassium

may rise about 0.5 mEq/liter/day, and anything that increases tissue breakdown, such as fever or injury, will increase the rate of potassium release and accumulation. Any of the manifestations of hyperkalemia, including muscle weakness and cardiac toxicity (Chap. 21) may develop.

Normal body metabolism produces about 1 mEq/kg/day of acid, and almost all patients with acute tubular necrosis experience a metabolic acidosis. If the acidosis becomes severe, coma, shock, and heart failure may supervene.

Phosphate is absorbed from the gut and released from the bone, and phosphate accumulation is enhanced by tissue (especially muscle) breakdown.

2. A combination of factors, including the presence of underlying illness and indwelling urinary and venous catheters, is responsible for a reported 35% to 70% rate of infection in patients with acute tubular necrosis. The urinary and respiratory tracts are common sites of primary infection. Sepsis accounts for a high percentage of deaths.

3. Virtually all the manifestations of the uremic syndrome, including pericarditis, anemia, bleeding tendencies, gastrointestinal disturbances, and central nervous system disorders can be present in patients with acute tubular necrosis. Peripheral neuropathies and renal osteodystrophy, however, are not seen in these patients.

Recovery. The recovery phase of acute tubular necrosis is heralded by the return of renal function. The serum levels of BUN and creatinine reach a plateau and then begin to fall. In patients with oliguric acute tubular necrosis, the urine output progressively increases, and some patients experience a diuresis with large daily urinary losses. Although the diuresis may be due to previous volume overload, care must be taken to avoid hypovolemia. A diuresis is usually not seen in patients with nonoliguric acute tubular necrosis.

The onset of recovery does not end the dangers of infection and electrolyte disorders, especially hyperkalemia. In addition, for unknown reasons, significant hypercalcemia may occur. Nevertheless, as renal function continues to improve, the patient's clinical condition becomes less precarious.

Renal function generally improves in 10 to 14 days. Mild renal abnormalities may persist, but these generally disappear during the ensuing year, and the patient is left with no residual renal impairment.

Prevention and Therapy

Careful medical management of the hospitalized patient can avert many cases of acute tubular necrosis. Thus, patients receiving potentially nephrotoxic drugs should have their serum creatinine checked every three days. It is necessary to maintain an adequate circulating volume in all patients, especially those undergoing major surgical procedures.

If a hospitalized patient suffers renal failure following a hypotensive episode, the primary therapeutic maneuver should be correction of the inadequate cardiac output. Intravenous diuretics, such as furosemide, are widely employed during the early stages of acute renal failure in the hope of maintaining renal function, but there are no studies that clearly support the effectiveness of this approach. Deafness is an occasional side-effect of high doses of intravenous furosemide.

The next step in managing the patient in acute renal failure is to match his fluid and salt intake to his daily output (the sum of urinary, gastrointestinal, and insensible losses). Special attention should be paid to the possibility of water overload, reflected in the development of hyponatremia.

Because the loss of potassium can be expected to be negligible, dietary and intravenous potassium should be strictly limited.

(The signs and treatment of hyperkalemia are discussed in Chapter 21.)

The mild metabolic acidosis is usually well tolerated, but severe acidosis must be treated. It must be remembered that acidosis protects against the effects of hypocalcemia, and rapid correction of the acidosis may precipitate tetany and other manifestations of severe hypocalcemia. Oral aluminum hydroxide absorbs dietary phosphate and can forestall the development of hyperphosphatemia.

The metabolic requirements of the body demand about 800 calories per day. If this is not supplied exogenously, protein catabolism ensues, with consequent tissue breakdown and increases in nitrogenous wastes. A patient in acute renal failure should therefore be supplied with 1000 to 2000 calories per day of carbohydrate, with no potassium, and with only small amounts of protein (20 grams per day or less).

Any evidence of infection requires aggressive therapy and a thorough examination, including a chest x-ray and sputum, blood, and urine cultures. Treatment must be presumptive until the culture results are learned. Indwelling catheters and intravenous lines must be kept sterile.

Drugs that are excreted by the kidneys (or whose metabolites are excreted by the kidneys) must be used with caution. Particular care must be taken with digoxin and the aminoglycosides. All drugs should be given according to recommended dosage schedules for complete renal failure.

If these therapeutic precautions are taken, patients frequently do not require dialysis. However, dialysis may be needed in patients who develop (1) pericarditis, severe hyperkalemia, severe acidosis, or fluid overload that has not responded to conventional medical regimens or (2) severe uremic symptoms (especially central nervous system symptoms).

Peritoneal dialysis is the most common mode of dialysis in patients with acute renal failure (Hemodialysis is discussed in Chapter 23). A catheter is inserted into the peritoneal cavity (usually by means of a midline abdominal approach to reduce the risk of injury to vasculature), and one or more liters of dialysis fluid is rapidly instilled. The fluid is allowed to "dwell" in the abdomen for 10 to 60 minutes and is then drained by gravity. The peritoneum serves as a semipermeable membrane across which solutes are exchanged. If volume overload is present, the dialysis fluid can be made hyperosmolar with 4.5% glucose to remove rapidly excess volume. The dialysis cycle is performed several times; the frequency is determined by the needs of the patient. The major complication of peritoneal dialysis is peritonitis. Aseptic techniques must therefore be rigorously observed during all phases of dialysis.

BIBLIOGRAPHY

Anderson RJ, Linas SL, Berns AS et al: Nonoliguric acute renal failure. N Engl J Med 296:1134–1138, 1977

DeTorrente A, Berl T, Cohn PD et al: Hypercalcemia of acute renal failure: Clinical significance and pathogenesis. Am J Med 61:119–123, 1976

Dossetor JB: Creatininemia vs uremia. Ann Intern Med 65:1287–1299, 1966

Dunnill MS: A review of the pathology and pathogenesis of acute renal failure due to acute tubular necrosis. J Clin Pathol 27:2–13, 1974

Elkin M: Radiology of the urinary tract: Some physiological considerations. Radiology 116:259–270, 1975

Finn WF, Arendshorst WJ, Gottschalk CW: Pathogenesis of oliguria in acute renal failure. Circ Res 36:675–681, 1975

Flamenbaum W: Pathophysiology of acute renal failure. Arch Intern Med 131:911–928, 1973

Levinsky NG: Pathophysiology of acute renal failure. N Engl J Med 296:1453–1458, 1977

Stein JH, Lifschitz MD, Barnes LD et al: Current concepts on the pathophysiology of acute renal failure. Am J Physiol 234:F171–181, 1978

Thomson GE: Acute renal failure. Med Clin North Am 57:1579–1589, 1973

23

Chronic Renal Failure

The term chronic renal failure embraces a large number of pathologic processes, all of which are characterized by the gradual loss of renal function. Renal destruction progresses slowly, sometimes over many years. During this time, the kidney is able to compensate for the gradual loss of functioning nephrons, presumably by amplifying the response of each remaining tubule. Renal compensatory mechanisms are adequate until more than 90% of the total nephron mass is destroyed.

The major clinical manifestations of chronic renal failure are diminished glomerular filtration and the loss of tubular function. In addition, the loss of renal endocrine activity (erythropoietin) and enzymatic activity (the systhesis of ammonia, the conversation of 25-OH-vitamin D to active 1, 25–(OH)$_2$–vitamin D) may eventually contribute to the clinical syndrome of chronic renal failure.

RENAL FUNCTION IN CHRONIC RENAL FAILURE

As already noted, the intrarenal compensation for chronic nephron loss is adequate to maintain function until most of the parenchyma is destroyed by disease. The earliest functional deterioration is the kidney's progressive inability to sustain its normal extremes of solute conservation and excretion. As the disease advances, the kidney becomes more and more inflexible, and water and electrolyte regulation is maintained within an increasingly narrow range. Adaptation to sudden shifts in intake occurs slowly, and such shifts are poorly tolerated.

Water and Sodium The first clinical sign of deteriorating renal function is often a diminished capacity to conserve water fully and thereby excrete a maximally concentrated urine. The patient becomes susceptible to dehydration, especially in the hospital, where access to water may be restricted. Excretion of a maximal water load is similarly impaired.

Most patients with early renal insufficiency also have a tendency to lose sodium in the urine. The loss of sodium may be consistent with or out of proportion to the amount of water lost. This inflexibility of Na$^+$ homeostasis impairs Na$^+$ conservation as well. Since the time required to regain a steady-state of Na$^+$ balance is also prolonged in renal insufficiency, the injudicious restriction of Na$^+$ intake can lead to serious volume contraction and, consequently, to additional loss of function as renal perfusion declines.

With further progression of renal insufficiency, patients become unable to conserve or excrete dietary and metabolic salt and water to any significant extent. Volume overload (contributing to hypertension and congestive heart failure) and water intoxication become serious problems.

Potassium. The normal potassium load can usually be excreted by the failing kidney until the glomerular filtration rate (GFR) becomes markedly diminished; the distal tubule is able to secrete sufficient potassium to avert hyperkalemia until oliguria develops. Increased loads of potassium, however, can cause hyperkalemia earlier in the course of chronic renal failure. Potential sources of excessive potassium include inappropriate oral and intravenous administration of potassium, and the release of potassium from cells due to acidosis or cell injury.

Acid-Base Homeostasis. In healthy individuals, the acid-base balance is preserved because the daily endogenous load of acid is excreted into the urine with filtered phosphate or sulfate (titratable acid) or with ammonia (NH_3). Tubule cells generate ammonia themselves, as needed, by hydrolysis of glutamine. As the kidney fails, the remaining tubules maintain the arterial pH within the normal range until the glomerular filtration rate is reduced about 50%. With further compromise, the tubular excretory capacity for H^+ ions is eventually overwhelmed, largely because renal production of ammonia becomes inadequate. In its early phases, the resultant acidosis will probably have a normal anion gap. In later phases of acidosis, with progressive renal deterioration, metabolically derived acids (sulfates and phosphates) are no longer adequately filtered, and their accumulation leads to an increase in the anion gap. The

manifestations of acidemia include anorexia, nausea, weakness, fatigue, and, eventually, Kussmaul respirations.

Calcium and Phosphate. Severe bone demineralization is common in patients with renal failure. Alterations in calcium and phosphate metabolism occur as the filtration of phosphate diminishes and as the loss of renal 1-hydroxylase activity leads to a deficiency of active vitamin D and reduced intestinal absorption of calcium. Alkaline salts are leached out of the bone to buffer the accumulating H^+ ions. The development of secondary hyperparathyroidism leads to osteitis fibrosa and metastatic calcification (see Chap. 28).

Creatinine Clearance

The renal excretion of certain solutes is governed solely by the rate of their filtration at the glomerulus. Creatinine is the most frequently measured substance because its rate of generation (from muscle) is fairly constant, and because it is neither secreted nor reabsorbed by the tubules. The correlation of creatinine clearance with glomerular filtration is used to quantitate the impairment of glomerular function. As renal function deteriorates, the elevation of serum creatinine correlates well with the extent of renal deterioration.

Blood Urea Nitrogen (BUN)

The levels of urea, like those of creatinine, reflect the glomerular filtration rate, so that a diminution in filtration results in elevated levels of urea. Because urea undergoes some passive back diffusion from the tubule, and because its level is affected by protein intake, catabolic rate (the latter influenced by infection and trauma), and urine flow rate, it is a less precise guide to the extent of renal compromise than the creatinine. Historically, however, uremia has been designated as the rubric for encompassing all the clinical manifestations of chronic renal failure.

The serum levels of substances such as sodium, potassium, and water cannot be used to quantitate the glomerular filtration rate. This is because as renal failure progresses, the remaining tubules compensate by increasing their reabsorptive and secretory functions for these substances.

UREMIC SYNDROME

Although it appears that elevations in the BUN do not directly compromise bodily function, the widespread systemic disorder associated with chronic renal failure has been designated the uremic syndrome.

The pathogenesis of this syndrome is unknown. The accumulation of metabolic byproducts may be responsible, but no particular systemic toxin has been identified. Nevertheless, the beneficial effects of hemodialysis in patients with uremia suggest that retention of small (300–1000 daltons) filterable molecules may be responsible, especially for the neurologic dysfunction and the anemia.

The uremic patient typically has a sallow complexion, shows signs of wasting, and has skin lesions of purpura and excoriation. He complains of pruritis, polydipsia, nausea, and vomiting. Examination of the urine is often noteworthy for the findings of isosthenuria, proteinuria, and an abnormal sediment, which includes the broad tubular casts of renal failure. Isosthenuria means that the kidney can no longer form urine with a specific gravity higher or lower than the protein-free plasma, and the specific gravity of the urine becomes fixed at approximately 1.010.

Neurologic Manifestations. Both peripheral and central nervous system derangements are prominent in uremia. A sensory polyneurop-

athy is almost always present. A bilateral foot drop may precede the appearance of a characteristic distal motor dysfunction, which is often progressive and disabling. Initial central nervous system derangements include insomnia and difficulty with concentration or train of thought. In more advanced disease, the onset of clonus (autonomous rhythmic contractions of muscle groups) and asterixis may herald the terminal obtundation of uremic encephalopathy. Seizures, both focal and nonfocal, may also occur.

Cardiopulmonary Manifestations. Hypertension is primarily, but not always, related to volume overload. Life-threatening arrhythmias accompany intracardiac metastatic calcification, which frequently begins within the specialized conduction fibers of the heart. In later stages, diffuse cardiac calcification occurs, as well as a cardiomyopathy with congestive heart failure. The causes of uremic congestive heart failure are legion, and include hypertension, the high output state of anemia, accelerated arteriosclerosis, and possibly a toxic cardiomyopathy.

Pleuropericardial inflammation may be the most devastating cardiopulmonary manifestation of uremia. Acute pericarditis is common and cardiac tamponade is an ever-present danger. Pericarditis usually resolves following dialysis. Chronic constrictive pericarditis is rare.

Pulmonary function is impaired by pulmonary edema, which is due partly to volume overload and partly to increased capillary permeability. Pulmonary calcifications are common and may to some extent account for the interstitial fibrosis that is seen. Uremic patients also suffer from large pleural effusions.

Hematologic Manifestations. All three of the circulating cell lines are affected by uremia. One of the hallmarks of chronic renal failure is the insidious onset of a normocytic, normochromic anemia, an almost inevitable development after loss of more than 50% of the glomerular filtration rate. Anemia can result from progressive impairment of erythropoietin production, circulating uremic toxins that induce mild hemolysis and inhibit erythropoiesis, and iron deficiency, aggravated by the propensity for gastrointestinal bleeding.

Although platelet production and survival are unaffected by uremia, there is a demonstrable defect of platelet function, manifested by a markedly prolonged bleeding time and abnormal platelet aggregation. This may be due to the accumulation of guanidinosuccinic acid. The uremic bleeding diathesis, when present, is mild.

The effect of uremia upon the white blood cells is complex. Lymphocyte number and function are reduced, and neutrophil chemotaxis and phagocytosis are impaired. These alterations may explain the increased susceptibility of these patients to infection.

Gastrointestinal Manifestations. Patients frequently complain of anorexia, nausea, and vomiting. Sometimes these symptoms may be due to electrolyte disturbances, but gastrointestinal symptoms are common even without significant electrolyte imbalances. Some patients develop mouth ulcers and parotitis, believed to result from the irritating effects of ammonia that is produced by the breakdown of urea by mouth flora. Mild gastrointestinal bleeding is common.

Metabolic Manifestations. The metabolic consequences of uremia are extensive and still poorly understood. Anorexia and vomiting contribute to inadequate caloric intake. Elevations in the serum triglyceride level are common and probably reflect complex alterations in hepatic lipid metabolism. There is also a form of glucose intolerance in uremia (deriving, in part, from insulin resist-

ance), characterized by an exaggerated insulin response following a meal and distinguished from true diabetes mellitus by a normal fasting blood glucose.

CAUSES OF CHRONIC RENAL FAILURE

The causes of chronic renal failure are numerous. Chronic renal failure can result from disease extrinsic to the kidney (obstructive uropathy, see Chap. 24) or from systemic disease (diabetes mellitus, connective-tissue diseases, sickle cell anemia, amyloidosis, advanced hypertension, and others). The intrinsic renal diseases may be broadly classified into interstitial diseases and glomerular diseases.

Interstitial Disease. Interstitial nephritis results when inflammation and fibrosis of the tubules predominate over the loss of glomeruli. These diseases are therefore marked by an impairment of tubular functions. Sodium wasting is characteristic. Failure of urinary concentration leads to a large urine volume with nocturia. Hyperchloremic acidosis reflects deficient tubular H^+ ion excretion, and the tubular handling of uric acid, amino acids, and glucose may be impaired. Anemia is often severe because of the loss of erythropoietin-producing tissue. On the other hand, significant proteinuria and red blood cell casts in the urine sediment—all signs of glomerular damage—are minimal or absent.

Interstitial nephritis with papillary necrosis may be caused by long-term ingestion of analgesics, first noted with medications containing phenacetin. Papillary necrosis frequently presents with acute lumbar pain and fever. It is often associated with renal infection. Besides analgesics, other predisposing conditions include diabetes and sickle cell anemia. The finding of sloughed papillary tissue in the urine aids in the diagnosis. The semisynthetic penicillins can produce an interstitial nephritis, initially accompanied by fever and eosinophilia. Environmental exposure to heavy metals may also produce interstitial nephritis.

Any disease that produces hypercalcemia or hypercalciuria can lead to the renal deposition of calcium, nephrocalcinosis, and renal failure (see chap. 28). Acute uric acid nephropathy is most frequently seen in the setting of chemotherapy and rapid cellular lysis (see Chap. 49). The intratubular deposition of uric acid leads to acute obstruction and acute renal failure. There is also another type of renal disorder caused by urate, in which the chronic deposition of monosodium urate crystals produces the insidious onset of interstitial nephritis.

Glomerular Disease. In contrast to interstitial nephritis, glomerular disease is associated with a relative sparing of tubular functions. Thus, the urine volume and the ability to conserve sodium are preserved until late in the course of disease. On the other hand, hypertension, proteinuria, and urinary sediment abnormalities figure prominently in the clinical presentation.

Chronic glomerulonephritis is the most common of the renal glomerular diseases. Perhaps 10% of these patients have unresolved, long-standing poststreptococcal glomerulonephritis. In the remaining 90%, the pathogenesis is obscure. Glomerulonephritis causes the insidious progression of hypertension, microscopic hematuria, and excretion of urinary red blood cell casts. Although the clinical course is often protracted, the ultimate appearance of anemia, progressive renal insufficiency, and uremia is almost inevitable. Biopsy reveals diffuse cellular proliferation and sclerosis in the glomeruli. Later in the course, tubular atrophy and interstitial fibrosis may accompany glomerular hyalinization and scarring.

Rapidly progressive glomerulonephritis is a form of acute glomerulonephritis marked by an extraordinarily rapid progression to uremia. This disease, which may follow streptococcal infection, has two identifying features on biopsy: the uniform destruction of glomeruli is accompanied by epithelial cresent formation in Bowman's space, and, on immunofluorescence microscopy, linear IgG deposition can often be seen along the glomerular basement membrane. The prognosis is poor. No therapy has been shown to slow the rapid renal deterioration, although the use of systemic heparin has been advocated.

Goodpasture's syndrome is a rare autoimmune disease also marked by linear immunofluorescent staining of the basement membrane on renal biopsy. In addition to glomerulonephritis with progressive renal insufficiency, the syndrome includes hemoptysis and diffuse pulmonary infiltrates due to hemorrhagic alveolitis. The renal and pulmonary lesions appear to be caused by antiglomerular basement membrane antibody that cross-reacts with the basement membrane of the pulmonary alveolus. Untreated, the disease is rapidly fatal. However, bilateral nephrectomy reduces the "antigenic load" and can be life-saving. Plasmapheresis has been shown to be beneficial. Renal transplants have been successful, although recurrence of the disease in the transplanted kidney has been reported.

Immune complex diseases exhibit an irregular "lumpy bumpy" pattern of IgG and complement (C3) deposition along the basement membrane. This granular pattern of immunofluorescence corresponds to the dense extraepithelial deposits seen on electron microscopy. These deposits represent the accumulation of circulating immune complexes within the basement membrane. Complement activation may be responsible for the glomerular destruction. The deposition of immune complexes seems to be important in the pathogenesis of many disorders that produce chronic glomerulonephritis, including acute poststreptococcal glomerulonephritis, membranous nephritis, and hypocomplementemic nephritis.

Focal glomerular sclerosis is a pathologic diagnosis made by renal biopsy. The characteristic lesion is an obliterative glomerulosclerosis (scarring of the renal glomeruli) that, initially, at least, involves only a limited number of glomeruli throughout the kidney. Deposits of IgM and complement can be detected in involved glomeruli by immunofluorescence. All patients present with proteinuria, and many have microscopic hematuria. Most patients develop hypertension and manifest evidence of renal insufficiency sometime during the course of their illness.

Focal glomerular sclerosis has been described in both children and adults. The initial presentation is generally more severe in adults, and the disease appears to progress more rapidly, occasionally culminating in severe chronic renal failure and death. In approximately 50% of adults, a partial resolution of the proteinuria can be obtained with corticosteroids; complete remissions have been described in children. The addition of other immunosuppressive agents appears to have little effect.

The *nephrotic syndrome* is the clinical expression of any glomerular lesion that produces massive proteinuria (more than 3 grams of protein excreted in the urine per day). All of the diseases that cause the nephrotic syndrome enhance the permeability of the glomerulus to plasma proteins. When the urinary loss of protein exceeds 3 to 4 grams per day, the resultant hypoproteinemia leads to the decline of plasma osmotic pressure with consequent edema and serosal effusions. Hyperlipidemia of unknown origin is frequently observed; the serum becomes lactescent, and polarized light examination of the urine sediment reveals the characteristic "maltese crosses" of urinary cholesterol crystals. The differential diagnosis of the nephrotic syndrome is vast, covering virtually all classes of intrinsic and systemic renal pathology.

Several systemic causes of the nephrotic syndrome merit special comment. *Renal vein thrombosis* can occur in association with disorders of hemostasis, malignancies, and trauma. Enlarged kidneys and heavy proteinuria are seen. In some cases, membranous glomerulonephritis may coexist with renal vein thrombosis. The diagnosis is confirmed by inferior vena caval and renal venography. Treatment includes systemic heparinization. Renal vein thrombosis can also complicate *amyloidosis*. When renal amyloidosis occurs secondary to an underlying disorder, such as a malignancy or tuberculosis, treatment of the primary disease process often alleviates the renal impairment to some degree. In *sickle cell anemia*, medullary and papillary damage is thought to occur because the hypertonic medullary interstitium causes the red blood cells to sickle within the vasa recta. Sickle cell anemia can cause the nephrotic syndrome and may also lead to a urinary concentrating defect as well as to recurrent bouts of papillary necrosis. *Diabetes mellitus* also predisposes to the nephrotic syndrome and to acute papillary necrosis. The nephropathy of *multiple myeloma* is characterized by the development of proteinuria in the majority of patients sometime during their course. Many of these patients have Bence Jones proteinuria (immunoglobulin light chains or their breakdown products in the urine). Other features of myeloma nephropathy are discussed in Chapter 48.

Renal Biopsy. The specific etiology of chronic renal failure in a given patient can usually be made by obtaining a renal biopsy. A combination of a light microscopic examination and immunofluorescence studies generally defines the specific renal lesion. In certain illnesses associated with several types of renal disease, such as systemic lupus erythematosis, a biopsy can reveal which lesion is present and thus provide important information about the patient's expected course and prognosis.

Because there are no specific therapeutic regimens that will clearly treat the basic pathologic lesions for many causes of chronic renal failure, a renal biopsy contains more diagnostic and prognostic rather than therapeutic information.

CONSERVATIVE MANAGEMENT OF RENAL DISEASE

Regardless of the etiology of renal damage, at some point in his clinical course the patient will usually require therapeutic intervention.

The extent of functional impairment must first be ascertained. A 24-hour creatinine clearance may be used initially to estimate the glomerular filtration rate. Thereafter, serial determinations of the serum creatinine are sufficient to follow the course of the disease: each 50% reduction in the glomerular filtration rate produces a doubling of the serum creatinine. This calculation only holds true in patients without significant muscle wasting, since muscle is a source of serum creatinine. The BUN is a useful adjunct but a less reliable measure of pure nephron loss. At any level of renal function, when volume contraction slows tubular flow, back diffusion of urea is increased and the BUN rises disproportionately to the serum creatinine. In addition, urea concentrations are elevated by the increased catabolism that accompanies fever, infection, and therapy with corticosteroids or tetracycline.

At any level of renal function, the precarious maintenance of a steady state can be upset by urinary obstruction, infection, electrolyte imbalances, or compromised renal perfusion. Initial evaluation should therefore include a urinalysis, electrolytes, BUN, creatinine, urine culture, a plain abdominal x-ray, and, when necessary, contrast nephrotomography to exclude the diagnosis of radiolucent stones. Hyperkalemia, hypercalcemia, and hyperuricemia are easily diagnosed and treated. The nephrotoxicity of numerous drugs, such as the aminoglycoside antibiotics, is well established, and they must be used with great caution and avoided whenever possible.

Pericardial tamponade and congestive heart failure are reversible causes of impaired renal perfusion and often require immediate therapy. Volume contraction is a more insidious cause of renal ischemia. Overzealous sodium restriction, rigorous diuresis, and uremic vomiting can lead to diminished total body sodium stores. These losses may exceed the limited capacity of the diseased kidney to conserve sodium. A trial of sodium chloride supplementation may be necessary to determine whether increased extracellular volume will lead to symptomatic improvement. Hypertension may contribute to arteriosclerosis and congestive heart failure and may be very difficult to treat.

After the extent of renal impairment is established and reversible factors are excluded, attention must be devoted to the amelioration of symptoms and prevention of further systemic deterioration. If there is a systemic cause for renal failure, specific treatment is often dictated by the nature of the underlying disease, but otherwise therapy is conservative and directed toward the management of diet, fluid, electrolytes, and calcium/phosphate balance.

Diet. The advent of uremic symptoms frequently signals the need for dietary modification. Acidosis, azotemia, and uremic nausea may improve substantially with modest protein restriction. It is imperative, however, that excessive catabolism be avoided through adequate caloric intake.

Fluids and Electrolytes. Even though weight gain, edema, and pulmonary congestion eventually necessitate sodium restriction in patients with renal failure, care must be taken to avoid depletion of salt and water. The response of daily urine volumes, body weight, and serum creatinine to dietary salt limitation should be measured. Restriction of potassium is rarely necessary until very late in the course of renal failure.

Calcium and Phosphate. Prevention of hyperphosphatemia early in renal insufficiency can often minimize the sequelae of uremic osteodystrophy. This can be accomplished by limiting the intake of phosphate-containing foods (especially dairy products) and by administering nonabsorbable aluminum-containing antacids, which bind intestinal phosphate and prevent its absorption from the gastrointestinal tract. Magnesium-containing antacids should be avoided because of the danger of hypermagnesemia. Later in the course, hypocalcemia may necessitate calcium supplementation with or without vitamin D. In some patients, hypercalcemia or painful osteitis fibrosa can be remedied only by parathyroidectomy.

Hemodialysis

The availability of dialysis therapy in chronic renal failure has enabled patients to overcome the potentially fatal complications of uremia. Hemodialysis is a potent clinical tool with many indications, many complications, and tremendous psychosocial consequences.

Absolute indications for hemodialysis include uremic pericarditis with or without cardiac tamponade, progressive motor neuropathy, intractable volume overload, and life-threatening acidosis or hyperkalemia. Otherwise, the decision to institute hemodialysis should probably be dictated by the recognition of those features of uremia that respond favorably to chronic dialysis. These include fluid and electrolyte imbalances, volume-dependent hypertension, central nervous system abnormalities, neuromuscular irritability, anemia, bleeding diathesis, anorexia, nausea and vomiting, pruritis, ecchymoses, glucose intolerance, and weight loss.

Chronic dialysis is not a panacea for uremia; many of the features of uremia will progress despite therapy. Accelerated atherosclerosis, with all its complications, is a well-recognized phenomenon in dialysis patients. Refractory pericarditis and hypertension are also occasionally seen. Hypertension refractory to dialysis frequently responds only to bilateral nephrectomy. Dialysis also fails to impede the progression of renal osteodystrophy, so that the incidence and severity of bone disease may be substantially greater in dialyzed patients. Finally, although the hematocrit does improve in many patients, some patients experience a persistent anemia; hemolysis and blood loss in the dialysis coils may be partially responsible.

There are a substantial number of undesired side-effects that must figure prominently in the decision to implement hemodialysis. Antecedent vascular disease often poses difficulties in the creation of a vascular access site, and revision of these sites becomes increasingly difficult after destruction of the vessels by thrombosis or aneurysmal dilatation. The two most commonly employed vascular access sites are (1) an artificial shunt introduced between an artery and a vein into which dialysis needles are placed, and (2) an arteriovenous fistula, usually created in the forearm, in which the engorged veins provide a ready access. Because of the frequent instrumentation and the patient's impaired immunity, shunt infection is an ever-present danger. These infections are often readily controlled with appropriate antibiotics, but subacute bacterial endocarditis and other sequelae do occur.

Other dialysis complications include an increased risk of viral hepatitis, chronic hepatitis, and chronic hepatitis B surface antigenemia due to the administration of blood products. More serious is the recently recognized "dialysis dementia," which may occur during chronic dialysis. It is manifested by seizures, psychosis, dementia, and even death.

Finally, it should not be forgotten that dependence upon dialysis for survival imposes an enormous psychological burden upon the patient. The financial cost to the patient and society is also substantial.

RENAL TRANSPLANTATION

For younger patients who fail to respond to conservative management of uremia, renal transplantation has become a reasonable alternative to chronic hemodialysis. Transplantation immunology is complex and constantly evolving, but the methods now exist for adequate antigenic matching of the allograft to the recipient.

Renal transplantations are routinely performed in many centers. All centers now routinely HLA type donors and recipients. The HLA antigens are gene products of a large genetic region that has been termed the Major Histocompatibility Complex (MHC). The MHC codes for many different products involved in various aspects of immune function. Although the physiologic function of the HLA antigens is not understood, they (or gene products that may be closely linked to them in the MHC) appear to determine the success or failure of tissue grafts in much the same way that the ABO blood group antigens determine the compatibility or incompatibility of a blood transfusion. HLA identity among siblings gives a reasonably good assurance for the success of a transplant. Among unrelated persons, HLA matching is a less reliable guide to success, indicating that other antigenic factors are also involved in transplant rejection. Other *in vitro* tests, which measure the activity of recipient lymphocytes in the presence of donor cells, appear to offer some hope of better guaranteeing host-donor compatibility.

Selection criteria for transplant recipients vary. Absolute contraindications now include active infection, a major blood group incompatibility, and prior sensitization to donor antigens. Less rigid contraindications include malignancy, advanced age, and systemic vascular disease.

Medical Management. Following transplantation, the mainstay of medical management is continuous immunosuppression to avoid destruction of the allograft by the patient's cellular and humoral responses. Most therapeutic regimens now combine high-dose corticosteroids with azothioprine.

Transplant Rejection. Despite effective immunosuppressive techniques, allograft rejection remains the major complication of renal transplantation.

Hyperacute rejection ensues within minutes of transplantation. It is due to preformed cytotoxic antibodies directed against the donor antigens. Allograft ischemia and necrosis occur, and the organ cannot be salvaged.

Acute rejection occurs within hours of transplantation. Many immune mechanisms are involved, but acute rejection appears to be primarily a T cell-mediated immune reaction. Symptoms of acute rejection are fever, malaise, hypertension, oliguria, and swelling and tenderness of the graft. Acute rejection must be differentiated from *acute tubular necrosis*, which can develop from pretransplantation ischemia. In acute tubular necrosis, isosthenuria and urinary sodium wasting are seen, whereas rejection is characterized by a concentrated urine, sodium conservation, and proteinuria. Radioisotope and arteriographic studies are sometimes useful in documenting the increase in allograft size that accompanies rejection. Episodes of acute rejection can often be controlled by large increases in steroid dosage followed by gradual tapering to maintenance levels.

Chronic rejection evolves over months to years. The etiology is uncertain, and humoral (antibody) mechanisms may be involved. Treatment involves immunosuppressive drug regimens, but ultimately the physician must decide when to abandon the allograft and revert to dialysis therapy.

Other Medical Problems. A primary medical complication of renal transplantation remains the increased susceptibility of these immunosuppressed patients to infection. Recipients are not only predisposed to common bacterial pathogens, but also to the entire array of viral, fungal, and parasitic agents (see Chap. 58).

A second major problem is recurrence of disease in the transplanted kidney. This is not unexpected in patients with systemic causes of renal failure, but it has also been regularly observed in membranous, proliferative, focal sclerosing, and rapidly progressive forms of glomerulonephritis.

Other complications of renal transplantation include proximal tubular dysfunction from ischemic graft damage, distal renal tubular acidosis, and persistent hypercalcemia from a continued excess parathyroid hormone levels after transplantation. The last problem is particularly threatening to the allograft because of the possibility of permanent impairment from parenchymal renal calcification.

BIBLIOGRAPHY

Anderson RJ, Gambertoglio JG, Schrier RW: Clinical use of drugs in renal failure. Springfield, Ill., Thomas, 1976

DeFronzo R, Andres A, Edgar P et al: Carbohydrate metabolism in uremia: A review. Medicine 52:469–481, 1973

Doolan PD, Alpen EL, Theil AB: A clinical appraisal of the plasma concentration and endogenous clearance of creatinine. Am J Med 32:65–79, 1962

Giordano C (ed): Uremia. Kidney Int 7(Suppl 3): S-267–S-435 1975

Gottschalk CW: Function of the clinically diseased kidney: The adaptive nephron. Circ Res 28:II-1–II-13, 1971

Higgins MR, Grace M, Ulan RA et al: Anemia in hemodialysis patients; changing concepts in management. Arch Intern Med 137:172–176, 1977

Lindner A, Charra B, Sherrard DJ et al: Accelerated atherosclerosis in prolonged maintenance hemodialysis. New Engl J Med 290:697–701, 1974

Maher JF, Nolph KD, Bryan CW: Prognosis of advanced chronic renal failure: I. Unpredictability of survival and reversibility. Ann Intern Med 81:43–47, 1974

Raskin NH, Fishman RA: Neurologic disorders in renal failure. N Engl J Med 294:143–148, 1976

Russell PS, Cosimi AB: Transplantation. N Engl J Med 301:470–479, 1979

Smith HW: From Fish to Philosopher. Boston, Little, Brown, 1953

Tyler HR: Neurologic disorders in renal failure. Am J Med 44:734–748, 1968

24

Obstructive Uropathy and Nephrolithiasis

OBSTRUCTION OF THE URINARY TRACT

The problems encountered with obstruction of the urinary tract include pain, infection, and renal failure. Medical or surgical alleviation can relieve pain, prevent or halt infection, and reverse uremia. If therapy is delayed, however, the kidney may scar irremediably, and it is therefore important to consider the possibility of obstruction in patients who develop renal insufficiency or pyelonephritis, as well as in patients with classic renal colic and hematuria.

Anatomic obstruction of the urinary tract can be caused by intrinsic blockage or extrinsic pressure, and can therefore occur with renal or ureteral stones, prostatic enlargement or neoplasia, pelvic neoplasia, adhesions from prior pelvic surgery or radiation therapy, pelvic inflammatory disease, Crohn's disease, endometriosis, genitourinary tuberculosis, carcinoma of the cervix, phimosis, or pregnancy.

Functional obstruction occurs secondary to an atonic, neurogenic bladder, and may be seen in patients with diabetes mellitus.

Pathophysiology and Clinical Manifestations

Because the kidney is encased within a fairly inflexible capsule, it has a limited capacity for expansion. When the lower urinary tract is obstructed, pressures throughout the urinary tract proximal to the obstruction begin to increase. The increased pressure is transmitted to the renal tubules. The functions of the distal segment of the nephron are affected first, and the inability to form a concentrated urine is therefore one of the earliest signs of obstructive uropathy. The capacity to excrete an acid urine is also diminished in the early phase of obstruction.

Intrarenal pressures eventually become so high that the renal blood flow and the glomerular filtration rate decline. Because the urine remains in the kidney for a longer time, increased quantities of urea are passively absorbed from the tubules, and the BUN may rise out of proportion to the creatinine. In complete obstruction, anuric renal failure ensues. Partial obstruction is far more common, however, and a dilute polyuria, caused by the concentrating defect, is the rule.

When the patency of the urinary tract is restored, a mild and self-limiting postobstructive diuresis occurs as the excessive water and solute that were retained during renal insufficiency are eliminated. Only rarely will the urinary losses be large enough to cause hemodynamic compromise.

Obstruction of a ureter may cause an ex-

173

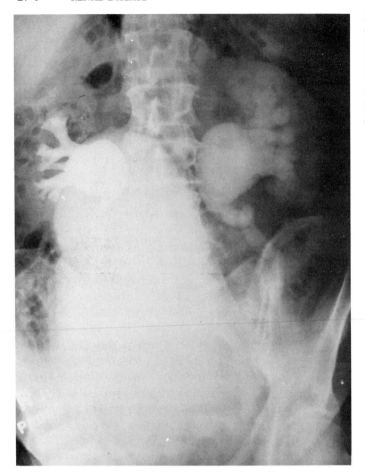

FIG. 24–1. Lower urinary tract obstruction with hydronephrosis. Benign prostatic hypertrophy develops in most elderly men. In this patient, prostatic enlargement produced an outlet obstruction. The large, radiopaque mass is the grossly dilated bladder. The ureters and calyces are also dilated and deformed.

cruciating, continuous but fluctuating flank pain as the ureter and renal capsule are stretched. This pain is known as *renal colic.* Classically, it is associated with hematuria and local flank tenderness. However, some patients with ureteral obstruction experience no pain. In these patients, obstruction may become evident only during the evaluation of uremia or pyelonephritis.

Obstruction of the lower urinary tract may result in infection, and ultimately in pyelonephritis (see Chap. 55). The risk of infection is markedly increased in patients who undergo invasive diagnostic tests.

The extent of recovery depends upon the severity of the renal injury. Infection developing in damaged kidneys may prove to be difficult to eradicate.

Diagnosis

The diagnosis of urinary tract obstruction can often be confirmed by *intravenous pyelography* (IVP). The obstructed kidney may be enlarged and its excretion of dye delayed. In chronic obstruction, the ureter may be tortuous (Fig. 24–1).

The obstructed kidney cannot be seen on

FIG. 24–2. Staghorn calculi. This patient had a history of chronic urinary tract infections. The pelvocalyceal system is filled with radiopaque calculi.

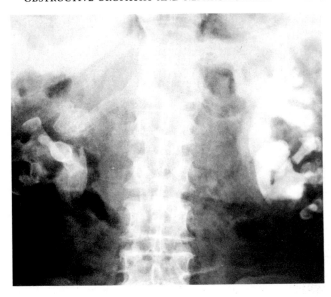

IVP if the tubular impairment is extensive enough to impede markedly the concentration of intravenously injected dye; in such patients, *retrograde pyelography*, an invasive procedure in which the dye is injected transurethrally, can be performed.

Recently, *sonograms* of the kidney and pelvis have proven to be useful in establishing the diagnosis of obstruction and may obviate the use of invasive procedures. Sonography reveals dilated ureters in patients with obstructive uropathy.

NEPHROLITHIASIS

Nephrolithiasis, the formation of renal stones, is the most common cause of urinary tract obstruction. Affected patients experience recurrent attacks of dysuria and a colicky flank pain that radiates to the groin. The urine contains red blood cells and protein.

Although surgical intervention is occasionally needed to relieve the ureteral obstruction, nephrolithiasis is often amenable to medical management with narcotic analgesia and diuresis to help dislodge the stone. Even without clinical intervention, however, more than three-quarters of all ureteral stones pass spontaneously; virtually all stones with a diameter of less than 0.5 cm eventually pass without medical assistance. Because renal colic is extremely painful and because urinary tract obstruction can lead to renal compromise and infection, prevention of further stone formation is the key to medical therapy.

A patient who presents in the emergency room with renal colic should receive narcotic analgesia and hydration. In most patients, a plain x-ray of the abdomen will reveal radiopaque stones (calculi); (Fig. 24–2). If a stone cannot be seen in this way, an IVP may reveal its presence. An IVP may also prove to be therapeutic, because the dye initiates a diuresis that can dislodge the stone from the ureter. All urine should be sieved to detect the passage of stones.

The formation of urinary tract stones is often associated with an abnormally increased urinary excretion of uric acid, cystine, struvite, calcium phosphate, or calcium oxalate. In some patients, however, no metabolic abnormality can be detected.

The mechanisms underlying stone formation are poorly understood. The patient's state of hydration and the urinary pH appear to be important factors in urinary crystal formation. Identification of the calculus material in the urine of a given patient often permits appropriate preventive measures to be taken against future stone formation. Regardless of the chemical identity of the stone or the pathophysiologic mechanism underlying its formation, a large daily fluid intake (more than 2 liters) may significantly decrease the incidence of recurrent stone formation.

Uric Acid Stones. Uric acid crystals are radiolucent, and unless present in a calculus of mixed composition, are not detectable on a plain abdominal x-ray. Hyperuricosuria, with or without hyperuricemia, is present in many patients (see Chap. 42). Hyperuricosuria may be caused by increased production, overexcretion, or decreased renal reabsorption of uric acid. Patients with hyperuricosuria may respond to chronic treatment with allopurinol, an inhibitor of uric acid synthesis. Uric acid is extremely insoluble in urine with a pH of less than 5, and uric acid crystals may form even in the absence of hyperuricosuria. Alkalinization of the urine is thus an important therapeutic adjunct.

Calcium Stones. Radiopaque calcium stones (mostly calcium oxalate or calcium phosphate) are the most common cause of nephrolithiasis. Three major risk factors for the formation of calcium stones are hypercalciuria, hyperuricosuria, and hyperoxaluria.

Hypercalciuria is often accompanied by hypercalcemia in patients with primary hyperparathyroidism, sarcoidosis, vitamin D intoxication, and the milk-alkali syndrome. In a number of patients, however, idiopathic hypercalciuria occurs despite a normal serum calcium:

1. In one group of patients with normocalcemic hypercalciuria, the serum parathyroid hormone is inappropriately high for the level of serum calcium. Some of these patients may have so-called "normocalcemic hyperparathyroidism." In this syndrome the serum calcium is only intermittently elevated, although it is usually on the high side of normal, and urinary cyclic AMP levels may be elevated. These hyperparathyroid patients respond to an oral calcium challenge with a marked increase in serum calcium. Nephrolithiasis is an indication for the removal of a parathyroid adenoma (see Chap. 28).

2. Some patients with idiopathic hypercalciuria absorb an abnormally high fraction of their dietary calcium. Some of these patients may be exquisitely sensitive to the effects of the active metabolite of vitamin D on intestinal calcium absorption. They have a normal serum calcium and decreased levels of urinary cyclic AMP. Patients with hyperabsorptive hypercalciuria should restrict their daily dietary intake of calcium.

3. A small number of patients have a defect in the renal tubular reabsorption of calcium. In these patients the serum calcium tends to be low. Low serum calcium results in a mild secondary hyperparathyroidism that may also cause hypophosphatemia. The synthesis of 1,25-OH-vitamin D is increased, and these patients hyperabsorb calcium from the intestine in order to compensate for the renal losses. Like patients with normocalcemic hyperparathyroidism, these patients also have increased urinary cyclic AMP and increased levels of serum parathyroid hormone. Thiazide diuretics impair the renal clearance of calcium, lower the urinary calcium, and have been used to diminish the incidence of stone formation in these patients.

Hyperuricosuria, the major contributing factor to urate stone formation, is also associated with calcium oxalate stones. It has been postulated that urate crystals may form the nidus upon which the calcium salt precipitates.

Increased intestinal absorption of oxalate leading to *hyperoxaluria* occurs most frequently in patients with severe ileal disease (*e.g.*, in patients with Crohn's disease or following ileojejunal bypass surgery in severely obese patients). Increased urinary oxalate is also found in patients with primary hyperoxaluria, a hereditary metabolic disorder. The reduction of dietary oxalate decreases the hyperoxaluria.

Cystine Stones. Patients with cystinuria, a congenital disorder of renal amino acid transport, are plagued by recurrent cystine stones. Cystine stones are radiopaque, and under light microscopy display a characteristic hexagonal shape. Increased fluid intake and alkalinization of the urine may diminish the incidence of future stone formation.

Struvite Stones. The precipitation of struvite (magnesium ammonium phosphate) in the urine occurs in patients with a chronically high urinary pH such as that produced by chronic urinary tract infections with urease-producing microorganisms. Antimicrobial therapy and acidification of the urine are successful in preventing recurrences.

BIBLIOGRAPHY

Broadus AE, Thier SO: Metabolic basis of renal stone disease. N Engl J Med 300:839–845, 1977

Coe FL: Treated and untreated recurrent calcium nephrolithiasis in patients with idiopathic hypercalciuria, hyperuricosia, or no metabolic disorder. Ann Intern Med 87:404–410, 1977

Falls WF Jr, Stacy WK: Postobstructive diuresis. Am J Med 54:404–412, 1973

Nemoy NJ, Stamey TA: Surgical, bacteriological, and biochemical management of "infection stones." JAMA 215:1470–1476, 1971

Pak CYC, Kaplan R, Boue H et al: A sample test for the diagnosis of absorptive, resorptive and renal hypercalciuria. N Engl J Med 292:497–500, 1975

Pak CYC, Sakhage K, Crowther C et al: Evidence justifying a high fluid intake in treatment of nephrolithiasis. Ann Intern Med 93:36–39, 1980

Smith LH: Medical evaluation of urolithiasis: Etiologic aspects and diagnostic evaluation. Urol Clin North Am 1:241–260, 1974

Yendt ER: Renal calculi. Can Med Assoc J 102:479–489, 1970

Endocrine Disease

25

Diseases of the Anterior Pituitary

PITUITARY GLAND

Anatomy

The pituitary (or hypophysis cerebri) is an endocrine organ that sits inside the skull within its own bony fossa, the sella turcica (Fig. 25–1). The sella is covered by a reflection of the dura called the diaphragma sella, which is pierced by the pituitary stalk and a portal vascular network. The sphenoidal sinuses lie just below the sella, and the optic tract and optic chasm lie above and lateral to the sella.

Because the pituitary gland is otherwise encased within bone, pituitary tumors expand mostly upward through the diaphragma sella and involve the optic nerve. Visual field deficits, especially bitemporal hemianopsias, are therefore often found in patients with pituitary tumors. Pituitary tumors can also erode the walls of the sella, and plain skull x-rays and polytomes of the sella may then show destruction of the sella or increased sellar volume (Fig. 25–2). The extent of pituitary enlargement is best evaluated by CT scanning.

The sella is also bordered by the cavernous sinus, which contains the carotid artery and the third, fourth, and sixth cranial nerves, and the ophthalmic and maxillary branches of the fifth cranial nerve. These structures are occasionally compromised by large pituitary tumors.

Physiology

The anterior pituitary receives a highly concentrated mixture of small peptide hormones from the hypothalamus through its portal system. These hypothalamic hormones stimulate the anterior pituitary to secrete its trophic hormones, and these in turn regulate much of the peripheral endocrine system. The anterior pituitary hormones include thyrotropin (TSH), luteinizing hormone (LH), follicle-stimulating hormone (FSH), prolactin (PRL), growth hormone (GH), and corticotropin (ACTH).

Hypothalamic Regulation. The concept that the brain can function as a secretory gland is a radical new paradigm. The brain synthesizes a number of peptide hormones that function as neurotransmitters or neuromodulators throughout the central and peripheral nervous systems. Among the best studied are the hypothalamic releasing hormones that regulate the activity of the anterior pituitary. At present, three have been fully characterized:

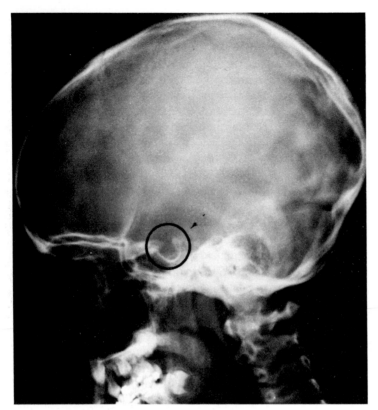

FIG. 25–1. The sella turcica is well seen on this lateral view of a plain skull radiograph.

1. Thyrotropin-releasing hormone (TRH) stimulates the release of both TSH and prolactin, although it is probably not the physiologic prolactin releaser. The neurotransmitter dopamine inhibits prolactin release at both the pituitary level and at higher central nervous system centers, and, hence, antidopaminergic drugs, like the phenothiazines, may cause hyperprolactinemic galactorrhea.

2. Gonadotropin-releasing hormone (GnRH or LHRH) stimulates the release of luteinizing hormone and follicle-stimulating hormone from the pituitary.

3. Somatostatin inhibits growth hormone excretion. It is also produced by the delta cells of the pancreas, and is thought to regulate the release of insulin and glucagon.

TRH has already been shown to have an important function in the laboratory evaluation of thyroid disease and hyperprolactinemia, and a somatostatin analogue may prove to be a useful adjunct in the treatment of diabetes mellitus. LHRH is now being used to treat infertility and hypogonadism.

• • •

Pituitary neoplasms are nearly always benign. They typically remain clinically silent for years, and only become apparent when the tumor encroaches on adjacent neural structures, begins to secrete excessive amounts of hormone, or produces pituitary insufficiency. Thus, disease of the anterior pituitary gland can present with visual field defects, neurologic symptoms, or endocrine hypo- or hyper-

FIG. 25–2. Abnormal sella turcica. This patient had a pituitary neoplasm. The sella is enlarged and partially destroyed.

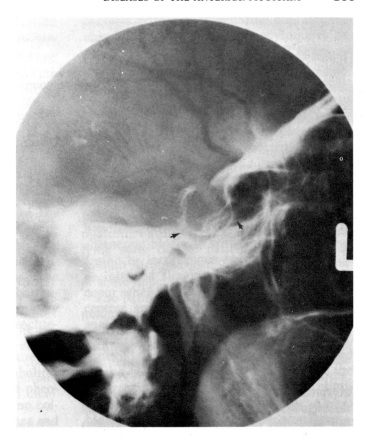

function. However, unless the signs of altered pituitary function are grossly apparent (*e.g.*, in the Cushingoid or acromegalic patient), the diagnosis of pituitary disease can be subtle. For example, chronic headache may be the sole presenting symptom. However, in patients who experience a vascular accident affecting the pituitary, the onset of symptoms may be sudden and catastrophic.

PITUITARY HYPERFUNCTION

Although autopsy studies have shown that 10% to 20% of people have pituitary neoplasms, the vast majority of these tumors are microscopic and asymptomatic. Pituitary neoplasms may be endocrinologically silent, may result in pituitary insufficiency, or may produce inappropriate amounts of any of the pituitary hormones. Whether these tumors represent primary pituitary disease or are the result of excessive hypothalamic stimulation of the pituitary is still a matter of debate.

Most pituitary tumors occur sporadically, but they may also occur in patients with the hereditary multiple endocrine neoplasia (MEN) type I syndrome. In MEN type I, the pituitary neoplasm may be accompanied by parathyroid hyperplasia and pancreatic islet cell tumors (*e.g.*, insulinoma).

Disorders of ACTH production are discussed in Chapter 29. TSH-producing tumors resulting in hyperthyroidism are extremely rare.

Acromegaly

Growth hormone is required for normal growth during childhood. Once the epiphyses close, however, the major physiologic role of growth hormone is apparently ended. In excess, the hormone is both diabetogenic and ketogenic. Growth hormone deficiency has no clinical manifestations in the adult.

Growth hormone has no specific peripheral target organ. Instead, its actions are thought to be mediated by a family of peripheral peptides known as the *somatomedins*. Like many other pituitary hormones, growth hormone is secreted in bursts, the largest bursts usually occurring early in the night's sleep. The amplitude of these surges declines in the elderly.

When growth hormone is secreted in excess before epiphyseal closure, the child grows to extreme heights (pituitary gigantism). If the growth hormone-producing tumor begins to function after epiphyseal closure, the patient develops acromegaly. His features coarsen and enlarge, the jaw becomes prognathic, and the teeth may loosen as the mandible grows. The head may enlarge, and frontal bossing becomes prominent. The tongue becomes thickened and the voice deepens. Hands and feet enlarge, and last year's hats, rings, and shoes may no longer fit. Growth hormone excess also causes glucose intolerance, and the patient may complain of any of the symptoms of diabetes mellitus.

Paresthesias, weakness, headache, amenorrhea, increased perspiration, arthritis, and arthralgias accompany the dramatic acral enlargement. A warm, moist, engulfing handshake is characteristic. The internal organs, including the heart, are also enlarged, but there is no distinct acromegalic cardiomyop-athy. Hypertension and other cardiovascular complications, especially congestive heart failure, are common. Patients may become debilitated from severe neuromuscular changes. The carpal tunnel syndrome (in which the median nerve is trapped by a thickened carpal ligament, causing pain, burning, or paresthesias in the hand) is often seen, and is typically bilateral. Visual field deficits may also develop.

Despite the dramatic presentation of the patient with full-blown acromegaly, the onset of the disease is insidious. The physical changes may take many years to develop and may not be conspicuous to family members. Patients are often diagnosed as having mild diabetes mellitus and hypertension several years before the entire acromegalic syndrome becomes obvious (Fig. 25–3).

Laboratory Findings. The plasma growth hormone is usually elevated. However, because growth hormone secretion is episodic, a random plasma growth hormone determination is not always diagnostic. Random somatomedin levels are nearly always high and thus more accurately reflect the disease state, but these are not generally available.

Acromegalic patients respond in a paradoxic manner to a variety of pharmacologic challenges: Glucose, which normally inhibits growth hormone release, may instead cause an increase in growth hormone levels, whereas L-dopa, normally a stimulating drug, can result in decreased levels. These abnormal responses may provide useful clues in making the diagnosis of acromegaly.

Characteristic x-ray findings include increased heel-pad thickness and large "spadelike" digits.

Treatment. Acromegaly is a chronic, progressive disease that does not resolve spontaneously except in rare instances of pituitary apoplexy. Surgery has been standard therapy

FIG. 25–3. Acromegaly can develop insidiously over a prolonged period of time. This is dramatically illustrated by the accompanying photographs of a patient which were taken over a period of more than 40 years. At age 25 (*A*), there was no evidence of the disease, but by the time the patient was 29 years old (*B*), some coarsening of the facial features was already apparent. By the time he was 42 (*C*), the acromegaly was quite pronounced. Nonetheless, he lived a vigorous, healthy life. Since the changes were so gradual and occurred over so many years, neither the patient nor his family were aware of the disease. Mild diabetes mellitus developed at age 56 (*D*). Frontal bossing is apparent by age 66 (*E*). When he was 76 years old, he had signs and symptoms of bilateral carpal tunnel syndrome and cardiac disease, and it was only then that acromegaly was diagnosed.

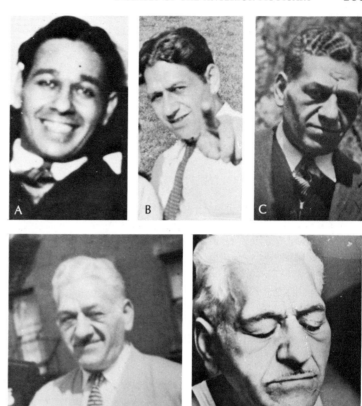

in the past. Medical intervention with the dopamine agonist bromocriptine has achieved only modest success, and the drug must be given in very large doses.

Transsphenoidal microsurgery has been effective, and some surgeons have added cryosurgical techniques. Radiation therapy using implanted pellets or cobalt beams is also frequently used. When the tumor does not extend beyond the sella turcica, proton beam therapy has been employed. Suprasellar extension of the tumor often requires a transfrontal surgical approach.

Long-term follow-up is needed to determine whether therapy has been effective. It may take many years before growth hormone levels return to the normal range. Many of the gross disfiguring changes resolve when the growth hormone levels decline, and glucose tolerance usually improves significantly.

Prolactin-secreting Tumors

For many years, it was believed that the most common pituitary tumor was a nonfunctioning chromophobe adenoma. However, with the advent of sensitive radioimmunoassays, it has been shown that a large number of these tumors actually secrete prolactin.

Prolactin appears to be under tonic inhibitory control by dopamine. Any tumor that compromises the hypothalamic-pituitary axis can block the activity of the prolactin "inhibitory factor" (which is probably dopamine), resulting in increased levels of plasma prolactin. The hormone is lactogenic and may be mammotropic, but in most men with prolactin-secreting tumors, there are no physical consequences of elevated hormone levels; in some cases, impotence has been ascribed to elevated prolactin levels.

The *galactorrhea-amenorrhea syndrome* is a common cause of infertility in women. Women lactate and fail to menstruate. The syndrome often occurs after pregnancy, but may appear at other times as well. Although the precise pathophysiology is not understood, the syndrome is frequently accompanied by hyperprolactinemia. The excess prolactin can be secreted by a pituitary tumor, but some of these tumors are too small to distort the sella turcica and are not radiographically apparent. Bromocriptine will reliably decrease prolactin levels and may actually cause shrinkage of the tumors. In many affected women, menses return and pregnancy becomes possible. Removal of the adenoma by a transsphenoidal approach may be necessary if the tumor enlarges while the patient is receiving bromocriptine or if headaches or visual field disturbances evolve.

Hyperprolactinemia can be caused by drugs that interfere with dopaminergic neurotransmission. The phenothiazines often increase prolactin levels by means of this mechanism and may cause galactorrhea.

PITUITARY HYPOFUNCTION

Pituitary Insufficiency

In most cases, pituitary insufficiency is an insidious, chronic disease that masquerades as depression. Since the pituitary has substantial reserves and the target glands maintain minimal autonomous function, the body usually suffers from a deficit rather than a total absence of endocrine function.

When all pituitary hormones are lacking, the syndrome is called *panhypopituitarism.* Patients are lethargic, sluggish, pale, and uncomplaining. Sexual interest is depressed and the sexual organs are atrophied. The absence of pubic and axillary hair, and an alabaster appearance of the skin are characteristic of the disorder. These patients may be borderline hypothyroid and Addisonian, and are subject to the problems of both of these illnesses. Failure of gonadotrophin secretion (LH, FSH) usually antedates the loss of TSH and ACTH.

The causes of panhypopituitarism are legion, including pituitary adenomas, nonpituitary tumors that impinge upon the hypothalamus or the pituitary, hypophysectomy (for the treatment of pituitary tumor, breast cancer, or diabetic retinopathy), trauma, postpartum pituitary necrosis, cerebral aneurysms, granulomatous diseases, and hemochromatosis. Some cases are idiopathic. Patients with sickle cell anemia or diabetes mellitus also have an increased incidence of panhypopituitarism. In the latter, glucose tolerance may be greatly improved as the hypopituitarism becomes manifest; this is probably caused by the decreased growth hormone levels.

A major concern in panhypopituitarism is hyponatremia, a common cause of coma in this syndrome. The etiology of hyponatremia is multifactorial in these patients, and is partly a consequence of decreased serum cortisol and thyroid hormone.

Patients with panhypopituitarism require hormone replacement with thyroxine, hydrocortisone, and gonadal steroids. Young children with panhypopituitarism also require growth hormone.

In treating patients with panhypopituitarism, several precautions must be taken. Restricting fluids in a hyponatremic patient with Addison's disease may cause cardiovascular collapse. Thyroid replacement increases the rate of metabolism of glucocorticoids, so unless exogenous steroids are also given, an Addisonian crisis may be triggered.

Selective hypopituitarism (lack of one or several pituitary hormones) can be seen in diseases of pituitary excess in which the pituitary neoplasm replaces normal glandular tissue. Thus, for example, patients with acromegaly may suffer from accompanying hypogonadotropic hypogonadism.

The most common form of selective hypopituitarism is the hypophyseal dormancy induced by therapeutic glucocorticoid administration. Large doses of daily steroids (approximately 20 mg prednisone daily for five days) or even smaller daily doses given for one to two weeks will suppress the hypothalamic-pituitary-adrenal axis for as long as two to three weeks. The axis may remain sluggish for a year or longer after the withdrawal of therapy. While there are numerous reports of patients who have tolerated major surgery without glucocorticoid coverage, most endocrinologists recommend that all patients who have had "suppressive" doses of glucocorticoids during the previous year receive supplemental steroids during major illness or surgery. Numerous protocols for withdrawing patients from steroid therapy have been devised, but all rely on a slow tapering schedule, changing to an every-other-day regimen and carefully monitoring symptoms of withdrawal—lethargy, anorexia, arthralgias, and orthostatic hypotension.

A rare but striking presentation of pituitary disease is the sudden, spontaneous infarction of a hypophyseal tumor. This event is referred to as *pituitary apoplexy* and carries a poor prognosis. The clinical picture is that of a subarachnoid hemorrhage, with severe headache, stiff neck, nausea, vomiting, and a depressed sensorium. Diplopia and blurred vision are common, and skull x-rays may reveal an enlarged or destroyed sella turcica. The cause of pituitary apoplexy is compromise of the nutrient vessels feeding the tumor at the notch of the diaphragma sella, resulting in ischemic necrosis and bleeding. When possible, an emergency transsphenoidal approach to hypophysectomy should be carried out in order to remove the debris and prevent further hemorrhage. This is especially important when the patient's vision is threatened. All patients with apoplexy should receive stress doses of parenteral glucocorticoids. Those patients who survive the acute event may subsequently suffer from hypopituitarism and hypothalamic dysfunction.

Empty Sella Syndrome

The empty sella syndrome is usually discovered when an enlarged sella turcica is seen on skull radiographs, which are routinely obtained in the evaluation of cranial trauma, chronic or severe headache, or visual field deficits, or when hypopituitarism is suspected. When enlargement or destruction of the sella turcica is noted, it becomes necessary to determine whether the sella is "empty" or whether a pituitary tumor is present.

Anatomically, the empty sella is defined as an extension of the subarachnoid space below the diaphragma sella. The pituitary gland is compressed into a small rim of tissue, but its endocrine function is usually entirely preserved. In most instances of the syndrome, the sella is symmetrically enlarged without gross distortion of the cortical bone. At present, the diagnosis can be definitively made by pneumoencephelography; cranial CT scanning performed after the intrathecal injection of dye is also sensitive and may soon replace the excruciatingly painful air study.

Although its etiology is unknown, it is thought that the syndrome is an acquired abnormality caused by transmission of cerebrospinal fluid (CSF) through a congenitally defective sellar diaphragm. Patients who have had cranial surgery with consequent destruction of the sellar diaphragm are said to have a "secondary empty sella."

The syndrome is quite common, with an incidence of between 5% and 20% in various autopsy surveys. Most patients do not have any symptoms referable to the pituitary gland. The majority of affected persons are obese women. Hypertension is often present. Only rarely is there evidence of papilledema, CSF rhinorrhea, or visual field abnormalities. Pseudotumor cerebri (benign intracranial hypertension) or mild degrees of pituitary dysfunction do rarely occur, but it must be emphasized that most patients have no pituitary symptoms. Headache is the most common complaint.

Unless there is evidence of visual field deficits, no therapy is required.

BIBLIOGRAPHY

Clemmons DR, Van Wyk JJ, Ridgway EC et al: Evaluation of acromegaly by radioimmunoassay of somatomedin-C. N Engl J Med 301:1138–1142, 1979

Jordan RM, Kendall JW, Kerber CW: The primary empty sella syndrome: Analysis of the clinical characteristics, radiographic features, pituitary function and cerebrospinal fluid adenohypophyseal hormone concentrations. Am J Med 62:569–580, 1977

Kleinberg DL, Noel GL, Frantz AG: Galactorrhea: A study of 235 cases, including 48 with pituitary tumors. N Engl J Med 296:589–600, 1977

Phillips LS, Vassilopoulou-Sellin R: Somatomedins. N Engl J Med 302:371–380, 438–446, 1980

Spark RF, Dickstein G: Bromocriptine and endocrine disorders. Ann Intern Med 90:949–956, 1979

Veldhuis JD, Hammond JM: Endocrine function after spontaneous infarction of the human pituitary: Report, review, and reappraisal. Endocrine Rev 1:100–107, 1980

Weisberg LA, Zimmerman EA, Frantz AG: Diagnosis and evaluation of patients with an enlarged sella turcica. Am J Med 61:590–596, 1976

26

Disorders of the Posterior Pituitary: Inappropriate ADH Secretion and Diabetes Insipidus

The posterior pituitary (neurohypophysis) is an extension of the hypothalamus. Peptidergic neurons, whose cell bodies reside in the supraoptic and paraventricular nuclei of the hypothalamus, send their axons into the posterior pituitary, where they release the small polypeptides, oxytocin and the antidiuretic hormone, vasopressin (ADH, also known as arginine vasopressin). Larger peptides, known as neurophysins, are also released with these hormones.

Oxytocin is involved in the ejection of breast milk, and possibly in the enhancement of uterine contractions during labor. It appears to have no physiologic activity in the human male. ADH is responsible for maintaining plasma osmolality and, to a lesser degree, plasma volume (see Chap. 21). Aberrancies of ADH secretion and function are being recognized with increasing frequency. Whether the neurophysins serve a specific endocrine role is not yet known.

PHYSIOLOGY OF ADH

Within the neuronal soma, the nonapeptide ADH is synthesized as part of a larger, prohormone complex. This larger polypeptide is packaged into granules and then transported to the axon terminals. *En route*, it is metabolized to smaller peptides; these include ADH and its neurophysin.

In a healthy, well-hydrated individual, ADH is secreted continuously. The chief stimulus for ADH synthesis and release is *increased serum osmolality*. The body strictly regulates its tonicity at approximately 285 mOsm/kg H_2O ± 2%; below a level of 280 mOsm, the secretion of ADH is entirely suppressed. At levels greater than 280 mOsm, the concentration of ADH increases linearly with the degree of hyperosmolality. Hypothalamic osmoreceptors can detect extremely small changes in osmolality, presumably by recognizing subtle changes in cellular volume, and signals are sent to the supraoptic-neurohypophyseal system, inducing ADH synthesis and secretion. The thirst center may be simultaneously stimulated by other mechanisms. ADH secretion remains elevated until free water conservation and water intake allow the body to return to its normal osmolality.

In very high concentrations, ADH is a potent vasoconstrictor, and is used therapeutically in the treatment of gastrointestinal bleeding (see Pitressin, Chap. 32). Synthetic chemical alterations in the structure of the

ADH molecule can nearly eliminate the pressor function of the hormone while preserving its antidiuretic properties.

ADH acts on the distal convoluted tubules and the collecting ducts of the kidney to produce a more concentrated urine. ADH increases the permeability of the renal tubular cells to water by binding to a specific receptor and activating the enzyme adenylate cyclase; the resultant rise in cyclic AMP is responsible for increasing the permeability of the cell membrane to water. Water then leaves the lumen because of the high osmolality of the renal interstitium surrounding the distal tubules and the collecting ducts. The binding of ADH to its receptors appears to be inhibited by calcium, and, thus, a dilute polyuria occurs during hypercalcemia.

The posterior pituitary is also stimulated to secrete ADH by hypovolemia, but in noncatastrophic conditions tonicity rather than volume is the primary regulator of ADH release.

Pain also stimulates ADH secretion. The endogenous morphine-like peptides, the endorphins, may also mediate a stress-induced release of ADH.

SYNDROME OF INAPPROPRIATE ANTIDIURETIC HORMONE SECRETION (SIADH)

Diagnosis. The syndrome of inappropriate antidiuretic hormone secretion is characterized by persistent hyponatremia and serum hypoosmolality despite an inappropriately concentrated urine that contains higher than expected amounts of sodium. Since the description of the disease in 1967, the diagnosis of SIADH has been made indirectly by simultaneous measurement of the osmolality and sodium content of the serum and urine. Hypouricemia is also frequently seen.

Dehydration must be ruled out before the diagnosis of SIADH can be made, since increased ADH secretion would be appropriate in such a situation. In addition, the diagnosis should not be made in the presence of renal, anterior pituitary, or adrenal disease, since water homeostasis is disturbed by altered kidney function, and because free water clearance is inhibited in the absence of cortisol. The clinical diagnosis of SIADH cannot be made in patients who are taking diuretics.

Patients with SIADH usually have normal total body sodium and increased total body water, but they rarely have edema.

It is important to realize that the chemical signs of SIADH will not be apparent if the patient is free-water restricted to the point at which his water intake is less than the sum of the obligatory renal water loss plus the insensible water loss.

Etiology. The excess ADH circulating in SIADH may be derived from the posterior pituitary or from an ectopic source. Lung tumors, especially small cell (oat cell) carcinomas, are frequent ectopic sources of ADH. Other tumors, including pancreatic islet cell tumors, can produce ADH.

Cranial trauma and any central nervous system infectious process may also produce SIADH. Aberrancies of pulmonary function, including tuberculosis, pneumonia, and the use of intermittent positive-pressure ventilation, are common causes of increased pituitary secretion. The hyponatremia of myxedema has been associated with SIADH.

Numerous drugs have also been found to initiate the syndrome. Oxytocin, often given to facilitate delivery of the placenta, has ADH properties. Chlorpropamide, an oral hypoglycemic agent, and carbamazepine, an anticonvulsant medication, potentiate the effect of ADH on the kidneys. There is also evidence that chlorpropamide and clofibrate release ADH from the pituitary. Several antineoplastic agents, most notably vincristine, have also been implicated in SIADH.

Complications. Although SIADH is usually mild, self-limiting, and asymptomatic, it can cause life-threatening neurologic crises when the serum sodium drops precipitously to dangerously low levels. Abrupt declines in the level of the serum sodium may result in brain edema, and hyponatremic patients may present with lethargy, headaches, seizures, and coma. With chronic hyponatremia, as can be seen in cases of SIADH due to carcinoma of the lung, symptoms are nonspecific and may mimic chronic organic brain syndromes; delirium, a depressed sensorium, and dementia may be evident.

Treatment. For most cases of SIADH, treatment should consist solely of free-water restriction. Since patients are generally not significantly salt depleted, sodium chloride supplementation is not required. By maintaining free water intake below the body's obligatory water loss, the patient's serum sodium osmolality will slowly rise.

When SIADH is a transient phenomenon (e.g., when associated with pneumonia), several days of fluid restriction, generally to between 1 and 1.5 liters per day, will suffice. It should be recognized, however, that fluid restriction does not cure the physiologic aberrancy, but only masks its clinical manifestations.

Chronic SIADH, as seen in paraneoplastic syndromes, may persist for months. It is unrealistic to expect outpatients to maintain strict fluid restriction, and these patients are thus liable to develop severe and even life-threatening hyponatremia. Demeclocycline, a derivative of tetracycline, inhibits ADH action at the level of the renal tubular cell, and may correct the hyponatremia on a long-term basis.

For patients who are comatose or actively seizing because of hyponatremia, emergency therapy aimed at elevating the serum sodium must be instituted. Hypertonic 3% saline solutions should be cautiously infused in conjunction with intravenous furosemide. The urine output should be carefully monitored. Fluid overload and pulmonary edema may complicate this therapy. When the serum sodium has increased beyond approximately 120 mEq/liter or when the neurologic disturbance has been corrected, fluid restriction should be instituted and the hypertonic saline should be discontinued.

DIABETES INSIPIDUS

Diabetes insipidus, a disease of ADH deficiency, is far less common than SIADH. Although there are rare familial and idiopathic forms of diabetes insipidus, it occurs primarily as a consequence of head trauma, cranial surgery, anoxic encephalopathy, and metastatic neoplasms, especially of the breast. A very mild, transient form of the syndrome can be simulated by drugs that inhibit ADH release. These include phenytoin and ethanol.

Patients with *idiopathic diabetes insipidus* complain of polyuria and polydipsia and produce astounding urine volumes, often more than 5 to 10 liters per day. These patients characteristically crave cold water and are often able to recall the precise moment that the disease commenced.

The diagnosis has traditionally been made in subtle cases by demonstrating a dilute urine despite an increased serum osmolality. This defect in urinary concentrating ability can be more clearly demonstrated by depriving the patient of fluid for 6 to 10 hours. A patient with an intact supraoptic–neurohypophyseal axis will increase his urine osmolality to 500 to 1400 mOsm/kg while keeping his serum osmolality below 295, but a patient with full-blown diabetes insipidus cannot protect his serum osmolality. Levels of serum osmolality greater than 320 with a urine osmolality less than 200 may then be seen. When this patient is given ADH intramuscularly, the urine osmolality will rise significantly.

Nephrogenic diabetes insipidus is a hereditary disease in which the renal distal tubular cells are unable to respond to ADH. It can be distinguished from central diabetes insipidus by showing that ADH administration does not increase the urine osmolality. The disease is treated with thiazide diuretics and strict salt restriction; these measures limit sodium delivery to the renal diluting segment.

Patients with *psychogenic polydipsia* (compulsive water drinkers) pose a difficult differential problem and present much like patients with diabetes insipidus. Their urinary concentrating mechanisms may be impaired by the washout of the concentrated renal medullary core by the large dilute urine flow. The diagnosis can often be made by depriving the patient of fluid for eight hours and then injecting ADH. A patient with diabetes insipidus should have a more concentrated urine after ADH administration than after water deprivation alone, whereas the compulsive water drinker will have maximally stressed his posterior pituitary by fluid deprivation, and thus will not increase his urine osmolality further with ADH.

Treatment. The treatment of central diabetes insipidus depends upon its etiology and the discomfort that it causes the patient. Diabetes insipidus secondary to trauma or surgery is frequently transient, especially if the pituitary stalk is sectioned, because hypothalamic secretion may commence soon thereafter. After section of the stalk, diabetes insipidus may be followed by transient hyponatremia (SIADH) as the ADH stored within the necrosing posterior pituitary is quickly released. If the hypothalamus itself is injured, permanent diabetes insipidus may ensue.

In patients in whom the release of ADH can be induced pharmacologically, chlorpropamide is an effective remedy for central diabetes insipidus. Hypoglycemia may result, however, especially during the fasting state (see Chap. 31).

In patients who have a complete lack of ADH, replacement hormone must be given. For some time, this has consisted of intramuscular vasopressin in oil or subcutaneous aqueous vasopressin. Recently, however, a new synthetic ADH analogue has been used in clinical practice with great success. 1-desamino-8-D-arginine vasopressin (DDAVP) is an ADH analogue with an antidiuretic/pressor activity ratio of 2000/1. It has a duration of action of 6 to 20 hours when taken intranasally. It requires only daily or twice daily administration, and is now the agent of choice for treating central diabetes insipidus.

In any treatment for diabetes insipidus, the patient must be warned to monitor his fluid intake in order to avoid water intoxication.

BIBLIOGRAPHY

Arieff AI, Llach F, Massry SG: Neurological manifestations and morbidity of hyponatremia: Correlation with brain water and electrolytes. Medicine 55:121–129, 1976

Bartter FC: The syndrome of inappropriate secretion of antidiuretic hormone (SIADH). DM 1–47, Nov 1973

Cobb WE, Spare S, Reichlin S: Neurogenic diabetes insipidus: Management with dDAVP (1-Desamino-8-D Arginine Vasopressin). Ann Intern Med 88:183–188, 1978

Coggins CH, Leaf A: Diabetes insipidus. Am J Med 4:807–813, 1967

Moses AM: Diabetes insipidus and ADH regulation. Hosp Prac 12:37–44, 1977

Robertson GL: The regulation of vasopressin function in health and disease. Rec Prog Horm Res 33:333–385, 1977

27

Thyroid Disease

Because of the thyroid's ready accessibility to physical examination, aberrancies of thyroid structure and function rank as the most commonly diagnosed of the endocrine diseases. In the 16th century, Paracelsus brought attention to the incidence of goiters in cretins, adding that the goiter "perhaps is not the characteristic of fools" only, "but also of others." As subsequent clinical observations have borne out, the presence of a goiter is merely a manifestation of thyroid pathophysiology and may be found in thyrotoxic, myxedematous, or euthyroid persons. Frequently, however, thyroid disease presents without goiter, or even without any palpable thyroid tissue at all.

Certain groups are at special risk: Thyroid disease is overwhelmingly an ailment of women between the ages of 20 and 60, and goiter has been associated with particular iodine-deficient geographic regions for thousands of years. Ultimately, a definitive diagnosis of thyroid malfunction depends upon a careful clinical examination and the intelligent use of a battery of biochemical function tests.

ANATOMY OF THE THYROID GLAND

The thyroid is a firm, vascular organ lying in the neck caudal to the cricoid cartilage. It is composed of two nearly equal lobes connected by a thin isthmus, and weighs approximately 20 grams. Rests of thyroid tissue are occasionally present in sublingual or retrosternal areas; a pyramidal lobe arising from the isthmus may also be present. Since any thyroid tissue can become hypertrophic or hyperfunctioning, the identification of ectopic thyroid tissue can be of importance during surgical exploration.

The parathyroid glands are embedded on the posterior surface of the thyroid, and the recurrent laryngeal nerves lie just medially to its lateral lobes. Vocal cord paralysis and hypoparathyroidism are thus the most significant postoperative complications of thyroid surgery.

The thyroid is composed of colloid-filled follicles that are storage compartments for thyroglobulin. Surrounding the follicles is an acinar epithelium which is capped by microvilli that project into the follicle. The height of this epithelium is indicative of the gland's state of activation. Parafollicular, or C, cells are found within the fibrous interstitium of the gland. These cells are believed to derive from the neuroectoderm and produce calcitonin, a hormone that causes hypocalcemia when given in pharmacologic doses, but whose physiologic function is not yet understood.

193

PHYSIOLOGY

The mechanisms for the synthesis and release of thyroid hormone have been carefully studied, and pharmacologic interventions have been devised to interrupt the metabolism of the hormone both within the gland and at its site of end-organ function.

The thyroid gland is able to concentrate the iodide ion against a concentration gradient. Once the iodide is transported into the gland, it is attached to tyrosine residues on the large thyroglobulin molecule. These iodinated tyrosine molecules then couple to form the thyroid hormones. The thyroid hormones are cleaved from this parent molecule and are released into the circulation. Most of the released hormone is in the form of thyroxine (T_4). Only a minimal amount of thyroglobulin finds its way into the blood under normal circumstances. However, during an attack of subacute thyroiditis, following thyroid surgery, or after an infusion of radioactive iodine, significant amounts of thyroglobulin may be extruded from the gland.

Circulating thyroid hormones are tightly bound to three plasma proteins—most are bound to thyroid-binding globulin (TBG), the remainder to albumin and, in the case of T_4, to thyroid-binding prealbumin. Only a tiny fraction remains unbound. Nevertheless, it is this free portion that constitutes the active hormone.

Although T_4 has intrinsic hormonal properties of its own, its primary function is to serve as a prohormone. After release from the gland, T_4 is deiodinated to form either 3,5,3'-triiodothyronine (T_3), the functional hormone, or 3,3',5'-triiodothyronine (reverse T_3 or rT_3), a molecule without any apparent biologic activity. In healthy people, approximately 80% of the circulating T_3 is derived from extrathyroidal T_4 catabolism. The deiodination of thyroxine represents a branch point in thyroid economy that may allow the body to regulate the amount of active hormone after the precursor has been released from the gland.

The levels of T_3 and rT_3 often change in opposite directions. Elevated levels of rT_3 with depressed levels of T_3 have been found in acute and chronic severe illness, in starvation and fasting, after glucocorticoid administration, and in the fetus. Although T_3 levels are often depressed in patients with nonthyroidal illness, the level of serum T_4 is usually within normal limits. In hypothyroidism, both T_3 and rT_3 levels are low.

Thyroid hormones interact with a variety of tissues by means of a mechanism that has only recently been explored. T_3 binds to specific nuclear binding sites and stimulates increased rates of RNA and protein synthesis. Thyroid thermogenesis is a result of increased ATP turnover, which is facilitated by the enhanced activity of sodium transport.

Although the normal thyroid gland is capable of significant autonomous function, the major control over thyroid homeostasis resides within the hypothalamic-hypophyseal axis. Thyrotropin-releasing hormone (TRH) is a tripeptide (pyro GLU-HIS-PRO NH_2) that is found throughout the central nervous system; it is especially highly concentrated in the hypothalamus. When it reaches the pituitary, TRH augments thyroid-stimulating hormone (TSH, or thyrotropin) synthesis and release. Thyroid hormone modulates the effects of TRH on the pituitary, inhibiting TRH-stimulated TSH release in states of thyroid hormone excess.

TSH, the pituitary hormone, circulates in the blood and stimulates growth of the thyroid gland, iodine uptake, and synthesis and release of the thyroid hormones. TSH release is markedly enhanced by depressed circulating levels of thyroid hormone and suppressed by elevated levels. In states of prolonged hypothyroidism of thyroid origin, the pituitary thyrotrophs (TSH-producing cells) hypertrophy impressively to the point at which a pituitary adenoma may result.

THYROID FUNCTION

A plethora of sophisticated biochemical tests now allow the clinician to determine the patient's thyroid status with far more assurance than in the past. Minimal deviations from normalcy can be discerned, and precise replacement therapy can be gauged.

Determination of Serum T_3 and T_4. The thyroid hormones, T_3 and T_4, exist in two forms in the serum, free and bound.

Total serum T_3 is measured by radioimmunoassay. Normal values usually range from 50 to 150 ng/dl.

Total serum T_4 is also measured by radioimmunoassay, with normal valves in the range of 4 to 12 µg/dl. A T_4 value above or below the normal range is not necessarily a sign of disease, since it can vary with fluctuating levels of the thyroid-binding proteins without concomitant changes in the free hormone level. Thus, with high levels of thyroid-binding globulin, the total T_4 may be elevated although the concentration of free hormone remains in the normal range. Causes of increased levels of thyroid-binding globulin include the use of estrogens and oral contraceptives, chronic heroin use, pregnancy, and hepatitis. Decreased levels of thyroid-binding globulin can be seen in patients with the nephrotic syndrome or with major illnesses associated with a general decrease in serum proteins, and in patients who are taking androgenic steroids or glucocorticoids. In these conditions, although the total T_4 is decreased, the concentration of free hormone is normal. Finally, there are hereditary syndromes of both increased and decreased levels of thyroid-binding globulin.

What clearly is needed is a measure of free hormone, but at most centers there is no clinically available, reliable test that directly measures free hormone concentration. Therefore, an estimate of protein binding is made. The concentration of thyroid-binding globulin can be measured directly, but this test is not widely available. Instead, the "T_3 resin uptake test" provides an adequate indirect estimate of thyroid hormone-binding capacity in the patient's serum. An aliquot of radiolabeled T_3 and a solid resin capable of binding free, but not bound, thyroid hormone are incubated with the patient's serum. The radioactivity bound to the resin is determined and is expressed as a percentage of the total radioactivity in the original aliquot of T_3. This percentage is inversely proportional to the available hormone-binding sites in the patient's serum. When the number of unoccupied binding sites is high (i.e., when the thyroid-binding globulin concentration is increased or when the endogenous thyroid hormone concentration is low), most of the tracer hormone binds to the serum protein and not to the resin, and, thus, the resin uptake is low. Conversely, the uptake is high when the number of binding sites is low or if the binding sites are occupied (i.e., with a decreased amount of thyroid-binding globulin or when there is excessive serum thyroid hormone).

A free T_4 or T_3 index can be computed by multiplying the resin uptake by the total T_4 or T_3. This value correlates well with the level of free hormone. In hyperthyroidism, both the T_3-resin uptake and the T_4 are elevated, whereas they are both depressed in hypothyroidism. An elevated total T_4 with a low T_3 resin usually indicates an increase in binding globulins, and a low total T_4 with a high T_3 resin is seen in thyroid-binding-globulin deficiency.

TSH Testing. Occasionally, in cases of borderline hypothyroidism, the serum thyroid hormone measurements may not provide a sensitive enough estimate of thyroid reserve. As thyroid hormone levels decline, the pituitary responds by secreting more TSH in order to maintain euthyroidism. As thyroid function continues to fail, higher levels of TSH are required. In general, when thyroid hormone levels are in the low normal range and the TSH is elevated, the patient may be considered to have incipient hypothyroidism.

When borderline hypothyroidism is of hypothalamic or pituitary origin, the TSH will be low or undetectable. The TRH stimulation test can then be helpful in confirming hypothyroidism. Patients are given an intravenous bolus of TRH, and serial samples are collected for TSH determination. Euthyroid patients show a significant increase in TSH within 30 minutes. Patients with primary hypothyroidism (i.e., intrinsic failure of the thyroid) start with an elevated TSH and have an exaggerated response after stimulation. In secondary hypothyroidism (i.e., primary disease of the pituitary with deficiency of TSH), the TSH level is undetectable and does not increase after TRH is given. In thyrotoxic states, TSH release is suppressed and a curve similar to secondary hypothyroidism is obtained. In cases of hypothalamic, or tertiary, hypothyroidism, the TSH response is delayed or sluggish.

Thyroid Scan. Radionuclide scanning with small doses of ^{123}I permits visualization of the thyroid gland. Thyroid scanning is useful in the delineation of palpated thyroid nodules and substernal thyroid tissue (Fig. 27–1).

Other Tests. With the advent of the modern biochemical tests discussed previously, less specific tests, such as the basal metabolic rate, radioiodine uptake, creatine phosphokinase (CPK), and serum cholesterol, are rarely used as primary diagnostic tools.

Drugs that Interfere with Thyroid Testing. Two commonly used medications interfere with these thyroid function tests. Euthyroid patients receiving phenytoin often have decreased measured total and free thyroid hormone, but pituitary testing and physical examination indicate that they are euthyroid. Heparin administration causes a spuriously elevated thyroid hormone level. It can also be difficult to make the diagnosis of hypothyroidism in a patient with concurrent chronic renal failure. Puffiness, hypothermia, and lethargy are common to both. The serum T_3 is often depressed in renal failure, although the T_4 is usually normal and the TSH normal or minimally elevated.

HYPOTHYROIDISM

Few clinical entities present in as dramatic and striking a manner as profound myxedema, and few diseases are as subtle as mild thyroid insufficiency. Nearly every organ system may be involved, and physicians have not missed the opportunity to apply alliterative and colorful labels to the various manifestations.

The skin is cool, coarse, rough, and dry, with a yellow-orange hue caused by elevated levels of serum carotene. Periorbital edema and nonpitting puffiness (so-called myxedema) are prominent throughout the body. Hair is brittle and alopecia may be present. Patients complain of feeling cold, lethargic, and depressed, and experience myalgias, arthralgias, arthritis, paresthesias, and distortions of taste and smell. Clinicians have long noted a bizarre sense of humor ("myxedema wit") and frank psychosis ("myxedema madness") in hypothyroid patients, and also an increased predilection for seizures. The relaxation phase of the deep tendon reflexes is visibly delayed. Moderate weight gain without significant change in appetite, and constipation are frequent complaints. Bradycardia and hypothermia are present in classic cases. A harsh deep voice is often more obvious to the physician than to the patient or her family.

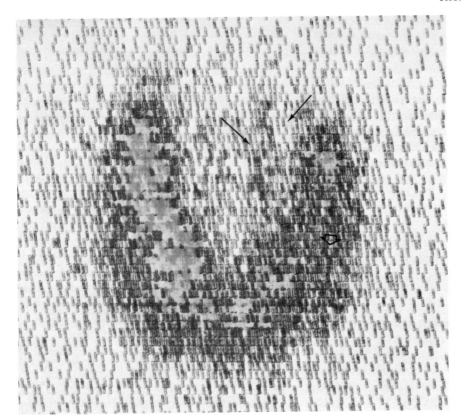

FIG. 27–1. Thyroid scan. This is a ^{123}I thyroid scan of a 19-year-old man who had a rapidly enlarging thyroid gland. The thyroid is diffusely enlarged, and a pyramidal lobe is present (arrows). An area of decreased uptake of radioactive isotope can be seen on the left. Biopsy revealed both Hashimoto's thyroiditis and papillary carcinoma of the thyroid.

Women of child-bearing age frequently cease to ovulate; menometrorrhagia is commonly present.

In moderate to severe hypothyroid disease, exudative effusions seep into many cavities: pericardial, pleural, and joint effusions are not uncommon, while ascites and middle ear effusions are less frequently seen.

Laboratory Findings. Anemia is present in at least one-fourth of hypothyroid patients; the etiology is often multifactorial. Pernicious anemia may occur in patients whose hypothyroidism is part of a syndrome of polyglandular failure.

Free-water clearance is impaired, and the serum sodium may be depressed, but significant hyponatremia is most frequently an iatrogenic blunder resulting from hypotonic intravenous infusions. A persistent, moderately elevated serum CPK should alert the physician to the possibility of hypothyroidism; "leaky" muscle cell membranes may be responsible.

The protein content of the cerebrospinal fluid (CSF) is elevated, and there is low-grade proteinuria.

The electrocardiogram of the hypothyroid

patient reveals low voltage throughout all leads. The serum cholesterol is usually elevated. Because of the known associations between hypercholesterolemia and myxedema and between hypercholesterolemia and coronary artery disease, the possibility that myxedema is a risk factor for arteriosclerotic heart disease has been raised. An autopsy study has shown, however, that hypothyroidism constitutes a risk factor only in patients who are also hypertensive.

Hashimoto's Thyroiditis

Hashimoto's thyroiditis, or chronic lymphocytic thyroiditis, is the most common cause of hypothyroidism in the United States. It was the first disease found to be associated with high titers of autoantibodies. These autoantibodies are directed primarily against thyroglobulin and thyroid microsomal antigens. Although the etiologic significance of these antibodies is still debated, it is likely that, in conjunction with cell-mediated immunity, they are responsible for many of the histopathologic changes.

Hashimoto's disease most commonly affects women in their third to sixth decades. Patients typically present with a diffusely enlarged nontender goiter and are usually hypothyroid or euthyroid. One biochemical lesion is a defect in organification of thyroid hormone, and TSH levels may be elevated despite normal free thyroid hormone indices. Many patients ultimately become permanently hypothyroid as the gland becomes fibrotic and shrinks, and the diagnosis can be confirmed by percutaneous thyroid biopsy. Treatment consists of lifelong replacement therapy.

Iatrogenic Hypothyroidism

The clinician may be an unsuspecting culprit in the genesis of thyroid insufficiency. The therapeutic use of ^{131}I for thyrotoxicosis generally leads to hypothyroidism, although often only after many years. It is necessary, therefore, to check thyroid hormone and TSH levels periodically in euthyroid patients who have received radioactive iodine in the past; a rising TSH may be the first indication of incipient hypothyroidism. Those patients who have received external radiation to the upper thorax and neck for lymphomas or head and neck tumors are especially in jeopardy of subsequently developing hypothyroidism. Lithium carbonate, a drug used primarily in the treatment of manic depressive disorders, has been shown to be a goitrogen, interfering at many points in the synthesis and release of thyroxine. Patients on lithium carbonate rarely become frankly hypothyroid, although approximately 4% of these patients on long-term lithium therapy develop an enlarged thyroid gland.

Iodine. The fact that iodine itself can be goitrogenic is now well recognized. Immediately after the administration of a large dose of iodine, glandular release of thyroid hormone is inhibited. Moreover, as the concentration of the iodide ion within the gland increases, the incorporation of iodide into the thyroglobulin molecule is shut down and hormone production declines markedly. This inhibition of thyroid hormone synthesis by iodide administration is known as the Wolff-Chaikoff effect. Normal patients usually escape from this inhibition and do not become hypothyroid even with chronic excessive iodide use. However, patients who have had previous thyroid surgery, who have received radioactive iodine, or who have Hashimoto's thyroiditis, may be unable to escape from the Wolff-Chaikoff effect and may eventually become myxedematous.

A common source of concentrated iodide is SSKI, a saturated solution of potassium iodine that is still used as an expectorant for asthmatics and for patients with chronic obstructive pulmonary disease. These patients may develop a goiter even in the absence of prior thyroid disease. Furthermore, SSKI may act synergistically with other goitrogens to depress thyroid function.

Dyes used routinely for pyelography, cholecystography, and angiography contain large iodide loads, and patients with thyroid disease may suffer an exacerbation of hypothyroid symptoms several days after the procedure.

Therapy

For most hypothyroid patients, oral administration of 100 to 200 micrograms of levothyroxine per day is sufficient replacement therapy, but the adequacy of the dose should be verified by a normal serum TSH in addition to a normal serum T_4. Since the thyroid target tissues themselves can convert T_4 to T_3, it is not necessary to prescribe T_3. Dessicated thyroid should no longer be used since the amount of T_4 and T_3 in each batch of pills is variable. In older patients, especially in those who have or are suspected of having coronary artery disease, treatment should begin with 25 to 50 micrograms per day, and then should be increased at a rate of approximately 25 micrograms each month until a replacement dose is achieved. Frequently, full replacement doses cannot be given without causing or severely exacerbating angina, and patients may need to be reconciled to a life of mild hypothyroidism. Recent experience indicates that some hypothyroid patients can withstand the stress of coronary artery bypass graft surgery, and that full thyroid replacement can subsequently be given without the recurrence of pain.

It is extremely important to obtain a serum TSH level before initiating therapy for hypothyroidism. If the TSH is not elevated, the patient probably has pituitary or hypothalamic disease and should be evaluated for panhypopituitarism. This patient must receive concomitant glucocorticoid replacement until this evaluation is completed.

Thyroxine has a half-life of seven days, and the serum level of thyroid hormone will diminish slowly when therapy is discontinued. Since thyroid hormone acts through the induction of new nucleic acids and proteins, the time course of hormone action also depends upon turnover of these latter molecules. The subsequent return of hypothyroidism after stopping therapy is therefore slow and insidious, and the patient is frequently not aware of any discomfort. Lethargy and forgetfulness are part of the hypothyroid syndrome, and patients who have stopped taking thyroid replacement therefore frequently do not seek medical help or remember to restart their thyroid medication.

Hypothyroid patients have decreased tolerance for most medications. Sedatives, for example, must be prescribed in lower than normal dosages. Sodium warfarin is one important exception; hypothyroid patients may require large amounts to maintain adequate anticoagulation in the face of decreased vitamin K turnover.

Myxedema Coma

The ability of hypothyroid patients to handle a number of various stresses is diminished. For reasons that are not at all clear, these patients may lapse into a stupor or coma when afflicted with even mild illnesses. In the classic descriptions, coma is precipitated by cold and exposure.

Myxedema coma is probably a potential danger for all patients who are significantly hypothyroid. Coma does not correlate with thyroid hormone levels, and replacement with levothyroxine alone does not reverse the neurologic state.

Medical intervention can pose a special risk to hypothyroid patients. Drug metabolism is slowed markedly in myxedema, making patients particularly sensitive to anesthetics and sedative hypnotics. An undiagnosed hypothyroid patient receiving a typical dose of a narcotic may suffer respiratory arrest.

Most critically ill hypothyroid patients who experience periods of unconsciousness are not comatose prior to hospitalization or even known to be hypothyroid upon admission to the hospital. Infection, particularly of the upper respiratory and urinary tracts, is a common precipitant of coma.

THYROTOXICOSIS

Patients with florid thyrotoxicosis (hyperthyroidism) complain of fatigue, weakness, heat intolerance, palpitations, dyspnea, polyphagia, insomnia, increased stool frequency, and weight loss. The skin is warm and moist, and outstretched hands reveal a fine tremor. The heart rate is rapid, usually greater than 90 beats per minute, and rapid atrial fibrillation is present in some cases. Increased metabolic demands lead to peripheral vasodilatation and an increased pulse pressure. A scratchy systolic flow murmur can be auscultated at the left sternal border. Frequently, the most dramatic findings are ocular; stare and lid-lag are prominent in most thyrotoxic states, whereas marked proptosis and exophthalmos are confined to Graves' disease. The thyroid gland itself may be diffusely enlarged or contain one or more nodules, and a bruit may be heard over the gland.

Nervous restlessness, hyperkinesis, and agitation are common. When these symptoms dominate the clinical picture, it can be difficult to distinguish thyrotoxic patients from those with primary neuropsychiatric disease.

Elderly patients may present very differently, appearing depressed and cachectic and complaining of anorexia and constipation. This so-called "apathetic" thyrotoxicosis may be marked only by mild tachycardia, but some patients also experience severe weakness and congestive heart failure. Ocular signs are rarely present.

The definitive diagnosis of hyperthyroidism is made by determining the free thyroid hormone index. In most cases, both T_4 and T_3 are elevated. In certain instances, however, T_3 will be high while T_4 remains in the normal range; this can occur when the thyroid gland is preferentially releasing large amounts of T_3. There are no clinically specific or distinctive characteristics of this syndrome of "T_3 toxicosis." While some patients with T_3 toxicosis never show a rise in T_4, many progress to a state in which both thyroid hormones are elevated, and some investigators believe that T_3 toxicosis is a prodrome of the full-blown syndrome of thyrotoxicosis.

Graves' Disease

Graves' disease is the most common cause of thyrotoxicosis in the United States. It is a systemic disease and has been associated with a number of autoantibodies. These antibodies can bind to TSH receptors in the thyroid and stimulate hormone synthesis and release. The immunoglobulin known as long-acting thyroid stimulator (LATS), and a similar antibody called LATS-protector, have been implicated in the genesis of Graves' disease. With the advent of radioreceptor assays, several laboratories have reported the presence of thyroid-stimulating immunoglobulins (TSIg) in practically every case of untreated Graves' disease.

Since both Graves' and Hashimoto's disease are associated with autoantibodies, some investigators believe that they represent components of a spectrum of a single autoimmune disease. Supporting this contention is the finding of kinships whose members are afflicted with either Graves' or Hashimoto's disease, and the occasional finding of TSIg in patients with Hashimoto's thyroiditis. Evidence that ophthalmopathy can exist in the absence of hyperthyroidism, and that patients with Graves' disease can sometimes present with hypothyroidism, has further clouded the traditional distinctions. These thyroid disorders are seen in conjunction with a host of other diseases associated with autoantibody production, including Addison's disease, idiopathic hypoparathyroidism, pernicious anemia, ovarian failure, systemic lupus erythematosis, and Sjögren's syndrome.

Among all the signs and symptoms of thyrotoxicosis, the most striking finding in Graves' disease is exophthalmos. The exophthalmos can be unilateral or bilateral, and may occur before, during, or even years after the thyrotoxic phase of the illness. It has been postulated that thyroglobulin, antithyroglobulin antibody, and antigen-antibody complexes travel through lymphatic channels from the thyroid to the orbit and are bound by the extraocular muscles, initiating a lymphocyte-mediated cytotoxic response. The extraocular muscles swell, and venous and lymphatic vessels become compressed within the bony confines of the orbit. Increased pressure makes the eyeball protrude (proptosis) to the point where it may occlude retinal vessels and cause diminished visual acuity or even blindness. Diplopia occurs when the swollen extraocular muscles can no longer function properly. When proptosis is so severe that the eyelids can no longer fully close, corneal damage can result.

In its early stages, the ophthalmopathy may respond to corticosteroids or high-energy radiation, but when fibrosis occurs, surgery is necessary to decompress the orbit.

Some retroorbital tumors may mimic endocrine exophthalmos. Cranial CT scanning is useful in resolving this differential diagnosis.

Pretibial myxedema, another very striking aspect of Graves' disease, is seen only infrequently.

Subacute Thyroiditis

Subacute thyroiditis is a self-limited, nonsuppurative inflammation associated with giant cells and granulomas on histologic section. It presents with the abrupt onset of pain in the throat and thyroid that radiates to the ear, jaw, and neck. Fever, fatigue, and lethargy are common, and the symptoms of mild hyperthyroidism may be seen early in the disease. The thyroid is very tender and diffusely enlarged. The erythrocyte sedimentation rate is elevated. The 24-hour uptake of radioiodine by the thyroid gland is very low, in contrast to that seen in Graves' disease, where it is usually elevated. The thyroid in Graves' disease is not tender.

After a transient period of hyperthyroidism, a mild but transient hypothyroidism occasionally ensues; patients with subacute thyroiditis rarely require lifelong thyroid hormone replacement. However, patients should be warned that recurrent attacks are possible. Therapy for subacute thyroiditis is symptomatic with anti-inflammatory agents, which can include steroids during the acute painful phase. Brief periods of beta blockade followed by thyroid replacement may be needed. Although the etiology of subacute thyroiditis is unproven, it is thought to be a viral-induced illness.

Multinodular Goiter

Most patients with simple multinodular goiter are euthyroid and may come to their physician's attention only when the goiter begins to pose a cosmetic problem, when the persistence of a palpable nodule causes concern, or when the enlarged gland impinges on the trachea and causes respiratory embarrassment. Even when only a single nodule is palpable on physical examination, postmortem studies frequently reveal the presence of other nodules. It is thought that the nodules represent areas of thyroid tissue that are unusually sensitive to TSH stimulation. These patients are treated with exogenous levothyroxine in the hope that TSH will be suppressed and that the thyroid gland will then decrease in size.

In some patients, especially among the elderly, one or several nodules may begin to synthesize excessive amounts of thyroxine, and hyperthyroidism may develop. This is referred to as toxic multinodular goiter.

Euthyroid patients with multinodular goiters are susceptible to an iodide-induced thyrotoxicosis known as the Jod-Basedow effect. These patients should therefore avoid pharmacologic doses of iodide and should be watched carefully after radiographic dye procedures.

Single Follicular Adenomas

Single follicular adenomas can develop autonomous function in a gland that is otherwise histologically normal. If the nodule is able to satisfy the body's need for thyroid hormone, TSH synthesis will be diminished and the remainder of the thyroid gland will be suppressed. A nodule may sometimes produce excessive quantities of thyroid hormone and give rise to a thyrotoxic state. The diagnosis can be confirmed by a ^{123}I thyroid scan, which shows a single active nodule. If TSH is then administered parenterally for several days, a repeat scan will show the remainder of the suppressed gland.

Thyrotoxicosis Factitia

When exogenous thyroid hormone is taken in such excessive quantities that symptomatic hyperthyroidism occurs, the syndrome is called "thyrotoxicosis factitia." It usually occurs in patients given improper supraphysiologic doses of thyroxine for depression or obesity. (It can also be seen in medical personnel attempting to feign illness. The latter group usually vehemently denies their efforts at self-medication, making the diagnosis difficult.) Even if the patient is isolated from any source of exogenous thyroxine for several days, the hyperthyroid state persists because of the long half-life of the hormone. The measurement of radioactive iodine uptake has been recommended as an aid in making the diagnosis. Since TSH is entirely suppressed by the exogenous drug, the 24-hour uptake of iodine by the thyroid gland is very low. The same picture, however, can be seen in subacute thyroiditis, and although the absence of thyroid tenderness and other signs and symptoms of thyroid disease may lead one to favor the diagnosis of factitious disease, the possibility of "silent" painless thyrotoxic thyroiditis without goiter must be considered.

Ingestion of a large number of thyroid hormone tablets in a suicide attempt is usually quite harmless in a young person, but can have disastrous consequences in an older person with cardiac disease. When an older patient is brought to the emergency room immediately after the overdose, he may have an enormously elevated total serum T_4, but he almost never demonstrates any physical findings of thyrotoxicosis. Within four or five days, however, the patient may become grossly thyrotoxic and remain that way for up to two weeks (two half-lives of the drug).

Rare Causes of Thyrotoxicosis

Uncommon causes of thyrotoxicosis include ectopic thyroid hormone production by ovarian teratomas (struma ovarii), TSH-producing pituitary adenomas, and hydatidiform moles which produce HCG, a molecule with thyroid-stimulating properties.

Therapy for Thyrotoxicosis

There are three nonsurgical therapeutic options available for the treatment of hyperthyroidism: (1) drugs that inhibit thyroid hormone synthesis, (2) radioactive iodine, which destroys thyroid tissue, and (3) drugs that block the actions of catecholamines, thereby lessening the severity of the thyrotoxic symptoms.

Propylthiouracil (PTU) and methimazole prevent the incorporation of iodide into thyroid hormone. PTU also inhibits the conversion of T_4 to T_3. Symptomatic relief is usually not apparent for about two weeks, and a euthyroid state may not be achieved for six weeks. Agranulocytosis is the most common serious side-effect. Drug therapy may have to be given for many years.

High doses of ^{131}I can be given to treat thyrotoxicosis. The proper dosage to destroy just enough of the gland so that the patient will be rendered euthyroid can be calculated from the uptake of low-dose radioiodine. Unfortunately, patients who have had therapy with ^{131}I often become hypothyroid after several years, and if lost to careful follow-up can become severely myxedematous. An argument can therefore be made to treat patients initially with ablative doses of ^{131}I, followed by replacement doses of thyroid hormone. [131]I can cause transient thyroiditis in high doses. The effect of ^{131}I is not immediate, and SSKI is an effective short-term medication for patients with Graves' disease who have received radioiodine and are not yet euthyroid.

Surgery remains an effective treatment in the hands of a skilled thyroid surgeon.

Antiadrenergic medications have been useful in curbing many of the symptoms of thyrotoxicosis without correcting the underlying hypermetabolic state. The beta-blocking agent, propranolol, also inhibits the conversion of T_4 to T_3; although a useful adjunct to therapy, it is not curative.

Thyroid Storm

Thyroid storm is a medical emergency characterized by extreme manifestations of thyrotoxicosis: rapid supraventricular arrythmias, congestive heart failure, hyperpyrexia, and a dramatic diaphoresis. It may be precipitated by surgery, severe illness, or other stress, usually in a patient who is already thyrotoxic. Treatment should be initiated with propranolol and PTU (or methimazole), and then followed with a continuous infusion of sodium iodide, which immediately blocks hormone release. Glucocorticoids, which inhibit the conversion of T_4 to T_3, should also be prescribed. Propranolol must be used with caution, because it may worsen heart failure or precipitate hypotension in patients with underlying heart failure. Acute myocardial infarction may be precipitated in older patients by thyroid storm.

CARCINOMA OF THE THYROID

Statistics from postmortem examinations reveal that approximately 4% of the population has thyroid nodules and that up to 2% may harbor foci of occult thyroid carcinoma that were unsuspected prior to death. It is vital from the standpoint of time and cost effectiveness, therefore, to determine which populations are at risk for developing thyroid cancer, which types of thyroid nodules are likely to be malignant, which require biopsy, and which can safely be followed clinically.

Children and men under the age of 30 with cold nodules (i.e., nodules that do not concentrate isotope on a radioactive iodine scan) have an especially increased risk of carcinoma, although the large majority of these nodules will also prove to be benign. Only within the past decade has it been appreciated that patients who received low-dose external radiation to the head and neck for tonsillitis, eczema, acne, and thymus enlargement have a much greater risk of developing thyroid neoplasms. This enhanced susceptibility to both benign and malignant tumors persists for at least 20 to 30 years after the radiation therapy was administered. There is no increased risk of carcinoma in those patients who have received ^{131}I therapy for Graves' disease.

Nodules that concentrate ^{131}I better than the surrounding tissue (hot nodules) are almost always benign. Multinodular glands are also usually benign, as are cystic nodules and nodules in the elderly. On the other hand, nodules that have recently increased in size and do not take up radioiodine on scan (cold nodules) are more likely to be carcinomas.

Several histologic types of thyroid cancer are recognized, and the prognosis can be correlated with the specific pathology. *Papillary carcinoma* is the most common and carries the best prognosis. Metastasis is usually via the lymphatics, and when spread is limited to the thyroid gland itself or to the nearby cervical lymph nodes, untreated patients have the same survival as healthy age-matched controls. *Follicular carcinoma* occurs in a somewhat older age group, spreads hematogenously, and carries a slightly worse prognosis. The bone and lung are the most frequent sites of metastasis. Both follicular and papillary carcinomas are well differentiated, indolent, and slow-growing. Tumors may have mixed papillary and follicular elements. *Anaplastic tumors* are often locally invasive, resulting in vocal cord paralysis and tracheal compression. In contrast to the papillary and follicular neoplasms, anaplastic tumors are usually large and carry a rather grim prognosis. *Medullary carcinoma of the thyroid*, which may present as a multinodular goiter, is a malignancy of the thyroid C-cells. It is often familial, and may also occur in conjunction with pheochromocytoma in the multiple endocrine neoplasia type II syndrome. The hallmark of the disease is an elevated serum calcitonin. This tumor invades locally, metastasizes widely, and carries a poor prognosis. Rare causes of thyroid neoplasia include lymphoma of the thyroid, squamous cell carcinoma, and metastases from other primary tumors.

The metastatic lesions of thyroid carcinomas may be of a different histologic type than that of the primary tumor. Follicular elements, for example, are often present in metastases from primary papillary tumors. Conversion of a chronic slow-growing well-differentiated tumor into an anaplastic neoplasm is also well documented.

The diagnosis of thyroid cancer ultimately requires biopsy, and several centers have reported great success with percutaneous needle biopsy. Any suspicious nodule, especially in patients who have had prior exposure to low-dose neck irradiation, should be biopsied. Thyroidectomy has long been a mainstay of therapy. Since thyroid tissue is sensitive to the trophic effects of TSH, suppressive treatment with thyroid hormone is also recommended to inhibit further growth. When tumors or metastases containing follicular elements are able to concentrate radioactive iodine, the progress of the disease can be followed by total body ^{131}I scanning. In some patients, high doses of radioactive iodine can effectively reduce the metastatic tumor mass.

BIBLIOGRAPHY

Bough EW, Crowley WF, Ridgway EC et al: Myocardial function in hypothyroidism. Arch Intern Med 138:1476–1480, 1978

Brown J, Solomon DH, Beall GN et al: Autoimmune thyroid diseases: Graves' and Hashimoto's. Ann Intern Med 88:379–391, 1978

Davis PL, Davis FB: Hyperthyroidism in patients over the age of 60 years. Medicine 53:161–181, 1974

Favus MJ, Schneider AB, Stachura ME et al: Thyroid cancer occurring as a late consequence of head-and-neck irradiation. N Engl J Med 294:1019–1025, 1976

Hamburger J: Evolution of toxicity in solitary nontoxic autonomously functioning thyroid nodules. J Clin Endocrinol Metab 50:1089–1093, 1980

Hill CS Jr, Ibanex ML, Samaan NA et al: Medullary (solid) carcinoma of the thyroid gland: An analysis of the M.D. Anderson Hospital experience with patients with the tumor, its special features, and its histogenesis. Medicine 52:141–171, 1973

Kidd A, Okita N, Row VV et al: Immunologic aspects of Graves' and Hashimotos' disease. Metabolism 29:80–99, 1980

Kriss JP: Graves' ophthalmopathy: Etiology and treatment. Hosp Prac 10:125–134, 1975

Sanders V: Neurologic manifestations of myxedema. N Engl J Med 266:547–552, 599–603, 1962

Schimmel M, Utiger RD: Thyroidal and peripheral production of thyroid hormones. Ann Intern Med 87:760–768, 1977

Sterling K: Thyroid hormone action at the cellular level. N Engl J Med 300:117–123, 173–177, 1979

Vagenakis AG, Braverman LE: Adverse effects of iodides on thyroid function. Med Clin North Am 59:1075–1088, 1975

28 Calcium Regulation and Disease of the Parathyroid Glands

CALCIUM HOMEOSTASIS

Calcium is the most abundant divalent cation found in mammals. A 70-kg man typically has approximately one kilogram of calcium in his body. More than 95% of the calcium exists in bone, complexed as calcium phosphate apatites. Under normal conditions, only a very small fraction (about 1%) of bone calcium is freely exchangeable with the extracellular fluid. However, when calcium homeostasis is disturbed, as in patients with hyperparathyroidism, enormous amounts of calcium can be leached from the bone.

The serum calcium is carefully maintained within the normal range (8.5 to 10.5 mg/dl). In contrast, the serum phosphate fluctuates greatly throughout the day.

Approximately 55% of the calcium present in the blood is bound to serum proteins, primarily albumin. The percentage of calcium bound to albumin increases as the blood pH becomes more alkaline. The unbound (or "free") calcium exists as ionized calcium, and it is this fraction that is biologically active.

In states of hypoalbuminemia, the total calcium is also low, but the amount of ionized calcium remains in the normal range.

Calcium is absorbed in the small intestine both by diffusional transport and by an active transport mechanism that is dependent upon the active form of vitamin D and, to a lesser extent, upon parathyroid hormone. When a person is in calcium balance, the amount of calcium excreted equals the amount consumed. Approximately 80% of calcium is normally excreted in the feces, and the rest appears in the urine.

The calcium ion plays a major regulatory role in a large number of biologic systems. Calcium is required for the secretion of many hormones, the release of central and peripheral neurotransmitters, muscle contraction, the activation or inactivation of many enzymes, exocytosis, and so on. It has also been postulated that calcium acts as an intracellular messenger, conveying information from cell membrane receptors to the cell interior. Because of the great number of vital functions dependent upon calcium, it is not surprising that calcium metabolism is so carefully regulated. Two interrelated hormone systems, parathyroid hormone and vitamin D, are primarily responsible for maintaining calcium homeostasis.

Parathyroid Hormone. Parathyroid hormone (PTH) is a polypeptide that is normally secreted in response to decreasing levels of serum ionized calcium. There are four parathyroid glands, which are usually located behind the thyroid gland (occasionally embedded in the posterior thyroid capsule). The location of the glands is quite variable, however, and it is possible to find parathyroid tissue lower in the neck or in the mediastinum.

Parathyroid hormone has a variety of actions, all of which serve to increase serum calcium:

1. In the kidney, parathyroid hormone facilitates the excretion of phosphate and the retention of calcium. It also stimulates the enzymatic synthesis of 1, 25–$(OH)_2$–Vitamin D from 25–(OH)–Vitamin D.

2. Parathyroid hormone stimulates bone resorption, and, to some degree, bone formation;

3. In conjunction with the active metabolites of vitamin D, parathyroid hormone increases the intestinal absorption of calcium.

In individuals with properly functioning glands, increases in serum calcium above normal levels inhibit the release of parathyroid hormone.

HYPERCALCEMIA

Causes. Severe hypercalcemia is usually associated with an underlying malignancy and is especially common in patients with multiple myeloma. The many ways in which a malignancy can cause an increase in the serum calcium are described in Chapter 49.

Hyperparathyroidism is a common cause of hypercalcemia (see discussion to follow). A more unusual cause is sarcoidosis, in which there is increased intestinal absorption of calcium due to enhanced sensitivity of the small intestine to the active metabolite of vitamin D. Increased absorption is also seen in patients who have taken excessively large doses of vitamin D and in patients with

gastritis or peptic ulcer disease who consume large amounts of dairy products and calcium carbonate antacids (the milk-alkali syndrome).

Thiazide diuretics inhibit the renal excretion of calcium and can mildly elevate serum calcium levels. Prolonged immobilization may lead to hypercalcemia because of resorption of bone calcium. Hypercalcemia may also be seen in patients with hyperthyroidism or adrenal insufficiency.

Signs and Symptoms. Hypercalcemia causes a variety of nonspecific symptoms, including malaise, fatigue, headaches, and diffuse aches and pains. Specific renal symptoms include polyuria (due to inhibition of the renal tubular response to antidiuretic hormone) and, frequently, nephrolithiasis and the symptoms of acute urinary tract obstruction. Gastrointestinal manifestations are common and include nausea, anorexia, and vomiting. These may contribute, along with the renal concentrating defect, to dehydration. Neuropsychiatric symptoms range from lethargy to psychosis and, with severe hypercalcemia, to stupor and coma. Metastatic calcification may occur in the skin, cornea, conjunctiva, and kidney.

PRIMARY HYPERPARATHYROIDISM

Primary hyperparathyroidism is a syndrome of unknown etiology characterized by elevations in serum calcium and parathyroid hormone. The syndrome is occasionally familial, and may also occur in conjunction with multiple endocrine neoplasia syndromes. In most instances, only one parathyroid gland is enlarged and is responsible for the excessive secretion of parathyroid hormone. The function of the remaining glands is suppressed. Most of these tumors are benign adenomas. Under the microscope, an adenoma cannot be distinguished from hypertrophy, and the diagnosis of a solitary adenoma depends upon the coexistence of three other normal glands. Occasionally, all the parathyroid glands undergo hypertrophy and hyperplasia and secrete large amounts of hormone.

Several distinct clinical syndromes of primary hyperparathyroidism are encountered:

1. The most common presentation of primary hyperparathyroidism is *asymptomatic hypercalcemia*. In general, a mildly elevated serum calcium is discovered on a routine blood test.

2. Another group of patients with primary hyperparathyroidism has a variety of *nonspecific complaints*, including fatigue, weight loss, depression, abdominal distress, and back pain. The diagnosis is usually unsuspected until an elevated serum calcium is discovered.

3. The development of *renal stones* is one of the classic problems of primary hyperparathyroidism. Nephrocalcinosis may also be present. It is not unusual for these patients to have had renal symptoms for many years before the diagnosis is made.

4. *Osteitis fibrosa cystica* is the most severe complication of primary hyperparathyroidism. Patients often complain of severe back pain, and vertebral crush fractures may be present. Bone cysts are now seen only infrequently on x-ray (Fig. 28–1), and diffuse osteopenia, which can be quantitated with bone densitometry, has become more common. Subperiosteal resorption of the radial aspect of the middle phalanx of the second and third fingers is an early x-ray sign of primary hyperparathyroidism. Osteoporosis may also be present.

5. Patients with primary hyperparathyroidism may also develop the signs and symptoms of *hypercalcemic crisis*. Severe hypercalcemia causes polyuria and dehydration. As the serum calcium increases, mental function begins to alter and patients may become psychotic, obtunded, or comatose. The profound altera-

tions in consciousness may prevent the patient from drinking to replace his fluid losses.

Peptic ulcer disease, gout, and, in some studies, hypertension are associated with hyperparathyroidism. Symptomatic primary hyperparathyroidism has been called the disease of "bones, stones, abdominal groans, and psychic moans."

Laboratory Findings. Hypercalcemia is usually defined as a total serum calcium greater than 10.5 mg/dl. Although hypercalcemia is the hallmark of primary hyperparathyroidism, the serum calcium may be only mildly or intermittently elevated. Mild hypercalciuria is usually seen.

Because parathyroid hormone enhances the renal excretion of bicarbonate and phosphate, patients with primary hyperparathyroidism usually have a mild hyperchloremic acidosis and hypophosphatemia. The serum alkaline phosphatase (that fraction derived from bone) may be elevated. Parathyroid hormone stimulates the formation of cyclic AMP by the renal tubules, and, as a result, the urinary cyclic AMP/creatinine ratio is increased. Hyperuricemia and a normochromic, normocytic anemia may also be present.

The serum parathyroid hormone will be inappropriately high for the level of serum calcium. There is, however, some difficulty in interpreting and comparing the results of different parathyroid hormone serum assays. The circulating parathyroid hormone is a heterogeneous collection of active hormone and inactive fragments, and radioimmunoassays usually measure both. Moreover, because antibodies may bind to both the biologically active amino-terminus and the inactive carboxyl-terminus portion of the hormone, there is a great variability in parathyroid hormone radioimmunoassays. Some antibodies also recognize "parathyroid hormone-like" peptides that are secreted by some tumors; in

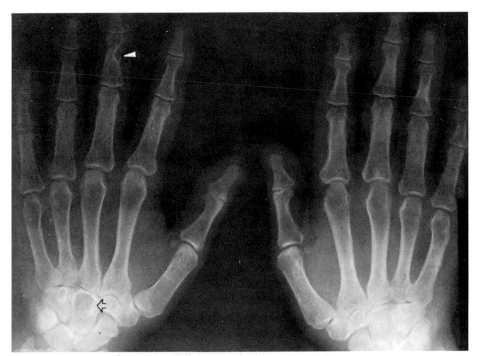

FIG. 28–1. Hyperparathyroidism. This patient had chronic renal failure and severe secondary hyperparathyroidism. The so-called "brown tumors" (arrows) are classic signs of hyperparathyroid bone disease.

these cases, radioimmunoassays are not helpful in distinguishing the hypercalcemia of malignancy from that of hyperparathyroidism.

Differential Diagnosis. Primary hyperparathyroidism can be mimicked by nonparathyroid tumors that produce ectopic parathyroid hormone-like substances. Hypercalcemia resulting from causes other than enhanced parathyroid hormone secretion inhibits secretion of the hormone, and can thus be distinguished from primary hyperparathyroidism by serum assays for parathyroid hormone that detect the active hormone. In these other diseases (see earlier discussion) the renal tubular reabsorption of phosphate is not suppressed, and, therefore, in contrast to primary hyperparathyroidism, serum phosphate levels tend to be normal or even elevated.

Therapy. The treatment of hypercalcemic crisis is discussed in Chapter 49.

In patients with symptomatic disease, surgical exploration and removal of the parathyroid adenoma is indicated. It is occasionally useful to perform preoperative angiography or venous catheterization with selective hormone assays in order to localize the source of the elevated parathyroid hormone. If there is hyperplasia of all four parathyroid glands, most surgeons remove three-and-one-half glands. Because hypoparathyroidism is so difficult to treat, some surgeons perform a total parathyroidectomy and retransplant a small amount of the tissue into the forearm in the hope of maintaining normal parathyroid function. The transplanted tissue is easily accessible for removal if hyperparathyroidism recurs.

Severe hypocalcemia may be seen after removal of a parathyroid adenoma, especially when there is pronounced bone disease. Removal of the tumor allows the osteitis to begin to heal, and thus the bones avidly take up calcium from the blood. An elevated preoperative alkaline phosphatase is a clue to the possible future development of "hungry bone disease."

All patients, symptomatic or not, should be investigated for evidence of renal or bone disease. If the patient is found to have a decreased creatinine clearance, urinary tract stones, or a significantly diminished bone mass, he should undergo parathyroidectomy. Surgery is also recommended for patients with severe hypercalcemia. Hyperparathyroid patients who lack any symptoms or signs of their disease should be carefully followed. No medical therapy should be given, but patients must be warned to avoid dehydration. Within four years, 20% of these patients develop signs and symptoms of hyperparathyroidism and will require surgery, but some patients can live for many years without symptoms and without requiring surgery.

SECONDARY HYPERPARATHYROIDISM

Patients with chronic renal failure almost always suffer from secondary hyperparathyroidism. The major clinical manifestations are bone pain and bone tenderness (especially in the pelvic girdle), proximal muscle weakness, severe pruritus, and soft-tissue ulcerations. Ultimately, diffuse soft-tissue calcification can affect the lungs and even the conducting system of the heart. These diffuse soft-tissue calcifications, which may be apparent on x-ray, are thought to be responsible for the associated pruritus and skin ulcers. Ectopic calcification is increasingly likely to occur when the product of the serum calcium and the serum phosphate (calcium × phosphate) is greater than 40 to 50 $(mg/dl)^2$.

Secondary hyperparathyroidism can also be seen in other disorders that are characterized by hypocalcemia, including malabsorption, anticonvulsant-induced osteomalacia, and a variety of disorders of vitamin D metabolism. In these disorders, hypophosphatemia may also be seen.

Pathophysiology. As renal tubular function fails in a uremic patient, the urinary excretion of phosphate declines and the serum phosphate increases. The rise in serum phosphate causes a fall in serum calcium and thereby elicits increased secretion of parathyroid hormone. Parathyroid hormone maximally stimulates the excretion of phosphate by each nephron, but as the number of functioning nephrons declines, the kidney becomes increasingly unable to excrete phosphate and the serum calcium remains low. Eventually, all the parathyroid glands hypertrophy and secrete large amounts of hormone in an attempt to increase the serum calcium. Most patients with chronic renal failure have a chronically low serum calcium and a high serum phosphate.

Calcium homoeostasis is further deranged by deficiencies in the synthesis of the active form of vitamin D. Vitamin D is both synthesized in the skin and acquired in the diet. The vitamin only becomes activated after two successive metabolic conversions: the liver converts vitamin D to 25-OH-vitamin D, which is then acted upon by a renal enzyme to form the active hormone, 1, 25-$(OH)_2$-vitamin D. The active hormone is essential for the normal intestinal absorption of calcium and phosphate; furthermore, in conjunction with parathyroid hormone, 1, 25–$(OH)_2$-vitamin D modulates bone resorption. In patients with chronic renal failure, renal 1-hydroxylase activity declines, and the body is unable to synthesize adequate amounts of active vitamin D. (Abnormalities in vitamin D metabolism are also seen in patients who take phenytoin or phenobarbital.)

Renal Osteodystrophy. The serum levels of parathyroid hormone are generally much higher in secondary hyperparathyroidism than in primary hyperparathyroidism, and very severe bony changes are more likely to occur.

Most patients suffer from a combination of four distinct disorders of bone metabolism in which the normal mineral content of bone is replaced with bone that is deficient in minerals. The clinical manifestations of these disorders include bone pain, fractures, and weakness.

1. *Osteitis fibrosa* is caused by parathyroid hormone-induced bone resorption, and is one of the earliest bone changes in renal osteodystrophy. It is found in most patients who have been on chronic dialysis for at least five years. Normal bone is replaced by fibrous tissue, primitive woven bone, and cysts.

2. *Osteomalacia* is associated with a deficiency of the active form of vitamin D; rickets is the result of vitamin D deficiency in childhood. The bone is replaced by poorly mineralized osteoid, and a bone x-ray reveals symmetric radiolucencies (pseudofractures, or Looser's zones) near the ends of long bones and at the edge of the scapulae. Bone pain is often localized to the pelvis, legs, ribs, and spine, and is often exacerbated by weight-bearing or by sudden movements. Skeletal deformities, muscle weakness, and hypotonia are characteristic.

3. In *osteoporosis* there is a decreased absolute volume of normal bone matrix and mineral that may not be apparent on x-ray until more than 30% of the bone volume is lost. Osteoporosis can be caused by the re-

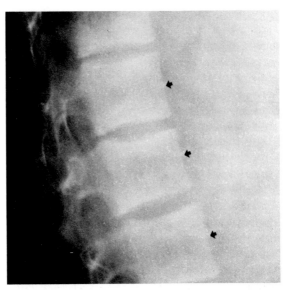

FIG. 28–2. Renal osteodystrophy. The "rugger jersey spine" is produced by the alternating regions of dense bone and areas of central vertebral radiolucencies (arrows).

sorptive action of parathyroid hormone, but is also seen commonly in postmenopausal women.

4. *Osteosclerosis* (increased bone density) may be noted in the long bones, pelvis, and vertebrae (rugger jersey spine) (Fig. 28–2). The sclerotic changes are caused by the anabolic actions of parathyroid hormone on bone.

Therapy. The bone disease of chronic renal failure is largely preventable. Secondary hyperparathyroidism can be significantly attenuated by avoiding severe hyperphosphatemia and hypocalcemia. All patients with chronic renal failure should therefore be given phosphate-binding aluminum hydroxide antacids early in the course of their illness in order to decrease the intestinal absorption of dietary phosphate. Calcium supplements may also be helpful, but only after the serum phosphate is lowered; the patient is otherwise at risk for ectopic calcifications. Vitamin D replacement with 1,25-(OH)$_2$-vitamin D can also increase the serum calcium (possibly by facilitating intestinal calcium absorption), and in this way lowers the serum parathyroid hormone. The use of the active vitamin D analogue is necessary since the kidney's 1-hydroxylase activity is markedly diminished in chronic renal failure. Bone biopsies in uremic patients given 1,25-(OH)$_2$-vitamin D replacement show amelioration of the parathyroid hormone-induced osteitis fibrosa, but surprisingly not of the osteomalacia; other vitamin D metabolites may be necessary to heal osteomalacia. The osteomalacia seen in patients who take anticonvulsant medications is reversible with vitamin D. All patients who require anticonvulsant therapy should also be given small doses of vitamin D supplementation in order to prevent the occurrence of osteomalacia.

Occasionally, subtotal parathyroidectomy may be required. Unrelenting osteitis fibrosa, pruritus, and soft-tissue or vital organ calcification are the major indications for surgery.

The complications of secondary hyperparathyroidism may be reduced by renal transplantation. With the return of normal renal tubular function, the serum phosphate declines and the serum calcium rises, thereby inhibiting further release of parathyroid hormone. The parathyroid glands usually regress to their normal size within several months. Occasionally, hypercalcemia occurs and persists long into the postoperative period. This occurs when the parathyroid glands, which had hypertrophied to such a great extent during renal failure, begin to function autonomously. This syndrome, formerly referred to as tertiary hyperparathyroidism, is dependent upon the persistence of a large mass of hypertrophied parathyroid tissue that apparently cannot be entirely suppressed. Subtotal parathyroidectomy may be required.

HYPOPARATHYROIDISM

Hypoparathyroidism may be idiopathic or it may occur when the parathyroids are removed surgically, when the glands fail to develop (as in the DiGeorge syndrome), when various target tissues are unresponsive to parathyroid hormone, or when there is severe magnesium deficiency. Patients with hypoparathyroidism suffer from symptoms of hypocalcemia.

Hypocalcemia may first become apparent as a tingling sensation in the lips and fingers. These paresthesias may soon progress to muscle cramps, spasm, and tetany. Anxiety, with consequent hyperventilation, respiratory alkalosis, and diminished serum ionized calcium may exacerbate the tetany. Tetany can be elicited by tapping the facial nerve at the zygomatic arch and observing involuntary contractions in the facial muscles, especially the orbicularis oris muscles (Chvostek's sign). Tetany can be elicited in the hand by placing a sphygmomanometer around the upper arm and inflating it to a level above the systolic blood pressure for two minutes (Trousseau's sign). Although tetany is unpleasant, it is rarely life-threatening. In patients with acute hypocalcemia, however, severe tetany may result in laryngospasm and respiratory compromise. Hypocalcemic seizures may also occur. Severe hypocalcemia may also cause hypotension.

Other manifestations of hypocalcemia include electrocardiographic abnormalities, notably prolongation of the QT interval (not present in all patients) and, in chronic conditions, lenticular cataracts.

Hypocalcemia is often very difficult to treat. Therapy consists of supplemental calcium salts and vitamin D analogues.

BIBLIOGRAPHY

Frame B, Parfitt AM: Osteomalacia: Current concepts. Ann Intern Med 89:966–982, 1978

Habener JF, Mahaffey JE: Osteomalacia and disorders of vitamin D metabolism. Annu Rev Med 29:327–342, 1978

Heath H III, Hodgson SF, Kennedy MA: Primary hyperparathyroidism: Incidence, morbidity, and potential economic impact in a community. N Engl J Med 302: 189–193, 1980

Mallette LE, Bilezikian JP, Heath DA et al: Primary hyperparathyroidism: Clinical and biochemical features. Medicine 53:127–146, 1974

Mundy GR, Cove DH, Fisken R: Primary hyperparathyroidism: Changes in the pattern of clinical recognition. Lancet 1:1317–1320, 1980

Myers WP: Differential diagnosis of hypercalcemia and cancer. CA: 27:258–272, 1977

Nusynowitz ML, Frame B, Kolb FO: The spectrum of the hypoparathyroid states. Medicine 55:105–119, 1976

29

Diseases of the Adrenal Gland

The adrenal gland consists of two distinct endocrine organs:

1. The *adrenal cortex*, which produces steroid hormones, is layered into three zones: the outermost zona glomerulosa produces mineralocorticoids, of which aldosterone is the most important, and the zona fasciculata and zona reticularis produce glucocorticoids and androgens.

2. The *adrenal medulla* synthesizes and secretes the catecholamines, epinephrine and norepinephrine. The medulla is fed by a portal venous system draining the cortex, and thus receives a rich flow of glucocorticoids that induces the enzymes responsible for catecholamine synthesis.

DISEASE OF THE ADRENAL MEDULLA: PHEOCHROMOCYTOMA

The adrenal medulla is not necessary for life, and no diseases of medullary hypofunction have been described. Studies of the gland's normal secretory function are somewhat complicated by the fact that a substantial fraction of the body's circulating catecholamines consists of norepinephrine derived from peripheral sympathetic nerve cells. Only the development of a pheochromocytoma, a rare catecholamine-secreting tumor, brings the adrenal medulla to clinical attention.

Clinical Manifestations. In its most exuberant expression, a pheochromocytoma erupts with paroxysms of catecholamine release, causing hypertension, palpitations, arrhythmias, headache, pallor, flushing, sweating, anxiety, and abdominal pain. The basal metabolic rate is increased.

Between paroxysms, most patients remain hypertensive. Because catecholamines stimulate glycogenolysis and, through α-adrenergic receptors, inhibit insulin release, glucose tolerance is impaired and mild diabetes mellitus may develop. A distinctive cardiomyopathy has also been described.

Surprisingly, many patients also suffer from orthostatic hypotension, perhaps because epinephrine may act upon vasodilatory β-receptors. Desensitization of the peripheral α-adrenergic receptors from chronic exposure to high levels of circulating catecholamines may also be partially responsible for the hypotensive episodes. After the tumor is removed, this relative insensitivity to catecholamines is dramatically exposed in the form of severe postoperative hypotension. Pheochromocytomas may also cause hypotension by stimulating the synthesis of vasodilatory prostaglandins or endogenous opiate peptides.

Diagnosis. The diagnosis of pheochromocytoma is often difficult; the symptoms can be nonspecific, and the patient's descriptions of the paroxysms may be more suggestive of an anxiety neurosis. The differential diagnosis and evaluation of hypertension is discussed in Chapter 10.

Pheochromocytomas may also occur in conjunction with medullary carcinoma of the thyroid in patients with the multiple endocrine neoplasia syndrome, type II. In the type IIb syndrome, patients also have mucosal neuromas and a Marfanoid body habitus. The presence of medullary carcinoma of the thyroid should therefore prompt a routine survey (see below) for the presence of a pheochromocytoma.

Several laboratory studies that measure the levels of catecholamines and their metabolites are available to make the diagnosis of pheochromocytoma. Twenty-four-hour urine collections are obtained for catecholamines and the amine metabolites, vanillylmandelic acid (VMA) and the metanephrines. The total urinary metanephrines is thought to be a more specific test, but it is fairly insensitive. To increase the diagnostic yield, it has been recommended that a 4-hour urine collection to measure catecholamines and their metabolites be obtained following a paroxysm. Plasma catecholamines may be chronically elevated in patients with pheochromocytoma even during periods of normotension, and plasma catecholamine levels may soon be an important ancillary test.

Once the diagnosis has been chemically confirmed, the tumor must be localized. Not all pheochromocytomas develop in the adrenal medulla; some arise in the sympathetic ganglia along the aorta or its major branches. Unfortunately, demonstrating that the tumor

secretes primarily epinephrine does not reliably localize the pheochromocytoma to the adrenal gland. Ultrasound and CT scans are being used with increasing frequency, reducing the need for abdominal arteriography. Most patients have single pheochromocytomas, but when pheochromocytoma is part of a multiple endocrine neoplasia syndrome, bilateral tumors should be expected.

Treatment. Approximately 90% of pheochromocytomas are benign and are cured by surgical excision. In preparation for surgery, hypertension must be controlled. Alpha-adrenergic blockade with oral phenoxybenzamine or intravenous phentolamine should be initiated slowly, since hypotension may occur when the vasodilatory β-adrenergic receptors are acted upon without counterbalancing α stimulation. On the other hand, β-adrenergic blockade, which may be needed to control tachycardia, must never be attempted until α-blockade has been achieved since the hypertension may be worsened by the elimination of β-mediated vasodilatation. Alpha-blockade causes significant peripheral vasodilatation, and patients need to be vigorously hydrated. Alpha–methyl-paratyrosine, an inhibitor of catecholamine synthesis, may help control blood pressure in patients who have malignant metastatic disease and in whom surgical excision is not possible.

DISEASE OF THE ADRENAL CORTEX

Aldosterone

Mineralocorticoid production is largely under the control of the renin-angiotension axis; the regulatory effect of ACTH on the zona glomerulosa is minor. Aldosterone secretion is therefore normal in cases of pituitary adrenal insufficiency, but in primary adrenal insufficiency, there is usually an associated aldosterone deficiency.

Tumors or hyperplasia of the zona glomerulosa can cause hyperaldosteronism, characterized by hypertension and mild hypernatremia and hypokalemia (Chap. 10).

Aldosterone deficiency is part of the hyporenin-hypoaldosterone syndrome seen in diabetic patients (see Chap. 30).

Adrenal Androgens

The adrenal androgens are synthesized in the adrenal cortex, and their synthesis can be stimulated by ACTH. Because only glucocorticoids and not androgens feed back to inhibit ACTH secretion, ACTH levels are elevated in patients with certain uncommon diseases associated with enzyme deficiencies in the pathway of cortisol synthesis (e.g., congenital adrenal hyperplasia secondary to 21–hydroxylase deficiency). As a result, the synthesis of adrenal hormones uninvolved with or preceding the enzymatic block is increased, and hypersecretion of the adrenal androgens can occur. Elevated levels of adrenal androgens are commonly seen in Cushing's syndrome.

Augmented adrenal androgen production causes virilization. Although this is primarily a problem of childhood, hirsutism or infertility can occur in adulthood as a result of mild forms of adult-onset 21–hydroxylase deficiency. Replacement doses of glucocorticoids suppress ACTH secretion and thereby halt androgen production.

Addison's Disease

Clinical Manifestations. Adrenal cortical insufficiency, or Addison's disease, is an insidious syndrome characterized by a host of nonspecific symptoms that typically evolve over a prolonged period. Fatigue, weakness, and weight loss are common, and may be accompanied by hypotension, nausea, vomiting, and intermittent periods of abdominal pain. In women, there may be a marked decrease in sexual hair as the production of adrenal androgens declines. Hyperpigmentation of the skin and mucous membranes may become noticeable. Hyperpigmentation is seen only with adrenal (primary) Addison's disease, and is probably the result of elevated levels of ACTH or related peptides. In patients with pituitary Addison's disease, in whom ACTH levels are depressed, hyperpigmentation is not seen.

Since cortisol is required to maintain free water clearance and since aldosterone is needed to maintain potassium balance, patients with primary Addison's disease present with hyponatremia and hyperkalemia. In pituitary Addison's disease, only hyponatremia is seen, much as in SIADH. Dehydration is reflected in an increased BUN. The heart is small, probably because of the decreased intravascular volume. The characteristic elevation in the eosinophil count can provide an important clue to the diagnosis.

Etiology. Most cases of primary (adrenal) Addison's disease are either autoimmune or idiopathic. (Secondary or pituitary Addison's disease is discussed in Chapter 25.)

Primary Addison's disease is often part of one of the syndromes of polyglandular failure, and is therefore seen in conjunction with thyroiditis, diabetes mellitus, pernicious anemia, and hypoparathyroidism. In the past, adrenal tuberculosis was a common cause of Addison's disease, and striking adrenal calcification could be seen on an abdominal x-ray. Adrenal hemorrhage, especially in the septic or anticoagulated patient, has also been implicated, but such catastrophes frequently progress swiftly to death, and it has generally not been possible to document true acute adrenal insufficiency in these patients. Rarely, Addison's disease may be caused when tumor

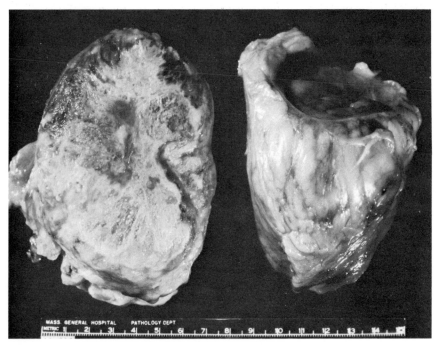

FIG. 29–1. Adrenal gland replaced with metastatic tumor. An elderly man with bladder carcinoma became weak and dehydrated. His serum sodium was 120, potassium 8.0, and BUN 110. He initially responded well to intravenous saline, glucocorticoids, and mineralocorticoids, but died of widespread carcinoma. At autopsy, both adrenal glands were massively enlarged and totally replaced by metastatic tumor.

metastases involve and completely replace the adrenal cortex (Fig 29–1).

Laboratory Diagnosis and Treatment. The diagnosis is confirmed by finding low levels of 24-hour urinary free cortisol and 17–hydroxycorticosteroids, and a diminished serum cortisol response to parenteral administration of ACTH or to insulin-induced hypoglycemia. Patients require daily glucocorticoid replacement and must be instructed to increase their normal dose of glucocorticoids during any illness or stress. Most patients also require mineralocorticoid supplementation.

Addisonian Crisis. Even a minor illness can initiate an Addisonian crisis in patients with Addison's disease. The patient in crisis typically presents in shock, with accompanying fever and, occasionally, hypercalcemia. The most common setting for Addisonian crisis is adrenal atrophy secondary to the use of exogenous steroids. Once the hypothalamic-pituitary-adrenal axis has been repressed by therapeutic glucocorticoids, the adrenal gland cannot respond to stress with the required outpouring of additional hormone for up to one year.

Emergency treatment with intravenous glucose, saline, and hydrocortisone is life-saving. Although any fever must be pursued with proper cultures, it is possible that the fever is part of the Addisonian crisis and will resolve solely with cortisol replacement and rehydration. In a patient not already known to be Addisonian, a serum cortisol obtained just before therapy is instituted can assist in the diagnosis. A random plasma cortisol of greater than 20 μg/dl is generally incompatible with the diagnosis of Addison's disease.

Cushing's Syndrome

Clinical Manifestation. Cushing's syndrome is an illness of glucocorticoid excess. Hypercortisolism causes glucose intolerance (and often frank diabetes mellitus), central obesity with a "buffalo hump" (an accumulation of fat in the back between the shoulders) and a supraclavicular fat pad, a moon facies, muscle weakness, easy bruisability, and striae. Hypertension is common. Mental changes, ranging from depression to euphoria, can usually be observed. Osteoporosis is characteristic, and vertebral fractures are commonly seen.

In women, serum androgens (of adrenal origin) are elevated, causing hirsutism, acne, and menstrual disorders. In men, the serum androgens may be low. Cortisol may have a suppressive effect on both the testes and the gonadotropins, and, as a result, men may suffer from impotence and loss of libido.

Laboratory Diagnosis. The best screening test for Cushing's syndrome is an overnight attempt to suppress serum cortisol levels with dexamethasone. At midnight, the patient takes 1 mg of oral dexamethasone, an extremely potent glucocorticoid. In normal people, ACTH secretion will be inhibited by this dose of dexamethasone. A serum cortisol is obtained approximately eight hours later. The serum cortisol will be suppressed to less than 5 μg/dl in normal people, but not in patients with Cushing's syndrome. Patients with unipolar depression or patients under unusual stress may also fail to suppress.

The diagnosis of Cushing's syndrome can be confirmed by finding elevated urinary levels of free cortisol or 17-hydroxycorticosteroids. Patients with Cushing's syndrome continue to have elevated urine test levels even after the administration of 2 mg per day of dexamethasone. In normal people, the levels of urinary 17-hydroxycorticosteroids fall dramatically on this regimen.

The normal diurnal variation in cortisol levels (highest at about 8:00 A.M. and lowest at midnight) is also absent in Cushing's syndrome. However, normal cortisol secretion is characterized by peaks and valleys occurring throughout the day, and random A.M. and P.M. serum cortisol determinations may fail to show diurnal changes simply because an A.M. valley or P.M. peak value was obtained.

Etiology. Cushing's syndrome can be caused by any of four disease entities, each with its own distinct etiology, pathophysiology, and spectrum of clinical manifestations.

1. Cushing's Disease. Bilateral adrenal hyperplasia secondary to a pituitary adenoma bears the eponym of Cushing's disease. It is a chronic, insidious disease especially common in women of child-bearing age.

Although the course of the disease is usually progressive, periodic fluctuations in symptomatology may be seen. Cushing's disease has long been associated with a myriad of central nervous system abnormalities, and some researchers have therefore suggested that the illness is of hypothalamic origin.

After the diagnosis of Cushing's syndrome has been confirmed, the specific diagnosis of Cushing's disease can be made by finding (1) a normal or elevated plasma ACTH (almost always inappropriately high for the degree of hypercortisolism) and (2) suppression of urine 17-hydroxycorticosteroids after a two-day, high-dose (8 mg per day) dexamethasone suppression test. Although patients with Cushing's disease fail to suppress on low dose

2 mg per day, dexamethasone, the pituitary gland usually retains a small degree of physiologic feedback regulation and responds to the higher dose.

Radiologic diagnosis can be difficult, since fewer than one-fourth of these patients have a pituitary tumor large enough to distort the sella turcica (see Chap. 25). These microadenomas often cannot be visualized on CT scanning.

In the past, bilateral adrenalectomy was the treatment of choice, but the mortality and morbidity of this procedure are formidable, and the syndrome can persist if adrenal remnants or ectopic adrenal rests are left behind. Moreover, after adrenalectomy, the pituitary corticotrophs become free from the feedback inhibition previously afforded by the very high levels of glucocorticoids. As a result, the pituitary tumor can grow, become locally invasive, secrete excessive amounts of ACTH, and cause increasing pigmentation (Nelson's syndrome).

Irradiation of the pituitary tumor has had only moderate success, and the initial wave of optimism for using centrally acting inhibitors of ACTH release (*e.g.*, cyproheptadine) has receded in the face of many treatment failures.

At present, hypophysectomy probably provides the best results for treatment of patients with Cushing's disease. In patients with small tumors that can be approached transsphenoidally, operative morbidity is low and postsurgical panhypopituitarism is rare.

2. Ectopic ACTH. The ectopic ACTH syndrome is most frequently associated with carcinomas of the lung, although numerous other tumors may also produce ACTH. Although only a few patients with oat cell carcinoma actually have Cushing's syndrome, elevated levels of radioimmunoassayable (though probably not bioactive) ACTH can be found in a sizable percentage of patients with lung tumors. In patients with Cushing's syndrome caused by ectopic ACTH production, the high levels of ACTH cause bilateral adrenal cortical hyperplasia. Because of the malignant nature of the underlying illness, these patients may experience rapid deterioration and some of the signs and symptoms of Cushing's syndrome may not have time to develop. Severe hypokalemic alkalosis and pedal edema are common in this form of Cushing's syndrome.

The diagnosis of the ectopic ACTH syndrome is usually not difficult, since most patients with ectopic disease manifest other severe effects of their malignancy. In some patients, however, Cushing's syndrome may be caused by an occult malignancy.

ACTH-secreting tumors are usually unresponsive to feedback regulation. ACTH levels are extremely high and generally cannot be suppressed with high dose dexamethasone. Unless the hormone-secreting tumor can be curatively resected, treatment is palliative. Inhibitors of steroid synthesis, such as metyrapone and aminoglutethamide, can ameliorate the patient's symptoms; ortho, para'-DDD, an adrenolytic agent, is also occasionally effective.

3. Adrenal Neoplasms. Adrenal tumors are usually unilateral, benign adenomas, and they can be cured by surgical resection. The tumors are best visualized by an abdominal CT scan or angiography. These neoplasms may produce any or all of the adrenal cortical hormones, causing syndromes of glucocorticoid excess, virilization, or feminization. Some carcinomas are endocrinologically silent; these neoplasms present late with the signs and symptoms of abdominal malignancy: weight loss, abdominal pain, hepatomegaly, and lymphadenopathy. In patients whose adrenal tumor is causing Cushing's syndrome, steroid production is autonomous and is not supressed by dexamethasone, even in high doses. ACTH levels are suppressed, and, thus, apart from the adenoma, the remainder of the adrenal cortex is severely atrophied. After removal of the tumor, supplemental gluocorticoids are therefore required for an indefinite period of time.

4. *Chronic Glucocorticoid Therapy.* Perhaps the most common etiology of Cushing's syndrome is the chronic use of exogenous glucocorticoids. Unlike the other varieties of Cushing's syndrome, patients with iatrogenic Cushing's syndrome usually lack hirsutism and other evidence of excessive adrenal androgen production. A variety of other signs, however, are seen almost exclusively in these patients, including pancreatitis, panniculitis, glaucoma, benign intracranial hypertension, and posterior subcapsular cataracts.

Pseudo-Cushing's Syndrome. Recently, a syndrome of pseudo-Cushing's syndrome has been described in the alcoholic population. Serum cortisol levels are increased, diurnal rhythms may be blunted, and dexamethasone suppression may be inadequate. All the classic signs of hypercortisolism may be present, but each of these abnormalities disappears within days of hospitalization as nutrition is improved and alcohol consumption is eliminated. The etiology of this syndrome is still unexplained. An extensive evaluation for Cushing's syndrome in a chronic alcoholic should be postponed until the pseudosyndrome can be excluded.

BIBLIOGRAPHY

Axelrod L: Glucocorticoid therapy. Medicine 55:39–65, 1976

Bravo EL, Tarazi RC, Gifford RW et al: Circulating and urinary catecholamines in pheochromocytoma. N Engl J Med 301:682–686, 1979

Crapo L: Cushing's syndrome: A review of diagnostic tests. Metabolism 28:955–977, 1979

Engelman K: Phaeochromocytoma. Clin Endocrin Metab 6:769–797, 1977

Gold EM: The Cushing syndromes: Changing views of diagnosis and treatment. Ann Intern Med 90:829–844, 1979

30

Diabetes mellitis is a chronic systemic disease capable of affecting virtually every organ system in the body.

At the cellular level, diabetes is a disease of insufficient insulin action, a result of either an absolute decrease in the amount of insulin or peripheral resistance to its effects.

Insulin is required for the efficient transport of glucose into muscle, adipose, and liver cells. Proper utilization of glucose within the liver cells is also dependent upon insulin.

In the absence of insulin, glucose cannot be effectively transported into cells and it accumulates in the blood. In addition, the liver begins to manufacture glucose from amino acids (gluconeogenesis). Additional glucose is thus secreted into the blood stream. The end result is hyperglycemia.

When the degree of hyperglycemia exceeds the kidney's capacity for tubular reabsorption of glucose, glucose appears in the urine, an osmotic diuresis ensues, and the patient experiences polyuria. Unless the diabetic patient compensates for this fluid loss by increasing his fluid intake (polydipsia), severe dehydration can result.

Under normal conditions, insulin also acts to inhibit lipolysis. With insulin lack, adipose cells degrade their store of triglycerides into fatty acids. Ultimately, ketone bodies are produced, and a metabolic acidosis (ketoacidosis) develops. The patient attempts to compensate for the acidosis by hyperventilating. The characteristic pattern of deep, rapid breathing is called Kussmaul ventilation.

• • •

The clinical spectrum of diabetes ranges from patients in coma with severe ketoacidosis and severe hyperglycemia to individuals with mild asymptomatic hyperglycemia.

A number of subcategories of diabetes have been delineated. *Clinical diabetes* refers to symptomatic illness in patients with elevated fasting blood sugars. Patients with *latent* or *chemical diabetes* have neither the signs, symptoms, nor late complications of clinical disease, but laboratory evaluation reveals an abnormal glucose tolerance test. The fasting glucose may be normal or only mildly elevated. In patients with *subclinical diabetes*, only major stresses (*e.g.*, pregnancy) cause glucose intolerance. Finally, *prediabetes* is a retrospective diagnosis that can only be made after one of the other three categories of diabetes has been diagnosed. Prediabetes describes the time prior to the onset of diabetes in a person with a strong genetic predisposition to the illness (*e.g.*, a person who has an identical twin with diabetes).

Clinical diabetes has been further subdivided. *Juvenile onset diabetes* (type I diabetes) is caused by the absence of insulin due to the destruction of insulin-producing cells. It most frequently occurs in persons under 40 years of age. These patients require daily insulin and are prone to ketosis. Islet cell antibodies may be present, and there is an association with the HLA-B 8 and Dw3 antigens. There is often a "honeymoon" period in juvenile onset disease one to two months after the onset of diabetes. During this time, insulin requirements decrease very dramatically; some patients may even become temporarily independent of insulin. This period, however, is short-lived, and these patients will require life-long insulin therapy.

Adult onset diabetes (type II diabetes) is commonly seen in obese persons. In contrast to the insulin-deficient type I, insulin levels are frequently elevated at the onset of the disease, although levels may also be normal or low. It is usually nonketotic. Adult onset diabetes is thought to be caused by insensitivity to the effects of insulin; for a variety of reasons involving the insulin receptor, the adipocytes of obese people do not respond normally to insulin. Most patients have a family history of adult onset disease. Because adult onset diabetes can usually be greatly or even completely ameliorated by weight loss and diet, these patients are said to be insulin-independent. However, insulin injections are often required, because many patients find it impossible to maintain weight loss.

• • •

The principal aims of therapy are (1) to ameliorate the symptoms of hyperglycemia (polydipsia, polyuria, polyphagia), (2) to prevent ketoacidosis and hyperosmolar coma, and (3) to prevent or delay the long-term complications of the disease (neuropathy, ret-inopathy, nephropathy, and cardiovascular disease).

In the light of the pathogenesis of diabetes described above, it would seem reasonable to assume that administration of insulin would cure the disease. Insulin was first put into clinical use in the 1920s and was found to aid greatly in the control of hyperglycemia and in the prevention of ketoacidosis. Nevertheless, insulin administration has not been found to prevent the chronic complications of diabetes. There are two possible reasons for this:

1. No method for the clinical administration of exogenous insulin has been found to regulate blood glucose as accurately as the pancreas.

2. Even if it were possible to mimic faithfully the insulin-secreting function of the pancreas, it is not clear that either insulin lack or hyperglycemia alone is responsible for all the chronic manifestations of diabetes.

Various oral hypoglycemic agents have been tried in an attempt to control diabetes by stimulating endogenous insulin release, but these drugs have not proved effective in maintaining a sustained lowering of blood glucose and are fraught with side-effects (see later discussion).

Patients with diabetes come to medical attention because of three categories of problems related to their disease:

1. because of the incidental discovery of an elevated blood glucose or the onset of mild symptoms, such as polydipsia, polyuria, and blurred vision,

2. because of the severe distress (or even coma) of ketoacidosis or a hyperosmolar state,

3. because of the chronic complications of the disease.

THE ONSET OF DIABETES

Early symptoms of diabetes include extreme fatigue, weight loss despite increased appetite and consumption (polyphagia), polyuria, polydipsia, and blurred vision. Women may complain of vaginal moniliasis. These patients are usually mildly dehydrated. Hyperglycemia and glycosuria without significant ketonuria are present.

All patients who are very ill, elderly, or unable to care for themselves at home should be hospitalized. Some physicians hospitalize all patients with newly diagnosed diabetes.

Hospitalization of these patients allows initiation of therapy and patient education:

1. *To plan diet therapy and to determine the extent of hyperglycemia.* Obese patients should be placed on a practical weight reduction diet high in natural fibers. Urine should be tested for glucose prior to meals and at bed time by the double void method (explanation later), and these values should then be correlated with a fasting and midafternoon (approximately 3 P.M.) blood glucose. In this way, the renal threshold for glucose can be determined so that home urine tests can be correlated with blood glucose levels.

At some centers, it is possible to use the level of a minor glycosylated hemoglobin (HgbA$_{1c}$) to provide an estimate of the extent of hyperglycemia during the preceding three months (the lifetime of a red blood cell). The extent of hyperglycemia and its duration correlate with the concentration of HgbA$_{1c}$.

2. *To begin insulin therapy.* All Type-I diabetics require insulin therapy. On the other hand, most adult onset diabetics do not require insulin if they lose weight and remain relatively lean. Patients who cannot maintain weight loss may require insulin to remain asymptomatic. Those who advocate tight control recommend insulin (or oral hypoglycemic agents) for all diabetics, symptomatic or not, who are hyperglycemic.

Nonketotic, adult onset diabetics should initially be treated with an intermediate-acting insulin, either NPH or Lente, given subcutaneously each morning. The intermediate insulins typically have a peak onset 6 to 14 hours after injection, and a duration of action of 18 to 28 hours. Patients should be started at low doses, approximately 10 to 20 units per day. The dose can be increased frequently to control hyperglycemia. If there is significant morning hyperglycemia, it may be convenient to divide the daily dose into two injections, one before breakfast and one before the evening meal. If there is hyperglycemia in the late morning or early afternoon, rapid-acting insulin (regular or semi-Lente) can be given with the morning NPH or Lente. The activity of regular insulin peaks in 3 to 4 hours and lasts up to 7 hours; semi-Lente peaks in 3 to 4 hours and lasts for 10 to 16 hours. In diabetics who have taken insulin chronically for several years, the peak activity of regular insulin may be prolonged to 4 to 6 hours, and its activity may persist for 9 to 11 hours.

Oral hypoglycemic agents (primarily sulfonylureas) are also used in the treatment of diabetes. However, there is considerable controversy concerning both their efficacy and safety. Many believe that the oral agents are effective hypoglycemic drugs when the dosage is properly tailored to each patient. Since the sulfonylureas are thought to work by increasing endogenous insulin secretion, they are appropriate only in the treatment of adult onset, type II diabetes.

In the 1960s, the University Group Diabetes Program (UGDP) conducted a study to determine whether diet therapy, insulin, or oral hypoglycemic medications could ameliorate or arrest the vascular complications of asymptomatic adult onset diabetes. The major finding was that patients taking a fixed dose of tolbutamide or phenformin had increased cardiovascular, but not overall, mortality when compared with patients treated with insulin or diet therapy alone. Furthermore, neither oral hypoglycemic agent was effective in maintaining sustained lowering of the blood sugar. Subsequently, phenformin was found to cause severe lactic acidosis and was taken off the market.

Oral hypoglycemic drugs have also been found to cause severe and prolonged hypoglycemia (see Chap. 31).

Sulfonylureas are most appropriately prescribed for overweight, type II diabetics who are unable to lose weight or maintain a proper diet and who refuse insulin therapy.

It is important to determine whether an underlying etiology of the patient's hyperglycemia can be identified. Cushing's syndrome and acromegaly must be considered. Hypokalemia can cause mild hyperglycemia; depressed levels of serum potassium inhibit insulin release, and potassium replacement may return the blood glucose to normal. Thiazide diuretics may also cause hyperglycemia.

3. *To teach the diabetic about his illness and how to care for it himself.* This is the most important part of the initial hospitalization. The patient must learn to inject the insulin by himself, or else the family must be taught to give the injections. Patients must be taught how to "double void"; that is, after emptying the bladder, the patient waits for 15 to 30 minutes and urinates again; only the second urine sample reflects the actual current blood glucose and should be tested for sugar. (Occasionally, it may be useful to test the first-voided morning urine as an "integrated" assessment of nighttime blood sugar control.) A diet must be planned and modified for the patient's tastes and budget. While overall caloric restriction is most important, recent studies indicate that the addition of large amounts of plant fiber may delay glucose absorption and significantly diminish glycosuria, serum cholesterol levels, postprandial blood sugar levels, and insulin requirements. The benefits of regular exercise for adult onset diabetics should also be stressed: in addition to promoting cardiovascular fitness and weight loss, exercise may lead to increased end-organ insulin sensitivity.

The patient's hospital stay should not be terminated until teaching is completed. Patients must be seen frequently thereafter to reassess the insulin dosage and reinforce diabetic teaching. The insulin dose that was optimal in the hospital is usually not optimal at home, since there will inevitably be changes in the patient's diet, and intermittent illnesses may necessitate an increase in the insulin dose. If renal failure develops, insulin requirements may decrease.

If, indeed, the chronic complications of diabetes are secondary to long-standing hyperglycemia, it would be important to aim for euglycemia in all diabetics. Aggressive therapy to maintain euglycemia is called "tight control."

DIABETIC CRISES

Ketoacidosis

Pathogenesis. Diabetic ketoacidosis is, first and foremost, a disease of insulin deficiency. It is greatly exacerbated by the actions of several counter-regulatory hormones whose normal homeostatic mechanisms are perturbed.

Peripheral lipolysis is normally inhibited by circulating insulin. In the diabetic on the verge of ketoacidosis, insulin levels are markedly reduced or absent and lipolysis is accelerated. Triglycerides are degraded into free fatty acids that are then released into the circulation. Upon reaching the liver, they are oxidized to the ketone bodies, *acetoacetate* and *β-hydroxybutyrate*.

Normally, ketone bodies are metabolized by cardiac and skeletal muscle; during starvation, the brain can also metabolize ketones. Lack of insulin, however, diminishes the body's ability to metabolize ketones, so that the ketone bodies accumulate.

With the initiation of insulin therapy, lipolysis ceases. Ketone production, however, does not stop immediately, since triglyceride stores are large and enzymes favoring ketone production have been induced. The elevated blood glucose in ketoacidosis is primarily the result of uncontrolled gluconeogenesis.

Lack of insulin by itself is probably sufficient for the initiation of ketoacidosis, but the presence of at least one of the counterregulatory hormones—glucagon, cortisol, growth hormone, and the catecholamines—may be needed for development of the full-blown syndrome. The importance of the counterregulatory hormones in ketoacidosis is indicated by several observations: (1) various stresses that precipitate diabetic ketoacidosis, particularly infection, also increase levels of the counterregulatory hormones; (2) glucagon levels are reciprocally related to insulin levels, and are greatly elevated as ketoacidosis develops; (3) these hormones are ketogenic when infused into diabetics; (4) in many animal models, the counterregulatory hormones are necessary for ketosis; and (5) removal or inhibition of these hormones in animal systems diminishes ketone production and delays acidosis.

Clinical Presentation. The typical prodrome of diabetic ketoacidosis consists of 12 to 24 hours of weakness, polyuria, polydipsia, Kussmaul hyperventilation, visual disturbances, and abdominal pain with vomiting. All patients are significantly dehydrated, and persistent emesis may greatly exacerbate the decrease in extracellular volume.

The abdominal pain can be caused by gastric distention, swelling of the hepatic capsule, neuropathy, or acidemia. It may be difficult to determine whether the abdominal discomfort is a symptom of ketoacidosis alone or whether it represents an underlying abdominal disorder that may itself have initiated the metabolic decompensation. This difficulty is intensified by the increased incidence of certain abdominal disorders in diabetics. These include cholelithiasis, atherosclerotic mesenteric insufficiency, pyelonephritis, peritonitis, and peptic ulcer disease. In patients with ketoacidosis who are over 40 years of age, one of these disorders is usually the cause of the abdominal distress.

Stupor and coma can complicate ketoacidosis. Recent studies have shown a good correlation between altered mental status and hyperosmolality.

The osmolality of the cerebrospinal fluid is often higher than that of the blood. When the blood osmolality increases rapidly, water is drawn out of the cellular portion of the brain. Cellular dehydration and, presumably, changes in consciousness ensue. Hyperglycemia eventually stimulates the intracellular production of large molecules that cannot diffuse outside the cell. These *idiogenic osmoles*, some of them polyols, allow the brain to resorb water from the extracellular space and become rehydrated.

Coma may also result from cerebral edema in the patient who has been receiving insulin therapy. With insulin therapy, the CSF glucose falls at a slower rate than the blood glucose. If the blood sugar declines too precipitously, water will flow from the plasma to the brain, and the brain cells, which have accumulated nondiffusible idiogenic osmols, will become edematous and swollen. Cerebral edema can be prevented by the judicious use of hypotonic fluids and by careful attention to the blood glucose level, making certain that it does not fall below 250 mg/dl during the first 10 to 12 hours of therapy.

The presence of coma in a diabetic whose initial serum osmolality is less than 340 mOsm/liter suggests that another disorder is also present. Intravascular coagulation and cerebral thromboses occasionally occur in diabetic ketoacidosis, but they are only infrequently the cause of an alteration in mental status.

Precipitants of Diabetic Ketoacidosis. In most series of patients with severe diabetic decompensation, *infection* ranks as the leading cause of ketoacidosis. Infection provokes a rise in the serum cortisol and other ketogenic hormones, and thus raises the body's insulin requirement. Patients who are debilitated and incapable of adjusting their daily insulin injection are at a special risk of developing ketoacidosis when infection supervenes.

It has long been suspected that diabetics are more prone to infection, and experiments showing that phagocytosis of certain gram-positive organisms is diminished in poorly controlled diabetics has added weight to the clinical observations. The possibility of infection must therefore be investigated in all cases of diabetic decompensation. Unfortunately, the typical signs of infection are often masked by the underlying illness. Hypothermia, however, is the rule in ketoacidosis, and a patient with even a normal temperature should be investigated for infection. A leukocytosis of approximately 15,000 with a left shift is common in acidosis uncomplicated by infection, and the tachycardia, hyperventilation, and acidemia of sepsis cannot be distinguished from those of the primary metabolic abnormality.

Other common precipitants of ketoacidosis include pregnancy and the failure to continue insulin therapy. Deliberate withholding of daily insulin is frequently encountered in rebellious adolescents. The stress of a myocardial infarction can induce ketoacidosis, but the infarct may be overlooked when classic anginal symptoms are not present (see Chap. 3). The mortality rate of persons with myocardial infarction and diabetic ketoacidosis is approximately 50% even at centers that specialize in diabetes mellitus.

Evaluating the Patient. When the patient arrives in the emergency room, an initial assessment should be made of the patient's clinical status, his past history—especially if the patient has already been diagnosed as a diabetic—and the testimony of family and friends. Blood should be obtained for arterial blood gases, blood glucose, electrolytes, BUN, creatinine, and a complete blood count. A sample of blood should be tested by Dextrostix for an immediate estimate of blood sugar. Cultures of blood, sputum, urine, and pleural and ascitic fluid (if any) should be obtained regardless of the patient's temperature or leukocyte count. Any alteration in consciousness is an indication for a lumbar puncture, and the CSF should be cultured for fungi and mycobacteria in addition to routine cultures. An electrocardiogram is mandatory to rule out myocardial infarction, and the patient should be placed on constant cardiac monitoring to detect arrhythmias or changes due to hypokalemia or hyperkalemia.

A blood sample should be tested with crushed nitroprusside (Acetest) tablets for the measurement of serum ketones; the value should be expressed as the highest dilution giving a "large" reaction. The nitroprusside reaction measures only acetoacetate reliably. β-Hydroxybutyrate gives a negative test, and the extent of measured ketosis is therefore dependent on the ratio of acetoacetate to β-hydroxybutyrate. This ratio is low when a state of lactic acidosis coexists with ketoacidosis, because the reduced redox potential of lactic acidosis favors production of β-hydroxybutyrate. In this event, the level of ketosis as determined by the nitroprusside reaction appears to be inappropriately low for the degree of acidosis, and the additional diagnosis of lactic acidosis should be considered.

Therapy. The keystones of therapy for diabetic ketoacidosis consist of the prompt administration of intravenous fluids, potassium, and insulin and a thorough search for precipitating causes.

Fluids. Although patients in ketoacidosis are significantly dehydrated, it is not necessary to replace all of the fluid loss immediately. Half of the estimated fluid loss should be repleted within the first four to eight hours. Initially, isotonic saline (0.9%) should be administered in order to restore intravascular volume. Later in therapy, hypotonic solutions should be given since patients will have lost water in excess of sodium during the osmotic diuresis. In young patients without renal or cardiac disease, vigorous hydration should be pursued with careful monitoring of the urinary output.

The measured serum sodium concentration often underestimates the true sodium concentration. Sodium is excluded from the lipemic portion of the serum, which is often substantial in diabetic ketoacidosis. Since "whole" serum is measured, the concentration of sodium in the water phase is artifactually diluted by the lipemic layer.

Potassium. Although potassium losses can be enormous, the serum potassium upon presentation may be above normal. This is often true when the patient is first seen in the early stages of acidosis. Hydrogen ions are buffered intracellularly with a concomitant exchange of potassium ions into the extracellular space, and for each 0.1 unit decline in pH, the serum potassium may be expected to increase by 0.5 to 0.6 mEq/liter. Later in the patient's course, renal compensatory mechanisms result in a large kaliuresis, exacerbated by the elevated levels of aldosterone seen in diabetic ketoacidosis. Acidotic patients who present with normal or low levels of potassium are actually severely total-body depleted, and even those with hyperkalemia at presentation require potassium replacement during the course of therapy. Because of the dangers of cardiac arrhythmias, some clinicians recommend starting potassium replacement with the first liter of fluid. In general, it is safe to withhold

potassium until the initial serum level has been determined or until the second liter of intravenous fluid has been given. By that time, dilution, insulin, and the improving acid-base balance have had time to lower the potassium from potentially dangerously high levels. The electrocardiogram can be useful in diagnosing hyperkalemia (large peaked T waves, widened QRS complex) or hypokalemia (flat T waves, U waves).

During the course of therapy, potassium enters the cells as the pH rises, and potassium levels continue to fall. Potassium retention is facilitated by bolus insulin therapy and bicarbonate administration, but if a low-dose insulin protocol is used, much of the potassium that is administered will be excreted in the urine. Patients therefore require several days of oral potassium supplementation following the restoration of their metabolic balance.

Insulin. Insulin therapy should be instituted as soon as the diagnosis of diabetic ketoacidosis is made. Previously, it had been recommended that a patient in diabetic ketoacidosis receive 50 to 100 units of regular insulin intravenously and a similar amount subcutaneously upon presentation; additional large boluses of insulin would then be given every one or two hours until the ketoacidotic state cleared. This regimen was effective, and patients in diabetic ketoacidosis tolerated such enormous doses well. However, recent studies of the effectiveness of low-dose insulin protocols indicate that such massive doses are not necessary.

Whether given by constant intravenous infusion or by hourly intramuscular injections, low-dose insulin therapy has several advantages over high-dose therapy:

1. The incidence of hypoglycemia is greatly diminished. In the first hour of therapy, the blood sugar will fall approximately 50 mg/dl with hydration alone. A steady decrease of 75

to 100 mg/dl/hour usually can be achieved with a constant infusion of insulin.

2. The risk of hypokalemia during the period of ketoacidosis is decreased. High levels of insulin cause an influx of potassium into cells, sometimes resulting in severe hypokalemia. Patients treated with low-dose insulin are usually spared this danger, but they do require larger amounts of supplemental potassium in the days following recovery from the ketoacidotic state.

3. Therapy is greatly simplified. Once an hourly dose of insulin has been shown to be effective, it can be continued unchanged, since each patient's rate of fall of blood sugar is fairly constant.

Recommended therapy consists of a low-dose constant infusion of insulin given by a pediatric infusion drip. The plastic tubing should first be rinsed with 50 ml of the insulin-containing solution in order to saturate the nonspecific insulin-binding properties of the plastic. Insulin should then be administered at a rate of 5 to 10 units per hour. Some authorities recommend preceding the infusion with a bolus intravenous injection of 10 to 20 units of insulin in order to bring the blood level of insulin immediately to a maximally effective range, but others argue that a high blood insulin level can trigger the release of counterregulatory hormones and exacerbate the ketosis.

Repeated measurements of serum ketones should be made during the course of therapy. The failure of measured ketonemia to decline in the face of a rising pH and falling blood sugar should not necessarily be cause for alarm. β-Hydroxybutyrate levels fall rather rapidly, but this change is not detected by the nitroprusside reaction. In addition, β-hydroxybutyrate can be metabolized into acetoacetate, giving the false impression that the ketosis is worsening.

Where constant infusions are impractical and where intensive monitoring cannot be achieved, the intramuscular approach offers a good alternative. An intravenous loading dose of insulin is necessary, and should be followed by hourly injections of approximately ten units of regular insulin.

Modified (NPH or Lente) insulin should not be employed in the initial treatment of ketoacidosis. Subcutaneous regular insulin is slowly and erratically absorbed in the dehydrated ketoacidotic patient, and this route of insulin administration should be avoided during the throes of ketoacidosis.

During the first hours of therapy, measurements of blood sugar, ketones, and pH should be made frequently. If treatment is not succeeding, the hourly dose of insulin should be increased. Intravenous insulin therapy should be continued for 24 hours or until the patient is able to eat. It is vital that insulin therapy not be discontinued when the blood sugar returns to the normal range, since the hormone is still required to reverse the ketotic diathesis. When the blood sugar falls to approximately 250 mg/dl, a dextrose infusion should be added to the fluid regimen in order to prevent hypoglycemia and should be maintained until the patient is able to eat. Subcutaneous modified insulin should be started on the morning that the patient begins to eat, while he is still receiving the low dose infusion. The constant infusion can be discontinued later that morning. If the insulin is not continued in this manner, the patient may again rebound and go into ketoacidosis.

Phosphate. Phosphate depletion can also complicate the therapy of diabetic ketoacidosis. Phosphate, a major intracellular anion, leaves the cells in acidemia and is excreted in the urine. The catabolic diathesis of diabetic decompensation further augments phosphate loss. Patients in diabetic ketoacidosis may have normal, low, or high serum levels of phosphate, but all are total body depleted. There are at present no studies supporting the value of early phosphate replacement in ketoacidosis. Phosphate repletion will be achieved within two to three days, when the patient resumes a normal diet.

Alkali. In most patients, bicarbonate administration is unnecessary. It can only be recommended in cases of severe acidemia (pH less than 7.1), or when its use is mandated by the development of cardiac arrhythmias or hypotension refractory to large volume replacement. If substantial exogenous bicarbonate has been administered, a rebound alkalosis can result after ketone production is halted and the ketoacids are metabolized. By forcing potassium to reenter the extracellular space, alkali therapy worsens hypokalemia. Bicarbonate therapy is accompanied by a large sodium load, a potential danger in patients with a history of congestive heart failure.

Bicarbonate therapy can also produce a paradoxic CSF acidosis even as the arterial pH is becoming normal. As the administered bicarbonate buffers the systemic acid, the peripheral stimulus for hyperventilation is diminished and the Pa_{CO_2} rises. Carbon dioxide diffuses readily into the brain, and the carbon dioxide tension of the CSF also rises, but without benefit of buffering from the exogenous bicarbonate, which crosses the blood–brain barrier only slowly. Thus, the elevated Pa_{CO_2} causes a CSF acidosis, which, it has been theorized, can result in diminished consciousness.

Additional Therapeutic Maneuvers. Infection is a principal source of morbidity in diabetic ketoacidosis. Meticulous intensive care and the availability of potent antibiotics have played a large part in limiting infectious complications. Catheterization of the urinary bladder is an obvious necessity in the comatose patient, but should be avoided in conscious patients unless they are truly unable to void. Thrombotic disease is now recognized as complicating the care of diabetic ketoacidosis, and infirm patients who will be bedridden for more than one or two days may benefit from some mode of anticoagulation.

Mortality. With the institution of intensive care for patients in diabetic ketoacidosis, the mortality rate has dropped to approximately 10% in major hospital centers. In smaller institutions, where constant surveillance is impossible, the mortality is higher. The prognosis for recovery is especially poor in the elderly and in those who are unconscious, hypotensive, or bradycardic. The levels of hyperglycemia, hyperosmalality, and azotemia correlate with increasing mortality, whereas the extent of ketosis and acidosis does not appear to carry a similar risk. With proper management, patients only rarely succumb to their metabolic abnormalities, and most deaths result from precipitating or coexisting illnesses.

Hyperosmolar Coma

In the elderly patient, diabetic decompensation can take a form quite different from ketoacidosis. Patients are extremely dehydrated upon presentation, and have enormously elevated blood sugars, with values sometimes exceeding 2000 mg/dl. Serum ketones, however, are absent or measurable only in trace amounts. Acidosis, if present, is mild.

Little is known about the etiology and pathogenesis of hyperosmolar coma. It has been postulated that the pancreatic beta cells are able to synthesize and release into the portal circulation only enough insulin to prime the liver (that is, sufficient to stimulate hepatic glycogen synthesis), and to guide free fatty acids into triglyceride rather than ketone synthesis, but insufficient to escape degradation in the liver. The peripheral circulation is thus left without adequate insulin levels; gluconeogenesis is stimulated, peripheral glucose utilization is inhibited, and serum glucose levels rise.

In contrast to the short prodome of ketoacidosis, patients with hyperosmolar coma usually have been ill for many days, complaining of polyuria and polydipsia. In most cases, a severe illness triggers the hyperglycemia; pneumonia and other infections, renal failure, and gastrointestinal hemorrhage are frequent precipitants. Numerous drugs, especially the thiazide diuretics and steroids, and the stress of surgery in conjunction with an increased glucose load have also been implicated as causes of hyperosmolar coma.

Diagnosis. The diagnosis of hyperosmolar coma is rarely obvious, and unless considered early may be missed for many hours. Kussmaul respirations and fruity breath are not present. The prolonged period of hyperglycemia and the consequent osmotic diuresis may result in profound dehydration and prerenal azotemia. Hemoconcentration results in an artifactually high hematocrit and promotes sludging and intravascular thrombosis. The dehydration may not be obvious, however, since the urine output may appear normal because of the osmotic diuresis.

Patients with hyperosmolar coma are often obtuded, confused, or stuporous, and focal neurologic signs are not unusual. As is true with diabetic ketoacidosis, the level of consciousness upon presentation is a function of the degree of hyperosmolality. Cerebrovascular accident is a common initial diagnosis suggested by the presence of paresis, aphasia, and Babinski signs. Focal seizures that are refractory to anticonvulsive therapy may fur-

ther complicate the diagnosis. If routine therapy with the anticonvulsive phenytoin is initiated, hyperglycemia may worsen, since phenytoin inhibits insulin release. A host of other neurologic signs have been described, and electroencephalographic abnormalities may also be found. With therapy and the return of serum osmolality to normal, most neurologic abnormalities vanish.

The serum osmolality in hyperosmolar coma is generally much higher than in diabetic ketoacidosis. The blood sugar is almost always greater than 600 mg/dl, a figure infrequently reached in diabetic ketoacidosis, and the serum sodium is also higher because of the greater water loss.

Therapy. The most important aspects of therapy for patients with hyperosmolar coma are rehydration and treatment for the underlying disease. Great caution must be exercised in the administration of insulin, since many of these patients are extremely sensitive to its action and are prone to hypoglycemia. Hyperosmolar coma is an ideal situation for low-dose insulin therapy. With volume replacement alone, the blood sugar drops dramatically and much more quickly than in diabetic ketoacidosis. Potassium depletion also occurs, but is not as profound as in ketoacidosis.

Mortality in hyperosmolar coma is high. Most deaths are attributable to the severe underlying illness.

Lactic Acidosis

Although lactic acidosis is not limited to the diabetic population, it has an increased prevalence among diabetics (see also Chap. 21). Treatment consists of volume replacement, administration of alkali, and a careful search for an underlying illness. If there is coexisting hyperglycemia or ketoacidosis, insulin use is mandatory.

CHRONIC COMPLICATIONS OF DIABETES MELLITUS

Renal Failure

Chronic renal failure is a major problem in adult onset diabetes, and it is the leading cause of death in juvenile onset diabetes. At autopsy, 25% of diabetic kidneys reveal the Kimmelstiel-Wilson lesion, a nodular glomerulosclerosis consisting of acidophilic, spherical, hyaline glomerular lesions. Diffuse hyaline thickening of the glomerular capillary basement membrane is also seen, and may be pathologically more significant. Anteriolarsclerosis, microaneurysms, and interstitial cellular infiltration may also be prominent.

Other causes of uremia in the diabetic include papillary necrosis and a neurogenic bladder. The latter is a common manifestation of diabetic neuropathy, and the consequent urinary stasis can give rise to urinary tract infections. An ascending, chronic pyelonephritis can develop, eventually leading to renal failure.

In patients with the Kimmelstiel-Wilson lesion, proteinuria, especially albuminuria, is usually the first clinical sign of renal pathology. Proteinuria occurs on the average of 15 to 17 years after the onset of diabetes, and the mean survival thereafter is less than 5 years. Although both dialysis and renal transplantation are feasible in diabetics, the prognosis with both modalities is somewhat worse than in nondiabetic patients with a comparable degree of renal failure.

Diabetics with only mild renal insufficiency face a host of potential iatrogenic catastrophes during hospitalization for other, unrelated problems. Diabetics with stable, mild, chronic renal failure are at a markedly increased risk of developing acute renal failure following routine radiologic angiographic procedures, including coronary angiography, aortography, and intravenous pyelography.

Juvenile onset diabetics, young patients, and those with severe renal failure (serum creatinine greater than 5 mg/dl) also have an increased risk from dye studies. The acute decompensation may be oliguric or nonoliguric and usually lasts three to five days. In a significant proportion of patients, however, the creatinine clearance does not return to baseline.

Special care should therefore be taken to monitor all diabetics with renal failure who must undergo angiographic procedures, especially those whose serum creatinine is greater than 5 mg/dl. The capability for emergency dialysis must be available.

Insulin, which is filtered, resorbed proximally, and then degraded by the kidney, has an increased half-life in renal failure, and insulin requirements decline during acute renal failure.

Neuropathy

A wide variety of neurologic lesions are included under the rubric of diabetic neuropathy. Many researchers believe that some forms of neuropathy can be alleviated by maintaining "tight" diabetic control. Others, however, have pointed out that neuropathy often occurs despite excellent control.

Neuropathy can be the initial presentation of diabetes. The most common lesion is a bilateral, symmetric sensory impairment usually found in the lower extremities. There is a decreased response to pin-prick and absent or diminished knee and ankle jerks. Patients complain of pain and paresthesias, particularly a burning sensation on the soles of the feet that commonly occurs at night. "Neuropathic" painless ulcers may appear on the soles of the feet. Because vascular insufficiency of the lower extremities is also very common in diabetes, these ulcers can easily become infected. The vascular and neuropathic insufficiency in the diabetic foot may make antibiotic therapy very difficult. Even "trivial" infections may not respond, and gangrene is a constant threat. Many patients eventually require lower extremity amputations. The critical importance of foot care must be emphasized, and the advice of a podiatrist should be sought for aged or infirm patients.

Because patients may unknowingly traumatize their relatively "anesthetic" feet, the tarsal and ankle joints may become destroyed, resulting in the dramatically puffy, but painless, *Charcot joints.*

Upper extremity lesions are less commonly seen in diabetes mellitus, although some patients may experience atrophy of the interosseous muscles of the hands. Radiculopathies have been known to mimic abdominal crises.

Mononeuropathy may present as a lesion of a single nerve (simplex) or of several nerves (multiplex). Mononeuropathy is caused by infarction of the blood vessels supplying the nerve. Any nerve may be affected. Mononeuropathy is heralded by the sudden onset of severe pain and there may be signs of muscle wasting. Involvement of the cranial nerves can cause Bell's palsy and extraocular muscle palsies. The third nerve palsy caused by diabetes classically spares pupillary function. Although recovery from mononeuropathy can take several months, the prognosis is excellent for full recovery of function.

The gastrointestinal tract can also be affected by neuropathy. In *gastroparesis diabeticorum,* emptying of the stomach is delayed, and patients may appear to have gastric outlet obstruction. Syndromes of hyperemesis and intractable diarrhea in diabetics have also been ascribed to autonomic neuropathy. Although 50% of diabetic men become impotent on the basis of diabetic autonomic neuropathy, diabetic women do not suffer any decrement in sexual interest or orgasmic performance. Cardiac neuropathies are discussed in a following section.

Retinopathy

Blindness is ten times more common in the diabetic population than in the normal population. Although diabetics have an increased incidence of open-angle glaucoma, the most common cause of blindness is retinopathy. Approximately 90% of patients develop retinopathy within 25 years of the onset of diabetes.

Any retinal lesion can cause some loss of vision. Ophthalmologists divide retinopathy into two broad categories: nonproliferative (background) and proliferative. Nonproliferative changes are seen earlier, and the first indication of retinopathy is the development of dilated venules and microaneurysms. Individual aneurysms can persist for months or years, and may be associated with small hemorrhages; the hemorrhages usually resorb within weeks. Retinal edema and exudates (shiny white or yellow lesions) may also be present.

Proliferative retinopathy is more likely to cause blindness: 25% of patients with proliferative changes are blind. Proliferative retinopathy is associated with diabetic nephropathy and coronary artery disease, and the average survival is less than six years from the onset of proliferative disease. Neovascularization is the hallmark of proliferative retinopathy. New vessels may sprout anywhere on the surface of the retina. These vessels have little supporting connective tissue, and are liable to hemorrhage. Glial proliferation about the new vessels soon follows. Eventually, the repeated hemorrhaging and subsequent fibrosis results in vitreoretinal traction and segmental retinal detachment, resulting in some loss of vision. Neovascularization of the optic disk carries a very poor prognosis.

Most lesions can be delineated with an ophthalmoscope, aided by slit-lamp examination. Fluorescein angiography, in which dye is injected intravenously and enlarged photographs are taken of the retina, can clarify the extent of retinopathy.

Ameliorative therapy is now available. Randomized controlled studies have shown that the application of xenon or argon laser photocoagulation to retinas with proliferative retinopathy can reduce the development of severe visual loss and inhibit the progression of the retinopathy. Laser therapy reduces the incidence of vitreous hemorrhages. Hypophysectomy is occasionally performed when photocoagulation has failed to halt the downhill course of retinopathy.

Although retinopathy is rarely present at the onset of diabetes, a baseline ophthalmologic examination should be scheduled within several months of diagnosis. The blurred vision that is commonly present in new onset diabetics is caused by osmotic changes in the lens and gradually resolves as the hyperglycemia is controlled.

Cardiovascular Complications

The major cardiovascular complications of diabetes mellitus derive from atherosclerotic vascular disease and autonomic neuropathy. Both large and small vessels are involved. Small vessel disease is most prominent in renal and retinal lesions. In the lower extremities, clinical syndromes of vascular insufficiency, such as claudication, are more often caused by small vessel disease in the diabetic than in the nondiabetic. As a result, surgical amelioration (peripheral bypass surgery) is more difficult.

Diabetics have an increased risk of coronary atherosclerosis, and approximately 50% of adult onset diabetics succumb to coronary disease or its sequelae. The increased risk of cardiovascular disease is twofold in men and nearly threefold in women. Diabetes in females is a more important risk factor for the development of cardiovascular disease than cigarette smoking, whereas diabetes is only

a minor risk factor in men; the normal male predominance in cardiovascular morbidity and mortality is not found in the diabetic population.

There are probably several reasons why diabetics are susceptible to atherosclerotic disease. Many diabetics, especially those with adult onset disease, have hyperlipidemia (no particular pattern predominates) and are obese. High-density lipoprotein, high levels of which are correlated with a decreased risk of coronary disease, is lower in diabetics of both sexes.

Diabetics also have abnormalities of platelet function, and it has been suggested that much of their coronary artery disease may be attributed to a hypercoagulable state. *In vitro* tests of platelets taken from diabetics show them to have a low threshold for aggregation and an accelerated aggregating response to adenosine diphosphate (ADP), collagen, and epinephrine. Platelet turnover is increased, and prostaglandin E secretion is elevated. Serum fibrinogen and Von Willebrand's factor also are frequently above normal.

Small vessel disease has also been implicated in diabetic cardiac illness. Microaneurysms, a hallmark of diabetic small vessel disease, have been found at autopsy in diabetic hearts. Diffuse small vessel disease of the coronary vessels has been implicated in the congestive heart failure of "diabetic cardiomyopathy."

The high proportion of myocardial infarctions in diabetics that are silent are probably due to neuropathy of the cardiac nerves. Autopsy reveals changes in both sympathetic and parasympathetic cardiac nerves that are similar to the neuropathic changes seen in the bladder and elsewhere. Diabetic autonomic neuropathy is manifested by a resting tachycardia and the absence of the normal beat-to-beat variation of sinus rhythm. Many patients lack the normal baroreceptor reflexes, and thus do not display the normal increase in heart rate after standing or slowing of heart rate after the Valsalva maneuver. As a result, hypotension and syncope may occur.

• • •

Tight control has been advocated in the hope of totally ameliorating and preventing the renal, retinal, neurologic, and cardiovascular sequelae of diabetes. Several centers are now experimenting with a pump that provides a constant low-dose infusion of regular insulin. The pump is worn on a belt and the insulin is delivered via a small-bore butterfly needle inserted into the subcutaneous tissue of the abdomen. The rate of flow can be adjusted so that more insulin can be administered prior to meals. Extremely tight control can be achieved with this pump, and abnormalities in serum amino acids, cortisol, and other hormones are nearly totally abolished. It is still too soon to know whether end organ damage can be lessened with this new therapeutic tool.

BIBLIOGRAPHY

Alberti KG, Hockaday TDR: Diabetic coma: A reappraisal after five years. Clin Endocrin Metab 6:421–455, 1977

Amery A, Bulpitt C, deSchaepdryver A et al: Glucose intolerance during diuretic therapy. Lancet 1:681–683, 1978

Boden G, Master RW, Gordon SS et al: Monitoring metabolic control in diabetic outpatients with glycosylated hemoglobin. Ann Intern Med 92:357–360, 1980

Ellenberg M: Diabetic neuropathy: Clinical aspects. Metabolism 25:1627–1655, 1976

Kannel WB, McGee DL: Diabetes and cardiovascular disease: The Frammingham study. JAMA 241:2035–2038, 1979

Kreisberg RA: Diabetic ketoacidosis: New concepts and trends in pathogenesis and treatment. Ann Intern Med 88:681–695, 1978

Kussman MJ, Goldstein HH, Gleason RE: The clinical course of diabetic nephropathy. JAMA 236:1861–1864, 1976

Miranda PM, Horwitz DL: High-fiber diets in the treatment of diabetes millitus. Ann Intern Med 88:482–486, 1978

Morse PH, Duncan TG: Ophthalmologic management of diabetic retinopathy. N Engl J Med 295:87–90, 1976

Pickup JC, Keen H, Parsons JA et al: Continuous subcutaneous insulin infusion: Improved blood-glucose and intermediary-metabolite control in diabetics. Lancet 1:1255–1257, 1979

Weinrauch LA, Healy RW, Leland OS et al: Decreased insulin requirement in acute renal failure in diabetic nephropathy. Arch Intern Med 138:399–402, 1978

31

Hypoglycemia

Hypoglycemia is a frequently encountered and readily treated metabolic derangement. Unfortunately, the diagnosis is often delayed because the symptoms may be vague, often appearing psychiatric in origin. The spectrum of symptoms is broad, ranging from palpitations and mild anxiety to coma.

Hypoglycemia may occur in both fasting and well-fed individuals. In patients presenting in the emergency room, drug overdose (including insulin) is the most common precipitating factor. In the hospitalized patient, overzealous administration of insulin is probably the prime offender. Hypoglycemic episodes may also stem from alcoholism or from insulin-secreting tumors. Patients critically ill with hepatic insufficiency, congestive heart failure, or Addisonian crisis may also demonstrate symptomatic hypoglycemia. Other patients have alimentary or "functional" hypoglycemia, both of which are characterized by low blood sugar in the postprandial state.

THE NORMAL REGULATION OF GLUCOSE LEVELS

The liver is responsible for maintaining euglycemia between meals. Within 8 hours after a meal, elevated blood levels of glucose, amino acids, and lipids have returned to baseline levels. In order to maintain euglycemia during prolonged fasts, the body requires active gluconeogenesis, since the liver provides at most only a 24-hour store of glycogen. The liver's ability to manufacture glucose depends upon the availability of nutrient substrates—primarily amino acids—and the proper hormonal milieu, especially the balance between insulin and glucagon. Thus, hypoglycemia may occur (1) when adequate substrates are not ingested (or are not presented to the liver), (2) with hepatic dysfunction, when glycogenolysis and gluconeogenesis are impaired, and (3) as a result of a hormonal imbalance.

A precise definition of hypoglycemia has not been established. Although most laboratories consider 65 to 70 mg/dl the lower limit of normal for blood sugar, healthy subjects frequently maintain blood sugars far lower without noting any symptoms of hypoglycemia. Women in particular are unable to maintain their blood sugars in the "normal" range while fasting. A recent study has suggested that the lower limit of normal blood sugar after a 24-hour fast should be 30–40 mg/dl for women and 50 mg/dl for men. (The plasma glucose is 10–15% higher than the corresponding level of blood glucose.)

235

SIGNS AND SYMPTOMS OF HYPOGLYCEMIA

The symptoms of hypoglycemia often depend upon the rate of fall of the blood sugar and the duration of hypoglycemia more than upon the actual level. Patients with islet cell tumors frequently tolerate blood sugars that are chronically in the range of 30 to 40 mg/dl without apparent ill effects. On the other hand, diabetics who are accustomed to blood sugars in the hyperglycemic range may demonstrate symptomatic hypoglycemia when the blood sugar falls precipitously into the normal range.

As the blood sugar plummets, there is an immediate release of the counterregulatory hormones, epinephrine, cortisol, glucagon, and growth hormone. This stage of hypoglycemia, the *adrenergic stage*, is characterized by palpitations, tachycardia, diaphoresis, anxiety, hyperventilation, shakiness, weakness, hunger, and nausea.

When the hypoglycemic episode is prolonged and the brain is receiving less than the required 80 mg of glucose per minute, neuropsychiatric symptoms predominate. In this *cortical stage*, disorientation, hallucinations, bizarre behavior, and fugue-like states are seen. Convulsions, hypothermia, paresis, and abnormal and primitive reflexes, such as the Babinski sign, may appear next and mimic primary neurologic disease. Focal neurologic deficits can resemble a stroke. If the low blood glucose is allowed to persist, extensive permanent neurologic sequelae can result. Repeated hypoglycemic episodes can cause severe intellectual impairment and progressive dementia, and unless the diagnosis of hypoglycemia is considered, the opportunity for effective treatment and cure will be lost.

With prolonged and profound hypoglycemia, a *medullary stage* eventually ensues, consisting of bradycardia, diminished respiratory rate, pupillary dilatation, coma, and, eventually death.

• • •

Hypoglycemia is encountered in patients who are fasted (or malnourished) as well as in patients who are eating normally. In considering the etiology of low blood sugar, the patient's general nutritional status must be carefully determined. Patients with diabetes mellitus, alcoholism, severe systemic diseases, and malignancies may experience hypoglycemia after a period of fasting or starvation, but these patients may also suffer hypoglycemic episodes soon after they are fed. On the other hand, those patients with reactive and alimentary hypoglycemia have symptomatic low blood sugars only in the postprandial (fed) state.

HYPOGLYCEMIA IN THE DIABETIC PATIENT

Causes

Insulin. Hypoglycemia in the insulin-dependent diabetic may be seen in both the fasting and the fed states. It is usually the result of skipping a meal or of failing to titrate the insulin dose downward on a day when the patient is engaging in vigorous exercise. Diabetics who attempt to achieve "tight" control (see Chap. 30) should expect frequent hypoglycemic attacks. These can usually be aborted in the adrenergic stage with a carbohydrate snack. However, patients with severe diabetic neuropathy may fail to manifest anxiety or tachycardia, and thus may not recognize the early warning signs of hypoglycemia. In most cases, the etiology of hypoglycemia in a diabetic is obvious. The patient can be treated with a rapid intravenous infusion of a 50% dextrose solution, sent home, and advised to consume an adequate diet. It is nevertheless important to obtain a careful history and determine why the patient failed to maintain a sufficient caloric intake; anorexia may be a symptom reflecting a serious underlying illness, particularly uremia or infection. The patient's visual acuity should be routinely tested to eliminate the possibility of inadvertent insulin overdose because of gradually worsening eyesight or a sudden major retinal hemorrhage.

A common iatrogenic cause of in-hospital hypoglycemia is failure to adjust the insulin dose in a diabetic with deteriorating renal function. As the glomerular filtration rate declines, so does the daily insulin requirement, in part because of the increased half-life of plasma insulin. The relationship between the glomerular filtration rate and insulin dose is by no means a linear one, and frequent sampling of the blood sugar is necessary. In patients with significant renal failure, estimates of urinary glucose become unreliable.

Sulfonylureas. Sulfonylureas are oral hypoglycemic agents that stimulate the islet cells to secrete insulin. Unlike the acute hypoglycemia of an insulin overdose, sulfonylurea-induced hypoglycemia can occur in patients who have been taking the medication in low doses for many months and who have neither increased their dosage nor decreased their caloric intake. The extreme danger of sulfonylurea hypoglycemia is twofold: the blood sugar is often greatly depressed, and the duration of action of these agents is extremely long. Chlorpropamide, the drug that has been implicated most often, has a serum half-life of approximately one and one-half days, and a duration of action that may extend beyond 60 hours. The hypoglycemia may be extremely refractory to treatment, and multiple ampules of concentrated intravenous dextrose solution may be needed. All these patients must therefore be hospitalized. The oral hypoglycemic agent should not be prescribed again, and insulin therapy, if necessary, should be instituted.

Propranolol. Propranolol is a β-blocking agent used in the treatment of hypertension, angina, thyrotoxicosis, and migraine. It has been reported to cause hypoglycemia in both the fasting and nonfasting states. Because of their increased incidence of cardiac disease, diabetics are frequently treated with propranolol. β-blockade can mask all the symptoms of the adrenergic stage of hypoglycemia, with the exception of sweating, and propranolol thus makes the diabetic vulnerable to the insidious onset of insulin coma.

HYPOGLYCEMIA IN THE ALCOHOLIC PATIENT

Alcoholics account for more than one-third of all drug-induced episodes of hypoglycemia. The precise pathophysiologic mechanism of alcohol-induced hypoglycemia is not fully understood. Ethanol does suppress hepatic gluconeogenesis by altering the availability of necessary cofactors within the hepatocyte. In addition, hepatic glycogen stores may be depleted in individuals who consume no nutrients other than ethanol. Although malnutrition may be a contributing factor in some instances, well-nourished individuals of all ages—whether chronic drinkers, binge drinkers, or simply occasional drinkers—are at risk of developing ethanol-induced hypoglycemia.

It is always important for therapeutic reasons to distinguish hypoglycemic coma from a drunken stupor (see Chap. 61). Alcohol-related hypoglycemia generally presents as stupor or coma several hours after drinking. The blood ethanol level is frequently below the intoxicating range of 150 mg/dl. Hypoglycemia can, however, occur in the midst of a drinking spree, and the presence of an alcoholic odor on an unconscious patient's breath does not rule out the possibility of hypoglycemic coma. Furthermore, the patient may pass imperceptibly from an alcoholic coma into a hypoglycemic coma.

Hypoglycemia may occasionally present as an agitated delusional state, and can then be confused with numerous syndromes frequently seen in the alcoholic patient: acute intoxication, alcohol withdrawal syndrome, the Wernicke-Korsakoff syndrome, hepatic encephalopathy, meningitis, subdural hematoma, and subarachnoid hemorrhage. Therefore, any alcoholic patient with altered mental status should receive intravenous glucose after a blood sample is obtained for a glucose determination, and after the patient has received 100 mg of intravenous thiamine. The latter will prevent the precipitation of an acute Wernicke's encephalopathy that can occur in starved patients who are given a glucose load. Rarely, alcoholic hypoglycemia is refractory, and prolonged intravenous infusions of dextrose are occasionally required. Thus, all patients suspected of having alcohol-induced hypoglycemia must be hospitalized.

HYPOGLYCEMIA IN PATIENTS WITH SEVERE SYSTEMIC DISEASE AND NON-ISLET CELL MALIGNANCIES

A hypoglycemic episode occurring in a severely ill, hospitalized patient may be the result of inadequate nutrition and depleted hepatic glycogen stores. It is not uncommon for patients to receive only 300 to 600 calories per day (in the form of 5% dextrose intravenous solutions) for a period of several weeks as they languish with acute or chronic illness.

Patients with certain severe illnesses are at special risk:

1. Severe liver disease results in a marked diminution or frank absence of liver glycogen stores and in the functional impairment of gluconeogenesis. Hence, the patient is unable to maintain an adequate fasting blood sugar. Although this difficulty is usually encountered with fulminant hepatic failure in patients with viral hepatitis, it may also be seen in the more common alcoholic and cardiac cirrhoses.

2. Hypoglycemia may be seen in severe congestive heart failure and uremia.

3. A glucocorticoid-dependent patient who fails to receive steroid replacement may have symptomatic hypoglycemia during an Addisonian crisis.

4. Nonpancreatic neoplasms have occasionally been associated with hypoglycemia. Most of these tumors are bulky sarcomas located in the abdomen, thorax, or retroperitoneal area, although numerous other tumors, including hepatomas, have also been implicated. The etiology of hypoglycemia is often multifactorial. Mechanisms include (1) the production of an insulin-like peptide, or a substance that interferes with hepatic gluconeogenesis, and (2) metastatic invasion of the liver.

INSULINOMA

Insulin-secreting pancreatic islet cell adenomas (insulinomas) are the most common of the pancreatic islet cell tumors. They may be seen in association with parathyroid and pituitary neoplasms in the familial multiple endocrine neoplasia, type I syndrome. The tumor, however, is very rare, with an incidence of less than 1 in 100,000. In more than 75% of patients, the insulinoma is not malignant.

Patients who have recurrent episodes of symptomatic fasting hypoglycemia should be suspected of having an insulinoma. Such patients occasionally have repeated hypoglycemic seizures.

The diagnosis is made by finding a depressed blood glucose and an elevated insulin level. Often, the patient must be fasted for 24 to 72 hours before symptomatic hypoglycemia is elicited; a two-hour exercise period at the end of the fast may uncover still other cases. An exaggerated insulin response can be provoked by an intravenous challenge of tolbutamide, leucine, or glucagon, but these tests can be dangerous and they are relatively nonspecific. The level of serum proinsulin is usually markedly increased.

Therapy involves surgical excision of the tumor. Frequently, however, widespread metastases, microadenomas, or severe β-cell hyperplasia are found at exploration. Diazoxide, in conjunction with a thiazide diuretic, has a demonstrable and persistent euglycemic effect in such patients. The most promising antineoplastic agent is streptozotocin, an antibiotic with destructive affinity for the islands of Langerhans.

Factitious hypoglycemia (pharmacologically self-induced hypoglycemia) should be suspected in patients who have access to insulin (especially medical personnel and diabetics) who present with a syndrome suggestive of insulinoma, *i.e.*, recurrent episodes of fasting hypoglycemia. When they are hypoglycemic, their insulin levels are also high. Repeated injections of insulin, which is of bovine or porcine origin, will usually result in the formation of serum antibodies to the foreign antigen. Thus, the presence of insulin antibodies in a non-insulin-dependent diabetic is strong evidence for insulin abuse, but there are patients who have antibodies to their own insulin who also have hypoglycemic attacks. Levels of serum connecting-peptide (C-peptide), a cleavage product of normal proinsulin metabolism, are increased in insulinoma but depressed in factitious disease; the hypoglycemia caused by the exogenous insulin inhibits endogenous insulin and C-peptide release. Bovine and porcine insulin C-peptides do not cross-react with the human peptide in the radioimmunoassay.

Hypoglycemia caused by sulfonylurea abuse is readily diagnosed by a toxic screen.

REACTIVE HYPOGLYCEMIA

It is not certain that reactive, postprandial hypoglycemia is a *bona fide* medical syndrome. Our understanding of this "disease" is obscured by the vagueness of its definition. In essence, the diagnosis is made when typical hypoglycemic symptoms, representing both the adrenergic and cortical stages, occur several hours after a meal and when a simultaneous blood sugar determination is low. As in fasting states, the precise definition of *low* is a matter of debate, since many people tolerate very low blood sugars (in the range of 35–40 mg/dl) without any symptoms at all. Some authorities use a blood sugar determination of 45 mg/dl as the cut-off point. Others have recommended that a further requirement for diagnosis should be the presence of elevated ("stress") levels of serum cortisol soon after the blood sugar has reached its lowest point.

The diagnosis is usually confirmed by a 5-hour oral glucose tolerance test (OGTT). A normal OGTT curve often shows a period of relative hypoglycemia (*i.e.*, a blood sugar below fasting levels, although often within the normal range) several hours after the glucose challenge. At that point, cortisol, epinephrine, and glucagon are released, and the blood sugar increases again. In reactive hypoglycemia, there is a discordance of insulin release and an exaggeration of the hypoglycemic portion of the curve.

The cause of postprandial hypoglycemia in most patients cannot be determined. A subset of patients with latent diabetes shows an early hyperglycemic phase after oral glucose, followed by late hypoglycemia secondary to a delayed output of insulin. This defect in the timing of insulin release may be a prodrome of frank diabetes mellitus.

The symptomatology of hypoglycemia has been discussed at great length in the lay press. More and more patients are recognizing these symptoms in themselves, making a self-diagnosis of reactive hypoglycemia, and treating themselves with the hypoglycemic diets (multiple small feedings) recommended in newspapers and magazines. In most patients, the symptoms are not due to hypoglycemia, but rather to anxiety or nervousness. This constellation of symptoms has been dubbed "non-hypoglycemia."

ALIMENTARY HYPOGLYCEMIA

Approximately one-third of patients who have undergone gastrectomy, gastrojejunostomy, or pyloroplasty and vagotomy, especially those with a Billroth II anastamosis, develop a *dumping syndrome*, consisting of abdominal fullness, nausea, weakness, and palpitations within the first hour of eating. These symptoms are occasionally followed over the next several hours by symptoms of the adrenergic stage of hypoglycemia. Without a normal pyloric sphincter mechanism, there is rapid emptying of food into the small bowel and premature unregulated absorption of glucose. An exaggerated insulin release potentiated by gut glucoreceptors and, perhaps, a gastrointestinal peptide hormone are thought to be responsible for the development of hypoglycemia. The majority of patients adjust and become asymptomatic within several months. Reconstructive surgery involving interposition of the reversed jejunal segment between the stomach and the duodenum has been successful in some refractory cases.

A high-protein diet of multiple small feedings that is free of simple sugars has been the mainstay of therapy. Anticholinergic medications may also alleviate some of the symptoms.

THERAPY

Hypoglycemia must be considered in every patient who presents in coma. In most instances, hypoglycemic coma can be distinguished clinically from other forms of coma. For example, the coma of ketoacidosis is marked by fruity breath and hyperventilation.

Occasionally, however, the diagnosis is difficult, and it has therefore become common practice to give all comatose patients an intravenous glucose challenge. The sugar in a standard 50 ml therapeutic test dose of concentrated dextrose does not cause a clinically significant increase in the blood sugar in a patient with hyperosmolar coma, but usually arouses the hypoglycemic patient.

The only patients at risk from a concentrated glucose infusion are diabetics who also suffer from hypoaldosteronism. These patients, who lack both sufficient insulin and aldosterone, can neither efficiently excrete potassium into the urine nor reabsorb it into the intracellular space. In the acute hypertonic state caused by hyperglycemia, there is an efflux of water into the extracellular space that is accompanied by potassium, and serum potassium levels in these patients can reach dangerously high levels. As a result, in these patients, glucose administration can cause or exacerbate hyperkalemia. It is therefore a sensible precaution to monitor the EKG while glucose is being administered, watching carefully for the peaked T waves characteristic of sudden elevations of serum potassium.

BIBLIOGRAPHY

Fajans SS, Floyd JC Jr: Fasting hypoglycemia in adults. N Engl J Med 294:766–772, 1976

Johnson DD, Dorr KE, Swenson WM, et al: Reactive hypoglycemia. JAMA 243:1151–1155, 1980

Madison LL: Ethanol-induced hypoglycemia. Adv Metab Dis 3:85–107, 1968

Merimee TJ, Tyson JE: Stabilization of plasma glucose during fasting. N Engl J Med 291: 1275–1278, 1974

Perlmutt MA: Post prandial hypoglycemia. Diabetes 25:719–733, 1976

Scarlett JA, Mako ME, Rubenstein AH et al: Factitious hypoglycemia. N Engl J Med 297:1029–1032, 1977

Seltzer HS: Drug-induced hypoglycemia: A review based on 473 cases. Diabetes 21:955–966, 1972

Yager J, Young RT: Non-hypoglycemia is an epidemic condition. N Engl J Med 291:907–908, 1974

Gastrointestinal Disease

32

Gastrointestinal Bleeding

A chronic slow ooze from colonic cancer or chronic gastritis is a straightforward problem of differential diagnosis that can often be evaluated on a leisurely outpatient basis. However, the rapid loss of blood in acute bleeding can be imminently life-threatening and requires emergency measures. This chapter will focus on acute gastrointestinal (GI) bleeding.

CARING FOR ACUTE GI BLEEDING

Initial Maneuvers. The presence of acute GI bleeding is usually apparent from a history of hematemesis, melena, or hematochezia. Melena is the passage of dark, tarry stools; hematochezia is the passage of grossly bloody stools. However, the patient may not have noted melena or may have attributed his black stools to oral iron therapy or Pepto Bismol. Any patient found to be anemic or to have the signs and symptoms of hypovolemia should have his stool examined for the presence of blood.

The maintenance of plasma volume (and, hence, cardiac output) is the first priority in an acute episode of GI bleeding, and takes precedence over all other diagnostic maneuvers. The adequacy of intravascular volume can be readily ascertained by obtaining orthostatic vital signs. Orthostatic hypotension and hematemesis are both generally associated with significant blood volume loss. The presence of hypotension and tachycardia in the supine position indicates approximately a 50% volume loss, and vigorous volume replacement must begin at once to avert death from hypovolemic shock.

Once the diagnosis of hypovolemia is established, a large-bore intravenous line must be started in order to administer large volumes of fluids rapidly. A central venous line for measuring the central venous pressure (CVP) can also be started. A single value of the CVP is not readily interpretable, but continual monitoring is useful. A rapidly falling CVP indicates significant ongoing blood loss, and a rising CVP suggests that therapy is effective. A CVP line also provides an access for emergency medication.

When the intravenous lines have been started, a variety of blood studies should be obtained. These include:

1. Blood bank samples for typing and cross-matching.

2. A prothrombin time and a platelet count. The latter may be estimated by an examination of the blood film.

3. Electrolytes.

4. Creatinine to evaluate renal function. The presence of renal failure indicates that the patient's course will be complicated in terms of volume and electrolyte replacement. Attention must be paid to the risk of hyperkalemia, a potential complication of massive blood transfusions. In addition, the patient may be unable to excrete a hypertonic dye load that he may receive in the course of the evaluation of his bleeding. Care must be taken in interpreting the BUN, because blood in the gut can cause a considerable elevation of the BUN that does not reflect either renal perfusion or intrinsic renal function. This is due to catabolism and absorption of blood protein, reflected by increased nitrogenous wastes.

5. Liver function tests. These tests may suggest the etiology of the bleeding (e.g., varices), and should alert the physician to the possibility of hepatic decompensation and the encephalopathy that can be precipitated in patients with marginal liver function who experience GI bleeding (Chap. 40). Hepatic decompensation probably results from impaired perfusion of the liver, and the encephalopathy may be due in part to the protein load of the intraluminal bleeding.

6. Hematocrit. The use of the hematocrit in evaluating GI bleeding is somewhat confusing. Because it is important to know the patient's oxygen carrying capacity, the hematocrit should be obtained. However, one cannot use the hematocrit to evaluate the amount of blood lost. There are several reasons for this: (a) the hematocrit is only the *percentage* of blood volume occupied by the red blood cells, and gives no information about the total blood volume; (b) the patient's baseline hematocrit is often not known, although it can sometimes be estimated, for example, when the presence of microcytic indices suggests chronic anemia; (c) when a person loses whole blood, there is no immediate change in the hematocrit. Hemodilution occurs gradually over the next 5 to 18 hours, and is brought about by the shift of extravascular fluid into the intravascular space. Because fluid continues to be absorbed by the gut, hemodilution can be more significant in GI bleeding than in an equivalent external bleeding episode. The rapidity of hemodilution varies with the speed and volume of intravenous (I.V.) crystalloid given. Despite these reservations, it is important to obtain the hematocrit. An adequate hemoglobin concentration must be maintained in order to supply the metabolic needs of the body. This is particularly true in elderly patients with coronary disease in whom an attempt should be made to maintain the hematocrit close to 30. Because of the kinetics of hemodilution, it is sufficient to follow the hematocrit every eight hours, although many choose to follow it more frequently.

Other parameters that should be followed include:

1. Urinary output. If there is any question about the adequacy of urinary output—that is, if the patient is severely hypovolemic or in shock—a Foley catheter should be inserted for constant monitoring of urinary output. Urinary output can be used as a valuable measure of intravascular volume and the adequacy of the replacement regimen.

2. An EKG should be taken in patients over the age of 40, in whom the risk of myocardial infarction is increased.

Finding the Source of Blood Loss. The next step in caring for acute GI bleeding is to find the source of bleeding so that measures can be taken to prevent further blood loss. Generally, bleeding is first identified as upper *versus* lower, which is taken to mean above or below the ligament of Treitz. Two aspects of the history can help to pinpoint the site of bleeding: hematemesis indicates bleeding from above the ligament, and melena indicates bleeding from any site above the colon.

The best way to localize the site of bleeding is to pass a nasogastric tube and infuse a small amount of saline. This is an easy and relatively safe maneuver. In the presence of active upper GI bleeding, bright red blood is present in the aspirate. The presence of only "coffee grounds" material suggests a recent bleeding episode that has stopped. If the patient is not actively bleeding, the nasogastric aspirate may be negative. In this case, it is probably wise to leave the tube in place for 30 to 60 minutes in case the bleeding is intermittent. The nasogastric aspirate may sometimes fail to detect blood coming from the duodenum, especially in the presence of a deformed or edematous pylorus, a common accompaniment of ulcer disease.

If active bleeding is found, the nasogastric tube should be left in place and an iced saline lavage should be initiated. Although there has been no documentation of the effectiveness of this maneuver, clinical experience suggests that it helps to slow down, and sometimes even to stop, upper GI bleeding. The presence of the tube also permits instantaneous monitoring of the regularity and rate of bleeding.

There are several potential problems associated with the use of a nasogastric tube. There is an increased risk of pulmonary aspiration due to the loss of competence of the lower esophageal sphincter. Studies also suggest that although the passage of a tube will not acutely rupture esophageal varices, variceal ulcerations may develop if a tube is left in place for more than several hours. Finally, overzealous nasogastric suction can itself produce gastric mucosal injury.

UPPER GI BLEEDING

If the source of bleeding has been localized to the upper GI tract, the next step is to define the specific etiology. In recent years, the number of therapeutic options for the treatment of upper GI bleeding has increased, and the precise approach varies according to the type of lesion.

In several large series, the major causes of upper GI bleeding have included varices, gastric and duodenal ulcers, gastritis, and Mallory-Weiss tears. Mortality depends more upon the nature of the lesion and the underlying state of the patient than upon the amount of blood lost. The overall mortality of acute upper GI bleeding is about 10%.

The patient's history is a notoriously poor predictor of the site of bleeding. Thus, only about 50% of upper GI bleeding in people with known varices is actually from the varices. The history can be of value in specific instances, however, as is discussed below.

After a history and physical examination have been obtained, there are three diagnostic techniques available: contrast radiology, endoscopy, and arteriography.

1. X-ray studies are easy to do and relatively risk-free. Unfortunately, most studies have shown them to be inferior to endoscopy for localizing the site of bleeding. According to several studies, x-rays can define the bleeding site in 15% to 50% of patients. The diagnostic problems with x-rays are twofold: x-rays cannot detect gastritis, duodenitis, or Mallory-Weiss tears, and they can reveal only whether structural abnormalities are present, *not* whether they are bleeding. Thus, x-rays are not unlike the history in that they can document the presence of a lesion but cannot indicate whether that lesion is bleeding. A further problem with contrast radiology is that the presence of barium in the stomach and duodenum obscures endoscopy and can make arteriography uninterpretable.

2. Endoscopy is a far more accurate tool. It provides a diagnosis in 70% to 90% or more of cases. Risks include aspiration, the use of intravenous sedation and the attendant danger of overmedication, and, rarely, esophageal rupture. Generally, however, endoscopy is a safe and easy procedure. Direct visualization allows accurate localization of the lesions and determination of those responsible for the bleeding.

Despite the great accuracy of endoscopy, it is still not clear whether identification of the source of the bleeding with early endoscopy as soon as the patient arrives in the emergency room affects mortality. There have been a handful of controlled, randomized, prospective studies, and all have failed to show an increase in survival with early endoscopy.

3. Arteriography has become increasingly valuable in both the diagnosis and treatment of patients with upper GI bleeding. It has been reported to localize the bleeding site in 85% of cases. When used only in diagnosis, it is generally employed either because endoscopy could not be performed or because endoscopy failed to provide the diagnosis.

The requirement for diagnostic angiography is active bleeding. Experimentally, 0.5 ml of blood per minute must enter the gut in order to be visualized as a radiopaque blush. The presence of hypovolemia or the persistence of bright red blood in the nasogastric aspirate are both indicators of significant ongoing bleeding, and thus suggest that angiography may be useful.

Most upper GI bleeding does stop. Nasogastric lavage alone controls bleeding in over 80% of patients within the first several hours. Perhaps 25% of these patients will bleed again while in the hospital, almost always within 48 hours. Varices and gastric ulcers are most likely to rebleed. The more abundant the initial blood loss, the more likely is rebleeding to occur.

It is perhaps surprising that early endoscopy has not been shown to improve the survival rate of patients with acute upper GI bleeding. It therefore, becomes pertinent to ask which patients or groups of patients die during bleeding. The majority of studies show that most deaths seem to be in patients over the age of 60. In addition, more than 50% of patients with upper GI bleeding have some significant underlying disease, such as coronary, renal, or hepatic disease, and most deaths occur in this group of patients. The various types of lesions also carry different mortalities, as will be discussed later. Other factors, such as the amount, persistence, and recurrence of bleeding, may also be involved in the question of survival. Glancing over this list of grim prognosticators, one can more readily appreciate that early diagnosis has only a minor impact on survival.

Each of the major upper GI lesions has its own special problems and requires a specific approach. These are considered in the following sections.

Varices

Bleeding from esophageal varices is one denouement to the ravages of alcohol, and in the United States Laennec's cirrhosis is the most common setting for variceal bleeding. There are two theories to explain why varices that may have been present for years suddenly bleed. One theory is that the thin-walled veins fail and break under the pressure/volume load. However, although the presence of varices has been correlated with elevated hepatic vein wedge pressure, there is as yet no correlation between the wedge pressure and bleeding. The second hypothesis is that gastric reflux ulcerates the wall of the esophagus and causes bleeding. Still other factors may be involved. Ascites often precedes and may precipitate bleeding; ascites raises intraabdominal pressure and diminishes the competence of the lower esophageal sphincter.

A history of liver disease or known varices raises the suspicion of variceal bleeding, but about 50% of upper GI bleeding in patients with cirrhosis is from other causes. Bleeding is more likely to be variceal in nonalcoholic cirrhosis patients than in patients with alcoholic cirrhosis, whose alcohol consumption constantly assaults their gastric mucosa, resulting in gastritis and ulceration that may lead to bleeding.

Although varices are frequently associated with hematemesis, it is not uncommon to see more protracted and less profuse bleeding, with the only evidence of bleeding being melena or guaiac-positive stools.

Mortality from variceal bleeding is high, and is often due to associated hepatic failure, renal failure, encephalopathy, aspiration, or sepsis, and not to exsanguination *per se*. Therefore, data concerning the mortality of the bleeding itself are hard to obtain and difficult to interpret; it is not surprising that the mortality of a single bleeding episode is reported to be anywhere from 10% to 75%. Much of the data concerns alcoholic liver disease; less information is available for other forms of cirrhosis.

The natural history of the varix is a dismal one. During the hospital stay, after the bleeding has been initially controlled, varices rebleed at a reported recurrence rate of 70% within the first 48 hours. After leaving the hospital, up to 50% of patients experience rebleeding within the first 15 months.

Treatment for variceal bleeding can be extraordinarily difficult and begins with conservative medical therapy with intravenous fluid, electrolytes, blood products as needed, and vitamin K. Antacid therapy is a reasonable approach in preventing the untoward effects of gastric reflux, but is of unproved benefit. Continuous intravenous infusions of low-dose vasopressin can often stop the bleeding. Vasopressin infusions reduce mesenteric blood flow to about 50% of baseline, and presumably

decompress the portal system. The success of vasopressin (Pitressin) in a given patient seems to be proportional to the severity of the underlying liver disease, with a 90+ % success rate in mild liver failure and 50% in severe liver disease. Other arteriographic methods, including transhepatic occlusion with an autologous clot, can be effective, but these techniques are too new to allow any final evaluation. In experienced hands, the Sengstaken-Blakemore tube can control bleeding in close to 90% of episodes. This tube contains a balloon that is placed in the stomach and a balloon that remains in the esophagus. The inflated gastric balloon anchors the tube while the inflated esophageal balloon tamponades the varices. Complications have discouraged its use in many centers.

As is true of all forms of GI bleeding, when medical management fails, surgery may become necessary. Portocaval shunts are very effective in stopping bleeding and reducing portal hypertension. However, the long-term mortality in patients with cirrhosis remains unchanged, with the mode of death shifted from bleeding to encephalopathy. The newer, more selective splenorenal shunts may prove to be a more attractive alternative, but the data are not yet available.

Mallory-Weiss Tears

The Mallory-Weiss lesion was initially described as a longitudinal tear at the gastroesophageal junction produced by forceful or repeated vomiting, and resulting in massive, often fatal hemorrhage. We now know that it accounts for 10% or perhaps 15% of upper GI bleeding and is not nearly as frightening as formerly believed. Vomiting initiates a complex series of pressure/volume changes and exerts a large transmural pressure gradient on the point of the GI tract passing between the high-pressure abdomen and the low-pressure thorax. In most individuals, this transition area is the gastroesophageal junction, but in patients with hiatal hernias, the Mallory-Weiss lesion is frequently seen in the cardia of the stomach.

Although 85% of patients present with hematemesis, only one-third give the classic history of repeated vomiting immediately preceding the production of blood. Most patients have a history of alcoholism. About one-half of patients present with significant hypovolemia, but this is generally corrected easily, and about 80% will stop bleeding spontaneously soon after their arrival at the hospital. The lesions heal rapidly and few rebleed. Angiography can define the site of bleeding and can be used to infuse vasopressin selectively; in the majority of cases, this stops the bleeding. Ultimately, only about 10% of patients require surgery, and the overall mortality is less than 5%.

Ulcer Disease

Ulcer disease is the most common cause of upper GI bleeding. For 20% of patients, bleeding is the first indication of their disease, and two-thirds of the patients, including those with a positive ulcer history, recall no recent dyspeptic symptoms. Conversely, a history of past ulcer disease cannot guarantee that an ulcer is responsible for a current bleeding episode.

The mechanism of bleeding in ulcer disease is felt to be erosion into a mucosal artery, and bleeding is believed to occur in spurts lasting 20 to 30 minutes. Gastric ulcers tend to bleed more profusely than their duodenal counterparts and seem to carry a higher mortality; this is probably due to their frequent proximity to the gastric artery.

Eighty percent of patients stop bleeding spontaneously or with medical intervention during their first episode. Their long-term outlook, however, is not encouraging. Rebleeding occurs in 25% to 40% of patients

treated medically and followed up for several years. Clearly, a patient who is bleeding to death needs emergency surgery, but surgery is not a guarantee against future bleeding.

Treatment for a bleeding ulcer includes iced saline lavage and neutralization or inhibition of acid secretion (see Chap. 33). The patient is transfused as needed. Arteriography with selective vasopressin infusion can stop bleeding from ulcers in over 50% of cases. The use of autologous clots may prove to be even more effective than vasopressin. There is no strict criterion for when a patient must go to surgery with this or any type of GI bleeding. Clinical judgment and good sense dictate that when medical therapy is failing, a nonmedical approach is needed.

Acute Gastric Erosions

The syndrome of acute gastric erosions includes a mélange of many etiologies, and accounts for 10% to 30% of upper GI bleeding. The two major causes are drug ingestion, including aspirin, ethanol, and indomethacin, and stress, including surgery, sepsis, renal failure, and burns. The pathology is one of diffuse hemorrhagic mucosal inflammation, often with one or more discrete, shallow ulcerous craters. Endoscopy is required to make the diagnosis. Drug-induced lesions generally stop bleeding within hours of the initiation of even conservative management and carry a low mortality. Stress-induced lesions are more persistent and carry a higher mortality, reflective of the often severe underlying illness. Clotting abnormalities may also be present and complicate the attempt to control bleeding. Antacids may facilitate control of bleeding in nondrug-related erosions, and cimetidine may also be effective.

LOWER GI BLEEDING

When there is no history of hematemesis and the nasogastric aspirate is negative, lower GI bleeding must be suspected. Generally, the bleeding is from the colon or rectum and presents as bright red blood per rectum. Rarely, melena indicates an unusual small intestinal site. The history is just as poor in defining the etiology of lower GI bleeding as it is in upper GI bleeding.

Diverticulosis

The most common source of massive lower GI bleeding is diverticulosis, small outpouchings of the intestine. Diverticulosis is generally asymptomatic and not coexistent with diverticulitis. (Diverticulitis, inflammation of diverticula, occurs when these small pouches become obstructed or perforate, leading to peridiverticular inflammation and, occasionally, local peritonitis.)

Diverticulosis is rarely seen before the age of 40. Seventy-five percent of the time, the bleeding is from diveritcula in the right colon. Most bleeding, which begins suddenly, stops completely after several hours. Perhaps 25% of patients continue to bleed, and another 25% of those that stop experience rebleeding while in the hospital. Bleeding can be halted in the majority of persistent bleeders with selective arterial vasopressin. Fifty percent of these patients, however, eventually require surgical therapy.

Angiodysplasia

Angiodysplasia is being diagnosed by angiography with increasing frequency. This lesion is believed to be an acquired defect in the veins in a localized area of the cecum and right colon. It is reported to have a 20% incidence in the elderly and is most often asymptomatic. Bleeding is the only clinical problem associated with angiodysplasia. It can be responsible for either chronic low-grade bleeding or episodic heavy bleeding. The heavy bleeding generally stops, but persistent

or recurrent bleeding may require surgical therapy or a right partial colectomy. Electrocoagulation by colonoscopy after the patient has stopped bleeding is sometimes effective.

Other Causes of Lower GI Bleeding

Both of the previously mentioned sources of significant acute lower GI bleeding are restricted to the older population. In younger people, *inflammatory bowel disease* (Chap. 36) or an anatomic anomaly such as *Meckel's diverticulum* are more likely to be responsible. In ulcerative colitis, bleeding is more likely to be massive than in Crohn's disease, and in either case, bleeding is rarely the only or first symptom. Meckel's diverticulum occurs in about 1% of the population and can contain ectopic, acid-secreting gastric mucosa that produces the same problems—including hemorrhage—that are seen in peptic ulcer disease.

Hemorrhoids rarely bleed massively. A bleeding site is usually recognized on anoscopy, but retrograde filling of the sigmoid with blood can obscure recognition of a distal source of bleeding.

Tumors of the small and large intestine can bleed, but, again, these rarely present as significant acute bleeding episodes. Malignant lesions are more apt to bleed heavily than benign tumors.

Bowel infarction generally occurs in the elderly within the setting of either a low flow state or arterial emboli. It presents with a clinical picture of abdominal pain, bloody diarrhea, and peritonitis; if surgical resection is not carried out, shock ensues. Although bloody diarrhea is common, large amounts of blood are unusual.

Pinpointing the site of lower GI bleeding is difficult. Anoscopy should be performed to find the unusual profusely bleeding hemorrhoid. Sigmoidoscopy may reveal a bleeding site, but sigmoidoscopy and, to an even greater extent, colonoscopy are very difficult to perform while significant bleeding is occurring. With ongoing bleeding, angiography is the next step, for both diagnostic and therapeutic reasons. If no diagnosis is available by the time that bleeding has stopped, a barium enema should be performed to document the presence of diverticula or tumors. If negative, repeat sigmoidoscopy and then colonoscopy with good visualization should be performed.

BIBLIOGRAPHY

Almy TP, Howell DA: Diverticular disease of the colon. N Engl J Med 302:324–331, 1980

Eastwood GL: Does early endoscopy benefit the patient with active upper gastrointestinal bleeding? Gastroenterology 72:737–739, 1977

Franco D, Durandy Y, Deporte et al: Upper gastrointestinal hemorrhage in hepatic cirrhosis: Causes and relation to hepatic failure and stress. Lancet 1:218–220, 1977

Graham DY, Schwartz JT: The spectrum of the Mallory-Weiss tear. Medicine 57:307–318, 1977

Northfield TC: Factors predisposing to recurrent hemorrhage after acute gastrointestinal bleeding. Br Med J 1:26–28, 1971

Palmer ED: The vigorous diagnostic approach to upper gastrointestinal tract hemorrhage. JAMA 207:1477–1480, 1969

Moody FG: Rectal bleeding. N Engl J Med 290:839–841, 1974

33

Peptic Ulcer Disease

An uncomplicated peptic ulcer is an outpatient problem that rarely requires hospitalization. Nevertheless, the high incidence of peptic ulcers in both the hospital and ambulatory populations, as well as the number of potentially serious and even life-threatening complications, necessitates a working knowledge of their diagnosis, evaluation, and treatment.

Much attention has traditionally been paid to the distinction between duodenal ulcers and gastric ulcers. Despite certain differences in their presentation and pathophysiology, the major clinical reason for distinguishing between them is the possibility that a gastric ulcer represents a gastric malignancy; the question of malignancy does not arise with duodenal ulcers.

SYMPTOMS OF PEPTIC ULCERS

Duodenal Ulcers

Eighty to eighty-five percent of peptic ulcers are duodenal. By far the most common symptom of an uncomplicated duodenal ulcer is pain. It is almost always confined to the epigastrium and is typically described as burning, aching, or gnawing. It is described more often as discomforting than excruciating. The pain typically occurs when the stomach is empty: before lunch or dinner, at bedtime, and in the very early hours of the morning. The pain often awakens the patient several hours after going to sleep. Because of the diminished secretion of gastric acid in the morning, the patient rarely complains of pain when he awakens.

One of the most reliable diagnostic symptoms of a duodenal ulcer is the relief of pain with food, generally within several minutes of ingestion. Although a duodenal ulcer is a chronic condition, the periods of active symptomatology fluctuate, and it is rare for a patient to complain of symptoms throughout the year. On physical examination, epigastric tenderness is the predominant finding.

Gastric Ulcers

The symptomatology of gastric ulcers is more variable. The pain can be indistinguishable from that of a duodenal ulcer, or may lack the characteristic daily rhythm of duodenal disease. In some patients, food exacerbates or even produces the pain.

DIAGNOSIS

In the absence of active gastrointestinal bleeding, an *upper GI barium x-ray* is the diagnostic test of choice. Several studies have shown that an upper GI series can detect as many as 90% of peptic ulcers. Anyone over the age of 30 with probable or possible ulcer symptoms warrants an upper GI series in order to determine the possibility of a gastric malignancy. In younger patients, in whom the likelihood of malignancy is very low, an upper GI series is not required, and the diagnosis of ulcer disease can usually be made by history and therapeutic response to antacids.

Two x-ray findings denote a *duodenal ulcer* (Fig. 33–1):

1. The presence of an ulcer crater. The ulcer is revealed as an immobile pocket of barium.

2. A deformed duodenal bulb. This reflects the existence of old ulcer disease with consequent scarring. Because duodenal ulcers are chronic, the finding of a deformed bulb in a patient with classic ulcer symptoms is accepted as sufficient evidence to make the diagnosis of active ulcer disease.

Several criteria have been established to determine whether the underlying etiology of a *gastric ulcer* is a *malignant* tumor. The diagnostic accuracy of these criteria exceeds 80%:

1. Benign ulcer craters project beyond the lumen of the stomach (Fig. 33–2), whereas malignant ulcer craters do not.

2. Benign ulcers are associated with a regular and smooth mound with normal rugae radiating at the ulcer base. Malignant ulcers exhibit an irregular base, and the ulcer is often eccentrically located.

3. Benign ulcers have a smooth bed, whereas malignant ulcers have a nodular bed.

4. Benign ulcers frequently exhibit a radiolucent line (Hampton line), representing the edge of normal mucosa. This finding is absent in malignant ulcers.

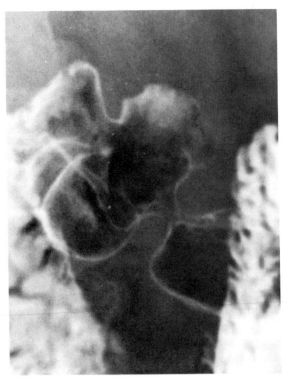

FIG. 33–1. Duodenal ulcer. This air contrast study depicts the classic "cloverleaf deformity" of the duodenal bulb. The increased density seen in the center of the cloverleaf is the ulcer crater.

The size, location, and rate of healing of an ulcer are, by themselves, unreliable as diagnostic criteria.

If the x-ray is in any way ambiguous, further evaluation is needed. The *fiberoptic endoscope* can increase the diagnostic accuracy to more than 98% when coupled with *gastric cytology* and *biopsy*.

Any gastric ulcer diagnosed as benign by a single upper GI series should be reexamined in two to three weeks. A benign ulcer under intensive medical therapy should show evidence of healing (a reduction in ulcer size), but, unfortunately, not all benign ulcers show radiographic healing. Nevertheless, the ab-

FIG. 33–2. Benign gastric ulcer. The arrow points to the ulcer crater, which lies along the lesser curvature of the stomach. The deformity surrounding the ulcer is caused by edema in the stomach wall.

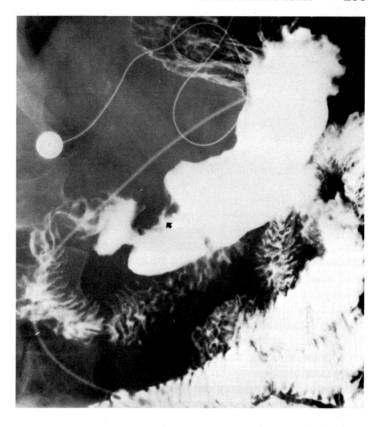

sence of any healing, enlargement of the ulcer, or detection of new "malignant" characteristics must prompt more vigorous attention to the possibility of malignancy.

The radiographic distinction between benign and malignant ulcers is difficult when the ulcer is in the antroduodenal area. If the bulb is markedly deformed, the distinction is even more difficult. The best way to be certain is by *gastroduodenoscopy*. Fortunately, ulcers in the antroduodenal area are usually benign.

THERAPY

The role of diet in ulcer therapy is uncertain, and no food has any proven correlation with pain relief. The patient should probably be encouraged to avoid eating highly acidic foods, such as orange juice or carbonated beverages. Many patients associate certain foods with exacerbations of pain, and these should be avoided.

The frequency of feeding, on the other hand, does correlate with pain relief. Food relieves ulcer pain because of its buffering effects. After a meal, however, there is a surge of acid release that persists several hours after eating, when the food is no longer available for buffering, and pain recurs. Frequent small feedings are thus extremely helpful in alleviating ulcer pain.

The mainstay of medical ulcer therapy is the *antacid*. An acute painful ulcer requires more vigorous therapy than a chronic ulcer. Rest is felt to be an important component of the treatment of acute ulcer pain, and many gastroenterologists enforce bed rest and the replacement of all foods with hourly skim milk and antacids. This regimen is generally effective. Pain occurring several hours after going to bed is treated with antacids just before bedtime.

Many antacids are currently available and, to some extent, the choice is arbitrary, although certain distinctions between the different agents can be made. Any given antacid is more effective in liquid than in tablet form. Calcium carbonate causes constipation and contributes to the milk-alkali syndrome of hypercalcemia (which, in turn, increases gastric acid secretion) and alkalosis. Magnesium-based antacids can counteract the constipation caused by other antacids. When given alone, they produce diarrhea. Some commercial antacid preparations have a high sodium content and should be avoided in patients who must restrict their dietary sodium. Aluminum hydroxide antacids can cause serious phosphate depletion, but an adequate dietary phosphate intake will prevent this complication. Antacids affect the absorption of certain drugs; thus for example, tetracycline absorption is inhibited in the presence of antacids.

A standard regimen uses antacids one and three hours after meals and at bed time. Once the acute episode has subsided, less vigorous antacid therapy can be instituted. In general, this regimen consists of frequent feedings and antacids one hour after meals and before bedtime.

The question whether medical therapy induces or hastens ulcer healing is still unanswered. One recent study employed endoscopy to evaluate duodenal ulcer healing, and found that antacid therapy does induce healing, although only in nonsmokers. There is no evidence that gastric ulcers heal more quickly with antacids. A drug that is available in Europe, *carbenoxelone*, appears to be effective in inducing gastric ulcer healing, but it is not particularly effective in treating duodenal ulcers. The drug frequently has an aldosterone-like effect, causing salt and water retention.

Cimetidine is a specific blocker of the H_2 histamine receptor, and is a recent addition to the medical treatment of peptic ulcers. Histamine receptors can be divided into two classes: (1) H_1 receptors are found in the skin, mucous membranes, and bronchi; and (2) H_2 receptors are found in the heart, uterus, and gastric parietal cells. Cimetidine can be given in oral or intravenous doses every six hours, and is extremely effective in reducing gastric acid secretion and ameliorating the symptoms of ulcer disease. Food-stimulated acid secretion is reduced 70% by cimetidine. Its effect on healing is better demonstrated for duodenal than gastric ulcers, and it may be helpful in the treatment of "stress" ulcers (see below). It is not an effective treatment for GI bleeding. Side-effects include disorientation in the elderly, gynecomastia and loss of libido in males, and reduction in the metabolism of warfarin and diazepam.

Anticholinergic drugs inhibit gastric acid secretion and delay gastric emptying. Unfortunately, these desired effects can only be achieved at doses that produce significant anticholinergic side-effects, including pupillary dysfunction, xerostomia, and bladder obstruction.

In patients in whom stress plays an important role in generating symptoms, the judicious use of sedatives and antianxiety agents can be helpful. These drugs should not, however, be used in place of antacids, and the danger of addiction must always be considered.

The above therapeutic modalities are all aimed at symptomatic relief, but their effectiveness has been questioned by several studies that show no difference between antacid therapy and placebos in reducing pain. For some patients, the psychological benefit of being on a treatment program may be of more importance in pain relief than the actual nature of the program.

Surgery is indicated in several circumstances: (1) uncontrolled bleeding, (2) perforation, (3) fixed obstruction, and (4) intractable pain. Most patients with peptic ulcer disease do not require surgery.

There are a large number of surgical options currently available. The most common surgical therapy is vagotomy. This procedure interrupts vagal stimulation to gastric acid secretion. It is combined with a drainage procedure (pyloroplasty) to allow emptying of the stomach in the absence of vagal innervation. Unfortunately, these procedures may be complicated by the dumping syndrome, diarrhea, and malabsorption. Partial vagotomy to selectively denervate the parietal cells has been introduced recently. Because it leaves vagal innervation to the antrum intact, this selective procedure obviates the need for a drainage procedure. It is slightly less effective but almost eliminates the untoward side-effects of operation.

STRESS ULCERS

A stress ulcer is the name given to an acute ulcer associated with other underlying serious illness, such as burns, central nervous system catastrophes, sepsis, or renal failure. Most stress ulcers are gastric, multiple, and shallow, although exceptions to this description are plentiful. They frequently do not present with pain, but rather with bleeding or perforation. The prophylactic use of intravenous cimetidine or antacids delivered by nasogastric tube in preventing stress ulcers in seriously ill patients has been advocated.

COMPLICATIONS

The complications of ulcer disease include gastrointestinal bleeding (Chap. 32), intractability, penetration, perforation, and gastric outlet obstruction.

Intractability and the Zollinger-Ellison Syndrome

Intractability is defined as the failure to control ulcer symptoms with standard medical therapy. When this occurs, surgical therapy should be considered.

It is important to be aware, however, that intractable ulcer symptoms can be part of the Zollinger-Ellison syndrome. This syndrome is caused by an ulcerogenic tumor of the pancreatic islets. The tumors secrete gastrin, which stimulates the antral cells of the stomach to produce excess acid. More than one-half of these tumors are malignant, and patients usually have multiple tumors at the time the diagnosis is made. The malignancy generally grows very slowly, and the major threat to the patient's health is the ulcer disease.

Recurrent, intractable ulcers, multiple ulcers, or especially ulcers in unusual locations should suggest the diagnosis. Diarrhea occurs in one-third or more of patients, and is often watery and profuse. Severe diarrhea and the presence of peptic ulcer disease should therefore also suggest the diagnosis.

The most common presentation of the Zollinger-Ellison syndrome, unfortunately, is a simple uncomplicated ulcer. Occasionally, the syndrome is part of a multiple endocrine neoplasia Type-I syndrome.

Once a Zollinger-Ellison tumor is suspected, the diagnosis is made by serum gastrin studies. Patients generally have elevated serum gastrin levels and show an exaggerated increase in serum gastrin to calcium infusion.

Serum gastrin levels also increase after intravenous secretin, whereas the normal response to secretin is a decrease in serum gastrin levels. Patients with pernicious anemia also have high serum gastrin levels, as do patients with a surgically removed gastric antrum. In both instances, this is due to the lack of acid feedback inhibition on gastrin secretion.

Therapy for Zollinger-Ellison disease is usually surgical. Surgery is directed at the end organ—the stomach—and not at the tumor; the tumor is often already metastatic, and it is the ulcer rather than the tumor that threatens the patient. The removal of the stomach in these patients carries a significant operative mortality, and the need for gastrectomy should be carefully assessed in each patient before surgery is performed. It has recently been shown that cimetidine can effectively control ulcer symptoms in the majority of patients with the Zollinger-Ellison syndrome.

Penetration

Posterior penetration of a duodenal ulcer is a common complication of peptic ulcer disease. When penetration occurs, the patient's pain usually changes to become more persistent and more resistant to food and antacids. The patient often notes the loss of the normal rhythmicity of the pain with respect to food intake. Penetration typically causes severe pain in the back, and may suggest a primary back disorder.

The diagnosis is most effectively made by visualizing the penetrating duodenal ulcer by means of either contrast x-rays or duodenoscopy. If the pancreas is involved, the serum amylase may rise, but acute pancreatitis is rare.

Treatment requires the same intensive medical management as acute ulcer disease. If medical therapy fails, surgery should be undertaken.

Perforation

Perforation of an ulcer presents as an acute abdominal catastrophe, with severe generalized abdominal pain that often radiates to the back and to the tip of the right shoulder.

The patient presents with all of the findings of acute pancreatitis (see Chap. 37). The loss of fluid into the peritoneal cavity can cause hypotension and shock. The white blood cell count is often elevated, and the hematocrit often rises because of hemoconcentration. The serum amylase is frequently increased, but the urinary amylase clearance—elevated in acute pancreatitis—is not increased.

Duodenal ulcers are much more likely to perforate than gastric ulcers. A history of symptomatic peptic ulcer disease is absent in almost one-fourth of patients.

The diagnosis is made by x-ray studies, which are especially important for making the distinction between perforation and pancreatitis. The finding of free air under the diaphragm suggests perforation (Fig. 33–3). To enhance the possibility of finding free air on the x-ray, the patient should be moved onto his left side for ten minutes. If no free air is seen, an upper GI series with a water-soluble contrast agent may delineate the perforation.

Definitive treatment of perforation usually requires immediate surgical correction. Postsurgical complications include the development of a subphrenic abscess.

Gastric Outlet Obstruction

Gastric outlet obstruction is a relatively common problem that results from narrowing of the gastric outlet. It may be caused by edema, spasm, and/or scarring and deformation. When the first two causes are responsible for the clinical symptoms, the obstruction is generally temporary and responsive to simple medical therapy.

Gastric outlet obstruction causes the char-

FIG. 33-3. Free air in the abdomen. After perforation of an ulcer, air can escape into the abdomen. A chest x-ray taken with the patient in an upright position reveals air under the diaphragm.

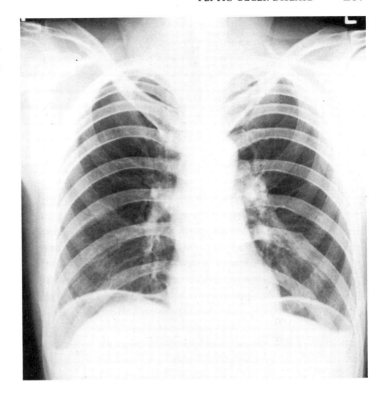

acteristic pain pattern of ulcer disease to be altered. The stomach is unable to empty its contents and dilates. Dilatation stimulates the antrum and results in further acid secretion; acid secretion further dilates the stomach. Because the stomach contents are always acidic, the pain is constant and no longer demonstrates daily rhythmicity. In addition, the volume of acid is too large to be buffered by antacids, and they therefore become ineffective. Early obstruction frequently presents only with these alterations in the pattern of ulcer pain.

Bloating and vomiting are more specifically suggestive of obstruction. The patient complains of feeling full, early satiety, and losing his appetite. Vomiting generally signifies far advanced obstruction. The patient characteristically vomits large amounts of gastric con-

tents one to two hours after eating. The vomitus may contain recognizable pieces of undigested food, sometimes from a meal eaten 12 or more hours earlier.

The only physical finding of obstruction is auscultation of a "succussion splash" over the distended stomach.

Two diagnostic maneuvers aid in the diagnosis of obstruction:

1. The patient should have a nasogastric tube inserted to remove all gastric contents, sometimes amounting to one or two liters. This procedure may rapidly alleviate the patient's symptoms.

2. A saline load test can assess the competency of gastric emptying. 750 ml of saline is placed into the stomach, and after 30 minutes the gastric contents are completely aspirated. The presence of more than 300 ml of

fluid in the stomach suggests obstruction. However, in mild gastric outlet obstruction, saline may pass more easily than food and not be retained.

Although the saline load test can confirm the diagnosis of obstruction, it does not answer the question of whether edema and spasm are responsible for temporary obstruction. The patient must be monitored over several days to see whether the obstruction resolves. If the patient can tolerate food, he should be permitted to eat dinner. Four hours after eating, a nasogastric tube is inserted and the quantity of gastric contents is assessed. If more than 200 ml can be obtained, gastric outlet obstruction is still present.

The first step in treating gastric outlet obstruction is to decompress the stomach. Decompression results in immediate symptomatic relief and breaks the cycle of distention that leads to increased acid secretion. Anticholinergic medication delays gastric emptying and should be discontinued. If the patient can tolerate food, frequent small feedings should be instituted, otherwise intravenous fluids are required. A diet of frequent small volume feedings may allow resolution of the obstruction after several days. If the patient has been vomiting profusely he may present with volume depletion and metabolic alkalosis.

When gastric outlet obstruction is due to edema and spasm, it generally resolves after a few days. One cannot, however, predict the likelihood of recurrences. Obstruction due to scarring may not resolve, and may require surgical correction.

BIBLIOGRAPHY

Bodemar G, Walan A: Cimetidine in the treatment of active duodenal and prepyloric ulcers. Lancet 2:161–164, 1976

Bynum TE, Hartsuck J, Jacobson ED: Gastric ulcer. Gastroenterology 62:1052–1060, 1972

Dunn JP, Etter LE: Inadequacy of medical history in the diagnosis of duodenal ulcers. N Engl J Med 266:68–72, 1962

Dwight RW, Schimmel EM, O'Hara ET et al: Controlled study of the surgical treatment of duodenal ulcers. Am J Surg 129:374–379, 1975

Fordtran JS: Placebos, antacids, and cometidine for duodenal ulcer. N Engl J Med 298:1081–1083, 1978

Goldstein H, Boyle JD: The saline load test—A bedside evaluation of gastric retention. Gastroenterology 49:375–380, 1965

Grossman MI, Guth PH, Isenberg JI et al: A new look at peptic ulcer. Ann Intern Med 84:57–67, 1976

Gudjonsson B, Spiro HM: Response to placebo in ulcer disease. Am J Med 65:399–402, 1978

Hofkin GA: Course of patients with perforated duodenal ulcers. Am J Surg 111:193–196, 1966

Littman A (ed): The Veterans Administration cooperative study on gastric ulcers. Gastroenterology 61:567–654, 1971

McCarthy DM: The place of surgery in the Zollinger-Ellison syndrome. N Engl J Med 302:1344–1347, 1980

Morrissey JF, Barreras RF: Antacid therapy. N Engl J Med 290:550–556, 1974

Peterson WL, Sturdevant RA, Frankl HD et al: Healing of duodenal ulcers with an antacid regimen. N Engl J Med 297:341–345, 1977

Rhodes J: Etiology of gastric ulcer. Gastroenterology 63:171–182, 1972

34

Most acute diarrheal illnesses are caused either by infection of the gut or by toxins released by infectious agents. Ingestion of the organism or its toxin disrupts normal bowel function by (1) reducing the rate of fluid absorption from the gut or (2) increasing the rate of fluid secretion into the gut.

Although treatment for diarrhea often is not necessary, identification of the etiologic agent can be important. Specific antibiotic therapy may be required, and the offending agent may pose a public health hazard.

BACTERIAL CAUSES OF ACUTE DIARRHEA

Staphylococcal Food Poisoning. Staphylococcal food poisoning is an acute illness caused by the ingestion of an enterotoxin elaborated by toxigenic *Staphylococcus aureus* organisms. This is the only common acute diarrheal illness caused by the ingestion of a preformed toxin. Many foods, especially precooked foods, support the growth of staphylococcus. The food gives no sign of contamination; its color, odor, and taste are unchanged. The illness begins one to six hours after the food has been eaten, and is charac-

terized by the sudden onset of nausea, vomiting, abdominal cramps, and, less often, diarrhea. The diarrhea can be explosive and voluminous. There is no fever. The syndrome abates within 12 hours and usually resolves completely within 72 hours.

Clostridial Food Poisoning. Heat-stable spores of type A *Clostridia perfringens* can survive inadequate cooking and are a common cause of food-related illness. The incubation period is longer than for staphylococcal food poisoning, ranging from 12 to 24 hours. The symptom complex is more restricted: nausea and vomiting are unusual, and the patient's complaints are limited to diarrhea and cramping abdominal pain. Fever is rare. The patient is usually well within 24 hours of the onset of the illness. Positive anaerobic cultures of the suspected source or the patient's feces will provide the diagnosis. No specific therapy is required.

Salmonellosis. When fever is a prominent part of the clinical picture, the most likely etiologic agents are salmonella or shigella. Salmonellosis may occur sporadically or in epidemics and is generally food-borne. Previous gastric surgery increases susceptibility to the illness. Within one to two days of exposure, gastrointestinal symptoms begin suddenly with nausea, vomiting, watery diarrhea, and cramping abdominal pain. Fever is common, sometimes rising to 102° F, but the peripheral white blood count usually remains normal. Salmonellosis is a self-limited illness and subsides without specific therapy within three to six days; in rare cases, it may persist for as long as two weeks.

Stool examination and culture may help to make the diagnosis. Polymorphonuclear leukocytes are usually present in the stool; they are even more prominent in shigellosis, but are not found in staphylococcal or clostridial food poisoning or viral gastroenteritis. Trace amounts of blood may be present in the stool, but this is true of all types of acute diarrhea. The stool culture is positive in more than 90% of patients during the early stages of the acute illness. This percentage decreases with time, and after one month less than 20% of patients have positive stool cultures. Some individuals continue to shed organisms for as long as six months after all symptoms have subsided.

Blood cultures are rarely positive. Antibiotic therapy is not indicated unless there is evidence of salmonella infection at a site other than the gastrointestinal tract. Some clinicians argue that antibiotics are contraindicated, since they can be responsible for prolonged excretion of the organism.

A variety of serotypes of salmonella can cause the syndrome previously described, but *Salmonella typhi*, the organism generally responsible for causing typhoid fever, is rarely isolated in the United States. *Typhoid fever* is an acute, systemic, febrile illness typically lasting three to five weeks. It begins with the gradual onset of fever, anorexia, malaise, and diffuse aches. Headache, abdominal pain, and constipation are common. The patient's condition worsens during the second week with high fever and mental apathy (occasionally

the patient may experience delirium). The symptoms gradually abate over the next two to three weeks, leaving the patient weak. A variety of physical signs accompany the illness, including a relative (for the degree of fever) bradycardia, splenomegaly, and a maculopapular skin rash (the so-called "rose spots") that is seen on the abdomen or chest.

The two major complications of typhoid fever are gastrointestinal hemorrhage and intestinal perforation. Gastrointestinal bleeding can be detected in 20% to 30% of patients, although only a small percentage experiences severe bleeding. Approximately 1% of patients experience perforation with the signs of acute peritonitis. Typhoid fever is treated with chloramphenicol or ampicillin, but the therapeutic response generally is not dramatic.

Shigellosis. Bacterial dysentery is most common in tropical regions, but it can and does occur in more temperate zones as well. Unlike gastrointestinal salmonellosis, transmission usually occurs directly from other infected persons. Within 48 hours of exposure, the disease begins abruptly with diarrhea, abdominal cramps, and tenesmus. Tenesmus is often prominent and is characteristic of shigellosis. Nausea and vomiting are absent or mild. Fever usually accompanies the abdominal symptoms. The stool is commonly filled with mucus and large amounts of blood, and microscopic examination reveals a large number of polymorphonuclear leukocytes. The diagnosis is made by stool culture. Blood cultures are virtually always negative. Shigellosis is a self-limited illness, lasting only a few days. A five-day course of ampicillin can be given to shorten the duration of the illness. Recently, *Campylobacter fetus* has been shown to be the cause of a similar diarrheal illness in a significant percentage of patients.

Staphylococcal Enterocolitis. Staphylococcal enterocolitis is a rare, life-threatening disorder, and represents a true infection of the bowel wall. It is seen in elderly, debilitated patients and often in patients following abdominal surgery. Frequently, the patient will have been taking antibiotics prior to the illness; partial sterilization of the gut has been implicated in permitting the staphylococcal overgrowth. Diarrhea begins suddenly and is profuse and often bloody. The patient rapidly becomes toxic with fever, abdominal pain, ileus, distention, dehydration, and shock. A gram-stain of the stool reveals many polymorphonuclear leukocytes and sheets and clumps of gram-positive cocci. The latter finding permits a presumptive diagnosis, and therapy with oral vancomycin should be instituted. Even with appropriate therapy, the severity of the illness coupled with the often serious underlying debility results in a high mortality rate.

Pseudomembranous Colitis. Like staphylococcal enterocolitis, pseudomembranous colitis affects debilitated patients and patients taking certain antibiotics. It is seen particularly after clindamycin and lincomycin therapy; ampicillin and cephalexin have also been implicated. Approximately 20% of patients taking clindamycin develop diarrhea. Of these, probably only a minority have pseudomembranous colitis. Ampicillin causes diarrhea in up to 10% of patients, but the incidence of pseudomembranous colitis is probably much less than 1%. Other settings of pseudomembranous colitis include postsurgery and uremia. The disease may also be seen in neonates.

Pseudomembranous colitis is a febrile, diarrheal illness with prominent abdominal symptoms. Once thought to be fatal in a large percentage of cases, studies of clindamycin-induced illness suggest that milder forms do exist. The diagnosis should be suspected when acute diarrhea develops in the appropriate setting. Sigmoidoscopy can confirm the diagnosis if either exudative plaques or pseudomembranes (actually a precipitate composed of fibrin and inflammatory cells) are seen on the mucosal surface. These lesions are most frequently found in the ileum and the colon, and therefore can be missed if sigmoidoscopy alone is carried out.

Recent evidence has implicated an overgrowth of a toxin-producing strain of clostridia as the cause of pseudomembranous colitis. Treatment involves supportive therapy and discontinuing the use of any ongoing antibiotics. Experimental evidence suggests a role for vancomycin in treating the disease.

VIRAL GASTROENTERITIS

Viral gastroenteritis, commonly and mistakenly referred to as intestinal flu, generally occurs in summer or winter epidemics. The enteroviruses and other unclassified agents have been implicated as causative agents. Suspicion of a viral etiology should be raised by the clustering of a common symptomatology in families and communities, as well as by the usual viral prodrome of myalgias and malaise. The syndrome itself is not unique: it persists for 24 to 48 hours with nausea, vomiting, abdominal pains, and diarrhea. Fever is mild or absent. The diarrhea can linger for days after the other symptoms have abated. A definite diagnosis is rarely made. In a patient with afebrile gastroenteritis preceded by a viral-type prodrome, a viral etiology is highly suspected. When low-grade fever is present, the epidemiology, viral symptomatology, and negative cultures make it the diagnosis of exclusion.

PARASITIC CAUSES OF ACUTE DIARRHEA

Giardia. *Giardia* is being recognized as a source of gastrointestinal distress with increasing frequency. The parasite is usually acquired during travel abroad—especially in the vicinity of Leningrad in the Soviet Union—but it can be acquired in the United States. The clinical manifestations of giardiasis run the gamut from acute watery diarrhea with fever to a chronic condition with recurrent diarrhea and malabsorption. A fresh stool examination reveals either trophozoites or cysts in fewer than 50% of patients. A duodenal aspirate gives a higher yield of organisms. Neither blood nor polymorphonuclear leukocytes are found in the stool. Treatment is with metronidazole.

Amebic Gastroenteritis. Acute *amebic gastroenteritis* is a very rare cause of acute diarrhea. The afflicted patient may have bloody stools and appear to have shigellosis. However, the stool of patients with amebic gastroenteritis does not have polymorphonuclear leukocytes. Rectal mucosal scrapings, preferably from an area of ulceration, provide the best chance for seeing the trophozoites and establishing the diagnosis.

TREATMENT

Hospital admission for acute diarrhea can generally be avoided unless severe fluid and electrolyte disorders or general toxicity complicate the picture. Elderly patients are especially susceptible to the danger of hypovolemia. Except where specific antibiotics or antiparasitic drugs are called for, treatment is symptomatic, and should include careful monitoring and replacement of fluids and electrolytes. Drugs that inhibit gut motility, such as the opiates, should be given cautiously or not at all, especially in invasive bacterial syndromes where they may lead to clinical deterioration.

BIBLIOGRAPHY

Bartlett JG, Chang TW, Gurwith M et al: Antibiotic-associated pseudomembranous colitis due to toxin-producing clostridia. N Engl J Med 298:531–534, 1978

Blacklow NR, Dolin R, Fedson DS et al: Acute infectious nonbacterial gastroenteritis etiology and pathogenesis. Ann Intern Med 76:993–1008, 1972

Drachman RH: Acute infectious gastroenteritis. Ped Clin North Am 21:711–737, 1974

DuPont HL, Formal SB, Hornick RB et al: Pathogenesis of Escherichia coli diarrhea. N Engl J Med 285:1–9, 1971

Nelson JD, Haltalin KC: Accuracy of diagnosis of bacterial diarrheal disease by clinical features. J Pediat 78:519–522, 1971

Plotkin GR, Kluge RM, Waldman RH: Gastroenteritis: etiology, pathophysiology, and clinical manifestations. Medicine 58:95–114, 1979

Sprinz H: Pathogenesis of intestinal infections. Arch Pathol 87:556–562, 1969

35 Malabsorption

Inadequate intestinal absorption can give rise to any of a large number of nutritional deficiencies. The symptoms of malabsorption fall into two categories, gastrointestinal and nutritional.

The *gastrointestinal symptoms* of malabsorption are nonspecific. They are identical with those found in other gastrointestinal diseases that are not associated with malabsorption, and are of no help in distinguishing among the various etiologies of malabsorption. Patients most frequently complain of abdominal distention and borborygmi (rumbling noises in the bowel produced by the movement of gas). The distention is usually not relieved by defecation. Diffuse, crampy lower abdominal pain is common. Frequent bulky, greasy stools are included in all classic descriptions, and are the result of fat malabsorption, but significant steatorrhea (the presence of stool fat) can be present without producing these findings.

Nutritional deficits dominate the clinical picture in patients with severe, chronic malabsorption, reflecting deficiencies of virtually all possible nutrients (see list). Vague complaints of weakness and malaise are most common, although the specific nutritional deficit causing these symptoms can be hard to identify. Weight loss results from poor caloric absorption and anorexia. Muscle wasting is related to a number of factors, including general caloric deprivation and the specific failure to absorb amino acids.

Sign or Symptom	Nutritional Deficiency
weakness, weight loss	fat, protein, carbohydrate
anemia	iron, vitamin B_{12}, folate
bone pain, fractures	calcium, vitamin D, protein
bleeding, bruising	vitamin K
tetany	calcium, magnesium
neuritis	vitamin B_{12}
glossitis	iron, vitamin B_{12}
edema	protein

Malabsorption must be suspected in any patient with gastrointestinal complaints, nonspecific complaints of weakness, weight loss, and fatigue, and evidence of vitamin or mineral deficiencies.

With the exception of patients with lactase deficiency (see discussion later in chapter), virtually all cases of malabsorption are characterized by steatorrhea, which can be quantitated by measuring the fat in a 72-hour stool collection. If a person consuming 100 grams of fat per day loses more than 7 grams per day in his stool, he is said to have steatorrhea. Unfortunately, this is a difficult test to perform on an outpatient basis and is expensive to perform in the hospital. Instead, most clinicians choose to screen a random stool sample for fat. The sample is mixed with saline, heated, and stained with Sudan III or IV. Microscopic examination then reveals the presence or absence of fat globules. Only rarely does the stool of a patient losing more than 20 grams of fat per day fail to reveal fat when stained in this manner. However, significant malabsorption can occur with less impressive steatorrhea, and the diagnosis may then be missed by this test. Oil-based cathartics give false-positive results. If malabsorption is strongly suspected and a random stool sample has failed to confirm the diagnosis, a 72-hour stool collection must be obtained.

ETIOLOGIES OF MALABSORPTION

The many causes of malabsorption can be divided into five categories:

1. Bile salt deficiency
2. Pancreatic insufficiency
3. Intestinal mucosal abnormalities
4. Lactase deficiency
5. Miscellaneous causes, including gastrectomy, drug use, infectious diseases, and endocrine disorders.

Bile Salt Deficiency

Bile salts solubilize fats and fat-soluble substances by means of the formation of micelles, which are then absorbed at the intestinal mucosal surface. Bile salts are synthesized in the liver and secreted into the gastrointestinal tract through the biliary system. They are conjugated to either glycine or taurine, and it is the conjugated salts that function to solubilize dietary fats. The bile salts are resorbed by the terminal ileum and returned to the liver, thus completing a single cycle of the enterohepatic circulation. Cholesterol and fat-soluble vitamins are highly dependent upon bile salts for absorption, but as much as 50% of fatty acids can be absorbed in the absence of bile salts.

The most common cause of malabsorption from an alteration in bile salt metabolism is intestinal overgrowth of anaerobic bacteria. These bacteria contain enzymes that deconjugate intestinal bile salts, thereby rendering the bile physiologically inactive.

Any disease or drug that interferes with the enterohepatic circulation of bile salts can cause malabsorption. The reutilization of bile salts is lost, and the liver cannot synthesize sufficient bile to satisfy the body's requirements in the face of the continued loss of bile salts.

Severe liver disease and extrahepatic obstruction of the biliary tract only rarely cause malabsorption. Biliary cirrhosis is an exception to this, and malabsorption and steatorrhea can be severe. Vitamin deficiencies—especially of vitamin D with consequent bone disease—are particularly common in this disease.

Intestinal Overgrowth. The absorption of fat and vitamin B_{12} are most significantly affected by the intestinal overgrowth of anaerobic bacteria. Bacterial enzymes deconjugate the bile salts and in this way prevent the formation of fat-absorbing micelles. The bacteria impede vitamin B_{12} absorption by utilizing the vitamin. Although absorption of fat-soluble vitamins A, K, and D may be impaired, clinical deficiencies of these vitamins are rare in this setting. The bacteria themselves may synthesize vitamin K, and this may account for the rarity of bleeding problems in these patients.

Bacterial overgrowth occurs in two settings: stasis, and contamination of the upper gastrointestinal tract with the bacterial flora of the lower gastrointestinal tract.

Stasis is the result of mechanical abnormalities or the failure of normal propulsive mechanisms. In elderly patients, bacteria can flourish in the stagnant pockets of jejunal diverticula. These are usually multiple and scattered, and surgery is therefore not the treatment of choice. Achlorhydria, the inability of the stomach to secrete acid, also occurs in a significant percentage of the elderly, and can exacerbate the problem because of the absence of the inhibiting effect of acid on bacterial growth. Bacteria can also thrive in blind loops, pouches of gut that have access to intestinal contents but fail to empty. Stasis resulting from abnormal peristaltic mechanisms occurs in patients with intestinal scleroderma and occasionally in diabetics with autonomic neuropathy.

Contamination of the upper gastrointestinal tract is most often caused by a fistula. The most common setting is granulomatous inflammatory bowel disease or peptic ulcer disease, where erosion extending through to the colon can create an abnormal enterocolic communication.

The diagnosis of bacterial overgrowth is made in two stages:

1. Identification of a lesion that may underlie bacterial overgrowth. A history of surgery, especially a Billroth II anastomosis, suggests the possibility of a blind loop. Granulomatous inflammatory bowel disease, especially if severe and long-standing, can produce enterocolic fistulae. Scleroderma is usually obvious from its other manifestations by the time bacterial overgrowth results. X-ray studies, including an upper GI and a barium enema, should be performed to locate any structural abnormalities, especially diverticula.

2. The bile acid breath test. The patient ingests the radio-labeled bile salt choly-1-^{14}C-glycine. When the bile salt is deconjugated, the labeled glycine is absorbed and metabolized to carbon dioxide, which can then be measured in the exhaled breath.

The treatment of bacterial overgrowth is with broad spectrum antibiotics.

Granulomatous Ileitis and Ileal Resection. Malabsorption can be caused by failure of the distal ileum to resorb bile salts. Granulomatous ileitis or surgical resection of more than two to three feet of distal ileum are usually responsible for this lesion. Failure to resorb bile salts can deplete the bile salt pool beyond the capabilities of the liver to replace it. Steatorrhea results. The passage of bile salts into the colon also inhibits colonic function and produces "bile salt" diarrhea. Since vitamin B_{12} is absorbed in the distal ileum, vitamin B_{12} deficiency usually accompanies this syndrome. Patients fail to absorb vitamin B_{12} even when given intrinsic factor. In a patient with known granulomatous disease, the increasing severity of diarrhea may be due solely to the inflammatory process and not to malabsorption. However, the presence of steatorrhea and vitamin B_{12} deficiency suggests that bile salt diarrhea may have developed. Bile salt diarrhea can be treated with cholestyramine, which binds the bile salts. Cholestyramine may, however, exacerbate the bile salt deficiency, and must therefore be titrated carefully in each patient.

Patients with granulomatous disease can be distinguished from those with bacterial overgrowth by a negative bile acid breath test.

Pancreatic Insufficiency

Pancreatic lipase hydrolyzes triglycerides. Absence of this enzyme inhibits fat absorption and produces steatorrhea. Absence of the pancreatic proteases contributes to concurrent protein malabsorption.

By far the leading cause of pancreatic insufficiency in the United States is chronic pancreatitis secondary to ethanol abuse. The disease can present as recurrent painful episodes of acute pancreatitis, or can present silently with slow, relentless destruction of the pancreas. An abdominal x-ray reveals diffuse calcification of the pancreas in many patients with chronic pancreatitis (see Chap. 37). Vitamin B_{12} levels are normal, but a blood film may reveal megaloblastic anemia from the folate deficiency that is common in alcoholics. The bile acid breath test is normal. Patients may have an abnormal glucose tolerance test.

A specific diagnosis can be made with a secretin test. A double-lumen tube is placed in the duodenum, and a baseline 20-minute aspirate is obtained for volume and bicarbonate concentration. Secretin is then given intravenously, and several more 20-minute aspirates are collected. The normal response to secretin includes the production of 2 ml of water per kg in one 20-minute aspirate and a bicarbonate concentration of 85 mEq/liter. Lower values indicate impaired pancreatic secretory capacity. Any person with alcoholism and steatorrhea should be suspected of having pancreatic malabsorption. Once the diagnosis is made, treatment with oral preparations of pancreatic enzymes is instituted.

Mucosal Abnormalities

The most common variety of mucosal abnormality that can lead to malabsorption is *celiac disease* (also called nontropical sprue or gluten-sensitive enteropathy). This disorder is probably due to an as yet undefined immunologic malfunction and is very highly correlated with the HLA antigen Dw 3. The disease is only active in the presence of gluten, a constituent of wheat. Patients exhibit both humoral and cell-mediated immunity to gluten, and bind gluten to their cells to a much greater extent than normal persons. Precisely how these observations fit together to produce the severe bowel mucosal pathology and the ensuing clinical problems is unknown.

The patient with celiac disease generally comes to medical attention with complaints of abdominal discomfort and diarrhea. He often has evidence of nutritional deficiencies and anemia. Fulminant cases may occur, and can be so severe that patients resemble victims of concentration camps. In these patients, the full impact of panmalabsorption is seen.

Celiac disease is usually a diffuse disease of the small intestine. The jejunum is more involved than the ileum, and vitamin B_{12} absorption is thus relatively spared. The presence of diffuse small intestinal mucosal disease can by measured by the D-xylose test. Ninety-five percent of patients with celiac disease show impaired D-xylose absorption. D-xylose is primarily absorbed passively by the mucosa, and is only minimally metabolized once absorbed. The patient is given a 25 g oral dose and, if his gastrointestinal mucosa is healthy, 4.5 to 7.5 g will appear in a 5-hour urine collection. Lower levels indicate small intestinal disease. The test is not abnormal in patients with bile salt deficiencies or pancreatic insufficiency.

Once an abnormal D-xylose test is obtained, a jejunal biopsy should be performed. A biopsy is necessary to rule out other mucosal diseases that may cause malabsorption. These include tropical sprue, Whipple's disease, intestinal lymphoma, and others. Unfortunately, celiac disease and tropical sprue can have identical histologies.

Celiac disease is treated with a gluten-free diet. Within eight weeks, the patient's symptoms should begin to abate, and his nutritional status, laboratory values, and histology should show improvement. Failure to respond to a strict diet is firm evidence against the diagnosis, and another mucosal disease should be sought.

Lactase Deficiency

Lactase is an enzyme that splits lactose into glucose and galactose. Lactase is a sugar most commonly found in milk and dairy products. Lactase deficiency is the one common cause of malabsorption not associated with steatorrhea (other diseases that cause malabsorption without steatorrhea, such as Hartnup disease and isomaltase deficiency, are extremely rare.)

Because lactase deficiency is missed by the stool fat screen, it must be recognized clinically. Lactase deficiency is very common, and the enzyme is deficient in 5% of adult whites and an even greater percentage of blacks. Not all these people are symptomatic, and only a minority have significant malabsorption. In general, lactase deficiency presents with gastrointestinal complaints and not with nutritional deficiency. Patients complain of bloating, distention, cramping abdominal pain, and watery diarrhea, occurring 45 to 60 minutes after eating. These symptoms are variable, and their severity depends on the lactose load and the enzyme level. Enzyme levels can be further reduced by inflammation of the gastrointestinal mucosa, as can occur with gastroenteritis, inflammatory bowel disease, and giardiasis, and these conditions exacerbate and sometimes unmask subclinical cases of lactase deficiency.

Lactase deficiency is diagnosed by a lactose tolerance test. One hundred grams of lactose are given orally, and in normal adults a rise of serum glucose levels of at least 20 mg/dl is seen. Patients with lactase deficiency show no rise in their blood glucose. Avoidance of lactose-containing foods successfully treats this syndrome.

Other Causes of Malabsorption

Gastrectomy, whether partial or total, may be associated with several syndromes of malabsorption due to a variety of causes:

1. An associated blind loop may result in bacterial overgrowth;
2. Some of these patients dump large volumes of food into the duodenum, producing a "dumping syndrome." Only rarely does this produce malabsorption. The pathophysiology of the dumping syndrome is not entirely understood, nor is it clear why many patients are spared. Patients with the dumping syndrome complain of epigastric discomfort, nausea, weakness and lightheadedness soon after eating. Some of these symptoms may result from the rapid "dumping" of food into the jejunum. Food is hypertonic with respect to serum, and fluid and electrolytes are rapidly drawn into the gut with resultant circulatory hypovolemia. The rapid absorption of glucose leads to hyperglycemia, and, rarely, these patients develop severe hypoglycemia after the sudden rise in blood sugar. Some of the symptoms of the dumping syndrome may also be due to the stimulation of gut hormone secretion.
3. For unknown reasons, gastrectomy may uncover dormant celiac disease and lactase deficiency.

Iron, calcium, and vitamin B_{12} malabsorption may be seen. Most postgastrectomy patients eventually become iron-deficient. Because the gastric mucosa is the site of intrinsic factor synthesis, total gastrectomy generally requires life-long parenteral vitamin B_{12} replacement. One-third of patients experience diminished vitamin D absorption, and may develop bone disease.

Drugs have been implicated in malabsorption, sometimes of just specific nutrients.

Birth control pills can lead to folate deficiency, and aluminum-containing antacids to a deficiency of phosphate. A few drugs, when used chronically, such as colchicine, cholestyramine, and laxatives can produce a more generalized malabsorption. Alcohol itself can cause malabsorption even in the absence of pancreatic insufficiency.

Several infectious diseases can cause malabsorption. *Tropical sprue* is a disease of the tropics that symptomatically and pathologically resembles celiac disease. Travelers and former residents of the tropics can develop the disease years after they have moved to more temperate zones. Although no organism has yet been identified, these patients respond to tetracycline. Unlike patients with celiac disease, they experience no improvement on a gluten-free diet. *Giardiasis* can uncommonly cause a malabsorption syndrome that resembles celiac disease. The organism appears in a duodenal aspirate in more than 50% of patients, but appears less commonly in the stool. A jejunal biopsy reveals the organism in a majority of patients. Therapy is with metronidazole.

Whipple's disease is extremely rare. It presents with abdominal distress, malabsorption, fever, lymphadenopathy, arthritis, and neurologic symptoms. It is probably caused by a bacillus, but the specific organism has not been identified. Diagnosis is made with an intestinal biopsy, which shows a lamina propria crowded with PAS-positive foamy macrophages. Response to antibiotic therapy can be dramatic.

It is not uncommon to see diarrhea and steatorrhea in patients with *endocrine disorders*. In patients with diabetes, malabsorption may partially derive from disordered intestinal motility. Interestingly, since an intestinal biopsy may reveal a pathology similar to celiac disease, symptoms may improve on a gluten-free diet. Steatorrhea occurs in some patients with hyperthyroidism and responds to treatment of the underlying thyroid disorder. Some patients with hypothyroidism also have malabsorption that appears to be due to mucosal disease.

DIAGNOSTIC FLOW SHEET

Evaluation of the underlying cause of malabsorption in a given patient is not as formidable as the extensive list of possible etiologies would suggest. A stool sample or 72-hour stool fat collection detects all but the patient with lactase deficiency, and a careful history, a trial of diet therapy, and a lactose tolerance test confirms or denies the possibility of lactase deficiency.

Once malabsorption is documented, the next step should be a complete series of GI radiologic contrast studies. If a lesion such as a blind loop, diverticulum, or fistula is demonstrated, the possibility of bacterial overgrowth should be explored with a bile acid breath test as well as a vitamin B_{12} level. If these are abnormal, a trial of antibiotics is then indicated.

If the GI x-rays reveal either a normal gastrointestinal tract or only nonspecific abnormalities, a D-xylose test should be performed for the evaluation of mucosal disease. If the D-xylose test is abnormal, a jejunal biopsy should be obtained. If the D-xylose test is normal, pancreatic function should be evaluated with a secretin test. If this is abnormal, the patient should be given a trial of pancreatic enzymes. If the secretin test is normal, especially when there is no history of alcoholism or pancreatic disease, a small intestinal biopsy is needed to look for rarer diseases, such as lymphoma, that may be present with a normal D-xylose test.

The added information that comes with the history of each patient will clearly shift the direction of the diagnostic work-up. A history of chronic relapsing pancreatitis should lead directly to a secretin test after steatorrhea is confirmed. Similarly, a history of surgery or ileitis allows certain steps in the overall scheme to be skipped.

The final step is to document the patient's nutritional deficiencies, not so much for diagnostic reasons, but to determine replacement needs. Thus, prolongation of the prothrombin time indicates a need for vitamin K, hypocalcemia a need for vitamin D, and so on. Folate, iron, and vitamin B_{12} levels should be measured and replacement given if needed. Oral administration may, of course, be futile.

BIBLIOGRAPHY

Bayless TM, Rothfield B, Massa C et al: Lactose and milk intolerance: Clinical implications. N Engl J Med 292:1156–1159, 1975

Hefner GW: Breath tests in gastroenterology. Adv Intern Med 23:25–45, 1978

Longstreth GF, Newcomer AD: Drug-induced malabsorption. Mayo Clin Proc 50:284–293, 1975

Phillips SF: Diarrhea: A current view of the pathophysiology. Gastroenterology 63:495–518, 1972

Symposium on Malabsorption. Am J Med 67:979–1104, 1979

Wilson FA, Dietsch JM: Differential diagnostic approach to clinical problems of malabsorption. Gastroenterology 61:911–931, 1971

36

Inflammatory Bowel Disease

The term inflammatory bowel disease encompasses a wide spectrum of clinical and pathologic entities. These are chronic illnesses that vary greatly in their severity, ranging from mild proctitis with tenesmus to fulminating, life-threatening intestinal inflammation with bowel perforation, hemorrhage, and shock.

The course of illness in most patients is punctuated by exacerbations and remissions, and the severity of the exacerbations and the completeness of the remissions vary unpredictably.

Symptoms may be limited to the gastrointestinal tract and typically include diarrhea, abdominal pain, tenesmus, and blood in the stool. When severe, diarrhea and inflammation can give rise to the systemic symptoms of anorexia, weight loss, malnutrition, and general debility. There are also a great many characteristic extraintestinal manifestations that may accompany inflammatory bowel disease, including liver disease, arthritis, and dermatologic and ocular disorders. In addition, patients have an increased risk of intestinal malignancy. Medical treatment is not curative, and multiple operations may punctuate the clinical course.

The etiology of inflammatory bowel disease remains unknown. No infectious organism has been identified despite an intensive search for a viral or bacterial agent. Various alterations in host immunity have been described, but these have not been successfully related to the onset or progression of disease. Early work that implicated psychosomatic factors has recently met with considerable criticism.

It has been useful to distinguish two types of inflammatory bowel disease, ulcerative colitis and Crohn's disease (also known as regional enteritis). In ulcerative colitis, inflammation is restricted to the colon, whereas in Crohn's disease, inflammatory lesions may be found throughout the gastrointestinal tract, from the mouth to the rectum. The radiographic and histologic characteristics of these diseases are also distinctive, as will be discussed below. Nevertheless, in practice, the distinction between ulcerative colitis and Crohn's disease of the colon is frequently difficult to make on clinical and even pathologic grounds. The extracolonic manifestations of inflammatory bowel disease can occur in both Crohn's disease and ulcerative colitis.

ULCERATIVE COLITIS

Clinical Presentation

Ulcerative colitis is an inflammatory disease of the colon that causes a diffuse mucosal inflammation. The rectum is virtually always involved, and, occasionally, proctitis is the sole manifestation of the colitis. In some patients, the entire colon may be inflamed (pancolitis). The clinical presentation of the disease is extremely variable. Mild abdominal cramps with tenesmus are characteristic. Watery, bloody diarrhea is usually present, and patients may describe an urgency at stool and nocturnal diarrhea. In more severe disease, systemic signs and symptoms such as fever, weight loss, and anorexia are also present. The disease pattern fluctuates: periods of remission are interrupted by flares of acute illness.

Sigmoidoscopy and Biopsy

Visual examination of the sigmoid colon must be undertaken in any patient suspected of having ulcerative colitis. Early in the course of the disease, the colonic mucosa is red, and the normal pattern of mucosal blood vessels is absent. The mucosa is said to be "friable," and bleeds easily when it is dabbed with a cotton swab. The mucosa may assume a blistering and granular appearance. Pseudopolyps (flat areas that appear to be raised because the surrounding mucosa has been eroded) can also be seen.

A biopsy of the rectal mucosa should also be obtained during sigmoidoscopy. In ulcerative colitis, an inflammatory infiltrate is seen in the lamina propria; microabscesses appear at the colonic crypts, but the submucosa is spared. If, however, granulomas are present, the diagnosis of Crohn's colitis is suggested. The biopsy can also aid in the diagnosis of

carcinoma or amebiasis. A stool sample should be obtained for culture to exclude the diagnosis of shigellosis or salmonellosis.

Radiographic Findings

A wide array of x-ray findings has been described (Fig. 36–1). In advanced ulcerative colitis, the colon appears as a foreshortened narrow tube, and the characteristic haustral markings are absent. Deep ulcerations, strictures, and pseudopolyps can also be seen. In mild disease, only the sigmoid colon may appear abnormal on x-ray.

Differential Diagnosis

In addition to Crohn's disease, a number of common illnesses can mimic ulcerative colitis:

1. *Ischemic colitis* secondary to atherosclerotic vascular disease is seen in elderly patients who present with lower abdominal cramps, rectal bleeding, and fever. The physical examination may suggest peritonitis, and lactic acidosis may be present. A barium enema may show the characteristic "thumb printing," which results from intramural intestinal hemorrhage and edema. Ischemic colitis has also been described in young women who take oral contraceptive medications.

2. The ameba *Entamoeba histolytica* causes a colitis that can have an insidious onset and a prolonged course. Amebic colitis must be considered not only in patients who travel, but also in those who have never left the United States. The diagnosis can be difficult. Fresh swabs or biopsies of ulcerative bowel are necessary to make the diagnosis. The organism is difficult to identify in stool specimens. Barium studies, bismuth, and antacids all interfere with detection of the ameba, and fecal leukocytes can be mistaken for the organism. Serologic confirmation of amebiasis

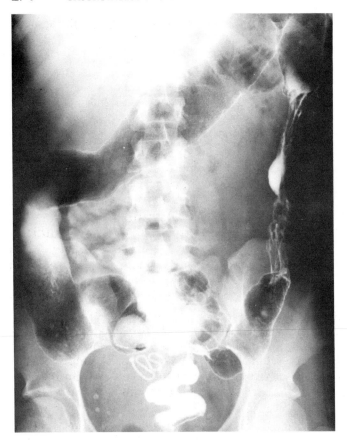

FIG. 36–1. Ulcerative colitis. An air contrast barium enema shows foreshortening of the colon in a patient with pancolitis. Note the absence of normal haustral markings. (The snake-shaped radiopacity in the pelvis is an IUD.)

should be sought. Amebicidal therapy is curative.

3. *Pseudomembranous colitis* (Chap. 34) must be considered in any patient taking antibiotics. Clindamycin and lincomycin are the most common offenders, but other antibiotics have also been implicated. Pseudomembranous colitis is caused by a toxin elaborated by *Clostridium difficile*, and has been successfully treated with vancomycin.

4. *Diverticular disease* of the colon can also be confused with ulcerative colitis. Diverticula are herniations of mucosa and submucosa through the muscular layers of the bowel, and are commonly found in the sig-moid colon in people over 60 years of age. They may occasionally cause mild rectal bleeding. In extreme cases, profuse rectal hemorrhaging may necessitate partial colectomy. When diverticula become inflamed (*diverticulitis*), a localized peritonitis can develop, causing pain and fever. Colonic obstruction, fistulae, and intra-abdominal abscesses can result. Diverticula can easily be seen on barium studies of the colon. Symptomatic disease is usually self-limiting, although diverticulitis often requires intravenous antibiotic therapy.

Other illnesses that may occasionally mimic colonic inflammatory bowel disease include appendicitis, shigellosis, and salmonellosis.

Clinical Course and Therapy

One-fourth of patients with ulcerative colitis have proctitis alone. The prognosis for these patients is good, and the overall mortality is similar to that of the general population. Few patients presenting with only proctitis develop pancolitis. On the other hand, many patients present initially with pancolitis, and they pursue a far graver course. Most of these patients require hospitalization.

In patients with mild ulcerative colitis, the goals of therapy are to reduce the abdominal discomfort, control the diarrhea, and decrease the inflammation. Sulfasalazine and, when needed, glucocorticoids are the mainstays of drug therapy in the treatment of mild flares.

Sulfasalazine is systemically absorbed, excreted with the bile, and then cleaved by bacteria within the colon to sulfapyridine, an antibiotic, and 5-aminosalicylic acid, an anti-inflammatory agent. It is not known which of these products is the active agent. In the patient who presents with a typical attack, sulfasalazine is often sufficient therapy.

In some patients, the anti-inflammatory effects of prednisone may prove helpful. Prednisone can be given as a suppository in patients with proctitis, or taken orally by patients with more diffuse disease.

Roughage should be eliminated from the diet. Antidiarrheal agents should be prescribed with caution, since their use can further the tendency to develop toxic megacolon (discussion later).

If a remission can be achieved, sulfasalazine should be continued, since it decreases the incidence of future flare-ups. Glucocorticoids are ineffective prophylactic agents, but chronic prednisone therapy may be required in patients who are unable to achieve remission or whose disease flares when the steroids are tapered.

Colonic Cancer

Patients with ulcerative colitis have an abnormally high incidence of colonic carcinoma. The risk of malignancy is increased in patients with pancolitis, in patients who experience the onset of disease in childhood, and in patients who have had ulcerative colitis for more than ten years. Long-term remission does not diminish the risk.

Early detection of colonic cancer is difficult and unsatisfactory. The use of elevated blood levels of carcinoembryonic antigen as a screen for the development of colonic cancer is severely limited by the observation that up to 50% of patients with ulcerative colitis uncomplicated by colonic cancer have elevated levels of the antigen, probably solely because of the inflammatory process itself. The development of intestinal obstruction or constipation in a patient with ulcerative colitis should raise the suspicion of carcinoma, but, at present, there are no clinical signs or symptoms that can be firmly relied upon to tell when cancer of the colon has developed.

The colonic tumors that develop in these patients are frequently small, flat, and difficult to distinguish from the inflammatory lesions. Dysplastic changes may precede frank malignancy, and frequent sigmoidoscopic and colonoscopic surveillance with biopsy is recommended, especially in patients with pancolitis. Colectomy is recommended when dysplastic changes are seen on biopsy. Colectomy is also the treatment of choice for unremitting colitis unresponsive to medical therapy.

CROHN'S DISEASE

Crohn's disease primarily affects young adults, and its incidence appears to be increasing. Patients typically present with mild diarrhea, abdominal pain, lassitude, and weight loss. Gastrointestinal bleeding is usually occult and gross lower gastrointestinal bleeding is seen only with significant colonic involvement. Because these symptoms are nonspecific, there is an average time lag of three years between the onset of symptoms and the diagnosis. Symptoms relating to the bowel may be absent altogether, and the disease can present as a fever of unknown origin.

Pathology

The inflammatory lesion in Crohn's disease is transmural, extending through the entire bowel wall. As a result, the formation of adhesions between adjacent loops of bowel and between bowel and other abdominal organs (*e.g.*, bladder) are common. Fistulae from bowel segment to bowel segment, bladder, abdominal wall, and skin also form. The inflamed areas of bowel occur in "skip areas," separated by segments of normal intestine. The involved areas are marked by submucosal thickening and fibrosis. Noncaseating granulomas are found in the serosa (thus, Crohn's disease is also called granulomatous enteritis). The inflamed bowel is entirely surrounded by rings of mesenteric fat. The presence of anal fissures is characteristic of Crohn's disease, even when the rectum itself is not affected. Fistulae opening to the skin may be present over the abdomen, flank, or in the perineum.

Radiographic Findings

The x-ray findings in a patient with Crohn's disease include the presence of numerous intestinal strictures, narrowings, and fistulae (Fig. 36–2). Areas of normal bowel intervene between the diseased areas. The inflamed bowel may assume a "cobblestone" appearance. The typical radiologic findings of toxic megacolon may also be seen in Crohn's colitis.

Clinical Course

As in ulcerative colitis, the clinical course of Crohn's disease is marked by exacerbations followed by relative periods of remission. Flares are characterized by anorexia, vomiting, weight loss, abdominal pain, and dehydration. Intestinal obstruction, partial or complete, is common, especially when the small bowel is extensively involved. Gastrointestinal hemorrhage is much less common than in ulcerative colitis. Patients with Crohn's disease have a higher incidence of small bowel carcinoma than the normal population.

Many patients with Crohn's disease ultimately require surgery for intractable disease, recurrent bleeding, external fistulae, intestinal obstruction, or intra-abdominal abscesses. In ulcerative colitis, the operation (colectomy) is curative, but surgery cannot cure Crohn's disease. New lesions evolve, and reoperation is the rule. As a result, many patients with Crohn's disease have most of their small bowel surgically removed over a period of years. Intestinal obstruction caused by strictures and adhesions remains a critical problem in these patients.

With extensive small bowel involvement, or after repeated surgical extirpations, *malabsorption* can become a significant problem. Bacterial overgrowth occurring in isolated loops of the small bowel compounds the problem. Even though remaining regions of healthy small bowel can adapt to absorb nutrients more efficiently, nutritional anemia can result from inadequate iron and vitamin B_{12} absorption. Vitamin D, magnesium, and calcium are also poorly absorbed. Malabsorption of fats, carbohydrates, and protein may also occur.

Decreased bile salt absorption has been blamed for the markedly increased incidence of gallstones in Crohn's disease. Kidney stones composed of oxalate are common in these patients. Oxalate is normally complexed with

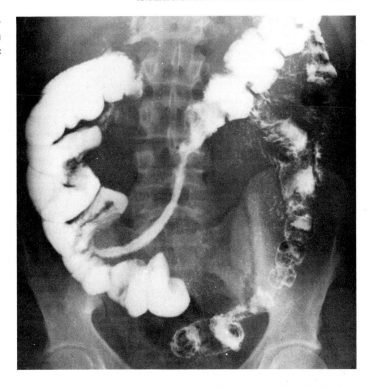

FIG. 36–2. Crohn's disease of the colon. A barium enema in a patient with Crohn's colitis shows the characteristic "string sign" in the transverse colon.

calcium in the gut to form a nonabsorbable salt. In patients with fat malabsorption, the intestinal calcium is saponified and is therefore unavailable to react with oxalate, which is then absorbed in the colon in abnormally high amounts. The formation of oxalate stones can lead to chronic renal failure. Other causes of renal insufficiency in Crohn's disease include amyloidosis and fistulae from the gut to the urinary tract.

The National Cooperative Crohn's Disease Study has recently completed a careful randomized investigation of therapy in Crohn's disease, and the inclusion of a placebo group has enabled them to outline the natural history of the disease. The typical patient has both small bowel and colonic involvement. The age of onset of the disease does not influence the severity of the illness. Clinical symptoms do not correlate with radiographic studies, and the study recommended against the routine use of x-rays for follow-up care.

Spontaneous remissions are part of the natural history of Crohn's disease. Both prednisone and sulfasalazine may help to induce remissions, but azathioprine is not effective. Patients with colonic involvement respond better to sulfasalazine then to prednisone. Patients whose disease is limited to the small bowel respond only to prednisone. Patients who take either sulfasalazine or prednisone and who do not achieve any therapeutic response also do not respond to a change in medication. In patients who have achieved remission, no drug has been shown to be effective as a prophylaxis against future flare-ups. Medical treatment does not affect extraintestinal manifestations, and the need for surgical intervention is also unaffected by medical treatment.

EXTRAINTESTINAL MANIFESTATIONS OF INFLAMMATORY BOWEL DISEASE

A large number of extraintestinal manifestations are seen in patients with ulcerative colitis and Crohn's colitis. Rarely, these manifestations may precede the onset of the bowel disease. The incidence of extraintestinal manifestations is independent of the site(s) of intestinal involvement.

Nearly 25% of patients with colitis have *arthritic* complaints during the course of their disease. Acute arthritis occurs with exacerbations in the colitis, and is commonly monoarticular, involving one large joint of the lower limbs. A chronic polyarthritis involving distal small joints is not correlated with the activity of colonic disease. Colitis increases the risk of ankylosing spondylitis in those patients who are positive for the HLA-B27 antigen.

Erythema nodosum occurs in up to 20% of patients at some time during their illness. It generally appears during active disease and may present as part of a triad with diarrhea and arthritis. It most often subsides in concert with remissions in the activity of the bowel inflammation. *Pyoderma gangrenosum* presents as poorly healing indolent ulcers that are generally confined to the extremities. Although it rarely occurs in the absence of inflammatory bowel disease, its appearance is not a measure of the severity of intestinal involvement.

Aphthous stomatitis, conjunctivitis, episcleritis, and *uveitis* are also occasionally seen. Although ocular inflammation is unusual, the development of ocular pain, photophobia, and visual impairment suggest uveitis, which may threaten vision and require ophthalmologic intervention. Steroids are generally effective in treating this condition and can be given locally.

Liver disease may occur in patients with ulcerative colitis, Crohn's colitis, and Crohn's disease of the small bowel. The etiology of hepatic dysfunction is not known; portal bacteremia resulting from bacteria infiltrating through intestinal mucosal lesions has been implicated. A careful histologic survey reveals some hepatic abnormality in up to 90% of all patients with inflammatory bowel disease. A wide variety of lesions has been noted, including *sclerosing pericholangitis* and *cirrhosis.* Sclerosing pericholangitis is rarely seen in the absence of inflammatory bowel disease. It may be clinically silent and only apparent through a rise in the serum level of 5'-nucleotidase. In some patients, however, the disease may be responsible for cholangitis (sometimes recurrent) with fever, abdominal pain, jaundice, and hepatic tenderness.

There are no controlled studies at present showing the effectiveness of steroids in the therapy of these extraintestinal manifestations.

FULMINANT COLITIS, HYPERALIMENTATION, AND TOXIC MEGACOLON

Fulminant Colitis

Patients with acute flare-ups of ulcerative colitis or Crohn's colitis may complain of more than abdominal cramps and blood-streaked stools. In *fulminant colitis,* patients are extremely ill, and days of severe bloody diarrhea and anorexia result in dehydration, anemia, and inadequate nourishment. Fever is often present, and patients may complain of severe abdominal pain. These patients require immediate hospitalization for rehydration, blood transfusion, correction of electrolyte imbalances, and monitoring for the development of toxic megacolon (see later discussion).

The possibility of an acute abdominal event, such as appendicitis, must not be overlooked. Furthermore, these patients, especially those with regional enteritis, are susceptible to acute intestinal obstruction. This must be treated with bowel decompression using a long tube and providing appropriate intravenous fluids and electrolytes.

An intensive medical regimen has been devised to treat these very severe attacks of colitis. No oral intake is permitted, thereby allowing the bowel to be "put to rest." Parenteral steroids are prescribed in high doses during an acute attack of colitis. In order for healing to begin, however, the body must obtain adequate nutrition. Most patients with severe inflammatory bowel disease are malnourished. Oral intake has been poor, electrolytes and minerals have been lost through chronic diarrhea, protein has been lost from gastrointestinal bleeding, and malabsorption may be present. Moreover, protein calorie malnutrition itself may decrease brush border enzyme activity and thereby diminish the absorptive capacity of the gut.

Hyperalimentation

In order to achieve adequate nourishment, therefore, many patients with severe inflammatory bowel disease receive *total parenteral nutrition* (TPN) through *intravenous hyperalimentation*. The primary goal of TPN is to achieve weight gain and to restore a positive nitrogen balance. After the patient has been rehydrated and his electrolyte imbalances have been treated by peripheral intravenous therapy, TPN is begun through a central intravenous catheter. The TPN solution consists of hypertonic dextrose, an amino acid solution, vitamins, and minerals (including trace minerals like zinc and copper). Exogenous insulin must be added to prevent hyperglycemia. Intravenous fat emulsions are also added if TPN is given for more than two to three weeks; otherwise, patients develop a deficiency of essential fatty acids. TPN usually improves the patient's general clinical status. If surgery is eventually required, sub-sequent wound healing will be facilitated by the improved nourishment.

Intravenous hyperalimentation is a very complex system of care, and it requires the presence of a specialized team of physicians, nurses, and dietitians. Complications of intravenous hyperalimentation include pneumothorax and hydrothorax, thrombosis of the central vein where the catheter has been placed, sepsis, electrolyte and mineral imbalances, and hyperosmolar, hyperglycemic coma. Interestingly, many patients experience gustatory hallucinations while receiving TPN. The sudden onset of fever in a previously afebrile patient mandates discontinuation of TPN. The catheter should be removed and the catheter tip should be cultured.

Toxic Megacolon

Although the lesions of ulcerative colitis are mucosal, inflammation may spread to the muscularis. As this layer becomes involved, the bowel loses its muscular support and dilates. All patients with acute flares of ulcerative colitis require plain x-rays of the abdomen. When colonic dilation is seen, frequent x-ray examinations must be performed in order to evaluate the course of dilation (Fig. 36–3). *Toxic megacolon* occurs when dilation becomes severe (more than 10 cm in diameter) and the patient becomes critically ill. The danger of colonic perforation and overwhelming peritonitis is immediate, and mortality is very high. The patient's abdomen is distended, tender, and painful. Bowel sounds are absent, except for occasional high-pitched sounds. Leukocytosis and hypokalemia are commonly seen. The use of steroids in the treatment of toxic megacolon is controversial, since it has been feared that these anti-inflammatory agents might mask the signs of colonic perforation. In addition, there have been no convincing studies documenting their effectiveness in these patients. However, the relatively

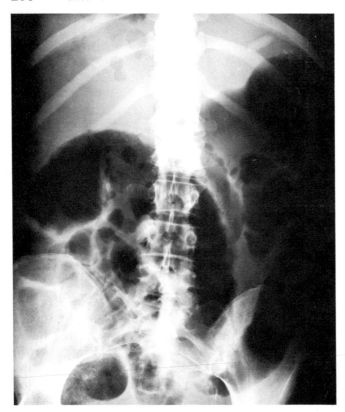

FIG. 36–3. Toxic megacolon. Enormous dilatation of the colon is readily apparent. Indentations in the bowel wall ("thumb printing") are caused by mucosal edema.

short-term steroid regimen used for toxic megacolon does not adversely affect surgical success. Furthermore, many patients with ulcerative colitis have taken glucocorticoids within the preceding year, and must therefore be presumed to have iatrogenic adrenal insufficiency and to require stress doses of glucocorticoids. Surgical advice should be sought early, since progression of dilation in the toxic megacolon and perforation are surgical emergencies.

BIBLIOGRAPHY

Dobbins, WO 3rd: Current status of the precancer lesion in ulcerative colitis. Gastroenterology 73:1431–1433, 1977

Fawaz KA, Glotzer DJ, Goldman H et al: Ulcerative colitis and Crohn's disease of the colon—a comparison of the long term postoperative courses. Gastroenterology 71:372–378, 1976

Goodman MJ, Kirsner JB, Riddell RH: Usefulness of rectal biopsy in inflammatory bowel disease. Gastroenterology 72:952–956, 1977

Greenstein AJ, Janowitz HD, Sachar DB: The extraintestinal complications of Crohn's disease and ulcerative colitis: a study of 700 patients. Medicine 55:401–412, 1976

Lennard-Jones JE, Powell-Tuck J: Drug treatment of inflammatory bowel disease. Clin Gastroenterol 8:187–217, 1979

Mekhjian HS, Switz DM, Melnyk CS et al: Clinical features and natural history of Crohn's disease. Gastroenterology 77:898–906, 1979

Waye JD: Colitis, cancer, and colonoscopy. Med Clin North Am 62:211–224, 1978

37

Pancreatitis

The hallmark of acute pancreatic inflammation is severe abdominal pain radiating through to the back and accompanied by peritoneal signs and fever. Only with chronic inflammation does the loss of pancreatic endocrine (insulin and glucagon) and exocrine function become a significant problem.

It is important to distinguish pancreatitis from other causes of an acute abdomen, including appendicitis, cholecystitis, and a perforating ulcer. Whereas these other diseases are generally curable by surgical intervention, pancreatitis—with very rare exceptions—is not.

Acute Pancreatitis. In the United States, biliary tract disease is the principal cause of acute pancreatitis. Other causes include hyperparathyroidism, hypertriglyceridemia, trauma, pancreatic carcinoma, birth control pills, thiazide diuretics, corticosteroids, and other drugs. In a small percentage of cases, no cause can be ascribed.

The pancreas possesses great regenerative ability, and acute pancreatitis is a reversible lesion. It is thus extremely unusual for multiple attacks of acute pancreatitis to lead to the irreversible destruction seen in chronic pancreatitis.

Chronic Pancreatitis. Alcoholism is, by far, the leading cause of chronic pancreatitis. Although alcoholic pancreatitis manifests itself by acute attacks that are indistinguishable from those of acute pancreatitis, the underlying pathology is most often that of chronic pancreatitis (Fig. 37–1). The lesion is irreversible (like alcoholic cirrhosis) and often calcified, and abstinence will not result in healing. An attack of alcoholic pancreatitis frequently begins the day after a debauch, and recurrent attacks are often increasingly painful and of longer duration. It is felt that even the first clinical attack should be considered chronic relapsing pancreatitis, since it invariably occurs against a background of several years of alcohol abuse.

PATHOPHYSIOLOGY

Mechanisms of Damage to the Pancreas

The precise biochemical reactions resulting in pancreatitis are still unresolved, and several theories have been advanced:

1. Ethanol is known to increase the concentration of protein in the pancreatic juices.

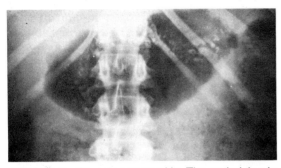

FIG. 37–1. Chronic pancreatitis. The underlying lesion of alcoholic pancreatitis is chronic calcific pancreatitis. This patient had malabsorption secondary to pancreatic insufficiency. The pancreas is outlined by diffuse, finely stippled calcifications, seen overlying the gas-filled stomach.

At high concentrations, the protein may precipitate in the pancreatic ducts and produce obstructive plugs, which may later calcify. It has been suggested that when the ethanol-abused pancreas is stimulated, the activated enzymes cannot be extruded through the blocked ducts. Trapped within the gland, the enzymes are activated and they then digest the pancreatic tissue.

2. Hypertriglyceridemia has been postulated as the final common pathway in the genesis of pancreatitis. Patients with type I and type V hyperlipoproteinemia have an increased incidence of pancreatitis, and alcohol is also known to stimulate triglyceride synthesis, (alcoholics often have elevated serum triglycerides.) Triglyceride metabolism produces free fatty acids, which, it is presumed, either are directly toxic to the pancreatic acinar cells or cause microthrombi in blood vessels that can lead to ischemic necrosis. It has thus been argued that the pancreatitis that develops secondary to the use of birth control pills may result from the increase in serum triglycerides that can accompany estrogen ingestion. The finding of increased triglycerides, however, is not a constant one in pancreatitis, and this mechanism may only account for certain cases.

SYSTEMIC MANIFESTATIONS

Hypotension and shock may occur in severe acute pancreatitis, although the pathophysiology is unclear. Some volume is lost in the protein-rich exudate surrounding the inflamed pancreas. In addition, myocardial depressant factors (and perhaps other vasoactive substances) are activated and released into the circulation. Peptic ulcer disease, commonly associated with acute pancreatitis, may cause bleeding and thereby exacerbate the loss of volume.

A significant number of patients with acute pancreatitis suffer acute respiratory distress. Severe abdominal pain causes splinting, with resultant atelectasis and pneumonitis. Sympathetic pleural effusions are common. In rare cases, patients with pancreatitis may suffer the adult respiratory distress syndrome.

A more unusual manifestation of pancreatitis is distal fatty necrosis with subcutaneous purple skin lesions. Lipases that are released into the circulation may be responsible. These skin lesions are pathognomonic for acute pancreatitis, and can occur in patients who lack all other symptoms of pancreatitis.

Decreases in serum ionized calcium are very common, and tetany or a positive Trousseau's or Chvostek's sign is occasionally seen. The reason for the hypocalcemia is unclear. Fatty necrosis and saponification result in the complexing and precipitation of calcium ions, thereby removing them from the circulation. Some investigators have also postulated a diminished response of the parathyroid gland to hypocalcemia, and others have proposed a decreased response of the bone to parathyroid hormone. Hypomagnesemia may also contribute to the persistent low serum calcium in alcoholics with pancreatitis.

DIAGNOSIS

The typical signs and symptoms of an acute attack of pancreatitis include abdominal pain radiating through to the back and hypoactive bowel sounds, often in conjunction with other peritoneal signs. X-ray findings may include pancreatic calcification, a widened duodenal sweep, or a sentinel loop.

The classic laboratory finding is an elevation of the serum or urinary amylase. Other organs, however, including the parotid glands, the fallopian tubes, the bowel, and the lung, also synthesize amylase, and severe abdominal pain with hyperamylasemia can occur with ruptured ectopic pregnancies, bowel obstruction, biliary disease, and peptic ulceration. In addition, the test for serum amylase may not be abnormal in patients with hypertriglyceridemia and lactescent (milky) serum, although the presence of lactescent serum in a patient with abdominal pain is in itself highly suggestive of acute pancreatitis.

Approximately 25% of serum amylase is filtered at the renal glomerulus and reabsorbed proximally. In pancreatitis, there is a marked decrement in proximal reabsorption, and, as a result, the urinary amylase is extremely high. Renal clearance of amylase may even be rapid enough to leave the patient with a normal serum level. It has recently become popular to calculate an amylase: creatinine clearance ratio by the following formula, using a random sample of urine:

$$\frac{\text{Urine amylase}}{\text{Plasma amylase}} \div \frac{\text{Urine creatinine}}{\text{Plasma creatinine}} \times 100\%$$

The greatly enhanced amylase clearance in patients with pancreatitis results in an increased ratio. A ratio of 5% or greater is considered to be diagnostic of pancreatitis. Patients with pancreatitis combined with hyperlipemia have a normal serum amylase, but may nevertheless have pancreatitis diagnosed by an increased clearance ratio, whereas patients with hyperamylasemia from other causes do not have altered tubular reabsorption and the ratio is normal.

There are recent reports of increased clearance ratios in patients with diabetic ketoacidosis and extensive burns. Although these patients had no obvious indication of pancreatitis, a mild subclinical pancreatitis could not be ruled out. Conversely, it is not known whether all cases of mild pancreatitis will demonstrate an increased clearance ratio.

In a small proportion of the normal population, circulating amylase is bound to globulin that is not filtered by the kidney, and this amylase does not appear in the urine in normal concentrations. These people are said to have *macroamylasemia* and manifest persistently elevated serum amylase levels.

THERAPY

Hypotension and shock must be treated promptly with appropriate volume, colloid, and crystalloid replacement. Symptomatic hypocalcemia requires the infusion of calcium gluconate. Relief of abdominal pain is best accomplished with parenteral meperidine. Morphine should be avoided since it can lead to spasms of the sphincter of Oddi and thus exacerbate the pancreatitis.

A primary goal should be to put the pancreas "at rest" by decreasing physiologic pancreatic secretions. This is generally accomplished by prohibiting all oral intake, removing gastric acid and fluid with nasogastric suction, and administering antacids to reduce gastric acidity. There is still some controversy over the value of nasogastric suction; one study of patients with *mild* pancreatitis failed to find any additional benefit from adding nasogastric suction to an NPO protocol.

The use of prophylactic antibiotics only serves to generate resistant organisms when infection does occur, and should be discouraged.

Careful conservative supportive care should be combined with monitoring of electrolytes and volume, and liberal use of analgesia. Feedings should be omitted until the pain resolves. The biliary tree should be investigated (Chap. 41) so that any surgically correctable obstruction (*e.g.*, gallstone, tumor) can be diagnosed.

COURSE AND MANAGEMENT

In uncomplicated attacks of pancreatitis, the pain and serum amylase resolve within three to seven days. If pain persists, the clinician should suspect the development of a pancreatic abscess or pseudocyst.

A *pseudocyst* is a loculation of pancreatic fluids that arises from a disruption of a pancreatic duct. It is called a pseudocyst because it is lined with fibrotic tissue, not epithelium. The symptoms of a pseudocyst are similar to those of pancreatitis, and the serum amylase may be elevated. An upper G.I. series may reveal the pseudocyst as an extrinsic mass displacing the stomach. Rarely, a pseudocyst may rupture and leak fluid into the peritoneum ("pancreatic ascites"). The elevated amylase in the ascitic fluid helps to distinguish pancreatic ascites from other causes of ascites (Chap. 39).

Eventually, in the alcoholic patient, the complications of end-stage chronic pancreatitis become the major management problems. Pancreatic insufficiency supervenes, with consequent failure of endocrine and/or exocrine pancreatic function. Destruction of the pancreatic islet beta cells results in diminished insulin reserve and often in overt diabetes mellitus. The control of glucose intolerance is complicated by the decrease in the counterregulatory hormone glucagon that follows the eventual destruction of the pancreatic alpha cells; many patients are therefore exquisitely sensitive to exogenous insulin.

Malabsorption results from failure of the exocrine pancreas. When 90% of the exocrine pancreas has been destroyed, steatorrhea and fecal protein loss becomes significant. Pancreatic enzyme tablets taken in large doses can supply sufficient enzyme activity to reduce those losses. The effectiveness of oral pancreatic enzyme supplements can, however, be greatly diminished by acid degradation in the stomach, and the concomitant use of the H_2 blocker, cimetidine (Chap. 33), allows more active enzyme to reach the duodenum.

There can also be malabsorption of the fat-soluble vitamins. Vitamin D deficiency may lead to hypocalcemia, hypophosphatemia, and osteomalacia (See Chap. 28; also see Chap 35 for the differential diagnosis and treatment of malabsorption).

BIBLIOGRAPHY

Arvanitakis C, Cooke AR: Diagnostic tests of exocrine pancreatic function and disease. Gastroenterology 74:932–948, 1978

Bourke JB, Mead GM, McIllmurray MD et al: Drug-associated primary acute pancreatitis. Lancet 1:706–708, 1978

Levitt MD, Ellis CJ, Meier PB: Extrapancreatic origin of chronic unexplained hyperamylasemia. N Engl J Med 302:670–671, 1980

Levitt MD, Johnson SG: Is the C_{AM}/C_{CR} ratio of value for the diagnosis of pancreatitis? Gastroenterology 75:118–119, 1978

Salt WB, Schenker S: Amylase—Its clinical significance: A review of the literature. Medicine 55:269–289, 1976

Sarles OH: Chronic calcifying pancreatitis—Chronic alcoholic pancreatitis. Gastroenterology 66:604–616, 1974

Strum WB, Spiro HM: Chronic pancreatitis. Ann Intern Med 74:264–277, 1971

38

Liver Disease

By virtue of its juxtaposition between the portal and systemic circulations, the liver is exposed to most ingested nutrients and drugs. The hepatocytes metabolize nutrients to prepare them for storage (i.e. glycogen synthesis) or for delivery to the rest of the body. The liver is also able to catabolize and detoxify a wide array of substances, ranging from therapeutic drugs to potential poisons. The liver is also a major biosynthetic organ, providing the body with proteins such as albumin, clotting factors, lipoproteins, and a wide variety of plasma protein components. The most important consequences of hepatic cell destruction are therefore a diminished capacity to utilize nutrients and to synthesize needed plasma proteins, and an inability to detoxify noxious substances.

During the early phases of liver injury—whether the precipitating cause of liver destruction is a toxin, a virus, or a metastatic neoplasm—the hepatocytes release bilirubin and their intracellular enzymes SGOT (serum glutamic oxaloacetic transaminase, also called aspartate aminotransferase), SGPT (serum glutamic pyruvic transaminase, also called alanine aminotransferase), and LDH (lactic dehydrogenase) into the circulation. A rising serum bilirubin leads to the appearance of jaundice.

Eventually, with severe or protracted injury to the liver, areas of the liver scar, resulting in cirrhosis. In addition to a loss of parenchymal cell function, cirrhosis is characterized by a damming up of the portal circulation, resulting in portal hypertension, ascites, and the development of portosystemic collaterals. The most clinically important collaterals are the esophageal varices, a source of frequent and sometimes fatal hemorrhage.

Fortunately, the liver has a remarkable ability to regenerate after injury, so that even a cirrhotic liver contains areas of viable hepatocytes. In patients with acute hepatic injury, liver function usually returns to normal.

JAUNDICE

Jaundice, or icterus, is a cardinal sign of disease of the liver and biliary tree. As the total serum bilirubin approaches 2 to 3 mg/dl, the sclera, skin, and mucous membranes acquire a yellowish hue, the plasma also becomes yellow, the urine becomes dark, and the stool often becomes light.

A small fraction of the healthy population maintains a chronic, low-grade hyperbilirubinemia due to inherited disorders of hepatic bilirubin uptake or conjugation (e.g., Gilbert's syndrome). In all other people, jaundice is an indication of disease and requires diagnostic evaluation.

Bilirubin Metabolism. When aging red blood cells are destroyed in the reticuloendothelial system, hemoglobin is liberated and catabolized. The heme moiety is converted to biliverdin and then to bilirubin. Bilirubin circulates bound to serum albumin and eventually enters the hepatocytes. Within the liver, bilirubin is further metabolized in order to facilitate its excretion from the body; it is conjugated with glucuronic acid to form bilirubin glucuronide. Only this conjugated form of bilirubin can be excreted into the bile and thus into the intestine where it can then be excreted in the stool (to which it imparts a dark-brown hue). It can be further degraded by gut flora into urobilinogen, which can be reabsorbed and may appear in the urine.

In patients experiencing severe hemolysis, the rate of bilirubin production may exceed the metabolic capability of the liver. The result is an unconjugated hyperbilirubinemia. Because unconjugated bilirubin binds to serum proteins, it is not filtered by the kidneys and bilirubinuria is not present.

Conjugated hyperbilirubinemia can result from liver disease or extrahepatic obstruction. With impairment of bilirubin excretion, conjugated bilirubin "leaks" back into the circulation and the serum concentration rises. Because conjugated bilirubin does not bind significantly to serum proteins, it can be filtered by the kidneys and excreted in the urine where it produces the characteristic dark urine of bilirubinuria. The feces, however, become less dark (acholic stools) as the amount of bilirubin reaching the intestine declines.

Differential Diagnosis

The most important diagnostic consideration is whether the jaundice associated with conjugated hyperbilirubinemia in a particular patient is caused by a disorder that can be remedied by surgery. Surgical jaundice is caused by extrahepatic obstruction of the biliary tree, and is most often a result of gallbladder disease, obstruction of the common bile duct by tumor, carcinoma of the ampulla of Vater, or carcinoma of the pancreas. Medical (nonsurgical) causes of jaundice include severe hemolysis, viral and toxic hepatitis, cirrhosis, infiltrative diseases of the liver (e.g., tumors which have metastasized to the liver and amyloidosis), and, rarely, sepsis. In most patients, a history, physical examination, and pertinent laboratory studies reveal the etiology of the jaundice.

Associated Symptoms. The signs and symptoms accompanying jaundice can occasionally aid in the diagnosis. *Epigastric pain radiating to the back* is characteristic of pancreatic carcinoma, although it also occurs in jaundiced patients with acute pancreatitis and hepatitis. *Colicky abdominal pain*, especially in association with an enlarged gallbladder, is seen in common bile duct obstruction. *Chills* and *fever* occurring in a jaundiced patient usually signify cholangitis and often accompany common duct obstruction. In patients with viral hepatitis, chills are usually part of the anicteric prodrome. Patients with severe alcoholic hepatitis may also have chills, fever, and abdominal pain, and thus appear to have a surgical disease.

Laboratory Tests. The most helpful laboratory test in distinguishing between medical and surgical causes of jaundice is the SGOT determination. The SGOT very rarely exceeds 300 IU in the absence of infectious or toxic hepatitis, and an extremely high SGOT is therefore suggestive of medical (nonsurgical) disease.

The ratio of the conjugated bilirubin to the total serum bilirubin can also be helpful.

FIG. 38–1. Anterior view of a normal liver–spleen scan. Homogeneous uptake of the radioactive tracer is seen in the liver. A small amount of uptake is also seen in the spleen (arrow).

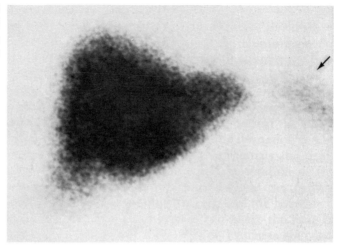

Unconjugated hyperbilirubinemia (ratio of less than 15%) is seen in patients with massive hemolysis or in patients with one of the benign inherited syndromes of hyperbilirubinemia. *Conjugated* hyperbilirubinemia (ratio of greater than 40%) can be seen in patients with either medical or surgical causes of jaundice.

A prolonged prothrombin time (PT) occurs in parenchymal hepatic disease (in which there is an inability to synthesize vitamin-K-dependent coagulation factors) and obstructive liver disease (in which oral vitamin K is not absorbed). If the prothrombin time is corrected by the administration of parenteral vitamin K, the defect is most likely to be obstructive.

Other Tests. It may be necessary to perform several specialized diagnostic tests in order to exclude the possibility of surgical jaundice. When the serum bilirubin exceeds 3 mg/dl, oral and intravenous cholangiography cannot be successfully performed. The biliary tree can, however, be investigated with (1) abdominal ultrasonography (which can show dilated intrahepatic or common bile ducts, seen in obstructive disease), (2) abdominal CT scanning (which can reveal the presence of an obstructing lesion), (3) endoscopic retrograde cannulation of the common bile duct and pancreatic duct, and (4) skinny needle cholangiography. A liver scan (Fig. 38–1) is often helpful as a screening test, and liver biopsy can delineate the etiology of medical jaundice.

In the event that the cause of jaundice remains occult, exploratory laparotomy must be undertaken to search for a resectable obstructing lesion.

ACUTE VIRAL HEPATITIS

Studies undertaken at the Willowbrook State School first demonstrated that there were at least two types of virally induced hepatitis—A and B—each with a distinctive clinical picture. This distinction was clarified by the discovery of the "Australia antigen," which has subsequently been shown to be a component of the hepatitis B virus and which at that time was responsible for most cases of blood-borne hepatitis. Subsequently, the cytomegalovirus (CMV), Epstein-Barr virus (EBV), and a "non-A, non-B" virus have been shown to cause acute hepatitis.

The nature of the viral agent determines (1) the route of interpersonal transmission, (2) the immune responses that are elicited, and (3) the prognosis regarding long-term hepatic injury. It is therefore important to determine the precise viral etiology in any given patient. It is also essential to rule out a toxic or pharmacologic etiology, since the treatment and prognosis of toxic hepatitis is far different from those for the various types of viral hepatitis.

Clinical Syndrome. Viral hepatitis is a common, exceptionally enervating illness. No therapy beyond rest and symptomatic care has been devised. Fortunately, the disease is usually self-limited and chronic sequelae are unusual.

Clinically, most patients with viral hepatitis experience a distinct prodrome. This lasts two to five days when the hepatitis is caused by the hepatitis A virus (HAV) and up to a month when the disease is caused by the hepatitis B virus (HBV). The prodrome typically includes arthralgias, myalgias, headache, photophobia, anorexia, nausea, vomiting, and weight loss, although some patients may complain only of malaise and weakness. Abnormalities of olfaction or gustatory function result in an aversion to cigarette smoke or certain foods. Just prior to the icteric phase, the patient may notice darkened urine and/or lightened stool.

The onset of jaundice is associated with increased anorexia, extraordinary fatigue, and, occasionally, mild pruritus. Some patients, however, remain anicteric throughout the duration of their illness.

The infected liver is large, flabby, smooth, and occasionally tender. Histologic examination at this stage reveals hepatic cell necrosis with a mononuclear inflammatory infiltrate. A sense of fullness or frank tenderness in the right upper quadrant may be accompanied by palpable splenomegaly in a small fraction of patients. Other signs of liver dysfunction, such as spider angiomas, may also appear.

The liver's ability to detoxify certain medications (*e.g.* barbiturates) may be greatly impaired, and an unintentional overdose may result when the patient takes a normal dose of a drug.

As jaundice diminishes over the ensuing month, other signs and symptoms of the disease also abate, and most patients recover fully within two to three weeks.

Laboratory Findings. Laboratory evaluation reveals dramatic elevations of the intracellular enzymes SGOT and SGPT. SGOT and SGPT activity may exceed 2000 IU and elevations may persist for several months, but the degree of enzyme elevation does not correlate with the severity of the clinical illness. The generalized impairment of hepatic uptake, conjugation, and excretion of bilirubin causes moderate elevations of serum bilirubin.

Alkaline phosphatase is released when hepatic excretory function is impaired, and small elevations are common during hepatitis. Dramatic increases are indicative of obstruction of the biliary tracts.

Rarely, hepatitis may result in a decreased synthesis of albumin and clotting factors. As a result, the serum albumin may be low and the prothrombin time prolonged. Hypoglycemia is uncommon but may occur, because these patients may be anorectic and have diminished glycogen reserves.

Fulminant Hepatitis. Rarely, the liver infection may evolve into a life-threatening fulminant hepatitis. The hepatitis B virus is usually responsible, but other viruses and agents, including drugs and hepatotoxic mushrooms, have also been implicated. Mild neuropsychiatric changes often herald severe hepatic decompensation: irritability and inappropriate behavior may quickly progress to coma (see Chap. 40). With rapid cellular necrosis, the liver actually shrinks. SGOT, SGPT, and bilirubin levels rise precipitously and subsequently fall just prior to death when the bulk of hepatocytes has been destroyed. Clotting factor levels decline, hemostasis is impaired, and the prothrombin time becomes prolonged. Mortality is extremely high.

Hepatitis A

In underdeveloped countries and in areas with poor hygiene, HAV infection is nearly universal during childhood. It is transmitted via the fecaloral route. Infection is asymptomatic and anicteric. As hygiene improves, however, the rate of childhood exposure declines, and the adult population becomes susceptible to infection.

In the United States, hepatitis A is now a disease of adults. Less than one-fourth of all children have detectable antibody to HAV. The prevalence of HAV antibody increases with age, and a majority of people over 50 have immunologic evidence of prior exposure. Adults in the higher socioeconomic strata, having had less opportunity for childhood exposure, are more susceptible to infection.

The incubation period of HAV ranges from 15 to 50 days. It is often contracted from food, water, or raw shellfish that have been contaminated by excreta from infected persons. Male homosexuals who engage in anal-oral sex have an increased risk for infection.

The hepatitis A antigen can be detected in the stool both during the incubation period and during the prodrome. By the time that jaundice has become clinically apparent, however, the hepatitis A antigen is generally absent from the feces. A mild, lower titer viremia may also occur during the early stages of infection, but it does not persist. Chronic carriers of HAV do not exist, and hepatitis A infection is not transmitted by blood transfusion.

Soon after infection with HAV, IgM antibody directed against HAV appears, followed by anti-HAV IgG. The IgG persists indefinitely, conferring long-term immunity.

The mortality of HAV infection is extremely low, and there is no evidence that this illness can progress to chronic active liver disease. Because of the very limited duration of viremia, hepatitis A is rarely a nosocomial hazard. Because the fecal antigen is absent once patients become jaundiced, health workers do not have a higher prevalance of HAV antibodies than the general population. Patients with hepatitis A who are hospitalized need no special enteric precautions. As a precautionary step, it is officially recommended that fecally incontinent patients be isolated. Immunoprophylaxis with standard immune serum globulin should be reserved for household contacts of patients with hepatitis A, since they will have been in contact with the patient during the contagious incubation period.

Hepatitis B

Like hepatitis A, most infections with HBV are asymptomatic. Nevertheless, the natural history of hepatitis caused by HBV differs in several important ways from hepatitis A, presumably because of the persistent and heavy viremia seen in hepatitis B.

In the past, blood transfusions have been a major source of HBV transmission. However, with the advent of sensitive radioimmunoassays for hepatitis antigens, it has become possible to screen blood donors, and the incidence of post-transfusion hepatitis B has declined dramatically. Drug abusers who share needles can transmit the virus to one another, and transmission has been described following tattooing, ear-piercing, hemodialysis, acupuncture, and sexual intercourse.

The blood, saliva, and semen of patients infected with HBV have been shown to be infectious, and viral antigen has been isolated from many other body fluids. Jaundice appears two to three months after exposure, but viral antigens can be detected in the blood much earlier. One to two weeks after exposure, a specific viral surface antigen (HB$_s$Ag) becomes detectable in the blood. Soon thereafter, another viral antigen, HB$_e$Ag, can be found in the blood; its presence may be indicative of increased infectivity. Subsequently, anti-HB$_e$ antibody may appear. Antibody to a core antigen (anti-HB$_c$) also appears in the blood.

In approximately 90% of infected patients, HB$_s$Ag disappears during or after the episode of acute hepatitis. Six to twenty weeks later, antibody to the surface antigen (anti-HB$_s$) can be detected, and it persists indefinitely. Some patients, however, never develop anti-HB$_s$ and remain chronic carriers of HB$_s$Ag; these patients incur an increased risk of chronic liver disease.

The immunologic response of the patient is responsible for many of the extrahepatic manifestations of hepatitis B. These responses can be divided into two categories. In the first, an exuberant host response during the early viremic phase causes formation of antigen–antibody complexes. These complexes activate the complement system and result in arthritis, urticaria, and angioedema. The second category of immune response occurs in chronic carriers of HBV. These individuals develop the manifestations of chronic immune-complex disease, most notably chronic glomerulonephritis

Careful blood precautions must be maintained in the hospital and in the clinic for all seropositive patients. Hepatitis B is an occupational hazard for health care personnel, and there is also a question of the possibility of

HB$_s$Ag seropositive workers posing a risk to their patients.

An immune globulin preparation with very high titers of anti-HB$_s$ has recently become available and is effective when administered within seven days of exposure. Immunoprophylaxis is not needed for casual, work, or nonsexual family contacts. This "hyperimmune" globulin is recommended for patients who inadvertently receive HB$_s$Ag seropositive blood products, for anti-HB$_s$ negative health workers who sustain accidental percutaneous or mucosal exposures to HB$_s$Ag positive material, and for seronegative sexual contacts of patients with acute hepatitis B. Infants of HB$_s$Ag seropositive mothers may also require prophylaxis.

With the advent of extremely sensitive radioimmunoassays for detecting HB$_s$Ag in blood products, the incidence of post-transfusion hepatitis B has fallen. Hepatitis still occurs in transfusion recipients, and has been attributed to an as yet unidentified set of viruses (Chap. 44). Although these viruses tend to cause a milder illness, this so-called "non-A, non-B" hepatitis closely resembles hepatitis B in its mode of transmission and its capacity to be carried chronically.

Management of Acute Hepatitis

For public health considerations, acute viral hepatitis is generally best managed on an outpatient basis, since hospital personnel and other patients who come in contact with a patient with infectious hepatitis or with that patient's blood or secretions may be at risk for contracting the disease. Treatment is symptomatic, and patients should be advised to rest. Because of the diminished detoxifying capability of the liver, medications must be cautiously prescribed. Alcohol must not be consumed by any patient with acute hepatitis.

Certain patients, however, will require admission to the hospital. Hospitalization is necessary for patients whose hepatitis is so severe as to result in a low serum albumin, a prolonged prothrombin time, or hepatic encephalopathy (see Chap. 40). Elderly patients and individuals who are severely anorectic may also benefit from a short hospital stay, where nutrition and hydration can be maintained.

TOXIC HEPATITIS

A variety of drugs and toxins can cause an acute hepatitis that is symptomatically indistinguishable from viral hepatitis. It is critical to consider a pharmacologic etiology in any patient with acute hepatitis, so that the offending agent can be identified and its use discontinued.

Some agents are directly toxic to the liver and predictably cause hepatocellular damage in every individual who is exposed. Included in this group are carbon tetrachloride, certain mushrooms, and acetaminophen in high doses (see Chap. 61). Signs of hepatic injury become evident within one to two days of exposure.

Other drugs, such as halothane, isoniazid, methyldopa, and phenytoin, produce liver injury in an unpredictable and idiosyncratic manner. Approximately one in ten patients who takes isoniazid develops elevated levels of SGOT. This elevation is transient and asymptomatic and does not mandate cessation of drug therapy. A much smaller percentage of patients (about 1%) go on to develop acute symptomatic hepatitis with markedly elevated serum transaminase levels during the first four to eight weeks of treatment; isoniazid should be discontinued in these patients.

Rarely, a patient who receives the general anesthetic halothane will develop acute hepatitis within two weeks of exposure. Liver damage is often severe and mortality is high.

CHRONIC HEPATITIS

When an inflammatory hepatic lesion does not resolve after three to six months, the diagnosis of chronic hepatitis may be made and a liver biopsy should be performed. The diagnosis of chronic hepatitis may be based purely on a biochemical abnormality (*i.e.,* persistent elevation of SGOT or SGPT) even when there are no physical findings and even when the patient is without symptoms.

Two types of chronic hepatitis are recognized: chronic persistent hepatitis (CPH), by definition a nonprogressive and benign disorder, and chronic active hepatitis (CAH), a progressive and often precirrhotic lesion.

Chronic persistent hepatitis is usually preceded by acute viral hepatitis, but drugs and inflammatory bowel disease may be responsible. Patients are usually asymptomatic, although they may complain of fatigue, anorexia, and right upper quadrant discomfort. There are few associated physical findings. Biopsy reveals a slowly resolving hepatitis with persistent portal inflammation; the overall architecture of the liver, however, remains intact.

Chronic persistent hepatitis resolves spontaneously without treatment. Since inactive chronic active hepatitis may mimic chronic persistent hepatitis on biopsy, frequent follow-up examinations are important. Deterioration in the patient's clinical situation mandates a repeat liver biopsy to rule out active chronic liver disease.

As its name implies, *chronic active hepatitis* is a far more serious illness. Precipitants include hepatitis B, non-A, non-B hepatitis, drugs, and various autoimmune diseases. Chronic active hepatitis is often, though not always, symptomatic. Hepatosplenomegaly, jaundice, and spider angiomas are frequent findings. The biopsy is usually dramatic: in addition to the changes of chronic inflammation in the portal areas, there are patches of hepatic cellular necrosis that may extend to adjacent lobules ("bridging necrosis").

The clinical course and histologic picture of chronic active hepatitis are useful prognostic indicators and guides to therapy. Most patients have mild disease and should be followed closely without therapy. A subset of patients with severe chronic active hepatitis who have an extremely poor prognosis has been identified. Severe chronic active hepatitis exists either (1) when bridging or multilobular necrosis is found on biopsy or (2) when symptomatic patients have an SGOT that is ten times normal or a serum gammaglobulin level that is twice normal in conjunction with an SGOT that is five times normal. A number of studies have shown that high-dose prednisone therapy (with or without the addition of azathioprine) can, in this group of patients, relieve symptoms, decrease the incidence of cirrhosis and the attendant complications of portal hypertension, and lower mortality. Treatment is continued for 6 to 18 months until a full remission is obtained. The patient should become asymptomatic, the SGOT should be within two times normal, and the piecemeal necrosis should heal. A sizable percentage of treated patients suffer drug toxicity; azathioprine is a hepatotoxic drug and has been associated with the development of hematologic malignancy.

Drug-induced chronic hepatitis has a good prognosis. The disease usually abates after the offending drug has been discontinued. Chronic hepatitis may also be seen as a precirrhotic lesion in Wilson's disease and in α-1 antitrypsin deficiency.

ALCOHOLIC HEPATITIS

Although alcoholic hepatitis and cirrhosis are commonly seen in individuals who are malnourished, it is the alcohol consumption itself that is the prerequisite for alcoholic liver disease. Alcoholic hepatitis, therefore, occurs in affluent and well-fed individuals as well as in the derelict population. Approximately 160 grams of alcohol per day is severely hepatotoxic, and will cause cirrhosis in 50% of persons who drink at that rate for 25 years.

Diagnosis. The definitive diagnosis of alcoholic hepatitis is made by history and liver biopsy. The presence of malnutrition, hepatosplenomegaly, and ascites supports the diagnosis. Patients can present with any of the manifestations of alcoholism, and hepatitis is usually a secondary diagnosis (see Chap. 61).

On occasion, however, hepatitis may be the presenting illness. The patient then complains of abdominal pain, jaundice, nausea, vomiting, and fever. The leukocyte count is elevated and all liver function tests may be abnormal. The aminotransferases rarely are extremely high. Hypoalbuminemia and prolongation of the prothrombin time after vitamin K supplementation indicate a significant loss of hepatic synthetic function and predict a poor outcome. A bilirubin of greater than 20 mg/dl also indicates a poor prognosis.

Histology. Fatty infiltration of the liver is a very early sign of alcoholic liver disease and may account for much of the patient's hepatomegaly. Biopsy reveals on-going hepatic injury. Cytoplasmic "alcoholic hyaline" (or Mallory bodies) is present, the mitochondria are swollen, and the endoplasmic reticulum is increased. Hepatocellular necrosis and a polymorphonuclear inflammatory infiltrate are pronounced, especially in the centrilobular regions.

Treatment. For most patients with alcoholic hepatitis, abstinence, rest, and proper nutrition lead to resolution of their inflammatory lesions. Eighty percent of patients who continue to drink after a bout of alcoholic hepatitis can expect to develop cirrhosis within five years. The presence of ascites, encephalopathy, renal failure, and severe leukocytosis are all poor prognostic signs. For very sick patients, especially for those with encephalopathy, a course of high-dose prednisone may offer some benefit.

A fatty liver is a universal concomitant to excessive alcohol consumption. However, clinical bouts of alcoholic hepatitis are relatively uncommon. Although alcoholic hepatitis is probably a predecessor to cirrhosis, many patients with alcoholic cirrhosis have never experienced a clinical episode of severe hepatitis.

CIRRHOSIS

Cirrhosis is the third leading cause of death in young men age 35 to 54, and its incidence is increasing. Although in the United States there are fewer female alcoholics than male alcoholics, women who do drink to excess appear to develop cirrhosis at a greater rate than men.

The cirrhotic liver is shrunken, scarred, and fibrotic, but nevertheless contains patchy, nodular areas of hepatocyte regeneration. In persons with cirrhosis who continue to drink alcohol, areas of alcoholic hepatitis and fatty infiltration may also be found. The two principal pathologic types of cirrhosis are (1) micronodular, or Laennec's cirrhosis, which is usually associated with alcoholism, and (2) macronodular or postnecrotic cirrhosis, which is often seen following chronic active hepatitis.

Alcohol is the most common cause of cirrhosis, but any severe chronic hepatitis or nutritional deprivation such as that accompanying jejunoileal bypass can lead to cirrhosis. Prolonged right-sided congestive heart failure can cause hepatic congestion and, eventually, cirrhosis. Hemochromatosis, primary biliary cirrhosis, and Wilson' disease are less common causes.

Cirrhosis can be totally asymptomatic and may become apparent only at autopsy. More often, cirrhosis becomes obvious late in the life of a chronic alcoholic, manifesting itself as encephalopathy (Chap. 40), ascites (Chap. 39), portal hypertension, or hepatic insufficiency. In patients with portal hypertension, a system of collateral veins is formed. Increased pressure in the plexus of veins in the esophagus results in the formation of dilated and fragile vessels referred to as varices. Esophageal varices become symptomatic only when they rupture and cause gastrointestinal hemorrhage (Chap. 32).

Assessment. Physical examination reveals a firm, shrunken liver, although an enlarged liver may be present in alcoholic patients with fatty infiltration. Splenomegaly, a result of portal hypertension, is not uncommon, but the enlarged spleen may be difficult to palpate in patients with ascites. Spider angiomas (small telangiectasias that radiate from a central point and blanch when pressure is applied), palmar erythema, gynecomastia, and testicular atrophy are prominent. Clubbing of the digits and Dupuytren's contractures (fibrosis of the palmar fascia that presents with flexion contractures of the fingers) are among the other characteristic signs.

Laboratory Findings. The evaluation of hepatic function in cirrhotic patients depends upon a battery of blood tests. Several serum tests provide a measure of the number of dysfunctional but still living liver cells. A patient with end-stage cirrhosis has relatively few functioning liver cells and may therefore have normal serum aminotransferases, while a patient with early cirrhosis and concomitant hepatitis may have increased serum enzymes.

A decreased BUN (less than 4 mg/dl) is characteristic of cirrhosis, indicating a decreased protein intake and an inability to synthesize urea. In the cirrhotic population, a BUN in the "normal" range of 15 to 20 mg/dl may indicate renal insufficiency.

A liver biopsy should be obtained in any patient suspected of having cirrhosis, in order to confirm the diagnosis, establish the etiology, and stage progression. Early in the disease, hemochromatosis may respond to desferoxamine or phlebotomy, and Wilson's disease to penicillamine; thus, the biopsy can also have therapeutic implications.

Complications. In addition to the catastrophic consequences of variceal hemorrhage and encephalopathy, the cirrhotic patient is faced with a large number of other difficulties. Nutrition may be compromised even if the patient abstains from alcohol, since malabsorption can result from portal hypertension, associated pancreatic insufficiency, or the loss of bile acids (see Chap. 35). Chronic neomycin or lactulose therapy, which are used to treat encephalopathy, can also cause a mild, usually asymptomatic steatorrhea.

Most cirrhosis patients have excessive sodium retention. Urinary diluting capacity and the glomerular filtration rate may also be decreased.

A common complication of cirrhosis is the onset of renal failure. Occasionally, the etiology of the accompanying renal failure is clear, for example, when renal hypoperfusion is exacerbated by diuretic therapy for ascites or by gastrointestinal hemorrhage. More often, however, the onset of renal failure in these patients is a spontaneous and unexplained event. Those patients in whom dehydration, obstruction, or other causes of renal failure cannot explain the oliguria are said to have the *hepatorenal syndrome.* It is marked by oliguria (less than 500 ml/day), progressive azotemia, an unremarkable urinary sediment, and a urinary sodium of less than 1 mEq/liter. No morphologic changes are apparent in the kidney, and the kidneys work well if they are transplanted to another host. It is essential to rule out hypotension, volume depletion, and other treatable causes of renal failure, especially drug-induced interstitial nephritis and urinary tract obstruction, before making the diagnosis of hepatorenal syndrome, which carries a dismal prognosis.

Mortality. Survival with cirrhosis is comparable to that of patients with untreatable lung cancer: approximately 8% of patients with cirrhosis are alive five years after the diagnosis is made. Those who abstain from alcohol have a somewhat better prognosis. The onset of jaundice is a particularly ominous sign, and only about 25% of these patients are still alive a year later. Varices, encephalopathy, ascites, spider angiomas, hypoalbuminemia, and a severely prolonged prothrombin time are also poor prognostic signs.

Primary Biliary Cirrhosis. Primary biliary cirrhosis is an uncommon, insidious cause of cirrhosis in middle-aged women (only 10% of affected patients are male). It most often presents with anicteric pruritus. Laboratory hallmarks include an elevated alkaline phosphatase and the presence of antimitochondrial antibodies, both of which may appear prior to any symptoms. On biopsy, a chronic cholangitis is seen early in the disease. Bile stasis and granulomas are also characteristic. Ultimately, periportal fibrosis and end-stage cirrhosis appear. The sicca syndrome, rheumatoid arthritis, and thyroiditis all are associated with primary biliary cirrhosis. Jaundice does not usually appear until several years after the onset of the pruritus. The course of the disease is inexorably downhill. Patients suffer from xanthomas and severe osteoporosis in addition to the complications of cirrhosis. Cholestyramine effectively treats both the itching and the xanthomas, but there is no cure at present for the illness itself. Current experimental therapies include penicillamine, azathioprine, and corticosteroids.

Wilson's Disease. Wilson's disease is a rare autosomal recessive illness characterized by copper deposition within the brain, liver, kidneys, and cornea. In adulthood, it often presents with neuropsychiatric signs, including lack of coordination, tremors, hypersalivation, masked facies, neuroses, psychoses, and dementia. All patients with neuropsychiatric signs have the characteristic Kayser-Fleischer rings at the limbus of the cornea in Descemet's membrane. Although these copper deposits may be visible to the naked eye, a slit-lamp examination may be needed. In younger patients, hepatic disease may predominate, and Kayser-Fleischer rings and neuropsychiatric signs are often absent. Wilson's disease must therefore be considered in all patients under the age of 30 who have chronic active hepatitis or cirrhosis.

Wilson's disease results from a deficiency of the copper-binding protein ceruloplasmin, and an abnormally low serum ceruloplasmin is the best single test to make the diagnosis. Because the concentration of ceruloplasmin is diminished, the total serum copper is also decreased. The urine and hepatic copper, on the other hand, are increased, but these abnormalities in copper metabolism can also occasionally be seen in a variety of cholestatic illnesses. Penicillamine, a drug that chelates copper, removes copper from the body and reverses much of the disease process. Wilson's disease is one of the few treatable and preventable causes of both dementia and liver disease.

HEPATOMA

Malignant hepatomas develop in cirrhotic livers three times more often than in patients who do not have cirrhosis. The diagnosis is usually made late, often after widespread metastasis has occurred. The diagnosis of hepatoma should be considered in cirrhotic patients who suffer sudden deterioration, such as an increase in liver size, weight loss, abdominal pain, or new or worsening ascites.

Alpha-fetoprotein, a serum protein that is found in high concentrations in the fetus, but which does not appear in significant concentrations in normal adults, is elevated in patients with hepatoma. This "tumor marker," however, is not specific for hepatocellular neoplasms.

Several paraneoplastic syndromes have been described. For example, patients who have an elevated hematocrit should be suspected of harboring an erythropoietin-producing hepatic tumor.

Unless the entire hepatoma can be resected, the prognosis is very poor, since neither radiation nor chemotherapy has much success.

Benign hepatic tumors have been reported with the use of anabolic steroids and with the use of oral contraceptives.

BIBLIOGRAPHY

Aach RD, Kahn RA: Posttransfusion hepatitis: Current perspectives. Ann Intern Med 92:539–546, 1980

Boyer JL: Chronic hepatitis: A perspective on classification and determinants of prognosis. Gastroenterology 70:1161–1171, 1976

Cartwright GE: Diagnosis of treatable Wilson's disease. N Engl J Med 298:1347–1350, 1978

Favero MS, Maynard JE, Leger RT et al: Guidelines for the care of patients hospitalized with viral hepatitis. Ann Intern Med 91:872–876, 1979

Krugman S, Overby LR, Mushahwar IK et al: Viral hepatitis, type B: Studies on natural history and prevention re-examined. N Engl J Med 300:101–106, 1979

Lieber CS: Pathogenesis and early diagnosis of alcoholic liver injury. N Engl J Med 298:888–893, 1978

Maddrey WC, Boitnott JK, Bedine MS et al: Corticosteroid therapy of alcoholic hepatitis. Gastroenterology 75:193–199, 1978

Sherlock S, Scheuer PJ: The presentation and diagnosis of 100 patients with primary biliary cirrhosis. N Engl J Med 289:674–678, 1973

39 Ascites

Ascites, the accumulation of fluid in the peritoneal cavity, is always a symptom of underlying disease. Treatment should ideally be directed at the primary disturbance, but often this is not possible. The most common causes of ascites are cirrhosis and advanced neoplasms, situations in which effective therapy is often not available. Other diseases associated less frequently with ascites include the nephrotic syndrome, constrictive pericarditis, pancreatitis, ovarian tumors, obstruction of the hepatic veins, and myxedema.

Even in patients in whom no final cure can be obtained, there are several reasons for reducing ascites. A therapeutic paracentesis can greatly palliate a patient with a tense, painful abdomen or severe dyspnea. Because the physiologic disruption caused by ascites can be great, even the compensated, uncomplaining patient may benefit from a reduction in ascitic volume.

If severe, ascites increases the intra-abdominal pressure, reduces venous return to the heart, and thus reduces cardiac output. It may also restrict diaphragmatic movement. Lung volume is diminished as the fluid-filled abdomen pushes the diaphragms upward. Ascites is also a prerequisite for the development of spontaneous bacterial peritonitis (discussion later in chapter). Patients experience an increased incidence of bleeding from fragile esophageal varices. The danger of gastroesophageal reflux, a potential cause of aspiration, is enhanced.

Mechanisms of Ascites Formation. The presence of ascites indicates that more fluid is being exuded into the abdomen than can be removed by the lymphatics. In some instances, the underlying mechanism of ascites formation is readily apparent. Malignant disease can cause ascites by destroying the abdominal lymphatics; lymphatic fluid spills into the abdomen and cannot be reabsorbed. In diseases characterized by severe hypoalbuminemia, such as the nephrotic syndrome, reduction in intravascular oncotic pressure allows fluid to be lost from the intravascular space because of a shift in the Starling equilibrium.

In patients with intrinsic hepatic disease, however, the etiology of ascites is still controversial. It is not known, for example, whether the liver alone leaks fluid (through its capsule), or whether the intestines and vessels also contribute a significant share.

Forces that favor extrusion of fluid in patients with cirrhosis include elevated intrahepatic pressures and a diminution in serum albumin.

Although the cirrhotic patient has a greatly increased extra-cellular volume, the kidney behaves as if the "effective volume" were decreased. The renin-angiotensin-aldosterone axis is stimulated and sodium is reabsorbed. The ascites compartment shares in this volume expansion.

PARACENTESIS

All patients with newly discovered or worsening ascites require diagnostic studies of the ascitic fluid. Even when the cause of ascites seems obvious, the possibilities of infection or an occult malignancy cannot be dismissed.

The fluid is removed percutaneously with a small-bore needle, a procedure known as paracentesis. Prior to initiating a paracentesis, the platelet count, prothrombin time, or bleeding time must be determined. Cancer patients and patients with cirrhosis frequently have abnormalities in one or all of these parameters. If necessary, platelet transfusions or fresh frozen plasma should be administered just prior to paracentesis. Intraabdominal bleeding, heralded by a falling hematocrit minutes to hours after the procedure, is a potentially lethal complication and may require surgical intervention.

In performing a paracentesis, it is vital to avoid puncturing blood vessels and bowel. Accidental puncture of an abdominal vein can result in catastrophic, uncontrollable hemorrhage, and perforation of the bowel can cause peritonitis.

Diagnostic paracentesis rarely requires needle bores wider than 20 or 22 gauge; with these needle sizes persistent leakage of the ascites from the paracentesis site is unusual. The midline or flank approach should be used, but care must be taken to avoid the epigastric vessels. Abdominal scars should also be avoided, since they may be overlying sites of bowel adhesions to the peritoneum. As a precaution, all patients with cirrhosis should be presumed to have a caput medusa (prominent varicose veins around the umbilicus), and the needle should therefore be inserted approximately 5 cm below the umbilicus. The patient should first empty his bladder.

The ascitic fluid should be carefully examined, and several laboratory studies are performed routinely:

1. The gross appearance of the ascitic fluid can be helpful. If, for example, the ascitic fluid appears chylous, lymphatic obstruction caused by malignancy or trauma should be suspected.

2. An ascitic protein content exceeding 2.5 to 3.0 mg/dl is frequently interpreted to mean that the fluid is an exudate, and is often taken as an indication of malignancy, infection, or hepatic vein obstruction. However, many patients with uncomplicated cirrhosis also have an elevated protein. A protein below 2.5 mg/dl signifies a transudate and is frequently seen in cirrhosis and nephrosis.

3. Very low glucose is associated with an infection or malignancy, but is also seen in patients with cirrhosis who are malnourished and hypoglycemic.

4. A high amylase in the ascites usually indicates *pancreatic ascites* (Chap. 37). However, the ovaries and intestines also produce amylase, and diseases of these organs can also cause ascites.

5. It was initially hoped that an elevated ascitic white cell count would be a sensitive and specific indicator of bacterial peritonitis. However, whereas over 90% of patients with spontaneous bacterial peritonitis have more than 300 white cells/mm³, approximately 50% of patients without peritonitis also have a leukocytosis. Nearly all patients with spontaneous bacterial peritonitis have more than 75 polymorphonuclear leukocytes/mm³, but

this finding may also be present in sterile ascites.

6. In all patients with ascites, whether or not infection is suspected, cultures should be obtained, acid-fast and gram stains performed, and a specimen examined in the cytology laboratory for possible malignant cells.

SPONTANEOUS BACTERIAL PERITONITIS

Spontaneous bacterial peritonitis is a recently described, catastrophic complication that occurs only in patients with ascites. It occurs primarily, but not exclusively, in patients with Laennec's cirrhosis, and carries an extremely high mortality. Fever, abdominal pain, shock, and peritoneal signs are its hallmarks. The infection may occasionally present in a more insidious manner, and the stress may cause the patient to gradually become encephalopathic.

The ascitic fluid is cloudy, but a gram stain is positive in less than 25% of patients. In general, therefore, antibiotic therapy must be started empirically when clinical suspicion of peritonitis is high. The pneumococcus and the enteric gram-negative rods are the most common organisms. Nearly all common antibiotics penetrate into the ascitic fluid in concentrations high enough that direct intraperitoneal installation is not needed.

The syndrome is referred to as "spontaneous" because no inciting element can be immediately identified. It is likely that the organisms reach the ascitic fluid by way of the bloodstream. The edematous bowel and overtaxed lymphatics of the cirrhotic patient are thought to predispose to bacterial penetration.

An intermediate period of asymptomatic bacterial ascites exists in which the patient is free from peritoneal symptoms, but in which the ascitic fluid is culture-positive. Although the patient could conceivably clear the bacteria spontaneously, this state is probably a prelude to peritonitis.

TUBERCULOUS PERITONITIS

Alcoholics are also especially predisposed to tuberculous peritonitis. The illness is usually heralded by abdominal pain, fever, weight loss, and, frequently, by increasing ascites. Although the patient can present with an acute abdomen, more commonly the symptoms have been present for weeks to months.

Extraperitoneal tuberculous foci are the rule, but the diagnosis is nearly always cryptic and rarely made without aggressive investigation. The disease is more common in women than in men, probably because of the ease of spread from tuberculous salpingitis.

Tuberculosis skin tests are usually negative. An acid-fast stain of the ascites is usually unrevealing, and cultures, which require several weeks to grow, are positive in only 50% of patients. A monocytosis in the ascitic fluid may provide a clue to the diagnosis. The diagnosis often depends on laparotomy and omental biopsy. Once diagnosed, tuberculous peritonitis is treatable with conventional antituberculous medicines. Although an uncommon disease, it carries a high mortality if the patient is untreated.

REDUCING ASCITES: THERAPY

Because of the debilitated nature of the population of patients who develop ascites, and because of the need for careful observation, therapy should be initiated in the hospital.

With the use of loop diuretics and aldosterone antagonists, it has become possible to reduce ascites successfully with diuresis. After restricting sodium and fluid intake, small doses of the aldosterone antagonist spironolactone are prescribed, and the dosage is increased every few days until diuresis begins. If necessary, furosemide can be added. Nearly all patients achieve a reduction of ascites on this protocol, but reduction must be pursued cautiously. The maximal capacity for the reabsorption of ascites is less than one liter per day, and attempts to reduce ascites too vigorously by diuresis will result in intravascular fluid volume depletion and eventual cardiovascular collapse. In patients with ascites and concomitant peripheral edema, weight loss of one kilogram per day can be tolerated safely, but in patients *without* edema, weight loss should not be allowed to exceed 200 to 300 grams per day. The hyponatremia that is often found in patients with ascites may worsen at first with diuretic therapy, and hypokalemia, which may accompany furosemide administration, can exacerbate hepatic encephalopathy.

In order to assist diuresis, many physicians advocate infusing salt-poor albumin or reinfusing the patient's own ascites to increase intravascular volume and oncotic pressure. No carefully controlled studies evaluating these modes of therapy have been performed.

Manual removal of ascites was for a long time the mainstay of therapy, and is still the most popular treatment for ascites related to malignancy. In patients with tense ascites associated with cirrhosis, one or two liters can be removed slowly and cautiously with consequent improvement in hemodynamic measurements and relief of pain as the intra-abdominal and intrapleural pressures diminish. Paracentesis performed too rapidly may cause circulatory collapse soon after fluid removal as fluid leaves the intravascular compartment and reenters the peritoneal cavity.

In ascites secondary to carcinoma, however, repeated paracenteses may represent the sole available therapeutic option. In patients with ascites caused by ovarian carcinoma, for example, many liters of fluid can be rapidly withdrawn from the abdomen by suction or drainage without concern that a sudden fluid shift will lead to hemodynamic compromise. Paracentesis is only palliative, however, and the fluid usually reaccumulates.

In patients with refractory ascites who cannot tolerate a diuretic regimen, it is now possible to reinfuse the patient's own ascites by surgically implanting a silicone catheter that connects the abdominal cavity to the superior vena cava (the LaVeen shunt). A one-way, pressure-sensitive valve allows ascitic fluid to drain into the vena cava when the intrathoracic pressure falls with each inspiration. The shunt can achieve total removal of the ascites. Complications include a universal, but usually mild, disseminated intravascular coagulation, as well as pulmonary edema from too rapid reinfusion, and sepsis.

BIBLIOGRAPHY

Donowitz M, Kerstein MD, Spiro HM: Pancreatic ascites. Medicine 53:183–195, 1974

Gregory PB, Broekelschen PH, Hill MD et al: Complications of diuresis in the alcoholic patient with ascites: A controlled trial. Gastroenterology 73:534–538, 1977

Mallory A, Schaefer JW: Complications of diagnostic paracentesis in patients with liver disease. JAMA 239:628–630, 1978

Shear L, Ching S, Gabuzda GJ: Compartmentalization of ascites and edema in patients with hepatic cirrhosis. N Engl J Med 282:1391–1396, 1970

Weinstein MP, Iannini PB, Stratton CW et al: Spontaneous bacterial peritonitis. Am J Med 64:592–598, 1978

40

In severe acute or chronic liver disease normal hepatic detoxification mechanisms are impaired. Collateral vessels allow shunting of portal blood away from the liver directly into the systemic circulation. Metabolites that are ordinarily detoxified by the liver therefore remain in the circulation. Their penetration of the blood-brain barrier results in a metabolic encephalopathy characterized by deteriorating mental function, a flapping tremor, myoclonus, and hyperventilation with respiratory alkalosis.

The decline in mental status seen in patients with hepatic encephalopathy is usually insidious. Family members typically describe increasing lethargy, irritability, and deteriorating judgment. Hepatic encephalopathy may become a chronic and recurring condition. Although the initial episodes usually respond to therapy, repeated bouts can leave permanent neurologic sequelae. These include dementia, seizures, paranoid thought disorders, a Parkinsonian-like syndrome, and progressive paraplegia.

The flapping tremor, or asterixis, reflects the patient's inability to maintain a posture, and is also seen in uremia and carbon dioxide narcosis. It is caused by momentary interruptions in the stream of electrical impulses required for muscular contraction. Asterixis can be elicited by asking the patient to pronate his arms in front of his body and bend his wrists upward; the patient will be unable to maintain this position, and his hands will begin to "flap" downward. This tremor may also be seen in the dorsiflexed foot or the protruding tongue. Myoclonus (sudden, rapid muscle jerks) is caused by spontaneous, erratic electrical discharges.

Hyperventilation can occur with even mild encephalopathy, but its presence should alert the physician to the possibility of early sepsis.

No physical signs specifically distinguish hepatic encephalopathy from other metabolic encephalopathies. Meningitis, subdural hematoma, alcohol withdrawal, uremia, and carbon dioxide narcosis can all mimic hepatic encephalopathy.

ETIOLOGY OF HEPATIC ENCEPHALOPATHY

The specific metabolic poisons responsible for hepatic encephalopathy are still unknown.

Ammonia (NH_3) and other nitrogenous products have been studied the most extensively, and an elevated arterial ammonia is at present the most specific test to distinguish hepatic encephalopathy from other forms of metabolic encephalopathy. Even so, 10% of patients with hepatic encephalopathy have a normal arterial ammonia, and the concentration of ammonia does not correlate with the severity of central nervous system involvement. Further, it has not been possible to induce coma reproducibly in patients with cirrhosis by experimentally increasing ammonia levels. Ammonia itself does not appear to be toxic to the reticular activating system. Nevertheless, therapeutic manipulations aimed at reducing arterial ammonia are usually effective in ameliorating coma.

Increases in serum *short chain fatty acids* have also been implicated in hepatic encephalopathy, but little convincing evidence has thus far been marshalled.

The relative concentrations of circulating *amino acids* are profoundly altered in liver disease. The aromatic amino acids tyrosine, phenylalanine, and tryptophan are precursors of the biogenic amines dopamine, norepinephrine, and serotonin. Since most aromatic amino acids are catabolized by the liver, their concentration rises in liver disease.

The biogenic amine tyramine is produced by gut microorganisms, and—if not detoxified by the liver—can enter the central nervous system and be metabolized into octopamine, a compound structurally similar to norepinephrine. It is thought that tyramine and its metabolites are able to replace the endogenous amines and become "false neurotransmitters," interrupting or confounding the brain's normal channels of communication. Thus, several studies have reported increases in serum and urinary octopamine in patients with deep hepatic coma. Other studies have demonstrated elevated levels of the amino acid glutamine in the cerebrospinal fluid.

PRECIPITANTS OF HEPATIC ENCEPHALOPATHY

The immediate cause of hepatic encephalopathy is usually apparent. As in myxedema coma, *sedative and tranquilizing medications* are common precipitants. Many of these drugs require hepatic metabolism for their clearance, and thus have greatly prolonged serum half-lives in all diseases with portal-systemic shunting. Drugs that are normally bound to proteins may have an increased "free" or unbound concentration, since the circulating levels of albumin are diminished; the concentration of unbound drug may thereby approach the toxic range. Whether there is a concomitant cerebral supersensitivity to such medications, most of which also effect neurotransmitter homeostasis, is not known. Unfortunately, sedatives are often prescribed for some of the symptoms of occult, impending coma, such as insomnia and anxiety, and benzodiazepines are sometimes mistakenly prescribed when the symptom complex is wrongly diagnosed as incipient delerium tremens.

Failure to maintain a low protein diet may be the most common cause of relapse; amino acids are a rich source of nitrogen, and ammonia is among the products of amino acid breakdown. Constipation and bacterial stasis in the gut also exacerbate encephalopathy.

Infection of any kind is an especially common cause of worsening coma, partly because of increased protein catabolism.

Gastrointestinal hemorrhage can be catastrophic in patients prone to or already suffering from hepatic encephalopathy. Since portal hypertension and variceal formation are common accompaniments of hepatic disease, subclinical bleeding from the gut must be sought in all patients with hepatic encephalopathy. Catabolized erythrocytes in the bowel enhance the nitrogen load.

Iatrogenic factors may contribute to the

genesis and worsening of hepatic encephalopathy. Rapid blood transfusions present a large protein load that can overwhelm the limited hepatic detoxification machinery. Diuretics, prescribed to rid the patient of ascites and peripheral edema, present a multifaceted management problem. First, a too-rapid diuresis can result in relative hypovolemia and decreased liver perfusion. Second, severe hyponatremia may complicate and exacerbate hepatic encephalopathy. Third, and most important, hypokalemia and alkalosis, two common sequelae of diuretic therapy, may trigger or greatly enhance the encephalopathic state.

Even a modest deficit of potassium or hydrogen ions may affect the sensorium in a patient with portal-systemic shunting. The kidneys respond to hypokalemia by generating significant amounts of ammonia through the deamination of glutamine to glutamate. The alkaline state also favors the reaction:

$$NH_4^+ \rightarrow H^+ + NH_3$$

NH_3 readily diffuses into the CNS; NH_4^+ does not.

TREATMENT

Treatment for hepatic encephalopathy must stress primary prevention, and patients should be encouraged to avoid heavy protein loads. Dietary protein should not exceed 40 grams per day. The patient's protein tolerance can be tested in the hospital by administering a known amount of protein. Potassium-sparing diuretics and/or potassium supplementation should also be used when appropriate. Vigorous attempts to prevent gastrointestinal hemorrhage with antacids and histamine (H_2) blockers should be instituted; in severe bleeding, Pitressin should be used (see Chap. 32).

In many cases, further measures are required to prevent recurrent episodes of encephalopathy. Nonabsorbable oral agents, such as *sorbitol*, cleanse the bowel of bacteria by stimulating multiple bowel movements per day. When used in conjunction with nonabsorbable antibiotics, which theoretically sterilize the gut of bacteria that produce nitrogenous material, hepatic encephalopathy can usually be well controlled. Oral or rectal neomycin has long been the mainstay of this form of therapy. At least 3% of neomycin is systemically absorbed through either route, making the drug particularly hazardous in patients with renal failure. Both ototoxicity and nephrotoxicity can occur with oral administration. Some researchers have suggested that neomycin does not act by sterilizing the intestine, but instead alters the gut flora in such a way as to cause a malabsorption syndrome, thereby eliminating the lower bowel as a source of ammonia.

Lactulose is a disaccharide that is neither absorbed nor metabolized in the upper intestine. In theory, it reaches the colon where bacteria degrade it into acidic metabolites. By decreasing the pH of the intestinal lumen, the drug allows ammonia to be trapped in its ionized form and thus excreted from the body. Since lactulose syrup is not metabolized in the small bowel, it presents an osmotic load to the large bowel, and therefore acts as a cathartic as well. Lactulose is just as effective as neomycin and is probably safer.

Experimental therapies have been designed in the belief that false neurotransmitters are ultimately responsible for the encephalopathy of hepatic disease. L-dopa (or the dopamine agonist bromocriptine) may improve hepatic coma by replacing the false neurotransmitters in the central nervous system.

Others have recommended removal of free ammonia by hyperalimentation with keto-acids. These non-nitrogenous homologues of amino acids react chemically with the ammonia to form amino acids.

BIBLIOGRAPHY

Fischer JE, Baldessarini RJ: Pathogenesis and therapy of hepatic coma. Prog Liver Dis 5:363–397, 1976

Gabuzda GJ, Hall PW: Relation of potassium depletion to renal ammonium metabolism and hepatic coma. Medicine 45:481–499, 1966

James JH, Jeppson B, Zuparo V et al: Hyperammonaemia, plasma amino acid imbalance, and blood–brain amino acid transport: A unified theory of portal-systemic encephalopathy. Lancet 2:772–775, 1975

Read AE, Sherlock S, Laidlow J et al: The neuropsychiatric syndromes associated with chronic liver disease and an extensive portal-systemic collateral circulation. Q J Med 36:135–150, 1967

41

Acute Gallbladder Disease

Gallstones are by far the most common cause of gallbladder disease (Fig. 41–1). Only very infrequently will a tumor or swelling caused by infection block the cystic or common duct and produce the same symptomatology as gallstone obstruction.

In the United States and other western countries, gallstones are composed chiefly of cholesterol that has precipitated out of solution. Cholesterol is normally solubilized by specific bile salts, and cholesterol stones result when there is an inadequate amount of these bile salts to keep the cholesterol in solution.

Most gallstones exist for years without causing any problems, but eventually about 30% of patients develop the symptoms of gallbladder disease. The most common symptom is pain, caused by obstruction of the cystic or common bile duct, and by the consequent inflammation.

Obstruction of the cystic duct produces *acute cholecystitis*. It is not known why obstruction leads to inflammation; the accumulated bile salts may cause irritation, or localized pockets of aerobic and anaerobic infections may form. The resultant pain can be extraordinarily severe, and often precipitates emergency admission to a surgical service. Clinical diagnosis can be difficult, and

radiographic confirmation is generally mandatory before surgery is undertaken.

The pain of biliary colic is severe, steady, and—despite the misnomer "colic"—prolonged, and may be accompanied by nausea and low-grade fever. If the right upper quadrant is not too tender to prevent careful examination, the swollen gallbladder may be palpated. Murphy's sign (inspiratory arrest upon palpation below the right costal margin) is classically associated with gallbladder inflammation. Leukocytosis accompanies the inflammation. Even if the common duct is unaffected, slight increases in serum bilirubin and alkaline phosphatase are characteristic.

If the gallstone has obstructed the common duct (choledocholithiasis), similar symptoms may develop, but the clinical picture may deteriorate even more acutely. In patients with obstruction, the entire biliary tree may be inflamed, including the portal tracts of the liver, producing an *acute cholangitis*. Increasing jaundice, spiking fevers, and biliary "colic" (Charcot's triad) should suggest the diagnosis of acute cholangitis, rather than cholecystitis. There is often an accompanying bacterial infection that may produce hepatic abscesses or develop into septicemia. Immediate surgical decompression is mandatory in patients with disseminated bacterial infection.

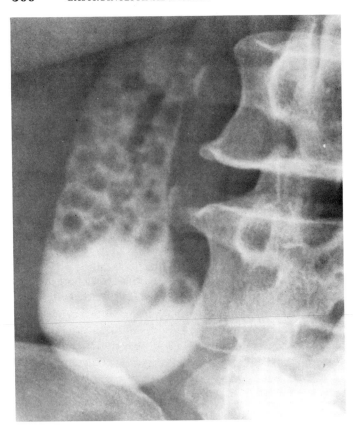

FIG. 41–1. Cholelithiasis. The gallbladder is filled with numerous, radiolucent stones.

Evaluation

Confirmation of biliary tract obstruction must be obtained prior to surgery, primarily to exclude hepatitis and pancreatitis; both of these diseases may be accompanied by pain and jaundice, and neither requires surgical intervention. In addition, severe bacterial infection elsewhere in the body (e.g., in the lungs or kidneys) may be associated with elevated bilirubin levels and may mimic gallbladder disease. Occasionally, an x-ray of the abdomen will reveal several radiopaque stones.

Oral cholecystography may not be successful in patients with biliary tract obstruction, and many centers use intravenous cholecystography. However, intravenous cholecystography is also frequently unsuccessful in patients with biliary tract obstruction, and virtually always fails to visualize the biliary tree if the bilirubin is greater than 4 mg/100 ml. There is also a significant incidence of side-effects that are generally dye-related with intravenous cholecystography.

Ultrasonography reveals stones in the gallbladder and, in patients with obstruction, dilated ducts, and can therefore preempt any further radiologic evaluation. However, if the diagnosis remains uncertain, direct visualization may be safely obtained with transhepatic cholangiography, in which contrast agents are injected directly into the biliary tract and liver through a thin needle. Alternatively, fiberoptic endoscopy permits catheterization of the ampulla of Vater and retrograde filling of the biliary tree.

Treatment

The definitive treatment for cholecystitis is removal of the gallbladder, and the key question facing the clinician is the timing of the operation.

Most patients enter the hospital with acute right upper quadrant pain and can be initially treated medically with narcotic analgesia (usually meperidine, a drug with less of the usual narcotic side-effect of spasm of the sphincter of Oddi), intravenous fluids, and cessation of all oral food intake. Most of these patients will respond within several hours with amelioration of pain and other acute symptoms. If the diagnosis of cholecystitis has not already been confirmed, further evaluation can then be pursued more leisurely. Surgery may be undertaken after several days. There is evidence suggesting that the operative mortality is improved when surgery is delayed until after the acute attack has subsided.

If, however, the patient continues to be acutely ill or shows evidence of developing any acute complication of cholecystitis, emergency surgery is required. Acute complications of cholecystitis include gallbladder perforation with bile peritonitis, cholangitis, or overwhelming sepsis. Signs and symptoms of clinical deterioration include increasing pain or fever, the development of peritoneal signs, a worsening leukocytosis, and hypotension. Diabetics with acute cholecystitis have a particularly high risk for developing gallbladder perforation and sepsis. These patients should therefore undergo surgery early in the course of acute cholecystitis.

Aerobic organisms (*Escherichia coli*, other coliforms, and enterococci) and anaerobic organisms (*Bacteroides fragilis* and *Clostridium perfringens*) can be grown from cultures of the bile taken at cholecystectomy. No antibiotic is effective in eliminating infection in an obstructed gallbladder. However, the threat of gram-negative septicemia requires prompt empirical coverage with ampicillin. In the severely ill or diabetic patient, gentamicin or cephalosporin are sometimes used.

There are some patients with documented acute cholecystitis who require emergency surgery but in whom advanced age or some underlying debility makes the risk of surgery and general anesthesia prohibitively high. These patients may be treated by surgical drainage of the gallbladder (cholecystotomy), which can be performed under local anesthesia. This procedure may be life-saving, but the majority of patients will continue to have recurrent attacks.

BIBLIOGRAPHY

Bismuth H, Malt R: Carcinoma of the biliary tract. N Engl J Med 301:704–706, 1979

Naitove A: When cholecystectomy? Hosp Prac June:121–128, 1978

Shimada K, Inamatsu T, Yamashiro M et al: Anaerobic bacteria in biliary disease in elderly patients. J Infect Dis 135:850–854, 1977

Thistle J, Hofmann AF, Ott BJ et al: Chemotherapy for gallstone dissolution 1. Efficacy and safety. JAMA 239:1041–1046, 1978

Vennes J, Jacobson JR, Silvis SE et al: Endoscopic cholangiography for biliary system diagnosis. Ann Intern Med 80:61–64, 1974

Rheumatology

42

Monoarticular Arthritis

Unlike the large number of systemic disorders that produce diffuse joint inflammation, monoarthritis presents a brief, discreet differential diagnosis. In the vast majority of patients, monoarthritis is the result either of infection (septic arthritis) or crystal-induced synovitis (gout or pseudogout). Other causes include trauma, hemarthroses (generally limited to patients with hemophilia), and single joint presentation of a polyarticular disease.

Whereas the chronicity of most polyarticular diseases usually permits a somewhat leisurely approach to diagnosis and management, the dramatic and acute inflammation of monoarthritis necessitates rapid intervention, both for the comfort and safety of the patient, and for protection of the affected joint. The course of monoarthritis is often readily reversible, and recurrences can frequently be prevented.

Diagnosis

Diseases that cause monoarticular arthritis may involve more than one joint at any given time. Although polyarticular systemic diseases may initially affect only a single joint, acute causes of monoarticular arthritis can usually be distinguished by their clinical presentation. Monoarticular diseases are characterized by the rapid onset of *pain, swelling,* and *joint effusion,* and by the appearance of *periarticular erythema.* Periarticular erythema is virtually unique to monoarticular disorders, and its presence is usually sufficient to exclude a consideration of systemic polyarthritis. (One must, however, be alert to the possibility that a monoarticular and a systemic polyarticular disease may coexist in the same patient.)

Synovial Fluid Examination. The volume of synovial fluid in a normal joint rarely exceeds several milliliters. In the knee, for example, the average amount of synvoial fluid is about 1 ml, and the upper range is about 3.5 ml. Inflammation increases the volume of synovial fluid and produces a joint effusion. An effusion can easily be removed by aspiration with a small-gauge needle and then be subjected to microscopic examination, chemical analysis, and culture.

Synovial fluid is normally clear, colorless, and highly viscous. All these properties are altered by inflammation. The fluid becomes xanthochromic and loses its clarity (assessed by attempting to read newsprint through a test tube containing the fluid). The concen-

Table 42–1

| | Normal | Synovial Fluid Analysis | | |
		I (noninflammatory)	II (inflammatory)	III (septic)
Appearance	colorless clear	straw clear	yellow translucent	opaque
Viscosity	high	high	low	
Mucin clot	good	good	poor	poor
White blood cell count	<200/mm³	200–2000	2000–100,000	>100,000
%PMN	<25	<25	>50	>75
Glucose	~ serum	~ serum	>25 mg/dl below serum	>25 mg/dl below serum

Adapted from Rodman GP (ed.): Primer on Rheumatic Diseases: Examination of joint fluid. JAMA 224(5):803, 1973. Copyright 1973, American Medical Association.

tration of hyaluronic acid declines, and the viscosity of the fluid, largely a function of the hyaluronic acid content, also diminishes. The mucopolysaccharide content also declines, and this can be measured qualitatively with a mucin clot test. A sample of synovial fluid is added to a small flask containing 5% acetic acid. Normal synovial fluid forms a firm mass within one minute, whereas abnormal fluid produces a clot that is friable and fragments when the sample is shaken.

The presence of microorganisms or large numbers of polymorphonuclear leukocytes lowers the glucose content of the fluid substantially below a simultaneously obtained serum glucose determination. A synovial glucose determination can therefore serve as a marker for infection and sterile inflammation. The total white blood cell count and the relative polymorphonuclear content can be assessed by conventional hematologic techniques.

A microscopic examination of the synovial fluid is crucial to the differential diagnosis of monoarthritis. Conventional gram stains of the fluid may reveal an infectious etiology. Unstained fluid may reveal the presence of crystals within neutrophils, which can confirm the diagnosis of gout or pseudogout. The intracellular monosodium urate crystals of gout appear as thin, needle-like refractile bodies. The crystals of pseudogout are composed of calcium pyrophosphate, and appear pleomorphic, blunt, and rectangular. Under a polarizing microscope with a first-order red compensator, monosodium urate has strong negative birefringence (yellow when the crystal is aligned parallel to the compensator axis), and calcium pyrophosphate is weakly positive (blue when aligned parallel to the axis). It is important to recognize that the presence of *extracellular* crystals within the synovial fluid is not sufficient to make the diagnosis of crystal-induced synovitis.

Three types of abnormal synovial effusions are recognized (Table 42–1). Noninflammatory effusions (Class I) are largely seen in degenerative and traumatic joint diseases, although crystal-induced diseases may also produce a noninflammatory fluid. Inflammatory effusions (Class II) are characteristic of virtually all the polyarticular diseases as well as the crystal-induced diseases. Septic effusions (Class III) necessitate a diligent search for the pathogen with appropriate therapy dictated by smears and cultures.

Gout

Gout is predominantly a disease of middle-aged and elderly men. Although the precise pathogenesis of gout is unknown, its prevalence is closely linked to the serum concentration of uric acid. Heritable abnormalities of purine metabolism therefore lead to gouty arthritis through chronic overproduction of uric acid. Secondary hyperuricemia also predisposes to gout, and can result either from increased cellular turnover, as seen in patients with psoriasis or myeloproliferative disorders, or from decreased renal excretion of uric acid, seen in patients taking certain drugs, such as the thiazide diuretics, or in patients with chronic interstitial nephritis. The latter is a common complication of the chronic lead intoxication that accompanies the ingestion of "moonshine" (saturnine gout).

The typical acute attack of gout takes the form of an exquisitely painful form of mono-arthritis. The periarticular swelling and inflammation that is characteristically seen may be mistaken for cellulitis. The most common initial site of involvement is the first metatarsophalangeal joint (podagra); (Fig. 42–1), but recurrent attacks may also involve the ankles, knees, fingers, wrists, and olecranon bursae. In long-standing disease, polyarticular attacks become more frequent. Other complications of chronic disease include bony erosions with joint deformities, renal insufficiency from parenchymal urate accumulation, and the deposition of tophi within tissues. Tophaceous deposits, typically found in the synovium, olecranon bursa, and periarticular locations, represent localized depositions of monosodium urate. These firm, irregular masses may occasionally be mistaken for rheumatoid nodules, but their tophaceous nature can be confirmed by microscopic examination of an aspirate, which shows the typical birefringent monosodium urate crystals in abundance.

Therapy for a patient with gout must be directed toward both the acute and chronic phases of the disease. Acute synovitis is treated with a high-dose, tapering regimen of

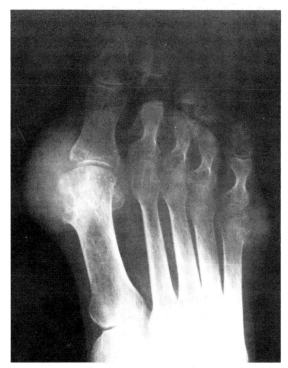

FIG. 42–1. Gout. Large tophi overlie the 1st and 5th toes. Destructive changes can also be noted in the joint spaces.

a nonsteroidal anti-inflammatory agent (phenylbutazone or indomethacin). This rapidly reverses the inflammation. The duration of the attack before therapy is initiated generally correlates with the time required for relief. All patients should be instructed in the use of indomethacin or phenylbutazone to abort new episodes of acute synovitis.

Because the use of anti-inflammatory agents may mask the signs of undiagnosed joint sepsis, these agents should never be employed without definitive crystal confirmation of the diagnosis. For patients in whom synovial analysis is not possible or inconclusive, a tentative diagnosis of gout can be made when hyperuricemia is present with the appropriate clinical presentation. (For unexplained reasons, the serum uric acid concentration frequently falls during acute gouty synovitis, and this may obscure the pre-existing hyperuricemia.) When the distinction between septic and gouty arthritis has not been firmly established, acute therapy with colchicine may be attempted. Colchicine frequently lessens the acute signs and symptoms of gouty arthritis, but will not mask the periarticular inflammation of joint sepsis.

Colchicine is a plant extract that has been used for centuries to treat arthritis. Its mechanism of action in treating gout is, nevertheless, still unknown. It can be given orally or intravenously, but therapy is limited by its profound, dose-related gastrointestinal side-effects of nausea, vomiting, and diarrhea. Upper gastrointestinal side-effects can be abolished by parenteral administration.

The chronic phase of therapy is dependent upon the underlying mechanism of the patient's hyperuricemia. When the acute synovitis subsides, the 24-hour excretion rate of uric acid should be quantitated on a normal purine diet. Patients who excrete more than 10 grams/day are considered *overproducers* of uric acid. They require treatment with allopurinol, a drug that blocks the enzymatic conversion of soluble xanthine to insoluble uric acid. Despite its potent effects on purine biosynthesis, allopurinol has remarkably infrequent side-effects. These include fever, skin eruptions, hepatic enlargement, and leukopenia.

All other patients are, by definition, *underexcreters* of uric acid, and may be treated with uricosurics such as probenecid or sulfinpyrazone. Allopurinol, however, is necessary to treat underexcreters who have (1) an impaired glomerular filtration rate, (2) a known intolerance to uricosurics, or (3) tophaceous gout (since allopurinol dissolves tophaceous accumulations of uric acid).

During the first year of either mode of therapy, daily doses of colchicine should be continued as a prophylaxis against recurrent attacks, because the chronic forms of therapy mobilize storage pools of uric acid and therefore may in themselves precipitate acute synovitis.

For patients with asymptomatic hyperuricemia, hypouricemic therapy should be undertaken only when the risk of incipient gout and uric acid nephropathy is high, for example, in patients with myeloproliferative disorders or in patients receiving chemotherapy for hematologic malignancies.

Pseudogout

Pseudogout is usually seen in elderly patients. The acute attacks of synovitis punctuate an articular disease that otherwise strongly resembles degenerative joint disease. Pseudogout is characterized by the fibrocartilaginous deposition of calcium salts (chondrocalcinosis), and the disease can be recognized on x-ray by linear, punctate calcification in the knee, hip, intervertebral disks, symphysis pubis, and other joints.

The acute synovitis of pseudogout is clinically indistinguishable from gout, except for its predilection for larger peripheral joints, particularly the knee. Involvement of more than one joint is not uncommon, and attacks can last up to two weeks when untreated. Diagnosis depends on the identification of synovial intracellular calcium pyrophosphate crystals. Therapy with indomethacin or phenylbutazone is usually beneficial.

Septic Arthritis

The differential diagnosis of acute monoarticular disease is primarily aimed at excluding the possibility of joint infection. Septic arthritis can masquerade as almost any other type of arthritis. If infection is allowed to go untreated, it will lead to certain loss of joint function.

The mechanism of joint infection is primarily through the hematogenous spread of microorganisms. The factors that predispose to pyarthrosis are therefore those that render the patient susceptible to any infectious agent. Notable among these are diabetes mellitus, chronic alcohol abuse, intravenous drug abuse, neoplasms, and immunosuppression. Joint sepsis commonly occurs in patients treated with corticosteroids, and the intercurrent immunosuppression may mask the inflammatory hallmarks of septic arthritis.

Neisseria gonorrhea, Staphylococcus aureus, and *Streptococcus pneumoniae* are the most frequently encountered bacterial pathogens. *Hemophilus influenzae* and other gram-negative organisms account for less than 5% of infections.

Joint sepsis is common in patients with rheumatoid arthritis and is almost always caused by infection with *Staphylococcus aureus.* In these patients, the diagnosis of septic arthritis is often hampered, because the signs of sepsis are masked by the presentation of generalized arthritis. Any disproportionate inflammation in a single joint (typically the knee) must be noted, and the appearance of a low-grade fever should arouse one's suspicion of infection.

In addition to the common bacterial pathogens, any microorganism can potentially invade the joint space. Thus, infections with both tuberculous and fungal organisms can produce a chronic monoarticular arthritis that will respond to appropriate therapy.

In patients with gonococcal arthritis, the diagnosis may not be apparent because of the relatively low synovial white blood cell count and the difficulty in growing the organism from the joint fluid. In these patients, the diagnosis can often be supported by a polyarticular pattern of joint inflammation coupled with the patient's young age, tenosynovitis, and characteristic skin lesions. Positive cultures may be obtained from sites of primary infection (mouth, genitalia, anus). The clinical picture of gonococcal arthritis must be distinguished from the gonococcal arthritis-dermatitis syndrome in which sterile polyarthralgia is accompanied by chills, fever, and a distinctive rash on the distal extremities. Blood cultures in this setting are often positive.

Confirmation of the diagnosis of septic arthritis requires documentation of an inflammatory synovial effusion, supported by positive gram stains and by culture. These bacteriologic procedures are most often diagnostic in the frankly suppurative joint effusions, such as frequently accompany staphylococcal and gram-negative infections. Other pathogens, notably *Neisseria gonorrhea,* may elude bacteriologic identification. Because joint sepsis usually occurs by hematogenous spread of microorganisms, simultaneous blood cultures may also be helpful.

In many patients, the diagnosis of septic arthritis may ultimately depend upon a salutary response to broad-spectrum antibiotic therapy. When morphologic evidence of infection is lacking, initial antibiotic coverage should be broad and subsequently modified according to the results of culture. Intrasynovial installation of antibiotics is not beneficial, but repeated complete aspiration of the joint effusion is necessary to minimize joint destruction. If this is not feasible, open surgical drainage may become necessary.

The prognosis for the return of joint function depends upon the patient's clinical status, the virulence of the pathogen, and, perhaps most importantly, upon the duration of infection prior to therapy.

BIBLIOGRAPHY

Boss GR, Seegmiller JE: Hyperuricemia and gout. N Engl J Med 300:1459–1468, 1979

Goldenberg DL, Cohen AS: Acute infectious arthritis: A review of patients with nongonococcal joint infections (with emphasis on therapy and prognosis). Am J Med 60:369–377, 1976

Handsfield HH, Wiesner PJ, Holmes KK: Treatment of the gonococcal arthritis-dermatitis syndrome. Ann Intern Med 84:661–667, 1976

Kelley WN: Current therapy of gout and hyperuricemia. Hosp Pract 11:69–76, 1976

Kelly PJ: Bacterial arthritis in the adult. Orthop Clin North Am 6:973–981, 1975

Klinenberg JR: Hyperuricemia and gout. Med Clin North Am 61:299–312, 1977

Liang MH, Fries JF: Asymptomatic hyperuricemia: The case for conservative management. Ann Intern Med 88:666–670, 1978

McCord WC, Nies KM, Louie JS: Acute veneral arthritis. Arch Intern Med 137:858–862, 1977

Resnick D, Niwayama G, Goergen TG et al: Clinical, radiographic and pathologic abnormalities in calcium pyrophosphate dihydrate deposition disease (CPPD): Pseudogout. Radiology 122:1–15, 1977

Ward JR, Atcheson SG: Infectious arthritis. Med Clin North Am 61:313–329, 1977

43

Polyarthritis and Vasculitis

Diffuse synovial inflammation and destruction is associated with many disorders, including rheumatoid arthritis, degenerative joint disease, multisystemic diffuse inflammatory disorders, and polyarthritis of the vertebral skeleton.

RHEUMATOID ARTHRITIS

The diagnosis of rheumatoid arthritis should be considered in any patient who presents with chronic, diffuse inflammation of the joints. The spectrum of presentation is broad. Many patients experience only moderate, slowly progressive polyarticular inflammation, whereas others display a relentless progression of joint destruction that leads to the loss of musculoskeletal function and to fixation and immobility of the affected joints. Rheumatoid arthritis is a systemic illness, and much patient morbidity is also due to extra-articular disease.

Pathology. The underlying joint lesion of rheumatoid arthritis is chronic inflammation of the synovial lining. Early in the course, inflammation produces synovial hypervascu-larity that causes edema, exudation, and cellular infiltration. Continuing inflammation induces hypertrophy of the synovium, which eventually produces much of the destruction and disability of the disease. This exuberant synovial thickening (pannus formation) erodes the articular cartilage and leads to eventual destruction of subchondral bone, laxity of tenoligamentous supports, and, ultimately, subluxation (incomplete dislocation) and ankylosis (stiffening and fixation) of the involved joints.

Pathogenesis. The etiology of rheumatoid arthritis is still obscure. Various theories proposing chemical or infectious causes for rheumatoid synovitis have been neither fully confirmed nor rejected. Although causal relationships cannot yet be established, it is nevertheless clear that immune phenomena are prominent in rheumatoid arthritis. Foremost among these is the presence of *rheumatoid factor*, a circulating IgM antibody that binds IgG. Its presence can be quantitated with several laboratory assays, including bentonite flocculation, latex fixation, and sheep red blood cell agglutination. Although rheumatoid factor can be detected in other inflammatory states, such as subacute infectious endocarditis, sarcoidosis, and most "connective tissue" diseases, high titers are more indicative of true rheumatoid disease when assayed with a less sensitive, more specific test, such as the sheep red cell agglutination. Furthermore, when present in rheumatoid arthritis ("seropositive rheumatoid arthritis"), a high titer of rheumatoid factor indicates that the disease is more likely to be relentless, progressive, and associated with extra-articular complications.

One component of rheumatoid arthritis that probably has an immune basis is vasculitis. The most common local manifestation of rheumatoid vasculitis is the *rheumatoid nodule*. This firm, round, rubbery mass is pathognomonic for rheumatoid arthritis, but must be distinguished from a gouty tophus. Although most frequently located in the subcutaneous tissue at sites of external pressure (*e.g.*, the olecranon), rheumatoid nodules, like other forms of rheumatoid vasculitis, can affect other organs. Rheumatoid nodules are seen almost exclusively in seropositive patients. Nodular, seropositive rheumatoid arthritis carries a grim prognosis.

Presentation and Clinical Course

Rheumatoid arthritis is predominantly a chronic, symmetric arthritis affecting synovial-lined joints. Early involvement is most often in the hands, with swelling, warmth, and tenderness affecting mainly the proximal interphalangeal and metacarpophalangeal joints. The patient complains of aching and stiffness. Maximal stiffness and pain upon awakening is a hallmark of rheumatoid arthritis. In most patients, the onset of the disease is slow and insidious, and many patients describe a prodrome of several weeks of weakness and fatigue. Vague aches and pains often precede the actual onset of arthritis. An occasional patient presents with acute polyarthritis and fever that may be confused with sepsis.

Although hand and foot involvement is most common, synovitis can be prominent in the large joints of the knee, ankle, and elbow, as well as in the intervertebral and temporomandibular joints. In most patients, more than one joint is involved, even at the onset of the disease, but rheumatoid arthritis occasionally begins as a monoarticular arthritis.

Joint inflammation in rheumatoid arthritis is generally symmetric and not migratory. Thus, when a joint becomes involved, it remains involved and does not return to normal when other joints become affected.

Clinical evaluation and follow-up must include a thorough evaluation of the articular system with documentation of the swelling, thickening, compression, tenderness, and pain of all peripheral joints. Nodules should be looked for since they confirm the clinical diagnosis and serve as markers for severe disease. They are most commonly found in the olecranon bursa and Achilles tendon, over the skull and ischial tuberosities, and along the extensor forearm. Radiographs of the hand, foot, and wrist may demonstrate fusiform soft-tissue swelling, muscle atrophy, juxta-articular osteoporosis, joint space narrowing, and characteristic bony erosions near the joint capsular attachments.

Aside from the tests for rheumatoid factor, laboratory evaluation can, at most, document the presence of an inflammatory disorder. Hyperglobulinemia, an elevated erythrocyte sedimentation rate, and the anemia of chronic disease are common. Synovial fluid analysis shows a poor mucin clot and may reveal rheumatoid arthritis cells. These cells are neutrophils that contain cytoplasmic inclusions of IgG and complement.

Mechanical Complications. If the synovial inflammation is allowed to proceed unchecked, a rheumatoid patient may experience disability from the mechanical effects of the joint involvement. In the hand, ulnar deviation and subluxation of the metacarpophalangeal (MCP) joints are the result of joint laxity. Sustained hyperextension of the proximal interphalangeal (PIP) joints with flexion of the distal interphalangeal (DIP) joints produces the characteristic "swan neck" deformity, whereas rupture of the flexed PIP joint through its extensor head results in the "boutonnière" deformity.

In the lower extremities, hallux valgus and metatarsophalangeal (MTP) joint subluxation occur. Spontaneous avascular necrosis of the femoral head can cause marked disability. Recurrent knee effusions provide the setting for popliteal (Baker's) cysts. Baker's cysts are formed from a herniation of the synovium or from rupture and communication with the bursae in the popliteal space. The cysts behave like one-way valves, so that use of the joint forces fluid into the cyst without any means of escape. When large, a ruptured Baker's cyst can dissect into the calf and mimic deep vein thrombophlebitis, producing local tenderness, a positive Homans' sign (pain in the calf or the back of the knee when the ankle is dorsiflexed), and pitting edema. This has been referred to as pseudothrombophlebitis. Diagnosis of a ruptured Baker's cyst should be considered when a previously swollen knee joint in the affected extremity shows apparent resolution. Cyst rupture must be confirmed and distinguished from deep venous thrombosis by arthrography; it responds to bed rest and intra-articular corticosteroids.

Peripheral nerve compression may result from synovial thickening, fibrosis, and nodule formation. The peroneal, ulnar, and median (carpal tunnel syndrome) nerves are most often affected. Surgical decompression may be required.

Potentially fatal mechanical complications may also occur. Synovitis of the cricoarytenoid joint, presenting as hoarseness, can result in sudden laryngeal obstruction. Inflammation of the synovial lining of the atlantoaxial joint produces erosion of the odontoid process with the consequent risk of atlantoaxial subluxation and spinal cord compression.

Localized Extra-articular Complications. Rheumatoid nodules may appear in many locations. In the eye, nodule formation can be complicated by a reactive scleritis and occasionally by thinning and perforation of the sclera. Other locations include the central nervous system, the lung, and the heart.

Rheumatoid disease can affect the lung in a number of ways. Pleural exudates are common and are marked by a high protein content and reactive multinucleated giant cells. Low or absent glucose is diagnostically helpful but is uncommon. Pulmonary nodules may resolve, persist, or cavitate. A solitary nodule in a patient with rheumatoid arthritis should not be assumed to be a rheumatoid nodule without a complete evaluation for malignancy. Nodular pulmonary involvement in patients with rheumatoid arthritis and silicosis (Caplan's syndrome) is common among coal miners. Chronic interstitial fibrosis is seen only rarely and is unaffected by steroids.

Cardiac lesions are common in patients with rheumatoid arthritis and can include granulomatous involvement of the myocardium and the mitral and aortic valves, a vasculitis of the coronary arteries, and pericarditis. These lesions only rarely become clinically apparent. Patients may then experience aortic insufficiency, heart block, or pericardial tamponade.

Systemic Complications. The debilitating systemic effects of profound inflammation produce malaise, inanition, and anemia. Amyloid deposits can be found in as many as 20% to 60% of patients with long-standing rheumatoid arthritis.

Two unique syndromes have been described

in patients with rheumatoid arthritis. In *Felty's syndrome*, the typical arthropathy of rheumatoid arthritis is accompanied by striking splenomegaly, neutropenia, and often leg ulcers. Patients may benefit from splenectomy when neutropenia is severe enough to threaten serious infection. *Sjögren's syndrome* is characterized by a lymphocytic infiltration of the lacrimal and salivary glands. The resulting dry eyes (keratoconjunctivitis sicca), dry mouth (xerostomia), and salivary gland swelling have been termed the sicca complex. Sjögren's syndrome occurs in perhaps 15% of patients with rheumatoid arthritis and can also accompany other forms of systemic inflammation, such as systemic lupus erythematosus, scleroderma, polymyositis, and primary biliary cirrhosis. In a significant number of patients no associated arthritis or other disease is present. The diagnosis can be established by a Schirmer test, in which diminished tear production is documented by insertion of a filter paper in the palpebral fissure. Biopsy of the minor salivary glands in the lower lip reveals a characteristic infiltration of lymphocytes and plasma cells. Malignant transformation of the cellular infiltrate to a diffuse histiocytic lymphoma has been reported. Less common features of Sjögren's syndrome include hypergammaglobulinemia, acute pancreatitis, renal tubular acidosis, and thrombotic thrombocytopenic purpura. The treatment for Sjögren's syndrome is generally similar to that for rheumatoid arthritis alone. Specific modalities include methylcellulose eyedrops for xerophthalmia, and immunosuppression with corticosteroids or cyclophosphamide for more profound cases of multisystemic inflammation.

Perhaps the most devastating complication of rheumatoid arthritis is the systemic vasculitis that develops in only a few patients. It frequently pursues a malignant course, involving the major medium-sized arteries of all systemic vascular beds. The clinical presentation most often includes fever, skin lesions, and chronic leg ulcers. Raynaud's phenomenon and microinfarcts in the nail fold and digital pulp are observed. If the nutrient arteries of the major nerves become involved, a particularly painful form of neuropathy, termed "mononeuritis multiplex," evolves. Many patients with this vasculitis display a unique, low-molecular-weight rheumatoid factor that may be involved in its pathogenesis.

Treatment

The therapy for rheumatoid arthritis is aimed at relieving mechanical disabilities and reducing the inflammation and pain. The involved joints should be put to rest, and exercises should be prescribed to strengthen muscles and increase the range of motion without undue joint strain. Light-weight splints have been designed for use during sleep to ensure alignment of the joints in positions of function. Complete joint immobilization, however, should be avoided. Patients with evidence of atlantoaxial disease must wear a hard cervical collar at all times. When preventive measures fail, surgical correction to improve function of the hands and knees is sometimes beneficial.

Aspirin must be taken continuously in doses that produce therapeutic levels. If remission or significant improvement is not attained after three to six months, other agents may be added.

The most common complications of aspirin use are gastrointestinal, including dyspepsia, gastritis, ulcers, and gastrointestinal blood loss. These complications can occur with either oral or parenteral aspirin. The precise mechanism(s) of gastrointestinal damage is unknown. Gastric erosions can be prevented with cimetidine.

The toxic effects of elevated aspirin levels include tinnitus and hearing loss; these effects are reversible when the drug is discontinued. Aural problems are often an early clinical manifestation of toxicity.

Potential allergic reactions to aspirin include (1) urticaria with angioedema and (2) precipitation of asthmatic attacks in patients with asthma. Frequently, these asthmatic patients also have allergic rhinitis and nasal polyposis.

Aspirin can also be hepatotoxic, resulting in elevated serum levels of liver enzymes and biopsy evidence of toxic hepatitis. This is generally a reversible problem and has been seen in patients with rheumatoid arthritis, Reiter's syndrome, and, perhaps most frequently, systemic lupus erythematosus. Children with juvenile rheumatoid arthritis are especially prone to aspirin-induced liver damage. The signs, symptoms, and treatment of aspirin overdose are discussed in Chapter 61.

Parenteral *gold* therapy, given in weekly doses for one year, produces remissions in many patients. If there is a beneficial response, monthly maintenance therapy should be continued. The toxic effects of gold include bone marrow depression and glomerulitis; patients should be monitored for these toxic effects with serial complete blood counts and urinalyses.

In some patients, the temporary addition of steroids and nonsteroidal anti-inflammatory agents is necessary to suppress flare-ups. A variety of these nonsteroidal anti-inflammatory agents are now available:

Indomethacin is commonly used to treat tendonitis, bursitis, and various inflammatory conditions ranging from ankylosing spondylitis to gout to the postmyocardial infarction (Dressler's) syndrome. It is also useful in treating osteoarthritis of the hip. The major side-effects of indomethacin include gastric ulcers and gastritis. Central nervous system symptoms may occur, including headache, dizziness, depression, and confusion.

Because it causes a high incidence of bone marrow toxicity, *phenylbutazone* is used much less frequently now that other agents are available.

Several compounds of the phenylpropionate family, including *ibuprofen* and *naproxen*, are good anti-inflammatory agents. Their effectiveness, when compared with that of aspirin, has yet to be fully evaluated; however, naproxen must be taken only twice daily, and it has a lower incidence of gastrointestinal side-effects than aspirin.

The effectiveness of nonsteroidal anti-inflammatory agents must still be evaluated for a wide variety of inflammatory states. It is also uncertain whether mixed drug regimens produce fewer side-effects for a given therapeutic effect and whether mixed regimens can enhance the overall therapeutic efficacy. It does appear that different persons with the same disease respond very differently to various drugs. A proper anti-inflammatory protocol must therefore be tailored to the responses and sensitivities of each patient.

The course of rheumatoid arthritis is variable, but up to 20% of patients may experience complete remission within the first year. Of the remainder, roughly one-half experience a stabilization of disease activity with appropriate treatment. It should be repeatedly stressed that rheumatoid arthritis is a chronic disease. In those patients who do not remit, either spontaneously or with drug therapy, the disease tends to persist in the initially inflamed joints and will generally spread in a symmetrical, slowly progressive fashion. Fortunately, only a small percentage of affected patients experience the highly destructive, incapacitating form of rheumatoid arthritis, and the debilitating extra-articular manifestations are even less commonly encountered.

DEGENERATIVE JOINT DISEASE

In patients with degenerative joint disease, also called osteoarthritis, destruction of the joints occurs without inflammatory changes. Weight-bearing and motion produce pain, and there are synovial effusions, but physical signs of active joint inflammation are ordinarily lacking. Nevertheless, long-standing degenerative disease of any joint can result in distortion and malalignment. Degenerative joint disease is a primary affliction of the articular cartilage believed to be caused by excessive wear and tear. Thus, the cartilaginous damage occurs in the weight-bearing joints of obese patients or in those joints unduly stressed by structural anomalies. Many metabolic diseases predispose to cartilaginous degeneration and joint disease, but aside from these obvious predilections, there does not appear to be a heritable tendency to the disorder.

Clinical evaluation of osteoarthritis reveals diminished range of motion, crepitation, and pain of the interphalangeal and large weight-bearing joints (knees and hips). Of special interest are the bony deformities of the DIP joints (Heberden's nodes) and PIP joints (Bouchard's nodes). These bony changes are readily palpable on examination and can be confused with the synovial thickening of rheumatoid arthritis.

Laboratory findings are of little use, except to exclude other diagnostic considerations. X-rays confirm the degeneration, with evidence of asymmetric joint space narrowing and bony overgrowth. The vertebral column is especially disposed to disease involvement, both in the apophyseal joints and in the intervertebral disk spaces, where narrowing is accompanied by the growth of laterally situated bony spurs, termed osteophytes.

A special category of joint degeneration is seen in patients in whom impairment of sensory innervation predisposes to repeated joint trauma. These neuropathic, or "Charcot," joints are seen in such disturbances as tabes dorsalis, diabetes, and syringomyelia. Radiographic examination often reveals dramatic destruction of the joint and subchondral bone with exuberant osteophyte formation.

Treatment of all degenerative joint disease is largely supportive, using mechanical assistance, analgesia, and local heat. Surgical correction of deformities and total joint replacement are sometimes beneficial in advanced, incapacitating illness.

SYSTEMIC DISEASES AFFECTING THE JOINTS

In patients afflicted with diseases of this category, diffuse joint involvement is usually one, and at times only a minor, manifestation of a widespread, multisystemic disturbance. These diseases were originally called the "collagen vascular" or "connective tissue" disorders, so named in the mistaken belief that they comprise the primary abnormality in the supporting framework of blood vessels and other tissues. They are now thought to arise largely through autoimmune mechanisms. Joint involvement appears to result from the deposition of immune complexes in blood vessel walls and supporting structures of the synovium.

Although this category of connective-tissue diseases comprises several discrete entities, there is a large degree of overlap in their clinical presentation, and the assignment of a particular diagnosis can at times be difficult.

Systemic Lupus Erythematosus (SLE). This disease is thought to result from the elaboration of antibodies to native DNA and nuclear proteins. Its spectrum of involvement ranges from mild impairment to fulminant life-threatening inflammation.

Ninety percent of afflicted SLE patients are

women, usually young to middle-aged. Most patients survive the first five years following diagnosis. The major causes of lupus-related deaths are renal failure, central nervous system disease, infection, and hemorrhage. The manifestations of lupus are protean, and there is no typical pattern of presentation or course. The problems that patients encounter can be broadly classified as due to (1) small vessel vasculitis, leading to renal, cutaneous, and central nervous system involvement and (2) polyserositis, leading to joint, peritoneal, and pleural symptoms.

This simple classification can be useful diagnostically in patients who present with what initially appears to be a bizarre combination of findings. Thus, a young woman who presents with joint symptoms and renal disease or with skin lesions and pleuritis may prove likely to have lupus. Patients with SLE also frequently have symptoms of weakness, malaise, or fever.

The clinical presentation of active lupus can involve all the major organ systems:

1. *Joints.* The joint involvement in SLE is common but usually not severe. It typically presents either as a migratory polyarthralgia or an asymmetric polyarthritis without joint deformity. Radiographic evidence of bony erosion is very uncommon. Articular involvement may be accompanied by popliteal cysts, tenosynovitis, and aseptic necrosis of the femoral heads (especially in patients receiving corticosteroid therapy).
2. *Skin.* Among the most characteristic findings in SLE is the "butterfly rash" that involves the malar areas with telangiectasias, erythema, and atrophy. Keratotic plugs are typical. There is also a localized form of the disease, known as discoid lupus, which produces similar cutaneous changes without accompanying systemic involvement. Although skin involvement in discoid lupus can be severe, it does not often progress to full-blown multisystemic involvement.

The skin rash of SLE is notably photosensitive. Exposure to sunlight can precipitate dangerous exacerbations of the visceral as well as the cutaneous components of SLE.

3. *Kidneys.* Morphologic evidence of renal involvement can be found in nearly all patients with SLE, but only one-half of these patients have clinical evidence of renal impairment, ranging in severity from mild proteinuria to complete renal failure. The nephrotic syndrome commonly accompanies renal lupus, and patients frequently display a "telescoped" urinary sediment, which includes erythrocyte, leukocyte, granular, and hyaline casts. Although repeated exacerbations of this glomerulonephritis are sometimes responsive to corticosteroids or immunosuppressive therapy, the progression to uremia is not uncommon. In addition, the susceptibility of lupus patients to infection includes urinary sepsis, which can further aggravate renal impairment.
4. *Hematologic.* Patients with lupus frequently exhibit hepatosplenomegaly, lymphadenopathy, and hematopoietic abnormalities. The latter include normochromic anemia, leukopenia, and thrombocytopenia. It is noteworthy that these patients can have a normal-to-low white blood cell count in spite of active infection.
5. *Serositis.* Sterile inflammation of the pleura, pericardium, and peritoneum is a hallmark of SLE. The latter at times can be confused with an acute surgical abdomen.
6. *Heart.* In addition to pericarditis, which occurs in one-third of patients at some point during the course of their disease, some patients develop small verrucous valvular lesions (Libman-Sacks endocarditis). Although the scarring may ulti-

mately result in valvular incompetence during life, verrucous endocarditis most often is a postmortem diagnosis.

7. *Lungs.* Pleurisy, with or without effusions, is common. Most pneumonias in patients with SLE are infectious, but acute lupus pneumonitis or diffuse interstitial lung disease occasionally develops without evidence of infection.

8. *Central nervous system.* Involvement of neural tissues can occur in up to one-half of patients, taking the form of seizures, peripheral neuropathy, or cerebritis. Inflammation of the brain is an ominous event in this disease, presenting as emotional lability, cognitive impairment, or psychosis. The EEG is abnormal and examination of the cerebrospinal fluid may reveal increases in lymphocytes and protein along with a depressed content of the C_4 component of complement.

Among the most characteristic findings in SLE are *serologic abnormalities* that accompany immune complex deposition. Perhaps the most specific serologic abnormality is the occurrence of antinuclear antibodies (ANA). These abnormal serum proteins can be detected by exposing the patient's serum to a frozen section of an animal tissue containing prominent nuclei, such as monkey kidney. After extensive washing, the section is overlayed with fluorescein-labeled anti-human immunoglobulin and examined microscopically under ultraviolet light. Immunofluorescence will be detected only if the patient's serum contains antinuclear antibodies that have bound to the nuclear constituents. Different patterns of nuclear immunofluorescence can be observed. A peripheral pattern correlates with the presence of anti-DNA antibodies, believed to be primarily responsible for the renal damage of SLE. A homogeneous pattern is caused by antibodies reacting with nucleoprotein, the same antibodies responsible for the LE cell phenomenon (see below). The presence of a peripheral or peripheral-plus-homogeneous pattern is virtually limited to SLE. Nucleolar and speckled patterns may also be observed, but these can also be seen in other connective-tissue diseases.

When anticoagulated blood from a patient with SLE is examined after incubation at room temperature, neutrophils containing phagocytosed eosinophilic material can be seen. The eosinophilic material represents free cell nuclei coated with IgG. These so-called LE cells can also be found in synovial and pleural effusions.

Serum can now be assayed directly to determine its titer of anti-DNA antibodies. The titer of anti-double-stranded (native) DNA appears to correlate well with the activity of visceral inflammation and can be used to follow serially the course of the disease. Antibodies directed against denatured DNA can also be detected, but these are also commonly seen in the drug-induced form of SLE produced by procainamide, hydralazine, isoniazid, and many other agents. The drug-induced form of lupus commonly abates following discontinuation of the offending atent.

Other serologic abnormalities of SLE include a false–positive test for syphilis, a positive Coombs' test, the presence of antimitochondrial antibodies, depressed levels of serum complement, cryoglobulinemia, and the presence of circulating anticoagulants that prolong the prothrombin time and partial thromboplastin time.

Therapeutic approaches to SLE vary. Salicylates and antimalarial medications are often effective in controlling some of the less severe aspects of the disease, such as joint pain and cutaneous involvement, but major complications, such as renal disease or cerebritis, require high-dose corticosteroids.

The use of steroids in SLE is not without complications. For example, lupus cerebritis can be difficult to distinguish from a steroid-induced psychosis. Furthermore, tapering of steroid doses must be approached with great caution to avoid flare-ups of the disease. Corticosteroid therapy has not been shown to affect the long-term outcome of the disease. In some patients who are resistant to corticosteroids, cytotoxic therapy can be beneficial in treating severe complications, such as nephritis and cerebritis.

The course of SLE varies and depends partly upon the pattern of organ system involvement. In general, the disease is characterized by relatively asymptomatic intervals that are punctuated by exacerbations of varying severity. Clinical deterioration of lupus patients is frequently precipitated by (1) stress, particularly induced by surgery, bacterial infections, and emotional upset; (2) exposure to sunlight; or (3) changes in the drug regimen. These underlying factors should always be sought and remedied when the patient's illness shows signs of worsening.

Progressive Systemic Sclerosis (PSS). This is a chronic debilitating disease of the connective tissue. Although various autoimmune phenomena have been identified, including the presence of antinuclear antibodies, it is unclear how these relate to the overall pathogenesis of the disorder.

Connective-tissue involvement is marked by inflammatory and vascular changes that stimulate an overexuberant sclerotic response. Sclerotic changes in the skin occur in 95% of patients and produce cutaneous thickening or swelling (scleroderma) that is especially noticeable over the digits (sclerodactyly). Loss of skin folds and gradual loss of facial motility are noticeable. These changes are frequently accompanied by a telangiectatic skin rash and diffuse, discrete subcutaneous calcinosis. Long-standing skin involvement eventually produces atrophy. Raynaud's phenomenon occurs in 90% of patients (Ray-naud's phenomenon is a cold-induced vasospasm associated with blanching, cyanosis, and erythema). It may be the earliest manifestation of PSS.

Joint stiffness and polyarthralgias are the major articular manifestations of PSS. Early skin involvement over the hands produces a sausage-like swelling of the fingers that can easily be confused with rheumatoid arthritis. Progressive disease ultimately leads to synovial fibrosis and joint contracture. Muscle weakness may sometimes be more troublesome to the patient than the polyarthralgias.

Visceral involvement in patients with PSS most often affects the gastrointestinal system. There is diminished peristalsis in the lower portion of the esophagus resulting in dilatation and reflux, which can produce an esophagitis, occasionally with stricture formation. Duodenal hypomotility predisposes to bacterial overgrowth and malabsorption. Wide-mouthed diverticula of the colon are common and pathognomonic of PSS.

Pulmonary involvement is common. Lower lung field fibrosis leads to restrictive lung disease with a diminution of lung volume and diffusion rate. Pulmonary vascular involvement may cause severe pulmonary hypertension and cor pulmonale.

Patchy fibrosis of the myocardium has been implicated as a cause of congestive heart failure and arrhythmias in PSS. Pericarditis may rarely lead to tamponade.

Involvement of the interlobular renal arteries in the disease process often progresses to malignant hypertension and progressive renal insufficiency.

Laboratory findings are largely nonspecific. Both speckled and nucleolar patterns of ANA immunofluorescence can be seen. High titers of antibodies with a nucleolar staining pattern are seen almost exclusively in patients with PSS.

There is no specific form of treatment for PSS. Conservative measures include good skin care, proper attention to espohageal reflux, and broad spectrum antibiotic coverage to minimize malabsorption. The prognosis is extremely poor in patients with significant visceral involvement, and malabsorption and limited gastrointestinal motility predispose to life-threatening inanition.

Polymyositis is characterized by profound inflammatory involvement of the skeletal muscle. When accompanied by cutaneous manifestations, it is referred to as dermatomyositis. Less common features include polyarthralgias, Raynaud's phenomenon, calcinosis, esophageal hypomotility, and pulmonary fibrosis.

The characteristic progressive, symmetric proximal muscle weakness and atrophy are presumed to be caused by a chronic inflammation of the muscles. The patchy erythematous rash may include the pathognomonic violet coloration of the upper eyelids, called the heliotrope rash.

The diagnostic approach to polymyositis is often predicated upon the patient's mode of clinical presentation. When the neurologist examines the patient for the insidious onset of muscle weakness, the initial evaluation is likely to include an electromyogram, which will reveal the diagnostic findings of spontaneous fibrillation, polyphasic and short-duration potentials induced by contraction, and repetitive high-frequency action potentials. The diagnosis, however, is most often confirmed by a skeletal muscle biopsy. Inflammatory cell infiltrates and a characteristic pattern of muscle fiber degeneration and regeneration will be seen. Some helpful, although less specific, laboratory determinations include an elevated erythrocyte sedimentation rate and elevations of serum creatine phosphokinase (CPK), SGOT, and aldolase, the intracellular enzymes released by degenerating muscle fibers.

Treatment for polymyositis requires high-dose corticosteroid therapy. Relapse of the disease during slow withdrawal from steroid therapy must be monitored with serum enzyme determinations. For unresponsive patients, other forms of immunosuppression, such as methotrexate, have met with success.

The prognosis of polymyositis is difficult to predict. In addition to the variable tempo of the disease, a significant percentage of patients develop malignancy. The causal relationship between polymyositis and cancer is disputed, but a rigorous examination for occult malignancy, especially in men over 50 years of age, is essential.

Mixed connective tissue syndrome is a clinical overlap of PSS, SLE, and polymyositis and is characterized by the production of antinuclear antibodies directed against a ribonuclease-sensitive extract of cellular nuclei. Elaboration of antibodies against this so-called extractable nuclear antigen is thought to predict a milder clinical course.

Vasculitis. Several disease entities have been described in which inflammation and necrosis of blood vessels occur in a diffuse, systemic fashion. These so-called *vasculitides* have diverse clinical manifestations, but because the synovia possess such an abundant blood supply, the joints provide a common focus for inflammatory changes.

Although clinical distinctions among the vasculitic syndromes are often subtle, the histopathology often proves to be more precise. Segmental inflammation in distinctive combinations of small muscular arteries, arterioles, capillaries, and venules segregates these disorders into recognizable pathological entities.

Despite the frequency of joint involvement in vasculitis, the patient's presentation is more often dominated by signs of vascular insufficiency or infarction. Involvement of the renal, mesenteric, coronary, and cerebral arteries can produce hypertension, renal insufficiency, gastrointestinal bleeding, angina, cardiac failure, and central nervous system dysfunction. Fever, myalgias, and asthma are also common findings. Leukocytosis with eosinophilia is sometimes observed. A biopsy can be used to document the presence of vasculitis, and angiography may reveal typical aneurysmal dilatations.

Several vasculitic syndromes merit special comment:

Polyarteritis nodosa tends to affect the medium-sized arteries of middle-aged men. It carries a poor prognosis. Characteristic features include (1) prominent systemic complaints of fever, chills, weakness, myalgias, and weight loss; (2) nodular arteritic lesions of the skin and mucous membranes; (3) congestive heart failure, arrhythmias, or pericarditis; (4) pulmonary infiltrates with cough and hemoptysis; (5) abdominal pain and gastrointestinal bleeding; (6) splenic or hepatic infarction; and (7) renal infarction or glomerulonephritis. Typical laboratory features include leukocytosis with prominent eosinophilia. Chronic hepatitis B antigenemia has been implicated in the pathogenesis of the syndrome. The diagnosis is suggested by the multisystemic pattern of involvement and can be confirmed by biopsy of the skin, muscle, or testes. Polyarteritis nodosa is often fatal, although both spontaneous remissions and corticosteroid-induced remissions do occur.

Giant cell arteritis (temporal arteritis) primarily involves the cranial vessels. Nodular obliteration of the temporal arteries produces severe headaches, and intracranial vascular lesions predispose to ischemic optic neuritis and blindness. The diagnosis must be vigorously pursued by temporal artery biopsy, because high-dose corticosteroid therapy can prevent retinal damage and blindness. The vasculitis can be accompanied by the painful muscle involvement of polymyalgia rheumatica. Temporal arteritis should be considered in older patients with a fever of unknown origin and elevated erythrocyte sedimentation rate.

Polymyalgia rheumatica, with or without concomitant cranial arteritis, is uncommon in patients under the age of 55. Proximal muscle pain, without weakness, is observed in conjunction with a markedly elevated erythrocyte sedimentation rate and systemic symptoms such as fever and weight loss. Temporal artery biopsy may reveal vasculitis even in the absence of symptomatic cranial arteritis. Occasionally, there may be evidence of widespread visceral involvement, with skin lesions, lymphadenopathy, articular inflammation, and polyneuropathy.

Polymyalgia rheumatica is responsive to low-dose corticosteroid therapy. Nevertheless, in the absence of concurrent giant cell arteritis, which requires high-dose steroids (see above), this disease is usually best managed with anti-inflammatory doses of salicylates.

Wegener's granulomatosis is marked by a unique mixture of granulomatous and vascular inflammation of the viscera. Although there is no pathognomonic clinical feature of Wegener's granulomatosis, several clinical features appear to be characteristic. Inflammation of both the upper and lower respiratory tract is common, and presenting features include purulent sinusitis, severe rhinorrhea, nasal mucosal ulcerations, purulent otitis media, cough, pleurisy, hemoptysis, and evanescent pulmonary infiltrates. These findings are often accompanied by systemic symptoms of fever, anorexia, and weight loss, along with evidence of cutaneous, ocular, and articular inflammation. A "localized" form of Wegener's granulomatosis has been described in which the respiratory tract inflammation is unaccompanied by the widespread, systemic involvement seen in patients with the systemic disease. In general, this variant does not carry the ominous prognosis of the more diffuse disorder.

The hallmark of generalized Wegener's granulomatosis is renal disease, which, by its severity, determines the outcome and prognosis of the disease. Renal involvement is characterized by a focal glomerulitis that progresses to generalized involvement and, if untreated, leads to death from end-stage renal failure. Early therapeutic attempts with high-dose corticosteroids were not found to alter the mortality of the disorder, but more recent trials with cyclophosphamide indicate that prolonged immunosuppression may be of great benefit in some patients.

Another group of vasculitic syndromes can be distinguished by the prominence of cutaneous involvement. These disorders, which involve the small vessels while sparing the muscular arteries, are called *hypersensitivity angiitis* and *Henoch-Schönlein purpura*. Skin inflammation takes the form of bilateral purpura, comprised of lesions in the dermis that vary from punctate petechiae to large ecchymoses. The purpura of vasculitis is distinctive in that it is most often palpable (*i.e.*, papular). Other systemic manifestations include fever, pericarditis, pulmonary infiltrates, and central nervous system involvement.

Hypersensitivity angiitis is thought, in many cases, to represent an allergic drug reaction, and many drugs, including antibiotics, anti-inflammatory agents, and vaccines have been implicated. In other cases, the disease is preceded by respiratory infection. Treatment is analogous to that for the other forms of vasculitis. In addition, where feasible, all possible offending antigens should be withdrawn.

If the typical presentation of hypersensitivity angiitis is accompanied by arthralgias, abdominal pain, gastrointestinal bleeding, and glomerulonephritis, the designation of Henoch-Schönlein purpura is applied. The disease most commonly affects children. In many cases, no inciting antigen can be identified.

POLYARTHRITIS WITH VERTEBRAL INVOLVEMENT

In polyarthritis with vertebral involvement, the typical rheumatoid joint involvement is characteristically overshadowed by the inflammation and destruction of the vertebral articulations.

Ankylosing spondylitis is predominantly a disease of young males. Chronic low-back pain from sacroiliitis frequently heralds the onset of spinal inflammation. Progressive involvement of the axial skeleton causes pain and restricts the motion of the cervical and lumbar spine. Spinal involvement can be diagnosed by sacroiliac tenderness, loss of normal lumbar lordosis, restricted lumbar flexion, and impaired chest expansion from costovertebral involvement. The final stage of ankylosing spondylitis is characterized by a fixed kyphosis with the head maintained in anterior flexion.

X-ray studies reveal sacroiliac involvement with symmetric joint space narrowing and subchondral sclerosis. Syndesmophytes are characteristic paravertebral ossifications that accompany intervertebral narrowing and erosions of the vertebral body. These progressive changes ultimately lead to the ankylosed "bamboo spine" (Fig. 43–1).

Systemic findings in patients with ankylosing spondylitis are also common. Weight loss and fatigue may be accompanied by iritis, first-degree atrioventricular block, and aortic valvular insufficiency. Peripheral joint lesions mimic rheumatoid arthritis, but subcutaneous nodules do not occur.

Although the pathogenesis is unknown, the HLA-B27 antigen is observed with greatly increased frequency in patients affected with ankylosing spondylitis, raising speculation

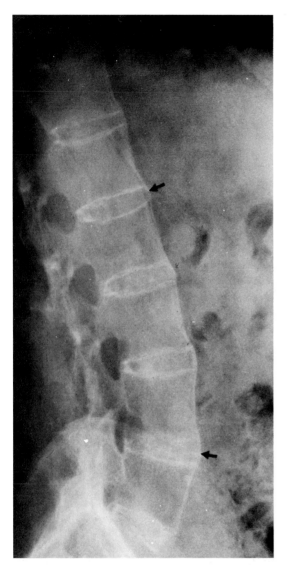

FIG. 43–1. Ankylosing spondylitis. The "bamboo spine" is produced by squaring of the vertebral bodies and calcification of the anterior spinal ligaments (arrows).

about an altered immune response in this disorder.

Treatment consists of physical therapy and a therapeutic salicylate regimen. There is no place for corticosteroids in treating ankylosing spondylitis, but at times a short course of a nonsteroidal anti-inflammatory agent, such as indomethacin, is indicated for the relief of articular pain.

Reiter's syndrome is also a disease predominantly of young men and is thought to be a postinfectious complication of gonorrhea or diarrheal pathogens (such as *Yersinia enterocolitica*). Patients with this syndrome suffer from urethritis and conjunctivitis and may also have spondylitis. Skin involvement may include oral ulcerations, penile or clitoral inflammation, and hyperkeratosis of the soles and fingernails, referred to as keratoderma blennorrhagica.

Several of the articular features seen in Reiter's syndrome are distinctive. The peripheral arthritis is asymmetric and involves the large joints, primarily in the lower extremities. Sacroiliitis is frequently unilateral. Spine involvement is also asymmetric. Despite syndesmophyte proliferation, generalized ankylosis is uncommon. Periostitis of the plantar calcaneus produces characteristic large calcaneal spurs.

Although the peripheral features often undergo spontaneous remission, relapse is common. Spondylitis, when present, can remain active for extended periods.

Psoriatic arthritis has many parallels with Reiter's syndrome. The spondylitis of psoriatic arthritis is virtually indistinguishable from that of Reiter's syndrome. The similarity between the diseases is underscored by the cutaneous hyperkeratosis and hyperkeratotic nail changes common to both. The disease activity varies with the severity of skin involvement, but in some patients the onset of peripheral arthritis can at times precede the development of the rash. Arthritis is far more prevalent in psoriasis patients with evidence of nail involvement.

Psoriatic peripheral arthritis mimics rheumatoid arthritis, but several distinguishing features merit comment. Unlike rheumatoid arthritis, asymmetric involvement of the DIP joints is almost pathognomonic. The classic x-ray pattern of DIP involvement is called the "pencil-in-cup" deformity. In general, this is a less destructive disease than rheumatoid arthritis; however, some patients display "arthritis mutilans," the most destructive polyarthritis that has been clinically described. Psoriatic arthritis does not respond to such standard antirheumatoid agents as gold and antimalarials, and is best managed solely with salicylates and conservative measures.

Inflammatory bowel disease (see Chap. 36) also produces progressive spondylitis. The arthritis may be punctuated by acute flare-ups of peripheral polyarthritis involving the large joints. As in the case of psoriatic arthritis, arthritis associated with inflammatory bowel disease can precede the underlying disease, but more frequently it accompanies active intestinal inflammation. Therapy of the bowel disease may produce ameliorations of the peripheral arthritis although the course of spondylitis is not generally affected by disease activity in the bowel.

BIBLIOGRAPHY

Baldwin DS, Gallo GR: Lupus nephritis. Clin Rheum Dis 1:639, 1975

Calin A: Reiter's syndrome. Med Clin North Am 61:365, 1977

Decker JL, et al: SLE: evolving concepts. Ann Intern Med 91:587, 1979

Engleman EG, Engleman EP: Ankylosing spondylitis: recent advances in diagnosis and treatment. Med Clin North Am 61:347, 1977

Fauci AS, Hynes BF, Katz P: The spectrum of vasculitis: clinical, pathological, immunologic and therapeutic considerations. Ann Intern Med 89:660, 1978

Feinglass EJ, et al: Neuropsychiatric manifestations of SLE diagnosis, clinical spectrum, and relationship to other features of the disease. Medicine 55:323, 1976

Fleming A, Crown JM, Corbett M: Early rheumatoid disease. Ann Rheum Dis 35:357, 1976

Goodman BW: Temporal arteritis. Am J Med 67:839, 1979

Healy LA, Witske KR: Manifestations of giant cell arteritis. Med Clin North Am 61:261, 1977

Hollingsworth JW, Saykaly RJ: Systemic complications of rheumatoid arthritis. Med Clin North Am 61:217, 1977

Kaye RL, Pemberton RE: Treatment of rheumatoid arthritis. Arch Intern Med 136:1023, 1976

Morkowitz RW: Management of osteoarthritis. Hosp Pract 14:75, 1979

Pearson CM, Bohan A: The spectrum of polymyositis and dermatomyositis. Med Clin North Am 61:439, 1977

Peyron JG: Epidemiologic and etiologic approach to osteoarthritis. Semin Arthritis Rheum 8:288, 1979

Pirotsky B, Bardana EJ: Immunosuppressive therapy in rheumatic disease. Med Clin North Am 61:419, 1977

Roberts MET, Wright V, Hill AGS, et al: Psoriatic arthritis. Ann Rheum Dis 35:206 1976

Rowell NR: the prognosis of systemic sclerosis. Br J Dermatol 95:57, 1976

Shearn MA: Sjögren's syndrome. Med Clin North Am 61:271, 1977

Wagner L: Immunosuppressive agents in lupus nephritis: a critical analysis. Medicine 55:239, 1976

Weissman BNW, Sosman JL: The radiology of rheumatoid arthritis. Orthop Clin North Am 6:653, 1975

Wolff SM, Fauci AS, Horn RG, et al: Wegener's granulomatosis. Ann Intern Med 81:513, 1974

Hematology/Oncology

44 Transfusions

Transfusions have become a mainstay of hospital therapy, and the clinician now has a wide range of component blood products at his disposal. The only remaining use for whole blood transfusions is in exsanguination, although even here adequate replacement can usually be achieved with IV crystalloid, red cells, platelets, and plasma as needed. Component therapy is better medicine, both for the safety of the patient and in the interest of economy.

RED CELL TRANSFUSIONS

One unit of blood represents the red blood cells from 500 ml of whole blood. It has been estimated that three units of blood are transfused each year for every 100 persons in the United States. It has also been estimated that up to one-half of these transfusions are unnecessary. The only indication for a red cell transfusion should be when the patient's clinical condition requires a higher hemoglobin.

A young, healthy person can lose 50% of his red blood cells but maintain O_2 delivery and do fine as long as his circulatory volume is maintained. On the other hand, a person with cardiopulmonary or vascular disease who cannot increase cardiac output or alveolar ventilation needs a hematocrit in the range of about 30. The acuteness of the insult also determines the minimum hematocrit that the patient can tolerate. Thus, a patient with chronic anemia and a hematocrit of 15 may note only fatigue and does not require an emergency transfusion. However, a patient who has suffered gastrointestinal bleeding, who has ST elevation on the electrocardiogram, and whose hematocrit has plummeted, does require blood replacement.

One unit of blood can be expected to increase the hematocrit by 3 points. Only rarely is there an indication for transfusion of a single unit. Occasionally, a patient on chronic dialysis may be symptomatic with the loss of one unit of blood and will improve significantly with replacement.

Red Cell Component Preparations

Several forms of red cell concentrates are available, including packed red cells, leukocyte-poor red cells, washed cells, and frozen red cells. Regardless of the preservative, different blood components have different shelf lives. Granulocytes are no longer viable for transfusion after 24 hours, and platelets after 72 hours. Clotting factors have variable lifespans. Factor VIII declines significantly after 2 days, Factor V after 4 to 5 days, and Factor XI after 6 to 7 days. The other components of the clotting cascade are stable for longer periods. Thus, in a patient with a massive acute hemorrhage for which a large transfusion is required, the use of blood that has been stored for longer than 1 or 2 days will fail to replete Factor VIII and platelets. However, units of blood that have been stored for several weeks can still be used if transfusions of platelets and plasma are given separately.

Packed red cells can be used to provide an especially concentrated transfusion. A unit of packed cells has a hematocrit of 60 to 90 in a volume of about 300 ml. Packed red cells are relatively inexpensive to use, since all the other preparations not only concentrate the red cells but purify them, removing platelets, granulocytes, and plasma proteins. Separation diminishes the allergic reactions that these components can cause.

Leukocytes and plasma components are removed from preparations of *washed red cells*, and this is probably the best way of removing allergens. Unfortunately, the saline washing introduces a potential source of bacterial contamination, and the cells must be used soon after processing.

Frozen red cells can be stored for years in the presence of glycerol with little biochemical degradation. The long shelf life makes this an excellent way to store rare blood types. The preparation is relatively poor in leukocytes and plasma proteins, and can be further purified by washing with saline. Studies suggest that the risk of hepatitis transmission is lower with frozen blood than with any of the other preparations, although the reasons are not clear. The major disadvantage of frozen red cells is expense. In hospitals where frozen red cells are available, the increased cost must be balanced against the decreased risk of hepatitis for each patient.

Adverse Effects from Transfusions

Adverse effects from red cell transfusions are not uncommon, and immediate problems include both transfusion reactions and complications.

Transfusion Reactions. Transfusion reactions can take three forms: (1) febrile and nonhemolytic, (2) hemolytic, and (3) immediate hypersensitivity reactions.

1. Febrile reactions are the most common. The risk of a febrile reaction in a given patient increases with the number of previous transfusions he has received. Febrile reactions usually begin during or just after the transfusion, but may occur up to 6 or even 12 hours later. These reactions are usually mild and can be accompanied by shaking, although rarely by significant rigors. Several studies have suggested that febrile reactions are commonly due to the presence of leukoagglutinins. A febrile reaction is believed to be the result of the interaction of recipient leukoagglutinins with donor white blood cells, inducing the release of pyrogens. In some patients, donor platelets, lymphocytes, and other plasma components may act as sensitizing antigens.

Febrile reactions are benign and can usually be prevented by the use of frozen, washed red cell preparations. Patients are treated with standard antipyretics. The transfusion does not have to be stopped, but the patient must be carefully observed.

Occasionally, a febrile reaction to a red cell transfusion is the first clue that the donor blood is contaminated by bacterial pyrogens. This type of reaction is usually more severe and may signify serious septicemia. Symptoms include pain, vomiting, decreased blood pressure, and circulatory collapse. Fortunately, these reactions are rare, since the mortality rate exceeds 50%. If contamination with bacterial pyrogens is suspected because of a marked febrile reaction, the transfusion must be stopped and two sets of blood cultures obtained from the recipient. The untransfused blood should be gram-stained and cultured. If the patient's condition continues to deteriorate, broad-spectrum antibiotic coverage should be initiated even before culture results are completed.

2. An acute hemolytic reaction is due to the transfusion of immunologically incompatible blood. The host's antibodies bind to the transfused cells and cause either intravascular hemolysis (as seen with ABO incompatibility) or destruction of the antibody-coated cells within the reticuloendothelial system. With careful crossmatching, hemolytic reactions are now rare.

The symptomatology of a hemolytic reaction is quite varied. Fevers and chills are typical early symptoms, and a hemolytic reaction can be indistinguishable from a common, benign febrile reaction. Thus, with the development of any febrile reaction following transfusion, all of the details of the crossmatching and identifications should be checked. It is wise to slow the rate of transfusion and carefully monitor the patient.

Development of the more florid symptoms of a hemolytic reaction—back and flank pain, hypotension, bleeding from intravenous sites, nausea, and vomiting—requires that the transfusion be stopped and steps taken to ascertain whether a hemolytic reaction has occurred. The patient's plasma should be examined visually for free hemoglobin (the plasma appears red), the type and crossmatch should be repeated (including an indirect Coombs' test with both the patient's and the donor's serum), and the urine should be examined for hemoglobin. A sample of the patient's blood should be sent for a hematocrit, haptoglobin, prothrombin time, partial thromboplastin time, and platelet count. Fibrin split products and fibrinogen levels should be quantitated to document the presence or absence of disseminated intravasular coagulation (DIC).

The antigen-antibody interaction that results in hemolysis produces a catastrophic chain of events that can include DIC, vascular collapse, and renal failure. DIC occurs in up to 50% of patients. In an anesthetized patient, bleeding due to DIC may be the first sign of a hemolytic transfusion reaction. Vascular collapse may be the result of activation of inflammatory pathways by antigen-antibody complexes. The renal failure presents a picture of acute tubular necrosis and may be caused by hypotension, the effects of the antigen-antibody complexes, or both.

After the transfusion is stopped, treatment consists of measures to support the blood pressure and maintain renal circulation. The urine output should be monitored. An intravenous bolus of 20% mannitol is usually given over 5 minutes in an attempt to elicit an osmotic diuresis and thus maintain the patency of the renal small vasculature, but this maneuver has not been proven to be effective.

3. Immediate hypersensitivity reactions to transfusions range from local urticaria to angioneurotic edema to anaphylaxis. These reactions are unusual and are generally mild. The transfusion is stopped, and the immediate hypersensitivity reaction is treated like any allergic reaction with antihistamines and sympathomimetics. IgA-deficient patients, who comprise up to 1 in every 500 people, are particularly disposed to allergic reactions. Some of these patients possess circulating anti-IgA antibodies, and the inclusion of even a small amount of IgA in a transfusion results in a hypersensitivity reaction. Transfusion of washed red cells is generally adequate prophylaxis in these patients.

Complications. Immediate complications of transfusions result from the physicochemical effects of the blood administration. Thus, circulatory overload in patients with cardiac disease can precipitate congestive heart failure. Because protein and salt are removed from washed, packed cells, circulatory overload is less likely to occur with these preparations. Slow administration of blood further diminishes the risk of overload, and diuretics can be given when required.

Rapid and massive transfusions of cold blood can cause significant hypothermia.

In patients with renal failure, large transfusions can deliver significant and dangerous potassium loads, and hyperammonemia can be dangerous in patients with marginal liver function. The concentration of free ammonia and potassium rises in nonfrozen blood the longer that it is stored.

PLATELET TRANSFUSIONS

Platelet transfusions can be very effective in stopping the bleeding in thrombocytopenic patients whose underlying disorder is inadequate platelet production. Platelets are stored at 22°F, and platelet concentrates can be stored up to 72 hours.

Platelet transfusions are usually restricted to several defined groups of patients. Patients with marrow aplasia or marrow failure due to infiltrative disease should have their platelet counts monitored, and transfusions should be given if the platelet counts fall below 10,000, when the risk of bleeding goes up markedly. Clearly, any thrombocytopenic patient who is bleeding should also be given a transfusion of platelets. The use of platelet transfusions in patients with immune thrombocytopenic purpura (ITP) is still uncertain, since the platelet count usually fails to rise after transfusion. It is not clear that transfusions help these patients, and platelet transfusions should be reserved for emergency situations with active bleeding.

For every unit transfused, the recipient's platelet count should rise about 10,000 to 20,000. If there is no source of platelet destruction, the infused platelets circulate in progressively smaller numbers for about a week. The most important determinant of transfused platelet survival time in patients without immune thrombocytopenic purpura is alloimmunization to HLA antigens carried on donor platelets. After four to eight weeks of regular platelet transfusion therapy from random donors, most patients show signs of allosensitization. These signs include a marked decrease in both the peak platelet response and the life span of the transfused platelets. The incidence of febrile transfusion reactions also increases. The use of HLA-matched donors decreases the likelihood of sensitization, and should be attempted in patients who are becoming refractory to randomly donated platelets. A more recent approach to this problem is the use of autologous frozen platelets, in which a patient donates his own platelets to be frozen before beginning chemotherapy. He can then be transfused with his own platelets when cytotoxic drugs cause marrow depression.

WHITE CELL TRANSFUSIONS

At present, neutrophil transfusions are expensive and hazardous, and the indications for their use are few.

The lifetime of stored white cells is measured in hours, and transfusions must therefore be given soon after the cells are collected.

Thus far, only patients with documented bacterial infections and persistent neutropenia seem to benefit from white cell transfusions. Generally, patients receive 10^{10} to 10^{11} granulocytes, and their peripheral white blood count rises anywhere from 0 to 1000 one hour following the transfusion. These data come from controlled, prospective trials, but the number of patients is too few to permit accurate generalizations about which patients may benefit from white cell transfusions.

Side-effects are common, and 20% to 60% of recipients have mild febrile reactions with or without chills. A few patients experience high fever, hypotension, and the adult respiratory distress syndrome.

HEPATITIS

With the virtual elimination of immediate hemolytic transfusion reactions, the major risk of transfusion therapy is the development of hepatitis. In several studies, the incidence of heptatitis ranges from 10% to 20%. The incidence varies with the source of blood, the screening procedures that are used, and the number of units that are received. Of those who contract hepatitis, about 20% become symptomatic.

Hepatitis B virus is still responsible for many cases of post-transfusion hepatitis. Donor blood is currently screened for hepatitis B surface antigen and this practice is contributing to a reduction in the incidence of hepatitis B antigen-positive hepatitis. Those cases that still occur are felt to represent situations in which the levels of hepatitis B surface antigen are too low to be detected by radioimmunoassay or in which the viral particles in the donor blood lack the B surface antigen.

Other potential causes for post-transfusion hepatitis include non-A, non-B hepatitis, cytomegalovirus (CMV), and Epstein-Barr virus (EBV). When CMV titers have been measured pre- and post-transfusion in prospective studies, no correlation has been found between a rise in CMV titers and evidence of hepatitis. Patients with post-transfusion hepatitis B are just as likely to exhibit a rise in CMV titers as patients without evidence of hepatitis B infection. A similar problem exists with Epstein-Barr virus titers, and many authors therefore feel that non-A, non-B hepatitis is the most likely etiologic candidate for most cases of post-transfusion non-B hepatitis.

The clinical syndromes of post-transfusion hepatitis are the same as those of viral hepatitis acquired through other modes of transmission (see Chap. 38). These include acute icteric symptomatic illness, anicteric asymptomatic hepatitis, chronic liver disease, and cirrhosis.

BIBLIOGRAPHY

Barry KG, Crosby WH: The prevention and treatment of renal failure following transfusion reactions. Transfusion 3:34–36, 1963

Collins TA: Massive blood transfusion. Clin Haematol 5:201, 1976

Goldfinger D: Acute hemolytic transfusion reactions: A fresh look at pathogenesis and considerations regarding therapy. Transfusion 17:85–98, 1977

Kay AB: Some complications associated with the administration of blood and blood products. Clin Haematol 5:165, 1976

Mitchell R: Red cell transfusion. Clin Haematol 5:33, 1976

45   Anemia

Anemia is defined as a reduction in the oxygen carrying capacity of the blood due to a decreased concentration of hemoglobin. Although anemia is virtually always reflected in a decreased hematocrit, an assessment of the hemoglobin concentration is a more accurate gauge of the adequacy or inadequacy of oxygen transport capacity.

The causes of anemia are legion, but the range of diagnostic possibilities can be greatly reduced by obtaining a reticulocyte count and examining a peripheral blood film (Fig. 45–1).

Reticulocytes are immature red blood cells, and they can be recognized on a blood film by the characteristic basophilic densities in their cytoplasm. Anemia stimulates their synthesis and release from the bone marrow. An increased reticulocyte count in a patient with anemia is a normal response and indicates that new red blood cells are being produced. An elevated reticulocyte count in a patient with anemia therefore indicates that anemia is the result of peripheral red blood cell destruction or blood loss. A low or even normal reticulocyte count in a patient with anemia indicates failure of red blood cell production, and the patient is then said to have a hypoproliferative anemia.

The morphology of the red blood cells permits further subcategorization. The red blood cell indices provide a quantitative description of the most important morphologic features:

1. The mean corpuscular volume (MCV) is a measure of the average size of the red blood cell, and is defined as

$$\frac{\text{vol of packed red blood cells per liter of blood}}{\text{number of red blood cells (millions per mm}^3)} .$$

The normal value is approximately $90\mu^3$/red blood cell.

2. The mean corpuscular hemoglobin (MCH) is a measure of the amount of hemoglobin per cell, and is calculated as

$$\frac{\text{hemoglobin (g/liter)}}{\text{numbers of red blood cells (millions per mm}^3)} .$$

The normal value is approximately 30 pg/red cell.

3. The mean corpuscular hemoglobin concentration (MCHC) is a percentage measure of how much of the red blood cell consists of hemoglobin. It is calculated as

$$\frac{\text{hemoglobin (g/100 ml)}}{\text{hematocrit}} \times 100.$$

The normal value is approximately 35%.

Among the hypoproliferative anemias, three morphologic types have been recognized,

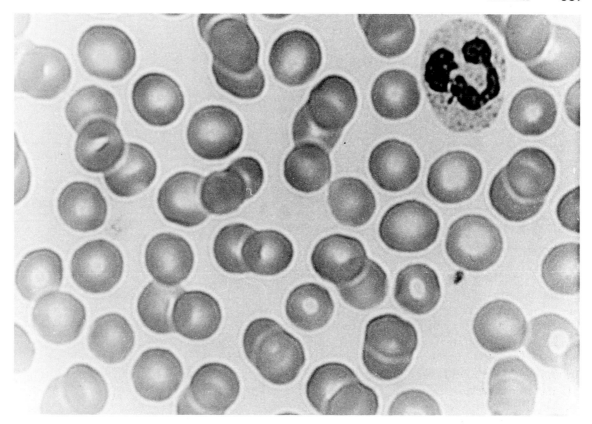

FIG. 45–1. Normal peripheral blood film. The red blood cells have a central lucency and are relatively uniform. The size of normal red cells (7 to 8 microns in diameter) can be compared with that of the polymorphonuclear leukocyte. The small dark cell is a platelet.

based on the mean corpuscular volume and hemoglobin concentration. *Macrocytic anemias* usually occur in patients who are deficient in vitamin B_{12} or folate. *Normochromic, normocytic anemias* are typically seen in patients with early iron deficiency, marrow aplasia, and underlying chronic disease. *Microcytic, hypochromic anemias* can also be associated with chronic disease, but are more often seen with iron deficiency and thalassemia.

In patients whose anemia is believed to be due to red blood cell destruction, a peripheral blood film may reveal the sickled cells of sickle cell anemia, the spherocytes of immune hemolysis, or the schistocytes (red cell fragments) of mechanical hemolysis (*e.g.*, in patients with prosthetic valves).

HYPOPROLIFERATIVE ANEMIAS

Macrocytic Anemia

Macrocytic anemia can result from alcohol abuse, liver disease, hypothyroidism, and the ingestion of certain drugs, but is usually caused by a deficiency of vitamin B_{12} or folate. The macrocytic anemias of vitamin B_{12} and

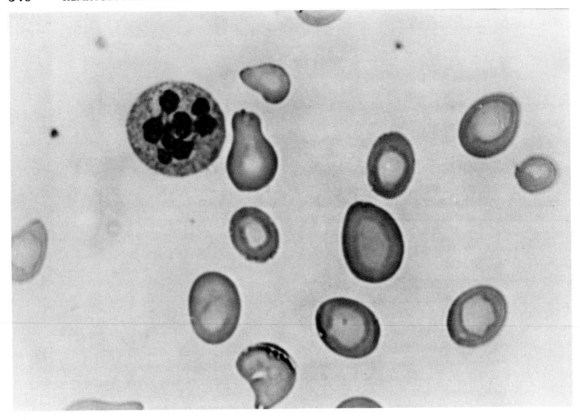

FIG. 45–2. Megaloblastic anemia. This film illustrates the large red blood cells in a patient with vitamin B₁₂ deficiency. Note also the hypersegmented nucleus of the leukocyte.

folate deficiency are termed *megaloblastic,* because a marrow examination reveals the cells of the erythroblast series to be exceptionally large. Large leukocytes and abnormal megakaryocytes are also found in the marrow. The polymorphonuclear leukocytes in the peripheral blood are larger than normal and often have an increased number of nuclear lobes. Cells with five or more lobes are said to be hypersegmented (Fig. 45–2). These white blood cell changes are characteristic of megaloblastic anemia and are not seen in the other forms of macrocytic anemia. The anemias of vitamin B_{12} and folate deficiency are identical. However, only vitamin B_{12} deficiency gives rise to neurologic problems.

Vitamin B_{12} Deficiency. In the adult, vitamin B_{12} deficiency can be caused by pernicious anemia, gastrointestinal bacterial overgrowth, or the loss of ileal function. In each of these diseases, vitamin B_{12} is poorly absorbed from the gut.

In *pernicious anemia,* poor vitamin B_{12} absorption is a result of the loss of intrinsic factor. Intrinsic factor is a glycoprotein that is normally secreted into the gut by the gastric parietal cells. It is responsible for binding vitamin B_{12} and facilitating its uptake by cells in the terminal ileum. The gastric parietal cells in these patients are also deficient in the secretion of hydrogen ions, and the presence of achlorhydria is therefore necessary for the diagnosis of pernicious anemia. Achlorhydria, the absence of acid secretion by the stomach, is tested by measuring the gastric acid output in response to histamine stimulation.

A variety of immune abnormalities are present in pernicious anemia. As many as 90% of patients exhibit humoral (antibody-mediated) or cellular autoimmunity against their parietal cells, and approximately 50% of patients possess anti-intrinsic factor antibodies. The gastric histology is also consistent with an immune process; biopsy of the gastric fundus reveals a lymphocytic infiltrate and an absence of parietal and chief cells. Nevertheless, the exact pathogenetic relationship of these findings to pernicious anemia is still uncertain.

Bacterial overgrowth syndromes are discussed in Chapter 35. Vitamin B_{12} deficiency is presumably the result of competition for the vitamin by the bacteria.

Inflammatory bowel disease or *ileal resection* can result in vitamin B_{12} deficiency because of the failure to absorb intrinsic factor-vitamin B_{12} complexes (see Chap. 35).

The diagnosis of vitamin B_{12} deficiency can be confirmed by laboratory measurement of serum B_{12} levels and urinary methylmalonic acid. (Patients with vitamin B_{12} deficiency characteristically have excessive amounts of methylmalonic acid in their urine.) The serum test for vitamin B_{12} is accurate. These tests should be ordered in any patient with megaloblastic anemia, or who presents with any of the neurologic symptoms of vitamin B_{12} deficiency. In addition to the abnormalities on the peripheral blood film, megaloblastic anemia is associated with glossitis, an elevated level of serum lactic dehydrogenase of erythrocyte origin (the LDH-1 isoenzyme frequently exceeds the LDH-2), and elevations of plasma bilirubin and iron.

The neurologic symptoms of vitamin B_{12} deficiency can be subtle or devastating. The pathologic syndrome of *subacute combined degeneration* consists of changes in both the dorsal and lateral spinal cord; symptoms include symmetric paresthesias, loss of proprioception, and ataxia. Cerebral function can be disturbed and may include what has been termed "megaloblastic madness." These neurologic syndromes occur not only as a late manifestation of vitamin B_{12} deficiency with severe megaloblastic anemia, but also with vitamin B_{12} deficiency in the absence of anemia. The course of the anemia and the neurologic decompensation are generally independent of one another.

Once the diagnosis of vitamin B_{12} deficiency is made, the cause of the deficiency can usually be ascertained from a clinical history and from the results of provocative testing for achlorhydria. A Schilling test can also be helpful: A test dose of vitamin B_{12} is administered, and intestinal absorption is measured with and without exogenous intrinsic factor. In pernicious anemia and severe ileal disease, a test dose of vitamin B_{12} alone will not be absorbed. Intrinsic factor corrects the malabsorption of pernicious anemia, but does not help the patient with ileal disease. A large test dose of vitamin B_{12} may be absorbed in patients with bacterial overgrowth syndromes, since the deficiency is probably the result of competition for available oral supplies of the vitamin.

Megaloblastic anemia responds dramatically to intramuscular injections of vitamin B_{12}. Blood and bone marrow abnormalities rapidly resolve. A reticulocytosis begins after 72 hours, the serum uric acid rises, and hypokalemia may develop as the new blood cells incorporate potassium. Large doses of folate may transiently improve or even correct the anemia, but folate does not prevent the progression of neurologic symptoms and may even accelerate them. Replacement therapy is generally started on a daily basis, and is gradually decreased to monthly intervals once the hematocrit returns to normal. Neurologic deficits caused by subacute combined degeneration probably are not reversed by subsequent vitamin B_{12} administration.

Folate Deficiency. Folate deficiency can also cause megaloblastic anemia, and the peripheral blood film can appear identical with anemia caused by vitamin B_{12} deficiency. Only vitamin B_{12} deficiency, however, causes the neurologic syndrome described above.

Folate deficiency can be caused by poor folate absorption in the presence of phenytoin or other drugs or by one of the malabsorption syndromes, but it is much more commonly the result of inadequate dietary intake. The most frequently seen patient with folate-deficient macrocytic anemia is the alcoholic. In the alcoholic, poor diet and the inability of the marrow to make use of folate combine to produce the anemia.

The distinction between megaloblastic anemia caused by folate deficiency and that caused by vitamin B_{12} deficiency is made in the laboratory. Serum folate levels generally reveal the deficiency, although the results can be confused by recent transfusions. In addition, many broad-spectrum antibiotics interfere with the bioassay for folate.

The anemia in an alcoholic patient may rapidly resolve upon admission to the hospital, when alcohol intake is halted and the patient begins to eat folate-rich hospital food. The anemia of folate deficiency is completely curable by oral replacement therapy.

Most anemias are not macrocytic. If a blood film presents an obvious microcytic hypochromic anemia, iron deficiency is the likely diagnosis. Other possibilities include thalassemia and certain cases of secondary anemia. A normochromic normocytic anemia can be caused by early iron deficiency, secondary anemia, and marrow aplasia or replacement.

Microcytic Hypochromic Anemias

Iron Deficiency. Iron deficiency is the most common cause of anemia, and is the result of blood loss combined with inadequate dietary iron replacement. Iron deficiency occurs most commonly in menstruating females. When iron deficiency occurs in males or nonmenstruating females, the most likely site of blood loss is the gastrointestinal tract, and the specific site and cause must be sought.

The diagnosis of iron deficiency is suggested by a microcytic hypochromic anemia on blood film (Fig. 45–3), a low or normal reticulocyte count, and a ratio of serum iron to total serum iron binding capacity (transferrin saturation) of less than 15%. The latter test, however, can be complicated by diurnal variations, the effects of underlying illness, and a whole host of drugs. The serum ferritin can be a helpful measure of total body iron stores, and is diminished in iron deficiency.

The constellation of noninvasive laboratory findings yielding a presumptive diagnosis of iron deficiency occurs only in moderate to advanced cases. Early in the course of iron deficiency, the anemia may be normochromic and normocytic. In a significant number of unexplained anemias, the bone marrow reveals iron deficiency despite the absence of peripheral blood findings suggesting the diagnosis. The bone marrow can therefore give a definitive answer. The marrow is stained to reveal iron; if the anemia is due to iron deficiency, iron stores are absent or markedly decreased.

Many clinicians begin a trial of oral iron therapy without a bone marrow diagnosis. This is appropriate in some situations, but the rapid and unambiguous results of a bone marrow examination favor the definitive approach, particularly when the diagnosis is in

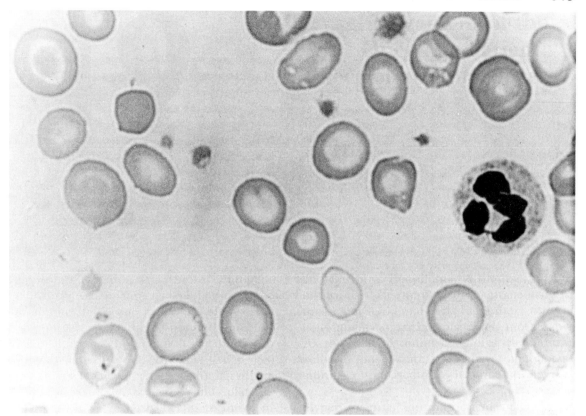

FIG. 45–3. Iron deficiency anemia. The most obvious characteristic of these erythrocytes is the hypochromia, with many of the red cells possessing only a thin rim of hemoglobin. The red cells are also small. Occasional "target cells" with a pigmented area within the central pallor (upper left) are seen. Generally, the erythrocytes have a varied and, at times, bizarre morphology.

any way uncertain and when significant future decisions (*e.g.*, intensive study of the gastrointestinal tract) are being made on the basis of the finding of iron deficiency.

A presumptive diagnosis of iron deficiency is sufficient to begin a trial of oral iron therapy in a menstruating woman who presents with microcytic hypochromic indices, a low reticulocyte count, a low transferrin saturation, and guaiac-negative stools. A menstrual source of blood loss can then safely be assumed. The earliest response to oral iron therapy is a reticulocytosis occuring within ten days, and this response confirms the diagnosis.

In a man or in a nonmenstruating woman in whom the source of blood loss is not clear, the situation is more complicated. If the patient's stool is guaiac-positive, it is reasonable to assume that the anemia is due to iron deficiency, and a search for the site of bleeding should be undertaken. If no blood loss is detected, despite laboratory findings compatible with iron deficiency, a bone marrow examination must be performed. The patient may or may not have a history suggesting a potential bleeding source (*e.g.*, alcohol abuse, the heavy use of aspirin, or peptic ulcer disease). In any case, an exhaustive search for a bleeding site is indicated if the bone marrow reveals a decrease in stainable iron stores.

The treatment of iron-deficiency anemia is oral iron replacement. Oral ferrous sulfate is inexpensive and well-absorbed. The majority of patients respond to oral iron therapy, but intramuscular or intravenous iron may sometimes be employed. Some patients receiving parenteral iron therapy experience severe allergic reactions, and all patients receiving parenteral iron should be carefully monitored.

Thalassemia. Thalassemia refers to any of several genetic defects in hemoglobin production. Patients may have deficient production of the hemoglobin β chain (β-thalassemia), α chain (α-thalassemia), δ chain (δ-thalassemia), and so on. Thalassemia minor is the clinical manifestation of patients who are heterozygous for a thalassemia gene. Thalassemia major is a severe disease occurring in patients who are homozygous for a thalassemia gene. It culminates in death *in utero* (α-thalassemia major), in childhood, or in early adulthood (β-thalassemia major).

The most common type of thalassemia is β-thalassemia minor. People with this disease have normal life expectancies. Depending upon the population under study, β-thalassemia minor may be second only to iron deficiency as the leading cause of microcytic hypochromic anemia. The population most at risk are people from the Mediterranean regions of the Middle East, Southern Europe, and Africa. Although the total red cell count is rarely elevated in iron deficiency, counts above 5.5 million red blood cells per milliliter are common in β-thalassemia minor. Also in contrast to iron deficiency, there is often a mild reticulocytosis. β-thalassemia minor is usually first suspected when a microcytic, hypochromic anemia fails to respond to oral iron therapy. Hemoglobin electrophoresis identifies thalassemia minor, revealing an elevated percentage of hemoglobin A_2. A bone marrow examination and staining for iron stores will resolve the differential. If β-thalassemia minor alone is the cause of the anemia, iron stores will be normal.

Other Causes. Other causes of microcytic hypochromic anemia include lead poisoning, sideroblastic anemia, and severe secondary anemia.

Normochromic Normocytic Anemias

Secondary Anemia. Secondary anemia, or the anemia of chronic disease, accompanies a variety of clinical states, many of which involve chronic inflammation. Chronic disease is the most common cause of normochromic normocytic anemias. The anemia is generally mild and only rarely is the hematocrit below 30. Occasionally, however, secondary anemia can mimic iron deficiency on the peripheral blood film. The transferrin saturation may then help to make the distinction: the transferrin saturation in iron deficiency is generally less than 15%, whereas in secondary anemia it is usually greater than 20%. In secondary anemia, the iron stores are normal or even increased.

Chronic inflammatory states such as tuberculosis, malignancies, and rheumatologic disorders can cause secondary anemia. Again, iron deficiency may also be present due to gastrointestinal blood loss. In rheumatoid arthritis, for example, 30% of patients are iron-deficient, probably due to chronic gastritis from the use of antiinflammatory agents.

Uremia is almost always associated with anemia, but the extent of anemia may be poorly correlated with the extent of renal impairment. The anemia is believed to be due to (1) the failure of the kidney to produce erythropoietin (a hormone that stimulates red blood cell production), and (2) the presence of toxins that suppress the marrow and shorten the life span of circulating erythrocytes. Patients with uremia also frequently have blood loss due to coagulation disorders or to uremic effects on the gastrointestinal tract. Thus, iron deficiency should always be considered as a possible contribution to anemia in renal failure. A severe hypoproliferative anemia in patients with uremia may therefore require a bone marrow examination to establish whether oral iron therapy will be sufficient therapy. Androgenic steroids will raise the hematocrit in many patients, but the side-effects, particularly in women, should be measured against the severity of the anemia. Hemodialysis generally improves the anemia, and transplantation may cure it.

Marrow Aplasia. Marrow aplasia is a far less common cause of normochromic normocytic anemia. Generally, marrow aplasia presents as pancytopenia, thereby immediately indicating total marrow failure. A bone marrow aspirate will be "dry" (no marrow is obtained), and a marrow biopsy will reveal hypocellularity and fatty replacement. *Pure red cell aplasia* is a rare disorder in which only the marrow erythroid forms are diminished. In both marrow aplasia and pure red cell aplasia, the serum iron is elevated and the transferrin saturation is high. The marrow reveals adequate or increased iron stores. Approximately one-half of all cases of marrow aplasia are traceable to marrow toxic drugs. Chloramphenicol is the most common offending agent, and the marrow aspirate reveals characteristic vacuolization of the marrow cells. Chemical exposure has also been implicated, and the list of probable offenders includes benzene, insecticides, and toluene. Viral hepatitis may also precede marrow aplasia. Infiltrative diseases of the bone marrow, including myelofibrosis and leukemia, can produce a picture of marrow failure.

The high transferrin saturation in many cases of marrow aplasia is of some clinical interest. On the assumption that a rise in transferrin saturation is an early sign of marrow toxicity, it has been proposed that the transferrin saturation be used as a sensitive screen for the development of drug-induced aplasia.

Whenever marrow aplasia is suspected, a bone marrow examination should be performed to determine whether there is infiltration of the marrow, as well as to assess the extent of precursor failure. Any potentially offending drug or chemical must be immediately stopped. The likelihood and rapidity of marrow recovery after toxic insult varies from patient to patient, and ranges from rapid and full recovery to no recovery at all.

ANEMIAS OF RED BLOOD CELL DESTRUCTION

An elevated reticulocyte count in a patient with anemia who has not experienced any acute blood loss implies peripheral red blood cell destruction. The elevated reticulocyte index indicates that the marrow is working normally and is attempting to compensate for the loss of red blood cells. There are four major causes of destructive anemias: (1) immune hemolysis, (2) mechanical hemolysis, (3) sickle cell anemia, and (4) glucose-6-phosphate dehydrogenase deficiency.

Immune Hemolysis

Etiology. Immune hemolysis is generally caused by warm-reacting (maximal reactivity above 31°C) IgG anti-red blood cell antibodies. In 20% to 30% of patients, immune hemolysis is not associated with underlying disease, and the disorder is termed idiopathic. Another 30% of cases occur in the setting of drug use. The drugs most commonly implicated in immune hemolytic anemia are quinidine, the sulfonamides, methyldopa, penicillin, and the cephalosporins.

The Coombs' test is the most common laboratory test for immune hemolysis. The direct Coombs' test can establish the presence of bound immunoglobulin or complement on a patient's erythrocytes by demonstrating agglutination of the erythrocytes with either anti-immunoglobulin or anticomplement antibody.

Recent work has elucidated some of the immunologic mechanisms that may account for drug-induced hemolytic anemia.

1. Penicillin attaches to the red cell membrane and serves as a hapten against which antibodies can be directed. Significant hemolysis is usually seen only when high doses of penicillin are given. In penicillin-induced immune hemolysis the patient's red blood cells are strongly positive in a direct Coombs' test.

2. Quinidine and many other drugs stimulate the production of antibodies, and drug-antibody complexes can nonspecifically attach to the surface of the red cell. This is the most common mechanism of drug-induced hemolytic anemia. The immune complexes can activate the complement pathway leading to acute hemolysis, and occasionally hemolysis may be so severe that it may cause renal failure. The antibody-drug complex can migrate from cell to cell, and hemolysis can therefore occur with low drug doses. The red blood cells show a positive direct Coomb's test to anti-complement antibodies.

3. Other mechanisms are more speculative. Methyldopa, for example, may alter red blood cell antigens so that they become immunogenic to the host.

Regardless of the specific mechanism of hemolysis and regardless of the specific drug, the anemia tends to remit when the drug is removed.

A large number of people with chronic lymphocytic leukemia or other lymphoproliferative diseases develop warm hemolysis during the course of their disease. An underlying lymphoproliferative disease should be suspected in any patient in whom warm-reacting autoimmune hemolytic anemia develops.

Certain infections are associated with immune hemolysis. These include mycoplasmal infections, infectious mononucleosis, and other viral illnesses.

Clinical Manifestations. The presentation of patients with immune hemolysis depends upon the acuteness and severity of the anemia. Patients with fulminant cases present with jaundice, pallor, and cardiopulmonary collapse. Other patients may be asymptomatic, and their illness is only noted incidentally during an evaluation for anemia, or because of the inability to find a compatible cross-match for transfusion. Hepatosplenomegaly occurs in one-third to one-half of patients. Thrombophlebitis is also frequently encountered.

A peripheral blood film classically reveals spherocytes. Spherocytosis is presumably the result of the ability of IgG molecules to opsonize the red blood cells, resulting in partial phagocytosis by the reticuloendothelial system. Progressive loss of the erythrocyte membrane renders the cell more rigid and it assumes a spherical shape. A direct Coombs' test will reveal either immunoglobulin, complement, or both on the patient's red blood cells.

Therapy. A patient with immune hemolysis should discontinue all drugs, and a thorough search for lymphoproliferative disorders should be carried out. Corticosteroids are usually successful in controlling the hemolysis. However, the evaluation of corticosteroid therapy (and all other drug therapy) is complicated by the episodic, relapsing course of the disease. Other immunosuppressants are often used in conjunction with steroids in

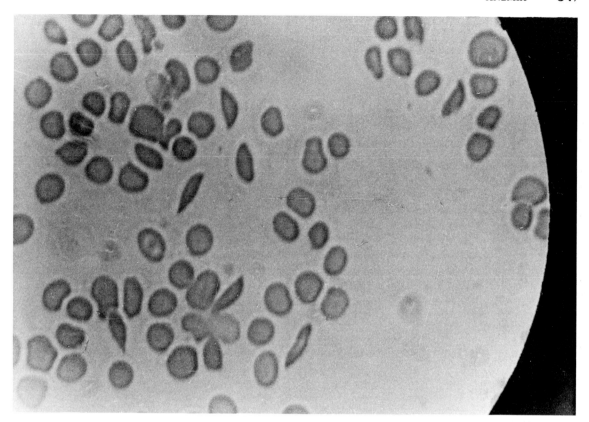

FIG. 45–4. Peripheral blood film from a patient with sickle cell anemia illustrating the numerous banana-shaped sickle cells.

order to lower the corticosteroid dosage. Splenectomy may be of benefit if drug therapy fails.

Mechanical Hemolysis

Mechanical hemolysis is most often caused by prosthetic heart valves. Disseminated intravascular coagulation, thrombotic thrombocytopenic purpura, and malignant hypertension can also cause anemia and produce the characteristic picture of mechanical hemolysis. The blood film is distinctive, re-

vealing schistocytes and other red cell fragments.

Sickle Cell Anemia

Sickle cell anemia is a genetic disease caused by the substitution of a valine for a glutamine in the sixth position of the β-hemoglobin chain. The altered hemoglobin, called hemoglobin S, has a strong tendency to form long crystalline aggregates when deoxygenated, and these crystalline structures distort the red blood cell into the typical sickle shape. A blood film of a patient with sickle cell anemia reveals elongated cells and target cells (Fig. 45–4), but the characteristic sickle cells may not be apparent unless the blood sample is first deoxygenated (e.g., with sodium metabisulfite).

Heterozygous persons are said to have *sickle cell trait*, and only very rarely experience any of the symptomatology of sickle cell anemia. Their red blood cells can be demonstrated to sickle when deoxygenated, but the concentration of hemoglobin S in their cells is sufficiently low that sickling does not occur at the oxygen tensions normally encountered in the body's vascular system.

The diagnosis of an adult with homozygous *sickle cell disease* is rarely difficult, since in most cases the disease will have been documented and followed for years before the patient leaves the pediatric age group. Sickle cell disease is far more common in blacks than in whites. It has been suggested that the geographic distribution of the hemoglobin S gene reflects the protection that it affords against malarial infection.

Patients with sickle cell disease experience a variety of chronic and acute problems. The patient's course reflects the chronic consequences of tissue infarction punctuated by acute, recurrent symptomatic periods referred to as sickle cell crises (see discussion below). Life expectancy is significantly reduced in these patients, who most often die before the age of forty.

Chronic anemia results in fatigue, but it is remarkable how well these patients adapt to even severe levels of anemia. They develop hyperdynamic circulations and almost always possess cardiac flow murmurs.

Most of the problems confronting these patients are not from the anemia *per se*, but rather from vascular sludging and thrombosis, which produce gradual but widespread tissue infarction, probably as a direct result of intravascular sickling.

Chronic Problems. Leg ulcers, especially around the ankles and anterior tibial regions, may be sites of infection. The chances for healing are increased if transfusions are given to maintain the hemoglobin level between 9 and 10 g/dl. Skin grafts may be required.

Chronic hematuria and hyposthenuria often occur, but these pose few problems for the patient. (These may also occur in patients with sickle cell trait.) Vascular sludging may be particularly marked in the kidney, where infarction and tissue necrosis may occur. The renal medulla is a region of low oxygen tension, and it is particularly susceptible to damage. Renal papillary necrosis with urinary obstruction may present as an acute, painful renal crisis with unilateral renal shutdown, hematuria, and chills.

The spleen is also a region of low oxygen tension and vascular stasis, and it is especially susceptible to intravascular sickling. Functional asplenism from repeated infarction contributes to the greatly increased susceptibility to infection.

There is an increased incidence of gallstones in patients with sickle cell disease, presumably due to the bilirubin released by hemolysis, and these may provide a source of sepsis. Many feel that the finding of gallstones in a patient with sickle cell disease should prompt elective cholecystectomy, often with an accompanying appendectomy. Surgery removes a possible source of sepsis and simplifies the differential diagnosis of an acute abdominal crisis.

There is an increased incidence of aseptic necrosis of the femoral heads seen in patients with sickle cell anemia, believed to be secondary to bone infarcts. When aseptic necrosis is far advanced, orthopedic advice must be sought and the possibility of total hip replacement must be considered.

Patients with sickle cell disease are also predisposed to develop osteomyelitis. Salmonella is frequently implicated, and its prevalence is believed to be due to a failure of the patient's immune system to opsonize the organism. The poor blood supply, vascular sludging, and (possibly) the presence of infarcts in the bone are felt to contribute to the predisposition to bone infection.

Sickle Cell Crisis. An acute painful attack, often with fever, is the most common type of sickle cell crisis. Among patients with sickle cell disease, it is the most frequent cause for hospital admission. The pain is usually located in the back and joints, and may migrate. Abdominal pain may accompany these other complaints, or the patient may present solely with a localized abdominal crisis. The abdominal pain can be severe and may simulate an acute surgical abdomen. Fever and decreased intake of food, along with the chronic defects in renal concentrating mechanisms may lead to dehydration.

Fever, leukocytosis, and acute debility always raise the question of infection, especially in sickle cell patients who are particularly susceptible to infection. However, most sickle cell crises do not involve infection, and the instinctive use of antibiotics for all crises is therefore not indicated. Blood cultures should be obtained, the urine examined for leukocytes and bacteria, and chest x-rays obtained. If any of these studies reveals evidence of infection, treatment should be instituted. In a patient whose illness is so severe that sepsis appears likely, cultures should be obtained and presumptive broad-spectrum antibiotic therapy begun.

In general, therapy for sickle cell crisis is symptomatic. Most painful crises begin to abate after several days. Narcotic analgesia must be provided for pain relief. Because narcotics are so often required, patients frequently become addicted.

Many precipitants have been associated with sickle cell crises, including cold, hypoxia, and acidosis. Any abnormalities of pH or oxygenation should be corrected during the crisis. However, the use of supplemental oxygen when no hypoxia is present does not seem to influence the course or severity of the crisis.

Pulmonary infarction, believed to be caused by clumps of sickled cells occluding the pulmonary vasculature, is a common problem and can produce acute symptomatology. The chest x-ray may reveal an infiltrate. Many of these infiltrates prove to be pneumonia (usually pneumococcal) and it is therefore proper to administer antibiotics to patients with pulmonary infiltrates while appropriate studies are obtained.

A different type of sickle cell crisis, less common than the one described above, is the hematologic, aplastic crisis. It is frequently precipitated by infection. Although usually short-lived (a few weeks), it can persist for much longer. The reticulocyte count should be closely monitored. Transfusions should be given until the marrow recovers.

Rarely, a third type of crisis may occur, characterized by hyperhemolysis.

Many therapeutic regimens have been tried in the past several years in an attempt to decrease the likelihood of the hemoglobin to sickle. However, these regimens have proven to be either ineffective or too risky. At present, only supportive therapy is available.

SC Disease. Some patients may present with a mild form of sickle cell disease, and many eventually are proven to have SC disease. These patients possess one gene for the β chain of hemoglobin of sickle cell disease, and one gene in which the normal glutamic acid at the 6th position of the β chain has been replaced by lysine. The latter is called the β^c gene.

Patients with SC disease share some of the clinical features of sickle cell disease, but pursue a less tragic course and have only a mild anemia (if any). The most common symptoms are episodic periods of pain in the abdomen, chest, bones, and joints. Chest symptoms of pain, cough, and fever are also common, and probably are caused by small pulmonary infarctions. The majority of patients have splenomegaly, unlike patients with sickle cell disease.

The diagnosis of SC disease should be considered in any black patient with the above symptoms or with symptoms suggestive of sickle cell disease, but without anemia and red blood cell sickling. The diagnosis can be confirmed by hemoglobin electrophoresis. Patients with SC disease have normal life expectancies.

Glucose-6-Phosphate Dehydrogenase Deficiency (G6PD)

The enzyme glucose-6-phosphate dehydrogenase is largely responsible for protecting the red blood cell from oxidative damage by maintaining intracellular levels of the reducing agent, NADPH. In patients with glucose-6-phosphate dehydrogenase deficiency, the red blood cells are unable to deal with oxidative stresses, and hemolysis can result. G6PD deficiency is extremely common and occurs in over 10% of black American males. Their abnormal enzyme is termed A-form, and it can be detected on serum electrophoresis. The most common type of G6PD in white populations is called Mediterranean type and is most often seen in Mediterranean and Middle Eastern peoples. Their abnormal enzyme is referred to as B-form.

Hemolysis is usually sudden and episodic. The degree of hemolysis is dependent upon the level of the oxidative stress, the type of enzyme abnormality, and the patient. The type A variety is generally milder and self-limited, whereas the Mediterranean type can be acutely fatal. The A-form is self-limiting because only the older red blood cells have significantly abnormal enzyme activity; as these cells lyse, the younger red cells that replace them are more resistant to oxidative hemolysis. Because abnormal enzyme levels are only detectable in older red cells, a quantitative test during or soon after a hemolytic episode may be normal due to the preponderance of young erythrocytes.

Heinz bodies (small densities in erythrocytes that probably represent denatured hemoglobin) can be seen before the onset and early in the course of hemolysis, but later there is nothing on the peripheral blood film that suggests G6PD.

Drugs are the most common initiators of hemolysis in these patients, typically producing hemolysis 24 hours following ingestion. Previous sensitization to the drug is not required. The sulfonamides are most frequently implicated. *Febrile illnesses* of almost any sort will also induce hemolysis. Hemolysis is then usually mild, but the absence of reticulocytosis in the presence of infection can exacerbate the red blood cell deficit. *Fava bean ingestion* can cause severe red cell breakdown in patients who are deficient in the enzyme, generally 24 to 48 hours after ingestion. The severity of hemolysis may demand aggressive transfusion therapy.

BIBLIOGRAPHY

Bainton DF, Finch CA: The diagnosis of iron deficiency anemia. Am J Med 37:62–70, 1964

Barrett-Connor E: Anemia and infection. Am J Med 52:242–253, 1972

Carmel R: The laboratory diagnosis of megaloblastic anemias. West J Med 128:294–304, 1978

Castle WB: Current concepts of pernicious anemia. Am J Med 48:541–548, 1970

Clegg JB, Weatherall DJ: Molecular basis of thalassemia. Br Med Bull 32:262–269, 1976

Dacie JV: Autoimmune hemolytic anemia. Arch Intern Med 135:1293–1300, 1975

Dean J, Schechter AN: Sickle-cell anemia: Molecular and cellular bases of therapeutic approaches.

N Engl J Med 299:752–763, 804–811, 863–870, 1978

Frank MM, Schreiber AD, Atkinson JP, et al: Pathophysiology of immune hemolytic anemia. Ann Intern Med 87:210–220, 1977

Garratty G, Petz LD: Drug-induced hemolytic anemia. Am J Med 58:398–407, 1975

Konotey-Ahulu FI: The sickle cell diseases. Arch Intern Med 133:611–619, 1974

Modell B: Management of thalassaemia major. Br Med Bull 32:270–276, 1976

Sears DA: The morbidity of sickle cell trait: A review of the literature. Am J Med 64:1021–1036, 1978

Sullivan LW: Differential diagnosis and management of the patient with megaloblastic anemia. Am J Med 48:609–617, 1970

46

Abnormalities of Hemostasis

Hemostatic defects are due to abnormalities of either platelets or coagulation factors. Bleeding that is due to a platelet disorder usually involves superficial small vessels and produces petechiae in the skin and mucous membranes. Coagulation defects are associated with more prominent bleeding in deep tissues; atraumatic hemarthroses, for example, are characteristic of severe coagulation abnormalities.

Virtually all bleeding disorders can be diagnosed with a few simple laboratory tests:

The *bleeding time* measures how long it takes a standardized skin incision to stop bleeding. The bleeding time is prolonged in all platelet abnormalities, but is normal in coagulation disorders.

The *prothrombin time* (PT) and *partial thromboplastin time* (PTT) detect almost all coagulation disorders. The coagulation cascade and the various tests used to screen for coagulation disorders are depicted in Figures 46–1 and 46–2.

The coagulation cascade is a complex series of biochemical reactions that ultimately leads to the formation of a fibrin clot. Each reaction generates an active product that in turn activates the next coagulation factor in the cascade, etc. All of the coagulation factors are

proteins, and most exist in an inactive form in the plasma. They are designated by Roman numerals according to the order of their discovery.

The final step in the cascade is the conversion of fibrinogen to fibrin, a reaction mediated by the protein, thrombin. Thrombin must itself be generated from prothrombin, and this conversion is mediated by activated Factor X (Xa). Activated Factor X can be generated by means of two pathways:

1. The *intrinsic pathway* is a true cascade initiated by the exposure of Factor XII to any of a variety of surface agents (e.g., collagen).

2. The *extrinsic pathway* involves only Factor VII. Factor VII complexes with calcium and a tissue factor and is then capable of activating Factor X.

The partial thromboplastin time measures the ability to form a fibrin clot by the intrinsic pathway. It therefore tests for all factors except Factor VII.

The prothrombin time measures the ability to form a fibrin clot by the extrinsic pathway. It is performed by measuring the time it takes to form a clot when calcium and a tissue extract are added to plasma. A normal prothrombin time indicates normal levels of Factor VII and those factors common to both the

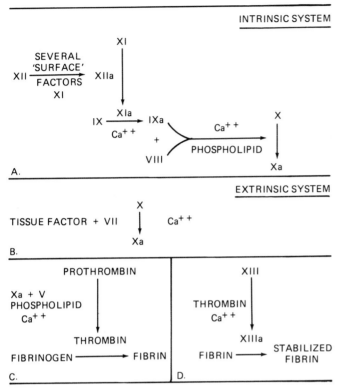

FIG. 46–1. The coagulation cascade. (*A*) The intrinsic system. (*B*) The extrinsic system. (*C*) The conversion of fibrinogen to fibrin. (*D*) The conversion of fibrin to stabilized fibrin.

intrinsic and extrinsic pathways (V, X, II, and fibrinogen).

PLATELET DISORDERS

Bleeding can result from thrombocytopenia or abnormal platelet function. The former is a much more common cause of significant bleeding.

The normal platelet count is approximately 250,000 per microliter of blood. Bleeding due to thrombocytopenia usually does not occur until the platelet count falls below 15,000 to 20,000. Thrombocytopenia of such severity

should be suggested by the scarcity of platelets on a peripheral blood film. An examination of the blood film should therefore be the initial screen for a platelet disorder. A peripheral platelet count should also be obtained.

If the platelet count is normal and if the prothrombin and partial thromboplastin times are normal, a bleeding time should then be performed. If the bleeding time is prolonged in a patient with a normal platelet count, an abnormality of platelet function must be considered. Several aspects of platelet function can be tested in the laboratory, including:

1. platelet adhesiveness—the ability of platelets to adhere to a foreign surface, and

2. platelet aggregation—the ability of several substances, including ADP, epinephrine, and collagen, to induce platelet aggregation.

The most common causes of thrombocy-

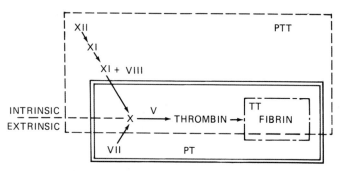

FIG. 46–2. Highly simplified scheme of the coagulation pathways. Shown are the factors involved in the intrinsic (top) and extrinsic (bottom) pathways. Also depicted by boxes are those aspects of the coagulation system tested by the three most common laboratory tests: (1) thrombin time (TT), (2) partial thromboplastin time (PTT), and (3) prothrombin time (PT).

topenia are (1) drug-induced thrombocytopenia and (2) immune thrombocytopenic purpura (ITP).

Drug-induced Thrombocytopenia. Drugs can cause thrombocytopenia either through marrow toxicity or platelet destruction.

Alcohol and the *thiazide* diuretics are the most common drugs implicated in suppressing the production of the megakaryocyte (platelet precursor) population in the bone marrow. In the alcoholic, folate deficiency and hypersplenism can also lead to thrombocytopenia. Thrombocytopenia is usually mild and chronic and only rarely results in bleeding. Platelet counts return to normal one to two weeks after alcohol ingestion ceases. The thiazides also produce a mild, chronic thrombocytopenia that resolves after discontinuation of the drug.

Peripheral platelet destruction, when drug-related, is usually due to an immunologic mechanism. Many drugs have been implicated, but the most common and best documented are *quinidine* and *quinine*. Others include heparin, gold, para-aminosalicylic acid, methyldopa, and the sulfonamides. Thrombocytopenia is typically sudden and severe and often results in bleeding. Patients with this condition should be admitted to the hospital, all drug therapy should be halted, and trauma must be scrupulously avoided. Corticosteroids are usually prescribed but their value has not been proven. Platelet transfusions fail to raise the platelet count. Fortunately, recovery is rapid and platelet counts return to normal within 7 to 10 days. Gold-induced thromobocytopenia, however, may last for months, probably because of the persistence of gold within the body. The use of BAL (dimercaprol), a chelating agent, is recommended to hasten the excretion of gold.

Immune Thrombocytopenic Purpura (ITP). ITP is a common disorder, and antiplatelet antibodies have recently been implicated in the massive peripheral platelet destruction that occurs in this illness.

Acute ITP can be seen in any age group, but it is predominantly a pediatric disease. The onset of bleeding is often acute, and the patient frequently remembers the moment of onset. The patient presents with petechiae and purpura that may be dramatic, but he is otherwise well. An enlarged liver and spleen can be palpated in only a small percentage of patients.

With the exception of marked thrombocytopenia, the laboratory findings are normal.

A bone marrow examination reveals normal-to-increased numbers of megakaryocytes. These are typically described as having a smooth contour.

When acute purpura and thrombocytopenia are present, the major diagnoses to consider are acute ITP and sepsis, notably meningococcemia. Patients with ITP have no symptoms of systemic illness and bear none of the other stigmata of sepsis.

Acute ITP is generally benign. The few fatalities are believed to be the result of intracerebral bleeding. Corticosteroids are standard therapy for a patient with acute ITP and are instituted from the time that the diagnosis is made. However, most studies have shown that approximately 80% of patients recover within six months whether or not therapy is instituted. Those who fail to recover may undergo splenectomy, which is usually effective. More recently, the immunosuppressive agents azathioprine and vincristine have proven successful in refractory cases. Platelet transfusion does not elevate the platelet count, presumably because of the presence of antiplatelet antibodies.

Chronic ITP is seen predominantly in adult females. The disease is characterized by an insidious onset, less severe bleeding problems than are seen with acute ITP, and a low rate of spontaneous remission. Chronic ITP is also associated with antiplatelet antibodies, and it is likely that acute and chronic ITP are manifestations of the same disorder presenting in different population groups.

Chronic ITP is also treated with steroids, splenectomy, and immunosuppression. It is frequently associated with an underlying illness, notably chronic lymphocytic leukemia (Chap. 47), and may be an early manifestation of lymphoma, systemic lupus erythematosus, sarcoidosis, and tuberculosis.

Thrombotic Thrombocytopenic Purpura (TTP). This is an uncommon syndrome seen mostly in young to middle-aged women. It is characterized by a clinical pentad of: (1) thrombocytopenic purpura, (2) anemia, (3) fluctuating neurologic signs, (4) renal deterioration, and (5) fever. Its cause is unknown. The anemia is a microangiopathic hemolytic anemia, and the finding of elevated fibrin split products suggests the presence of disseminated intravascular coagulation. Widespread arteriolar occlusion may be responsible for the renal dysfunction, the frequent occurence of abdominal pain, and for the neurologic signs and symptoms, which include headache, seizures, acute psychosis, and coma. The neurologic symptoms are notable for their rapid and often dramatic fluctuations. Hemorrhagic complications include skin purpura and gastrointestinal and genitourinary bleeding. TTP generally pursues an aggressive course terminating in death. A variety of treatment regimens have been reported, but none can be advocated as being of proven benefit.

Bone Marrow Failure. Patients with bone marrow failure develop thrombocytopenia with bleeding. Leukemia is frequently responsible, but other causes include aplastic anemia (Chap. 45), myelofibrosis, and drugs that are toxic to the bone marrow. The patient's history and an examination of a peripheral blood film and bone marrow aspirate or biopsy usually reveal the diagnosis. Other causes of thrombocytopenia include vitamin B-12 or folate deficiency and paroxysmal nocturnal hemoglobinuria.

COAGULATION DISORDERS

If a disorder of hemostasis is suspected and the platelet count is normal, the coagulation pathways should be investigated. A clinical sign that suggests a coagulation disorder is deep tissue bleeding in the absence of skin and mucous membrane petechiae.

Acquired Coagulation Disorders

Vitamin K deficiency is the most common of the acquired coagulation disorders. Factors II, (prothrombin), VII, IX, and X are made in the liver and require vitamin K for synthesis of their active forms. Specifically, vitamin K is a co-factor for an essential post-translational modification of these factors. Factor VII has the shortest half-life among the coagulation factors (3 to 5 hours), and thus a prolonged prothrombin time is the first laboratory evidence of vitamin K deficiency. Vitamin K deficiency can be caused by oral anticoagulants or intestinal malabsorption. Liver failure and other less common diseases can cause a deficiency of the vitamin K-dependent coagulation factors.

Oral Anticoagulants. Coumarin anticoagulants competitively inhibit the action of vitamin K and can cause bleeding through accidental or intentional overdose. These drugs are bound to albumin and metabolized in the liver. An accidental overdose can occur with simultaneous ingestion of agents that displace coumarin from albumin, thereby increasing the amount of free drug.

Patients taking the coumarin drugs who experience bleeding have a prolonged prothrombin time and partial thromboplastin time. Vitamin K returns these coagulation parameters to normal within 6 to 14 hours. The drawback of administering vitamin K is that the patient must be restarted on anticoagulants, and it may take several days to return the patient to a therapeutic level of anticoagulation. If bleeding is severe, replacement transfusions containing the missing factors (such as fresh frozen plasma) are necessary (See Chap. 44).

Malabsorption. Vitamin K is fat-soluble and requires bile acids for complete absorption. Any interruption of the normal cycle of bile acid synthesis, release, and re-uptake can lead to a deficiency of vitamin K and a bleeding disorder (see Chap. 35).

Because intestinal bacteria can synthesize vitamin K, a diet deficient in the vitamin rarely produces vitamin K deficiency unless the intestine has been sterilized with antibiotics.

Parenteral vitamin K is curative, and a therapeutic response should ideally permit one to distinguish these patients from those with an acquired coagulation disorder due to liver failure.

Liver Disease. When liver failure is responsible for deficiencies of the vitamin K-dependent coagulation factors, the liver disease is usually severe and the prognosis is grim. Patients with liver failure are usually hypoalbuminemic, and may have thrombocytopenia as a result of the hypersplenism that accompanies the portal hypertension. Parenteral vitamin K is not helpful, since the defect is not one of vitamin K deficiency but rather of the inability of the liver to synthesize the vitamin K-dependent coagulation factors.

Other Causes. Only rarely is a circulating anticoagulant responsible for an acquired coagulopathy. Up to 15% of patients with systemic lupus erythematosus acquire a circulating anticoagulant, usually directed against Factor VIII, but overt bleeding is rare. Patients with other autoimmune diseases and patients receiving transfusion therapy for hemophilia A may also develop a circulating anticoagulant.

Inherited Coagulation Disorders

Most inherited disorders of coagulation are very rare. A major exception is *hemophilia A*, which affects more than 10,000 people in the United States. Hemophilia A is acquired as a sex-linked recessive trait. It results in a deficiency of Factor VIII that, in some patients, is due to a complete failure to produce Factor VIII, and, in others, to production of an altered, nonfunctional Factor VIII.

The clinical severity of hemophilia A correlates inversely with the amount of normal Factor VIII activity in the circulation. Patients with mild hemophilia have up to 30% of normal Factor VIII activity. These patients experience abnormal bleeding only when exposed to a hemostatic stress, such as dental extraction or surgery. Bleeding after dental extraction is such a reliable hallmark of hemophilia that its absence by history generally rules out the diagnosis.

Patients with moderate to severe deficiencies in Factor VIII experience a variety of problems directly related to deep tissue bleeding, usually subcutaneous or intramuscular hemorrhages. These can be quite large with significant intravascular blood loss, and are often painful. Intramuscular bleeding may lead to serious contracture deformities. Hemarthrosis is also common and frequently involves the knee, although any large joint can be affected. Hemophiliacs most often enter the hospital because of hemarthrosis. Although episodes of hemarthrosis are frequently preceded by trauma or exercise, they often occur spontaneously. Hemarthrosis can produce an extremely painful, tender, and swollen joint, and repeated hemarthroses can destroy the affected joints. Destruction may extend to the adjoining bone with cystic subchondral changes and marked osteoporosis. Careful rehabilitative therapy and management can markedly reduce joint destruction.

Neurologic problems are common in patients with coagulation disorders. They usually result from the compression of peripheral nerves by local muscular hemorrhage and cause severe pain and sensory and motor deficits, and may eventually lead to muscle atrophy. These compression syndromes usually resolve spontaneously. Intracranial bleeding, however, is more serious, and frequently follows trauma. Intracerebral bleeding is often fatal. Any person with significant hemophilia who suffers head trauma must therefore be hospitalized for observation and should receive empirical Factor VIII replacement. Lumbar punctures should not be performed without adequate replacement therapy.

Hemorrhaging into deep tissues may produce a variety of syndromes, many of which mimic nonvascular problems. Retroperitoneal bleeding can produce a painful abdominal syndrome suggestive of appendicitis or some other acute surgical problem. Oropharyngeal bleeding can cause gradual or sudden airway obstruction. Periureteral bleeding can produce painful ureteral spasms and obstruction. Hematemesis and hemoptysis, however, are only rarely caused solely by hemophilia, and other causes, including tuberculosis and peptic ulcer disease, should be sought.

Hemophilia A should be suspected in any male with abnormal bleeding, especially if he has a family history of hemophilia. Certain clinical syndromes, especially hemarthroses not associated with major trauma, are highly suggestive of the diagnosis. Laboratory testing reveals a prolonged partial thromboplastin time, a normal bleeding time, and a normal prothrombin time. Specific assays for Factor VIII are available.

Therapy for ongoing bleeding involves replacement of Factor VIII. Therapy should be rapid and vigorous, especially if the bleeding is occurring in the central nervous system, pharynx, or abdomen. The goal of replacement therapy is to restore normal hemostasis; this usually requires a Factor VIII level of at least 25% of normal. Replacement must be continued for at least several days after the bleeding has stopped. The bleeding may otherwise resume due to the anatomic damage that produced the first bleeding. Any procedure that might produce or exacerbate bleeding should be preceded by replacement therapy.

Factor IX deficiency, or hemophilia B, is a

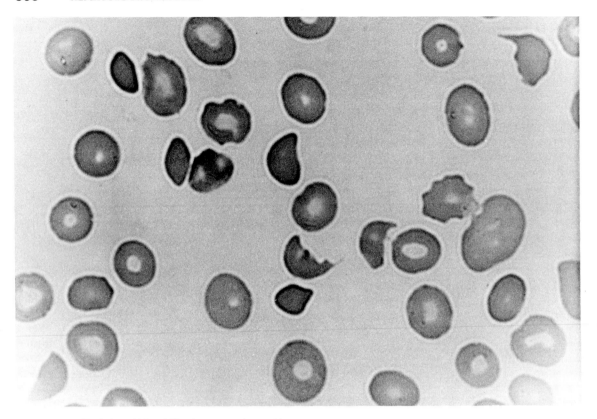

FIG. 46–3. Peripheral blood film from a patient with disseminated intravascular coagulation (DIC). The characteristic schistocytes (with pointed edges and crescent shapes) are apparent. Note also the absence of platelets in this field, consistent with severe thrombocytopenia.

sex-linked recessive disorder that is clinically identical to hemophilia A. It is much less common than factor VIII deficiency.

DISSEMINATED INTRAVASCULAR COAGULATION (DIC)

Disseminated intravascular coagulation is primarily a coagulation disorder, but severe thrombocytopenia can also be present and exacerbate the tendency to bleed.

Pathophysiology. DIC results from widespread activation of the coagulation system. The extent of clotting is so great that platelet and coagulation factors are depleted and bleeding results. Accompanying fibrinolyis yields high levels of fibrin split products (FSP), whose antihemostatic properties further enhance bleeding. Deposition of fibrin in the microvasculature leads to a characteristic microangiopathic hemolysis, and red blood cell fragments and schistocytes can be detected on a peripheral blood film (Fig. 46–3). The prothrombin time and partial thromboplastin time are prolonged, and the thrombin time is also prolonged due to decreased levels of fibrinogen. The effects of this massive derangement of hemostasis include small vessel emboli and thromboses, severe anemia, and tissue bleeding.

Etiology. Usually, the most common causes of DIC are (1) infection, (2) the abnormal production or liberation of procoagulant tissue factors, and (3) endothelial damage. In a given patient, any combination of these factors may be responsible.

Infection is probably the most common setting for DIC. Severe bacterial infections—either gram-positive or gram-negative—with sepsis are usually involved. A source of infection should be looked for, and, unless a clear-cut noninfectious cause of DIC is apparent, broad-spectrum parenteral antibiotics should be administered empirically.

Liberation of tissue factors is believed to be the cause of DIC in patients with tumors, fat emboli, massive acute hemolysis, and obstetric catastrophes. Endothelial damage can cause DIC in patients with heat stroke, burns, shock, acute glomerulonephritis, and Rocky Mountain Spotted Fever.

Therapy. Plasma and platelet transfusions are often given in an attempt to control severe bleeding in patients with DIC, but plasma transfusions provide more material for intravascular coagulation and can conceivably worsen the condition. Intravenous heparin has been advocated in order to interrupt the cycle of coagulation and fibrinolysis, but the difficulty in giving heparin to a patient with a severe bleeding diathesis is obvious, and studies of heparin therapy have produced mixed results. It has therefore been difficult to formulate a specific therapeutic approach beyond treatment of the underlying disorder.

VON WILLEBRAND'S DISEASE

Originally described as a bleeding disorder associated with an autosomal dominant mode of inheritance, von Willebrand's disease is now known to exist in several genetic variants. In addition, acquired forms of the disease have been described in patients with severe autoimmune or lymphoproliferative disorders. Patients experience severe mucous membrane bleeding, easy bruisability, and prolonged bleeding from wounds. Epistaxis is the most common manifestation, occurring in approximately 75% of patients. Women frequently complain of hemorrhagia. The bleeding tendency is often severe in childhood and adolescence but generally improves with age.

Laboratory testing reveals a number of abnormalities, and the diagnostic picture may be clouded by the existence of patients who satisfy only some of the laboratory criteria for diagnosis. In general, patients have evidence of both abnormal platelet function (a prolonged bleeding time) and a deficiency of clotting factor VIII. Platelet counts are normal. All of these abnormalities are corrected by infusions of factor VIII-containing preparations. The platelet activity is not abnormal in hemophilia, and hemophiliac plasma will correct the platelet defect in von Willebrand's disease. Cryoprecipitates of plasma fractions rich in factor VIII are the current therapy of choice.

BIBLIOGRAPHY

Arkel YS: Evaluation of platelet aggregation in disorders of hemostasis. Med Clin North Am 60:881–911, 1976

Bennett B: Coagulation pathways: interrelationships and control mechanisms. Semin Hematol 14:301–318, 1977

Bick RL: Disseminated intravascular coagulation and related syndromes. Am J Hematol 5:265–282, 1978

Gralnick HR, Coller BS, Shulman NR et al: Factor VIII. Ann Intern Med 86:598–616, 1977

Mueller-Eckhardt C: Idiopathic thrombocytopenic purpura (ITP): Clinical and immunologic considerations. Semin Thromb Hemostas 3:125–159, 1977

Rizza CR: Clinical management of hemophilia. Br Med Bull 33:225–230, 1977

Rosenberg RD: Biologic actions of heparin. Semin Hematol 14:427–440, 1977

47

Leukemia and Lymphoma

LEUKEMIA

Although the complex and rapidly changing diagnostic criteria and drug regimens for leukemia belong in the province of the specialized hematologist/oncologist, the general medical service still bears much of the responsibility for patient management and must be alert to the major clinical features and complications of the various leukemias.

Leukemia can be divided into acute and chronic forms. *Acute leukemia* is a fulminant disease, and, when untreated, is usually fatal within six to nine months. Immature leukocytes proliferate and accumulate in large numbers in the bone marrow and the circulation. The clinical manifestations are caused by the loss of normal marrow elements and by infiltration of the body's tissues by the malignant cells. *Chronic leukemia* is a proliferative disease of relatively mature leukocytes. It may follow a rapid and aggressive course or remain stable and asymptomatic for as long as ten to fifteen years.

ACUTE LEUKEMIA

Various cytological, cytochemical, immunologic, and, more recently, enzymatic criteria have been used to subcategorize acute leukemia. The subdivision into *acute lymphocytic leukemia* (ALL) and *acute myelocytic leukemia* (AML) is traditional and still useful. It may be difficult to distinguish ALL and AML on a peripheral blood film (Fig. 47–1). Cytologically, AML can be distinguished from ALL by the presence of granules and eosinophilic rods, called Auer bodies, that are present in the cytoplasm of the malignant cells of AML. Auer bodies are not present in the cells of ALL.

An enzyme that is normally confined to the thymus, terminal deoxyribonucleotidyl transferase, has recently been detected in the cells of nearly all patients with ALL. In approximately 20% of patients with ALL, the malignant cells possess T lymphocyte surface markers (*i.e.*, they are able to form rosettes with sheep red blood cells). In the remaining patients with ALL, the cells bear neither T nor B cell markers, and have been termed null cells.

The cells of AML stain positively with Sudan black and myeloperoxidase. Several subtypes of AML have been defined according to the morphologic resemblance of the malignant cells to various normal cells. These subtypes are thus termed myelomonocytic,

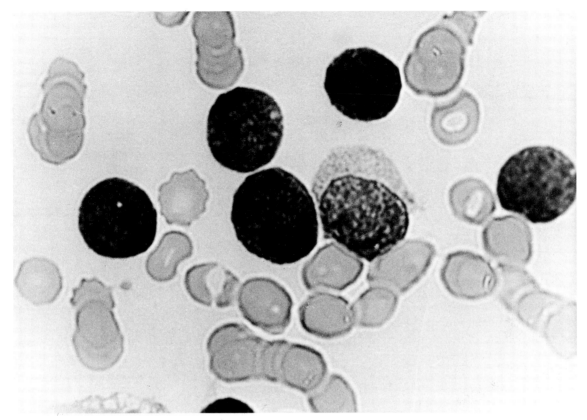

FIG. 47–1. Peripheral blood film from a patient with acute lymphocytic leukemia.

myelocytic, promyelocytic, monocytic, and erythroleukemia. Myelomonocytic leukemia is the most common form of AML. Pure monocytic leukemia is rare and is generally considered a variant of myelomonocytic leukemia. Promyelocytic leukemia is so named because of the presence of granule-containing leukemic cells resembling normal promyelocytes. They all carry similar prognoses.

Some acute leukemias do not fit any of the established classifications, and are termed acute undifferentiated leukemia.

Epidemiology. Most cases of ALL occur in children. Adult cases of ALL are more resistant to therapy, and the malignant cells in adults more frequently carry T cell markers. AML is mostly seen in the adult population.

Diagnosis. Fatigue is the most common symptom of leukemia. Bone pain occurs secondary to marrow infiltration and occurs most often in ALL. Most symptoms can be attributed to the replacement of normal marrow elements by the leukemic cells: anemia produces weakness, pallor, and, occasionally, cardiopulmonary compromise; neutropenia leads to frequent infections; thrombocytopenia causes purpura and hemorrhage.

Enlarged lymph nodes, splenomegaly, and hepatomegaly may occur. These are usually prominent in ALL and less obvious and less frequent in AML. Fever is common and is usually due to infection. Early in the course of disease, however, fever is more likely to be due to the leukemia itself.

The symptoms of leukemia at the time of presentation are usually nonspecific, but the patient's complaints of weakness, fever, infection, or bleeding usually prompt an examination of the peripheral blood. This is generally diagnostic. Only about 30% of patients present with white blood cell counts of greater than 50,000, and about 20% have counts of 5000 or less, but even in the latter group of patients, the majority of the white blood cells are leukemic cells. A bone marrow examination is confirmatory.

Management

Infection. Infection is the leading cause of death in adults with acute leukemia. Many factors, including neutropenia, cachexia, and immunosuppression due to the disease and especially to chemotherapy contribute to the greatly increased risk of severe infection. Infection and antibiotic therapy in immunosuppressed patients are discussed in depth in Chapter 58.

Bleeding. Bleeding is the second most common cause of death in patients with acute leukemia. In the majority of patients, bleeding is due to thrombocytopenia. In patients with very low platelet counts, care must be taken to avoid injury (especially head trauma). Intramuscular injections and toothbrushing should be carried out very carefully. Stool softeners should be given to minimize rectal trauma. In females, menstruation should be hormonally supressed.

In approximately 10% of patients, disseminated intravascular coagulation (DIC) is the cause of bleeding. DIC usually develops in patients with promyelocytic leukemia, although it occasionally occurs in patients with other forms of leukemia, often accompanying sepsis.

The cause of DIC in acute promyelocytic leukemia is believed to be the release of procoagulants that are present in the leukemic promyelocytic granules. Their release results in prolonged prothrombin, partial thromboplastin, and thrombin times, decreased Factor V and fibrinogen levels, and increased levels of fibrin split products. Patients with promyelocytic leukemia virtually always have a bleeding diathesis, evidenced by petechiae, hematuria, ecchymoses, epistaxis, and even gastrointestinal and intracerebral bleeding.

The bleeding abnormality may acutely worsen with the initiation of chemotherapy, presumably because of the increased granule release from cells destroyed by the cytotoxic drugs. Many clinicians now recommend that patients receiving chemotherapy should be put on continuous low-dose infusions of heparin at the time of diagnosis and before therapy is initiated; heparin should not be stopped until remission is achieved. A positive response is indicated by a rise in fibrinogen or Factor V levels and by a decrease in bleeding. Platelet transfusions are given during this time to maintain the platelet count at levels of 40,000 to 50,000.

Anemia. Most patients with leukemia develop anemia at some time during their course. The anemia is often acutely exacerbated by marrow-suppressive chemotherapy. Rapidly progressive anemia in the setting of acute leukemia suggests hemorrhage or DIC. Transfusion therapy is discussed in Chapter 44.

Leukocytosis. White blood cell counts of more than 100,000 (leukocytosis) pose the threat of fatal circulatory embarrassment and can be a medical emergency. The great mass of cells can cause sludging and thus lead to the occlusion of vessels. The cerebral vessels are particularly susceptible to intravascular leukostasis, and stroke and death can result. Symptoms of hyperviscosity include blurred vision, headaches, weakness, abdominal pain, and dyspnea from congestive heart failure. Treatment is aimed at rapidly reducing the white blood cell count. This is usually accomplished with cytotoxic agents, such as hydroxyurea, but leukophoresis has also been used with success.

Hyperuricemia. Hyperuricemia results from the turnover of the large number of malignant cells and the resultant increased breakdown of nucleic acids. Sudden and marked elevations of uric acid occur with the institution of cytotoxic chemotherapy and irradiation. Acute uric acid nephropathy can result, with obstruction and renal failure. Nephropathy can be prevented by treating these patients with allopurinol, a xanthine oxidase inhibitor.

Electrolyte Disturbances. *Hypokalemia* is the most common electrolyte disturbance. It is most often seen in AML, where it has been correlated with elevated levels of serum lysozyme, an enzyme released from the leukemic cells, that believed to damage the proximal renal tubules.

Hyperkalemia usually occurs during chemotherapy, when the large numbers of rapidly lysed cells release their stores of potassium into the circulation. Renal insufficiency and renal failure also lead to hyperkalemia. Genuine hyperkalemia must be distinguished from *pseudohyperkalemia*, which results from the release of potassium from the large number of damaged white cells and platelets in a drawn blood sample (see Chap. 49).

A transient *hypocalcemia* occurs during rapid lysis of the leukemic cells by chemotherapy, and is associated with marked *hyperphosphatemia*. Prolonged hypocalcemia may accompany renal insufficiency.

Other electrolyte abnormalities are more infrequent. The syndrome of inappropriate ADH with *hyponatremia* (Chap. 26) is occasionally seen, especially with leukemic meningitis, and may also accompany the use of vincristine and cyclophosphamide. The hyponatremia may be exacerbated by vomiting. *Hypercalcemia* is unusual, although it has been described in ALL. It carries a poor prognosis. *Lactic acidosis* is not infrequently reported in ALL and AML, and is always an indication of very severe illness. It is generally associated with a huge leukemic cell burden.

Central Nervous System Complications. Although any organ can be compromised by the proliferation of leukemic cells, the central nervous system (CNS) presents the widest range of symptom complexes and the greatest number of diagnostic difficulties. Only a minority of patients experience significant CNS problems, but these problems are potentially fatal.

There are three general types of CNS disease: hemorrhage, infiltrative disease, and infectious disease.

Three factors predispose to hemorrhage: (1) thrombocytopenia or DIC (2) very high leukocyte counts with leukostasis, and (3) trauma, coexistent with the other predisposing conditions. The site of bleeding is usually either subarachnoid or intracerebral; the latter produces stroke symptomatology.

Infiltrative disease can affect any part of the nervous system, from the cortex to the brainstem to the spinal cord. Vomiting, nausea, headaches, papilledema, cranial and spinal nerve palsies, lethargy, confusion, and loss of consciousness may occur. Some patients with infiltrative disease are asymptomatic. The diagnosis can be made by finding leukemic cells in the CSF.

Infectious complications of the central nervous system accompany the general loss of antimicrobial defenses and do not present unique findings in leukemic patients.

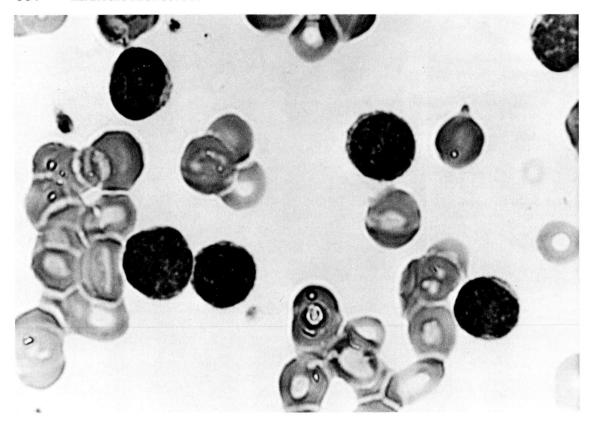

FIG. 47–2. Peripheral blood film from a patient with chronic lymphocytic leukemia. Note the normal-appearing small lymphocytes in contrast to the appearance of cells in the patient with acute lymphocytic leukemia.

CHRONIC LEUKEMIA

The two major forms of chronic leukemia are chronic myelocytic leukemia (CML, also referred to as chronic granulocytic leukemia, or CGL) and chronic lymphocytic leukemia (CLL). Except for the altered time course and often lessened severity, these entities present the same problems as the acute leukemias. Thus, early in the presentation of CML or CLL, there are symptoms of malaise, fatigue, and decreased appetite, as well as symptoms relating to bone marrow and organ infiltration, including anemia and thrombocytopenia. Thrombocytopenia in patients with CLL is often due to immune thrombocytopenic purpura (ITP). These patients may also have immune hemolytic anemia. In the majority of patients, CML eventually enters an accelerated phase or blast crisis; at that point, the problems encountered by the patient are essentially those of acute leukemia.

Chronic Lymphocytic Leukemia (CLL)

CLL (Fig. 47–2) is almost exclusively a disease of patients over 50 years of age. It is the most "benign" of the leukemias, in that it is most likely to pursue an indolent or slowly pro-

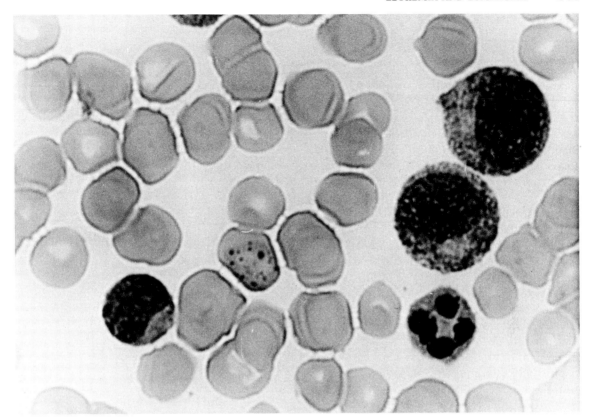

FIG. 47–3. Peripheral blood film from a patient with chronic myelogenous leukemia. Note the coexistence of mature white blood cells with leukocyte precursor cells at various stages of maturation.

gressive course. The clinical presentation reflects the consequences of small lymphocyte accumulation in lymphoid tissue, consisting of the enlargement, often dramatic, of the lymph nodes, spleen, and liver. The bone marrow is also gradually infiltrated and replaced by malignant cells. An altered immune system may provide a reasonable explanation for some of the other, variable manifestations of CLL, including recurrent bacterial infections, hypogammaglobulinemia, and a Coombs' positive hemolytic anemia. The causes of anemia may, however, be multiple,

related, at least in part, to the direct effect of bone marrow infiltration. Thrombocytopenia is also seen and is frequently accompanied by detectable antiplatelet antibodies.

CLL does not transform to an acute, accelerated form of leukemia. Nevertheless, hematogenous spread of the more malignant, immature lymphoid cells of lymphosarcoma may be difficult to distinguish from CLL.

In general, a remission from CLL is readily achieved with cytotoxic agents and corticosteroids.

Chronic Myelogenous Leukemia (CML)

The other form of chronic leukemia, CML (Fig. 47–3), presents a more aggressive profile than CLL. In this disease, bone marrow replacement by abnormal leukopoietic cells is characteristically accompanied by extensive peripheral release of circulating myeloid cells at all stages of development from myeloblast to mature granulocyte. The disease is therefore readily diagnosed, although differentiation from a *leukemoid reaction* (a nonmalignant, sustained white blood cell count above 30,000/mm³ from any cause) may prove difficult. It should be noted, however, that the bone marrow release of myeloblasts and basophils into the circulation is not ordinarily a feature of the leukemoid reaction. The leukemoid response rarely contains cells less mature than metamyelocytes, and the leukocyte alkaline phosphatase, in contrast to CML, is typically high.

Confirmatory laboratory tests for CML include a low leukocyte alkaline phosphatase level as well as cytogenetic identification of the "Philadelphia chromosome" (a partial long arm deletion of chromosome 22 in bone marrow granulocyte precursors) which is present in over 90% of patients.

Most patients, in particular those who have the Philadelphia chromosome, respond well to initial chemotherapy. The vascular occlusions that accompany leukostasis will occasionally necessitate prompt lowering of the dramatically elevated white blood cell count. In addition to cytotoxic agents, leukophoresis is often employed.

Despite the salutary initial response to treatment, an acute blastic transformation ("blast crisis") heralds the patient's rapid demise after a variable duration of remission. The blastic transformation is frequently preceded by the new appearance of fever, lymphadenopathy, bone pain, or myelofibrosis. CML in blast crisis is highly resistant to therapy.

POLYCYTHEMIA VERA

Polycythemia vera (PCV) is a profound disorder of the bone marrow that is classified as one of the preleukemic disorders. These disorders are known collectively as the *myeloproliferative syndrome*. PCV is typified by an uncontrolled, erythropoietin-independent increase in hematocrit.

The clinical characteristics of the disease are predicated upon the striking increase in total blood volume and viscosity. Symptoms consist of headache, tinnitus, pruritus, dyspnea, weakness, and nonspecific dyspeptic gastrointestinal complaints. The physical examination reveals ruddy facial cyanosis, ecchymoses, and hepatosplenomegaly. In addition to the elevated red blood cell mass, laboratory investigation may also reveal confirmatory evidence of generalized bone marrow hyperplasia: leukocytosis with prominent basophils and eosinophils, elevated leukocyte alkaline phosphatase, and hyperuricemia and hyperuricosuria.

The course of PCV is highly variable and is determined by the extent of extramedullary hematopoiesis and the occurrence of serious vascular hemorrhage and thrombosis resulting from the markedly increased blood viscosity. Myeloid metaplasia and myelofibrosis both tend to supervene in patients with ongoing disease activity. Acute leukemia develops in a small percentage of patients.

The chief diagnostic problem in PCV resides in its differentiation from secondary forms of erythrocytosis. These fall into several broad categories:

(1) Hypoxemia stimulates erythropoietin which in turn stimulates red blood cell production. This may occur in chronic lung disease, cyanotic congenital heart disease, and in persons living at high altitudes. A unique, familial variant of erythropoietin-mediated erythrocytosis occurs in patients in whom altered oxygen affinity is produced by heritable aminoacid substitutions in the β-chain of hemoglobin.

(2) Many tumors and other structural lesions can initiate inappropiate erythropoietin release. Among these are renal cell and ovarian carcinoma, hydronephrosis, and cerebellar hemangioma.

(3) Stress erythrocytosis (Gaisböck's syndrome) represents an example of *relative* polycythemia due to hemoconcentration in which, typically, a middle-aged, stocky male presents with hypertension, a normal-to-slightly-elevated red cell mass and a low or normal plasma volume. Its cause is unknown. Other mechanisms of hemoconcentration, such as diuretic therapy and protracted diarrhea, can produce a similar picture. A normal red cell mass and a contracted plasma volume exclude the consideration of PCV.

It should be stressed that, while these and other conditions can produce secondary erythrocytosis, the identification of PCV is facilitated by the concurrence of basophilia, splenomegaly, hyperuricemia, and an elevated leukocyte alkaline phosphatase with the erythrocytosis. On the other hand, erythrocytosis *cannot* be comfortably ascribed to PCV unless the arterial oxygen saturation has been documented to be normal. In the absence of hypoxemia, PCV can be assumed to be present if the plasma volume and hemoglobin electrophoresis are found to be normal and the red blood cell mass (measured by Cr^{51} labeling) increased. Other erythropoietin-dependent diseases should also be sought and excluded.

Therapy of PCV is primarily designed to reduce the elevated red blood cell mass. This is usually accomplished by repeated phlebotomy to a state of mild iron deficiency. Abrupt changes in blood volume should, however, be avoided, since acute hemoconcentration and a consequent increase in blood viscosity can result. The role of cytotoxic therapy for PCV is controversial, and its use is probably not indicated for most patients. Therapy for PCV reduces the risk of vascular accidents. Median survival now exceeds 15 years.

LYMPHOMA

Lymphomas are characterized by the neoplastic proliferation of cells within the elements of the reticuloendothelial system: the lymph nodes, bone marrow, spleen, and liver. Lymphomas are traditionally divided histologically into Hodgkin's and non-Hodgkin's lymphomas.

Hodgkin's Disease

The distinguishing histologic feature of Hodgkin's disease is the presence of giant multinucleated cells, called Sternberg-Reed cells, in affected lymph nodes. Many abnormal cells can be identified in addition to the Sternberg-Reed cell, and there is an accompanying—primarily lymphocytic—inflammatory reaction to these unusual cells. It is not clear which of the various cell types represents the malignant cell.

Four histologic types of Hodgkin's disease are recognized:

1. *Lymphocyte predominance.* Lymphocytes greatly outnumber the abnormal cells.

2. *Mixed cellularity.* The proportion of lymphocytes and abnormal cells is more balanced.

3. *Lymphocyte depletion.* The abnormal cells outnumber the small population of lymphocytes.

4. *Nodular sclerosis.* Bands of connective tissue surround islands of abnormal cells and lymphocytes.

Without therapy, the prognosis worsens as the number of lymphocytes decreases. Nodular sclerosis, found mostly in young women, has a good 5-year survival rate.

Hodgkin's disease is fairly common (about 6000 new cases each year in the United States) and has a bimodal age distribution, with peaks at age 30 and age 70. Patients usually present with painless lymphadenopathy in the supra-clavicular or cervical nodes. About 50% of patients also present with systemic manifestations, such as fever, night sweats, weight loss, and pruritis. A defect in cellular immunity leads to a propensity for infections such as candidiasis, tuberculosis, and disseminated herpes zoster.

Unlike the other lymphomas, Hodgkin's disease progresses in an orderly fashion from one lymph node region to a neighboring one. This has proved to be an important consideration in designing portals for radiation therapy.

For purposes of planning therapy, Hodgkin's disease has been divided into four stages:

Stage I: Disease of a single lymph node region or single extralymphatic site.

Stage II: Disease in two or more lymph node regions on the same side of the diaphragm. The disease may also involve an extralymphatic site on the same side of the diaphragm.

Stage III: Disease of lymph nodes on both sides of the diaphragm that may also involve the spleen (IIIs) or localized extralymphatic sites.

Stage IV: Involvement of more than one extralymphatic site (such as the bone marrow, liver, skin, or gastrointestinal tract).

Patients with Hodgkin's disease are further subclassified as A or B, depending upon the absence (A) or presence (B) of unexplained 10% weight loss, fevers, or night sweats.

Staging is carried out through a number of steps: (1) biopsy of the involved nodes, (2) a chest x-ray to search for hilar or mediastinal involvement or spread to the parenchyma of the lungs, (3) a bone marrow examination to detect extralymphatic spread, (4) liver function tests, (5) bilateral lower extremity lymphangiograms, and (6) if there is not already conclusive evidence of disease below the dia-phragm, a staging laparotomy, with sampling of the nodes, and splenectomy. The necessity of a staging laparotomy in all these patients, however, remains controversial.

Treatment for Hodgkin's disease is quite effective, but requires expertise in delivery of the extremely toxic therapies. Stages I and II are treated with high doses of radiation to the involved nodes and neighboring nodal regions. Stages III and IV are treated with chemotherapy, most notably the MOPP program, which includes nitrogen mustard, vincristine (oncovin), procarbazine, and prednisone given in cycles over six months. The major side-effects of MOPP therapy are myelosuppression from the nitrogen mustard and procarbazine, and neurotoxicity from vincristine. In patients treated with a combination of chemotherapy and irradiation, there are the potential late complications of developing acute monocytic leukemia and non-Hodgkin's lymphoma.

MOPP therapy has resulted in a 70% five-year survival for patients who begin therapy with widespread disease. Many patients have now been shown to remain disease-free for ten years. Radiation therapy for Stages I and II results in an 80% to 90% five-year survival.

Non-Hodgkin's Lymphomas

Lymphadenopathy is usually the initial complaint of patients with non-Hodgkin's lymphoma. The histologic classification is based on the overall appearance of the lymph nodes and the predominant cytologic types. The most important distinction is between patients with a nodular lymph node architecture and those with diffuse lymph node involvement. In general, nodular lymphomas carry a better prognosis than diffuse lymphomas. Further subdivision depends upon the morphologic appearance of the predominant neoplastic cell, that is, histiocytic, poorly differentiated lymphocytic, and well-differentiated lymphocytic.

The most common non-Hodgkin's lymphoma is nodular, poorly differentiated, lymphocytic lymphoma. The tumor is often widespread at the time of diagnosis even though the patient may complain only of localized adenopathy. Despite dissemination, the disease often runs an indolent course for several years before becoming more aggressive.

Of the diffuse lymphomas, the histiocytic type is most common. Patients often present while the disease is still localized to one group of nodes, usually in the neck. However, the malignancy is very invasive, compressing nerves and blood vessels and destroying nearby bone.

Staging for non-Hodgkin's lymphoma is done in a manner similar to that for Hodgkin's disease. Exploratory laparotomy and splenectomy are usually avoided, however, since they have little influence upon subsequent therapy. The nodular lymphomas are almost invariably first detected in Stages III and IV; the diffuse lymphomas are detected in Stages I or II only slightly more often. Radiation therapy is therefore rarely of value. No chemotherapeutic regimen has been developed for non-Hodgkin's lymphoma that is as consistently effective as MOPP is for Hodgkin's disease.

BIBLIOGRAPHY

Aisenberg AC: Malignant lymphoma. N Engl J Med 288:883–890, 935–941, 1973

Berard CW, Gallo RC, Jaffe ES et al: Current concepts of leukemia and lymphoma: Etiology, pathogenesis, and therapy. Ann Intern Med 85:351–366, 1976

Chabner BA, Johnson RE, Young RC et al: Sequential nonsurgical and surgical staging of non-Hodgkin's lymphoma. Ann Intern Med 85:149–154, 1976

Chang H-Y, Rodriguez V, Narboni G et al: Causes of death in adults with acute leukemia. Medicine 55:259–263, 1976

DeVita VT, Simon RM, Hubbard SM et al: Curability of advanced Hodgkin's disease with chemotherapy. Ann Intern Med 92:587–595, 1980

Gralnick HR, Galton DAG, Catovsky D et al: Classification of acute leukemia. Ann Intern Med 87:740–753, 1977

Jones SE, Fuks Z, Bull M et al: Non-Hodgkin's lymphomas: IV. Clinicopathologic correlation in 405 cases. Cancer 31:806–823, 1973

Levine AS, Schimpff SC, Graw RG et al: Hematologic malignancies and other marrow failure states: Progress in the management of complicating infections. Semin Hematol 11:141–202, 1974

Rosenthal S, Cannellos GP, DeVita, VT Jr et al: Characteristics of blast crisis in chronic granulocytic leukemia. Blood 49:705–714, 1977

Wolk RW, Masse SR, Conklin R et al: The incidence of central nervous system leukemia in adults with acute leukemia. Cancer 33:863–869, 1974

48

Multiple Myeloma

Multiple myeloma is a malignant proliferation of plasma cells originating in and primarily involving the bone marrow. Solitary accretions of myeloma cells (plasmacytomas) can occasionally be found at sites outside the bone.

Although multiple myeloma is an uncommon disease in the general population (approximately 3 out of every 100,000 hospital admissions), its varied and painful sequelae necessitate frequent and prolonged hospitalizations.

SIGNS AND SYMPTOMS

Multiple myeloma occurs primarily in the elderly; fewer than 5% of hospital patients with multiple myeloma are under age 40. Multiple myeloma should be suspected in any elderly patient with osteolytic bone lesions, pathologic fractures, unexplained renal failure or hypercalcemia, or signs of amyloidosis (e.g., carpal tunnel syndrome or nephrotic syndrome). In the United States, the disease occurs more frequently in blacks than in whites.

Severe bone pain, especially in the lower back and ribs, is the presenting symptom in two-thirds of patients with multiple mye-loma. This excruciating bone pain is the most disabling feature of myeloma. The central skeleton, the site of hemopoiesis (i.e., the red marrow), is most frequently affected. Although nearly any type of skeletal pathology may occur, osteolytic lesions (punched out circular defects) and osteoporosis are the most common. The cortex is thin and the trabeculae are destroyed.

Many patients also have vague systemic complaints, such as fatigue, malaise, and anorexia. Symptomatic renal disease often occurs during the course of myeloma, and some patients may develop uremia early in the disease. Anemia and neutropenia are common, and patients with myeloma have an increased risk of recurrent infections. More than one-fourth of patients have elevated serum calcium levels at the time of their initial evaluation for myeloma, although symptomatic hypercalcemia at this time is unusual.

DIAGNOSIS

Laboratory Findings

In the majority of patients, the malignant plasma cells of multiple myeloma appear to arise from a single clone of immunoreactive cells, and they secrete a single, homogeneous protein molecule. These monoclonal proteins can be detected as a sharp peak ("M-spike") on either serum or urine electrophoresis. These proteins are usually intact immunoglobulin molecules, but in 20% of patients, they are monoclonal light chains.

Two special tests, serum protein electrophoresis and immunoelectrophoresis, are employed to aid in the diagnosis of multiple myeloma and to quantify further and identify the monoclonal peak.

In serum protein electrophoresis (SPEP), a current is applied to a serum sample in an agar gel, and the proteins are separated by their characteristic mobilities in an electric field. The separated serum proteins can then be permitted to interact with antisera, and precipitin bands form whenever a specific antigen-antibody reaction occurs. This latter procedure, termed immunoelectrophoresis (IEP), allows for definitive identification of the immunoglobulins. In additon to its utility in diagnosing the monoclonal immunoglobin peak of myeloma, IEP can also clarify the broad polyclonal immunoglobulin peaks seen on SPEP in patients with infection, cancer, and connective-tissue or other inflammatory diseases.

In 70% of patients, the SPEP will reveal a monoclonal spike. If, however, the M-spike is small, it may not be detectable on serum protein electrophoresis, and IEP is needed to quantify and identify the monoclonal peak.

In some patients, no serum abnormalities will be found, although an M-spike may be found on urinary electrophoresis. The urine may reveal the presence of "Bence Jones proteins," which are immunoglobulin light chains (or their breakdown products).

Occasionally, patients with multiple myeloma lack evidence of an M-spike on either serum or urine electrophoresis. Because no abnormal protein can be demonstrated, these are considered to be cases of nonsecreting multiple myeloma.

Frequently, the non-"spike" immunoglobulins are found to be depressed. This hypogammaglobulinemia may be responsible for the increased incidence of bacterial infections.

Other diagnostic aids include a bone marrow biopsy, which may reveal large numbers of plasma cells, and skeletal x-rays, which may reveal osteolytic lesions and osteopenia (Fig. 48–1). Anemia is common, and rouleau formation of erythrocytes on a blood film may be present. A Wright's stain of a blood film characteristically shows a bluish background because of the increased plasma protein. Chemical signs of renal failure may also be present (see Chap. 22).

Once the diagnosis of multiple myeloma has been established, the progression of the disease and the response to therapy can be monitored by quantitating the M-spike on the SPEP or on whichever test the M-spike is most clearly delineated. It must be remembered that the myeloma-derived proteins are cationic, and therefore will not register on the dipstick test for urinary proteins.

DIFFERENTIAL DIAGNOSIS

A small monoclonal M-spike without additional evidence of pathology is not a sufficient criterion for the diagnosis of multiple myeloma. A small percentage of otherwise healthy elderly individuals possess a monoclonal protein spike without any evidence of myeloma, macroglobulinemia, or other illnesses. The erythrocyte sedimentation rate (ESR) is often elevated, but the patient's renal function, blood count, and serum electrolytes are within normal limits. This laboratory diagnosis, not truly a disease, is called *benign monoclonal gammopathy* (BMG). It is far more common than myeloma.

The natural history of BMG has been investigated by the Mayo Clinic. In more than half the patients under study, the size of the M-spike remained stable, and there was no evidence of disease. Only 11% of this population eventually developed a malignancy. Of these, two-thirds developed multiple myeloma after a median interval of five years from the time the M-spike was first noted. The size of the initial M-spike did not reliably indicate which patients would progress to myeloma. There is at present no reliable test that can distinguish the small group of patients that progresses to malignancy from the majority of patients who do not. It is therefore appropriate to follow carefully patients with monoclonal gammopathy of undetermined origin, but aggressive treatment of monoclonal gammopathy is clearly not warranted.

COMPLICATIONS

Bone

The severe bone pain of multiple myeloma can be exceptionally disabling, making ambulation impossible and thus increasing bone demineralization and hypercalcemia. Pathologic fractures, especially of the ribs, are common and present a major management problem. The rib pain causes splinting, thereby increasing the risk of pneumonia. Nerve root injuries can occur when vertebrae fracture. "Punched out" lesions can be seen on bone x-rays.

Electrolyte Imbalances and Hypercalcemia

Electrolyte imbalances and hypercalcemia in patients with malignancy are discussed in Chapter 49.

Kidney

The so-called myeloma kidney, a major cause of chronic renal failure in myeloma patients, is thought to be a light-chain-induced lesion. Renal histology shows marked tubular atrophy and protein casts obstructing both the proximal and distal tubules. Light chains are filtered, reabsorbed, and catabolized by the renal tubular cells. These Bence Jones proteins are probably nephrotoxic, and may cause tubular atrophy. There is evidence suggesting that this nephrotoxicity is the primary cause of myeloma kidney. Obstructing casts are a secondary phenomenon. The degree of Bence Jones proteinuria correlates with the extent of renal failure. The patient presents with defects in acidification (distal renal tubular acidosis), concentrating ability (nephrogenic diabetes insipidus) and proximal tubular reabsorption (adult Fanconi's syndrome).

The kidneys may also be affected by a number of other insults, including hypercalcemia and hyperuricemia. Pyelonephritis is a common complication and care must be taken that antibiotic treatment with nephrotoxic drugs (e.g., the aminoglycosides) does not further compromise renal function. Amyloidosis can cause the nephrotic syndrome, and plasma cell infiltration of the kidney has been seen.

The intravenous pyelogram (IVP) has long been considered especially hazardous for patients with myeloma. The osmotic diuresis induced by the dye load can lead to decreased renal perfusion and the precipitation of proteins within the tubules. Dye-induced intrarenal vasospasm has also been postulated as the mechanism of renal damage. If dehydration is avoided, however, an IVP can be performed safely in most patients.

Infection

Infection is the leading cause of death in patients with multiple myeloma. The patients' immunologic defenses against infection are usually depressed. Hypogammaglobulinemia may be present, and antibody

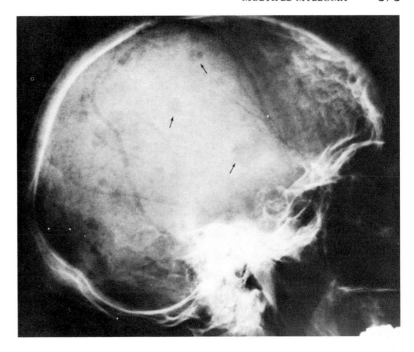

FIG. 48–1. Skull x-ray of a patient with multiple myeloma. The punched-out lesions of multiple myeloma (arrows) are evident. Diffuse osteopenia is also present.

production is usually inadequate. Leukopenia is present in approximately one-sixth of patients, and chemotherapy may further compromise the defenses against infection. The urinary tract and lungs are the most common sites of infection. Gram-negative pneumonias are now more common than the previously classic occurrence of pneumococcal pneumonia.

Hyperviscosity and Cryoglobulinemia

Serum viscosity is invariably normal when the serum IgG or IgA spike is less than 4g/dl. Higher levels may result in abnormally elevated serum viscosity. Signs and symptoms of hyperviscosity include mucosal bleeding, skin necrosis, blurred vision, and a variety of neurologic complications.

Cryoglobulinemia refers to the precipitation of antibodies or antibody-antigen complexes in the cold. Manifestations of cryoglobuline-mia include Raynaud's phenomenon, immune complex deposition in the kidneys (glomerulonephritis), skin (purpura), and joints (arthralgias), and the complications of hyperviscosity.

THERAPY

Bone pain is often the most disabling feature of multiple myeloma, and potent narcotic analgesia must be supplied despite the risk of addiction.

Chemotherapy consists of alkylating agents in concert with high-dose glucocorticoids. Radiation therapy has been used in the treatment of pathologic fractures and extraskeletal plasmacytomas that are impinging on vital structures. Although leukemia may be a late feature of the natural history of multiple myeloma, acute leukemia, especially acute myelomonocytic leukemia, is also a late side-effect of alkylating therapy. Leukemia occurs in less than 10% of treated patients, but the risk of leukemia must be considered a serious possibility. The distinction between multiple myeloma and benign monoclonal gammopathy is therefore crucial, since therapy has potentially lethal complications.

MORTALITY

Although the 5-year survival rate in myeloma is low, the disease affects an elderly population that is more likely to have other chronic and lethal illnesses. The period of survival after diagnosis is extremely variable; the presence of uremia and hypercalcemia are the worst prognostic signs. Neither the immunoglobulin type nor the height of the M spike is predictive of survival time.

BIBLIOGRAPHY

DeFronzo RA, Cooke CR, Wright JR et al: Renal function in patients with multiple myeloma. Medicine 57:151–166, 1978

Kyle RA: Multiple myeloma: Review of 869 cases. Mayo Clin Proc 50:29–40, 1975

Kyle RA: Monoclonal gammopathy of undetermined significance. Am J Med 64:814–826, 1978

Kyle, RA, Greippe PR: The laboratory investigation of monoclonal gammopathies. Mayo Clin Proc 53:719–739, 1978

49

Management of the Oncology Patient: Electrolyte Imbalances

Opportunistic infection, thrombocytopenic hemorrhage, and major electrolyte imbalances are among the most serious problems complicating the care of the hospitalized oncology patient. Recent refinements in antibiotic, antifungal, and antiviral therapy (Chap. 58), combined with new techniques for harvesting and transfusing leukocytes and platelets (Chap. 44) have recently begun to make inroads in the management of the first two problems. The tools for treating the electrolyte disorders, however, have, in large part, been available and familiar to physicians for several years. Nevertheless, significant morbidity and mortality still result from electrolyte imbalances, often because they are not anticipated and thus not recognized and treated. Electrolyte homeostasis in malignant disease can be upset by metastatic disease invading endocrine organs, by humoral substances released by the tumor, by treatment of the tumor, and by other as yet unexplained "distant effects."

CELL LYSIS

The phenomenon of massive cell lysis is usually observed in hematologic malignancy, particularly acute lymphoblastic leukemia and Burkitt's lymphoma. Although, on rare occasions, lysis may occur spontaneously in masses of leukemic cells, it is more often a consequence of antineoplastic chemotherapy. As the bulk of tumor cells dies, their intracellular ions—urate, phosphate, and potassium—are released into the circulation.

Hyperuricemia. Serum uric acid, an end-product of nucleotide metabolism, is often mildly elevated even before cytotoxic therapy is begun, because of the rapid turnover of cancerous cells. With cell lysis, uric acid levels can skyrocket to 20 to 30 mg/dl. The major danger of hyperuricemia to these patients is acute renal failure; acute gouty arthritis, on the other hand, is extremely rare. Fortunately, the nephropathy is reversible if the hyperuricemia is treated expeditiously. Renal dysfunction is believed to be caused by the precipitation of uric acid crystals in the distal tubules and collecting ducts. Diuresis may help to prevent tubular blockage.

Preventive measures should be taken prior to the administration of chemotherapy. Allopurinol, a competitive inhibitor of xanthine oxidase, decreases the synthesis of uric acid and should be given in relatively high doses. Allopurinol metabolites may themselves, however, form renal precipitates. The administration of sodium bicarbonate helps to maintain the urine in an akaline state and thereby increases the solubility of urate. Adequate diuresis must be maintained by fluid administration or by the use of loop diuretics or mannitol. If renal failure supervenes, peritoneal dialysis may ultimately become necessary.

Hyperphosphatemia. Massive cellular lysis can lead to the release of significant amounts of phosphate. The increased phosphate levels may cause symptomatic hypocalcemia, or lead to the ectopic precipitaton of calcium phosphate. Treatment consists of oral aluminum-hydroxide which will bind phosphate and prevent its intestinal absorbtion.

Hyperkalemia. During cell lysis, large amounts of potassium can be released into the extracellular space. If hyperkalemia occurs a patient with uric acid nephropathy, lethal levels of potassium may be reached before effective treatment can be instituted.

One must be careful in evaluating hyperkalemia associated with leukemia and other myeloproliferative states. When the blood sample clots or when the cells are not quickly separated from the serum, the malignant white blood cells and platelets can rupture (or undergo an increase in cell membrane permeability) and extrude potassium into the serum. All cells are rich in intracellular potassium. When the white blood cell count is greater than 100,000 or when the platelet count is greater than one million, there may be an elevation of the measured serum potassium. This phenomenon is called "pseudohyperkalemia." It can be verified by immediately analyzing a heparinized specimen of blood and finding a normal potassium concentration.

Hyperkalemia can appear very rarely in patients with solid tumors when metastatic invasion of the adrenal glands is extensive enough to cause Addison's disease.

HYPERCALCEMIA

Malignant disease is the principal cause of significant hypercalcemia in the hospitalized population. Tumors of the breast, lung, kidney, head, and neck are most frequently associated with an elevation in the serum calcium. Hematologic malignancies, especially multiple myeloma, have also been seen in conjunction with hypercalcemia. The symptomatology depends upon the rate of rise of the serum calcium, the presence of pre-existing renal disease, and the general physical health of the patient. Weakness, lethargy, polyuria, polydipsia, and anorexia predominate, but mental changes and, eventually, coma supervene in the absence of therapy.

The pathogenesis of hypercalcemia in cancer is multifactorial:

1. Bony metastases are seen in the majority of patients, and the mechanical pressure of the metastases may cause local resorption of bone mineral with the consequent release of calcium phosphate. In addition, multiple myeloma may produce a locally acting osteolytic polypeptide called *osteoclast activating factor.*

2. A tumor may produce parathyroid hormone or a peptide with similar properties. Ectopic parathyroid hormone is only rarely the cause of hypercalcemia. The finding of increased parathyroid hormone and hypercalcemia in a patient with a malignancy should therefore raise the possibility that the patient has primary hyperparathyroidism in addition to malignant disease.

3. Prostaglandins, presumably produced by certain tumors, stimulate bone resorption, and increased prostaglandin levels are responsible for hypercalcemia in some patients with solid tumors, especially renal cell carcinomas. Indomethacin, an inhibitor of prostaglandin

synthesis, may effectively lower the serum calcium in this setting.

Several factors aggravate hypercalcemia in cancer patients. Thus, for example, prolonged bed rest or immobilization results in bone resorption. The androgenic steroids used in the treatment of breast tumors can enhance hypercalcemia. Polyuria, secondary to the ADH resistant diabetes insipidus of hypercalcemia, in conjunction with anorexia, nausea, and lethargy, makes these patients susceptible to dehydration, which increases the serum calcium and thus results in a vicious circle.

Hypercalcemia is usually defined as a total serum calcium of 10.5 mg/dl or greater. However, although calcium is heavily bound to albumin, it is the unbound (ionized) calcium that is biologically active. Many patients with advanced carcinomas are cachectic and have decreased levels of serum albumin. As a result, the total serum calcium may be normal or even low, whereas the ionized calcium may be elevated. In hypoalbuminemic patients, the normal range of serum calcium must therefore be adjusted downward approximately 0.8 mg/dl of calcium for each 1.0 gram/dl of albumin below normal (4.0 g/dl).

Therapy. In-hospital management of severe symptomatic hypercalcemia (hypercalcemic crisis) is usually successful. Ambulation, if possible, should be encouraged. Intravenous normal saline in large amounts can replete the intravascular volume and initiate calciuresis. Furosemide may be required to maintain the diuresis; furosemide also promotes the urinary loss of calcium. Because potassium stores may already be depleted by the hypercalcemia and because saline and furosemide diuresis further augments urinary potassium losses, potassium replacement should be initiated early. Serum magnesium may also be low in malnourished patients, and it may not be possible to achieve normal potassium levels until magnesium stores are repleted.

Mithramycin, an antineoplastic antibiotic that inhibits RNA synthesis, should be tried if diuretics and saline fail to lower the serum calcium or if hypercalcemia recurs. By disrupting osteoclast activity, the drug reduces the serum calcium within 36 to 48 hours and maintains it at that level for up to two weeks. Mithramycin may cause thrombocytopenia, especially after repeated doses.

Glucocorticoids also have a hypocalcemic effect. They increase urinary calcium excretion and decrease the movement of calcium from the bone, but their effect may not be apparent for several days. *Salmon calcitonin* is an effective drug, but its action is not sustained and declines with repeated use. The simultaneous administration of glucocorticoids and calcitonin may result in a more prolonged decrease in the serum calcium than the use of either agent by itself. A trial of the prostaglandin inhibitor, *indomethacin*, may also be instituted, but it should be accompanied by antacids or cimetidine because of the risk of gastric hemorrhage; hypercalcemia itself is also considered a risk factor for peptic ulcer disease.

Once the patient's hypercalcemia has stabilized, outpatient control can be maintained by glucocorticoids or inorganic phosphate preparations. *Phosphate* enhances calcium deposition in bone and stimulates extracellular precipitation of calcium phosphate; however, there is the risk of further renal compromise by causing calcium phosphate to precipitate within the kidney.

OTHER ELECTROLYTE DISTURBANCES

Hypokalemia. Hypokalemia is seen in approximately one-third of patients with leukemia. In general, hypokalemia is due to a kaliuresis which reflects, in many instances, a generalized defect of tubular function. A

Fanconi-like syndrome, with aminoaciduria, glucosuria, and hyperphosphaturia has been variously attributed to direct renal parenchymal invasion by the leukemic cells and to increases in serum lysozyme, which may be toxic to the renal tubules. Therapy of hypercalcemia with saline and diuretics also causes a kaliuresis and may cause hypokalemia.

Hyponatremia. In many instances, hyponatremia derives from coexistent SIADH caused by ectopic secretion of antidiuretic hormone, ADH (see Chap. 26). The antineoplastic drugs vincristine and cyclophosphamide are also associated with SIADH.

Others. Other metabolic changes seen in malignancy include hypoglycemia, Cushing's syndrome, and the lactic acidosis of terminal widely metastatic cancer. Although aggressive therapy of these metabolic disorders may not be appropriate in severely cachectic or dying patients, successful treatment of these metabolic imbalances may increase the patient's comfort, and in some instances may allow the patient to survive the critical intervals of curative or palliative chemotherapy.

BIBLIOGRAPHY

Besarab A, Caro JF: Mechanisms of hypercalcemia in malignancy. Cancer 41:2276–2285, 1978

Binstock, ML, Mundy GR: Effect of calcitonin and glucocorticoids in combination on the hypercalcemia of malignancy. Ann Intern Med 93:269–272, 1980

Bronson WR, DeVita VT, Carbone PP et al: Pseudohyperkalemia due to release of potassium from white blood cells during clotting, N Engl J Med 274:369–375, 1966

Myers WPL: Differential diagnosis of hypercalcemia and cancer. CA 27:258–272, 1977

O'Regan S, Carson S, Chesney RW et al: Electrolyte and acid-base disturbances in the management of leukemia. Blood 49:345–353, 1977

Skrabanek P, McPartlin J, Powell D: Tumor hypercalcemia and "ectopic hyperparathyroidism." Medicine 59:262–282, 1980

Infectious Disease

50

Septic Shock

The prototypical patient with septic shock is the elderly male who becomes febrile following a urologic procedure. His blood pressure falls, but his skin becomes flushed. This peripheral vasodilatation distinguishes septic shock from shock due to hemorrhage or massive heart attack. If the patient is untreated or refractory to treatment, his blood pressure continues to fall and his skin becomes clammy. He becomes dyspneic, and a chest x-ray shows mottling with evidence of what has come to be referred to as "shock lung" (see Chap. 12). Myocardial and renal function swiftly deteriorate, and approximately 50% of such patients die.

It was hoped that with the advent of antibiotics the almost inevitably fatal outcome of septic shock might be averted. This has not proven to be true. The nature of septic shock has altered considerably, in part a result of the widespread use of antibiotics and because of technologic and pharmacologic innovations that have permitted patients to survive previously fatal illnesses, although often in a severely debilitated state.

THE ORGANISM

In the prepenicillin era, gram-positive organisms were responsible for most cases of septic shock. Today, about two-thirds of episodes of septic shock are due to virulent strains of gram-negative bacteria, most commonly E. coli, Klebsiella, Enterobacteriaceae, Serratia, and Pseudomonas. Gram-negative bacteremias appear to progress to shock more often than gram-positive bacteremias. The incidence of anaerobic and polymicrobial bacteremias is also increasing.

The appearance of these new organisms seems to be due to several factors:

1. The widespread and often careless dispensing of antibiotics

2. The introduction of these organisms into the host by new surgical procedures and by indwelling urinary, venous, and arterial catheters

3. The increasing number of elderly patients whose lives are being prolonged despite the presence of multisystem disease, and whose immune systems are often compromised by underlying illness or by corticosteroid or cytotoxic therapy.

It is not clear that bacteremia is the *sine qua non* for septic shock. Septic shock can occur with apparently localized infections. The negative blood cultures in such patients suggest either that the bacteremia is intermittent and the blood drawing ill-timed, or, more likely, that bacterial debris alone can be responsible for shock. In order to investigate this question, researchers have utilized a lysate of the blood cells of the horseshoe crab, limulus. This lysate gels upon exposure to the endotoxin component of gram-negative bacterial walls. It was hoped that this technique could be used to identify a subset of patients with endotoxemia without bacteremia, but frequent false-positive and false-negative results have left the limulus test with few proponents.

The state of host resistance profoundly affects susceptibility to sepsis and the nature of the offending organisms. *Hemophilus influenzae* and pneumococcal sepsis appear to be more frequent in patients who have undergone splenectomy. Sepsis with gram-negative or opportunistic organisms occurs in patients neutropenic from leukemia or cytotoxic therapy. In patients with severe burns, local thrombosis prevents the access of phagocytic cells to sites of infection and enhances susceptibility to sepsis. Local factors, such as the neuropathy of diabetes and the impaired mucociliary and glottic function following ethanol ingestion, combined with various chemotactic abnormalities, predispose to bacteremia in diabetics and alcoholics. Cirrhotic patients with ascites are prone to spontaneous peritonitis and bacteremia, often with E. coli or pneumococci. Surgery is frequently the precipitating event in sepsis, especially urethral manipulation, bowel surgery, and organ transplantation.

PATHOLOGY

Postmortem examination of a patient who has died of septic shock often reveals evidence of only a localized infection. In some immunosuppressed patients, even this is lacking. Evidence of disseminated intravascular coagulation, with diffuse thrombotic occlusion of small vessels and glomerular capillaries, may frequently be found in patients dying of septic complications of obstetric surgery. Occasionally, a mild intrahepatic bile stasis may be present; this may underlie the conjugated hyper-bilirubinemia and mild alkaline phosphatase and transaminase elevations found in some patients with septic shock. The lungs are often soggy and congested, exhibiting a nonspecific "shock lung" pathology. Other organs manifest focal necrosis and evidence of hypoperfusion.

PATHOPHYSIOLOGY

The body has two major defenses to limit bacteremia and its complications: (1) The reticuloendothelial system, with the mediation of the complement system, ingests invading organisms; (2) antibodies are produced against the organism. Of the latter, probably the most important are antitoxins that bind the endotoxin and block its activity.

The complement cascade can be activated either by antigen-antibody complexes or directly by the antigen through the properdin pathway. The complement cleavage fragments C3a and C5a release histamine from mast cells. Histamine may be partly responsible for the arteriolar vasodilatation seen in septic shock and histamine also makes the microcirculation leakier; plasma is lost into the interstitium, producing hemoconcentration and intravascular volume depletion.

Bacterial endotoxin activates the plasma kinin system through its interaction with granulocyte and plasma kallikrein. Kallikrein splits kininogen to bradykinin, a powerful vasodilator.

Activated Hageman factor initiates the clotting and fibrinolytic cascades. Fibrin degradation products appear in the serum, even when pathologic evidence of disseminated intravascular coagulation (DIC) is lacking.

White blood cells and platelets are lysed directly and as innocent bystanders, and they release their store of lysozomal enzymes and serotonin into the circulation. Granulocytopenia and thrombocytopenia may result and may also be caused by bone marrow suppression.

ORGAN SYSTEMS IN SEPTIC SHOCK

The result of all the elaborate biochemical activity discussed above is the first stage of septic shock, the warm stage. Vasodilatation reduces peripheral resistance. As a result, the cardiac output is high and the pulse bounding. Because of a reflex attempt to maintain an adequate blood pressure, the patient is tachycardic. Volume depletion, a result of vascular leakage into the interstitium, is reflected in low central venous and pulmonary capillary wedge pressures.

Blood is shunted past the tissues, oxygen is not extracted, and the A-VO$_2$ difference is narrowed. This is in contrast to the vasoconstricted state of hemorrhagic and cardiogenic shock, in which the venous oxygen concentrations are low and the A-VO$_2$ difference (the difference between arterial and mixed venous blood oxygen saturation) is high. Different vascular beds suffer to different degrees. Those affected most adversely by the shunting are unable to continue oxidative metabolism. Anaerobic metabolism supervenes and the cellular pH drops as lactic acid is produced. A metabolic acidosis of less than 7.10 reduces myocardial contractility and responsiveness to catecholamines.

The warm stage of shock is also accompanied by a respiratory alkalosis. Hyperventilation may be secondary to the stiff lungs of early pulmonary edema (endotoxin causes the bronchial venules to leak protein and water) or to the central nervous system effects of endotoxin.

The patient is generally febrile, warm to the touch, and tachycardic. Blood pressure is usu-ally maintained, but the central venous pressure is low. The respiratory alkalosis is usually more marked than the cellular metabolic acidosis, and the blood pH is therefore alkalotic. The white blood cell count is variable, and the clotting, fibrinolytic, complement, and kinin systems are activated.

As long as the cardiac output is maintained at the levels required by the febrile septic state—often two to three times the basal state—the prognosis is good. However, diminishing cardiac output eventually leads to organ failure. As the intravascular volume falls, the venous return becomes inadequate to maintain the cardiac output. In addition, the myocardium begins to fail; this is thought to be caused by a circulating *myocardial depressant factor* that is released by the pancreas. As the blood pressure falls, evidence of catecholamine activity becomes apparent: blood vessels constrict and the patient becomes cold, clammy, restless, and oliguric. The lungs stiffen and cyanosis ensues. Death from refractory metabolic acidosis becomes almost certain.

THERAPY

Immediate surgical intervention is mandatory if there are surgically remediable lesions: septic sites that are the source of infection, including abscess cavities and incomplete abortions, must be drained and necrotic and infected tissues, such as infarcted bowel, must be removed.

Treatment with large volumes of saline and colloid increases the venous return and the cardiac index. Many liters of fluid may be required, and the central venous pressure is often an inadequate guide to the function of the left ventricle. The pulmonary capillary wedge pressure should, therefore, be used as a guide to careful titration of volume replacement, allowing one to maximize the stroke volume and minimize the likelihood of iatrogenic pulmonary edema. If the blood pressure continues to fall despite fluid replacement and correction of metabolic acidosis with bicarbonate, sympathomimetic amines should be administered. Dopamine, because of its cardiotonic and renal arterial dilating properties, is currently the drug of choice.

Cultures should be obtained and antibiotic therapy should commence immediately, even if no etiologic diagnosis is available. In the immunosuppressed patient or in the patient in whom the source of sepsis is unknown, broad antibiotic coverage often includes (1) a penicillinase-resistant penicillin or a cephalosporin, (2) an aminoglycoside, such as gentamicin, and (3) carbenicillin. Carbenicillin is particularly important in patients with burns, who are highly susceptible to infections with Pseudomonas.

Treatment of a patient with intra-abdominal sepsis often includes an aminoglycoside for coverage of gram-negative coliform organisms, and chloramphenicol or clindamycin to protect against anaerobic infections (such as *Bacteroides fragilis*) that may cause local abscess formation. Some feel that a penicillin should also be used to protect against enterococci and clostridia. These organisms are frequently isolated from the blood of septic patients, but their importance in the pathogenesis of septic shock is still undetermined.

The treatment of urinary tract infections is discussed in Chapter 55, and the treatment of pulmonary infections in Chapter 52.

The use of massive doses of glucocorticoids has long been advocated to stabilize lysozomal membranes and reduce the permeability of the microcirculation. Recent studies support their clinical utility.

BIBLIOGRAPHY

Elin RJ, Wolff, SM: Biology of endotoxin. Ann Rev Med 27:127–141, 1976

Kreger B, Craven D, Carling P et al: Gram negative bacteremia. Am J Med 68:332–343, 1980

Lillehei RC, Longerbeam JK, Bloch JH et al: The nature of irreversible shock. Ann Surg 160:682–710, 1964

McHenry MD, Baggenstoss AH, Martin WJ: Bacteremia due to gram negative bacilli. Am J Clin Path 50:160–174, 1968

McKenna V, Meadows JA, Brewer N et al: Toxic shock syndrome: A newly recognized disease entity. Mayo Clin Proc 55:663–672, 1980

Schumer W: Steroids in the treatment of clinical-septic shock. Ann Surg 184:333–341, 1976

Shine K: Aspects of the management of shock. Ann Intern Med 93:723–734, 1980

Winslow EJ, Loeb HS, Rahimtoola S et al: Hemodynamic studies and results of therapy in 50 patients with bacteremic shock. Am J Med 54:421–432, 1973

Wolff SM: Biological effects of bacterial endotoxins in man. J Infect Dis 128 (Suppl):S259–S264, 1973

51

Infectious Meningitis

Although it is overwhelmingly a disease of young children, infectious meningitis also affects adults, especially the elderly and the debilitated. Approximately 1 out of every 1000 hospital admissions is for infectious meningitis. The overall mortality has declined sharply since the introduction of antibiotics, but the mortality rate for patients over 60 years old has shown little or no improvement.

The most common cause of infectious meningitis in the adult population is the pneumococcus. *Neisseria meningitidis* (the meningococcus) and *Hemophilus influenzae* are also frequently implicated as, with increasing frequency, are gram-negative organisms and fungi. The tuberculous bacillus remains a common cause of chronic meningitis.

PATHOPHYSIOLOGY

Meningitis is an infection of the pia and arachnoid meninges. The subarachnoid space, which separates the two membranes, contains cerebrospinal fluid (CSF) and is continuous from the cerebrum to the spinal cord. Organisms can infect the CSF and spread over the full extent of the meninges. Leukocytes migrate out of the inflamed meningeal vessels, producing a purulent exudate that covers the meninges and later the spinal and cranial nerves. If treatment is delayed, fibrosis of the membranes may cause adhesions to form between the pia and the arachnoid meninges that can block the subarachnoid space and produce hydrocephalus or permanent nerve damage.

Organisms reach the meninges in a variety of ways: by way of the bloodstream in septic patients with, for example, pneumonia or endocarditis, by direct invasion from cranial trauma or neurosurgery, or indirectly from parameningeal infections, such as sinusitis, mastoiditis, or otitis.

DIAGNOSIS

The presenting signs and symptoms of meningitis depend upon the route of infection, the etiologic organism, the age of the patient, and the presence of any underlying disease. Classically, the patient with meningitis complains of severe headache, a stiff neck, fever, and, occasionally, photophobia. In the elderly, however, the disease may cause only confusion and disorientation; fever may be minimal and nuchal rigidity absent. The diagnosis of meningitis must therefore be entertained in any elderly patient who presents with altered mental status.

Patients can present in coma, with focal neurologic signs, or with seizures. Focal signs may indicate an abscess, or they may occur transiently after a seizure (Todd's paralysis). Meningitis can therefore be confused with a cerebrovascular accident.

Nuchal rigidity is a striking physical sign that reflects the underlying inflammation of the pia and arachnoid membranes around the pain-sensitive spinal nerves and roots. The patient attempts to shorten and immobolize the spine, avoiding the added meningeal irritation caused by stretching. Forced neck flexion in a patient with meningitis results in flexion at the knee and hip (Brudzinski's sign). Pain in the back and hamstring muscles can be elicited by extending the knee with the thigh at right angles to the trunk (Kernig's sign). The presence of a characteristic rash suggests the possibility of meningococcal meningitis (discussion later).

Cerebrospinal Fluid

Examination of the CSF is obviously of utmost importance in the diagnosis and treatment of patients with meningitis. The only absolute contraindication to a lumbar puncture (LP) is a skin infection or subdural abscess directly over the LP site (L1–L4); it may then be necessary to obtain ventricular CSF.

Thrombocytopenia and hypoprothrombinemia should be corrected prior to LP. It may also be prudent to delay a lumbar puncture when papilledema or focal neurologic signs suggest an intracranial mass rather than meningitis, since a lumbar puncture may then very rarely result in herniation; an emergency CT scan should be obtained first in a patient with these signs. Skull x-rays have also been used to diagnose an intracerebral mass by revealing a shift of the calcified pineal from the midline. This sign is extremely unreliable, and the CT scan is now the most accurate and preferred method for evaluating intracranial lesions.

In order to obtain CSF, a small needle (21- or 23-gauge) should be inserted at L2–L3, and if the opening pressure is markedly elevated, a minimal amount of CSF should be removed. Some authorities have recommended a mannitol infusion if the CSF pressure is abnormally high, but such hypertonic solutions present a danger of late rebound intracranial hypertension. In infectious meningitis, the CSF pressure is nearly always elevated, but papilledema is infrequent, possibly because of the short duration of the increased pressure. The CSF should be routinely cultured for bacteria, tuberculosis, and fungi. A CSF cell count and differential should be performed, and protein and glucose levels (along with a simultaneous blood glucose) should be obtained. A Gram stain, Ziehl-Neelsen stain, and an India ink preparation (to detect the cryptococcus) should be prepared on the sediment in all cases; however, studies have revealed that the Gram stain is positive only when the concentration of bacteria exceeds 100,000 colony-forming units per milliliter. In some institutions, countercurrent immunoelectrophoresis has been used as a rapid detector of bacterial antigens in the CSF. Ancillary studies include skull x-rays to detect trauma, sinus films to diagnose a parameningeal focus, and chest x-rays. Blood cultures are mandatory.

CSF profiles have been delineated to aid in the differential diagnosis of meningitis. Normal CSF contains fewer than 5 leukocytes per cubic millimeter; these are usually all mononuclear cells. The protein content is less than 40 to 50 milligrams per deciliter, essentially all of it albumin, and the CSF glucose is usually 50% to 60% that of a simultaneous blood glucose.

In purulent meningitis, the CSF reveals

polymorphonuclear leukocytes, an elevated protein, and a decreased glucose (less than 40% of a blood glucose; note that the CSF level might appear to be abnormally high in a hyperglycemic patient). Most cases of bacterial meningitis present in this way, but just as meningitis can present with clinical signs suggestive of a cerebrovascular accident, a stroke patient may on rare occasions have a CSF profile suggestive of acute meningitis. In the stroke patient, the CSF pleiocytosis (white blood counts occasionally exceeding 1,000 per cubic millimeter) represents a reaction to cerebral infarction and peaks four days after the stroke, usually returning to normal within a week. Unfortunately, there is usually no way to resolve this differential diagnosis in the absence of positive gram stains or culture, and these stroke patients must be treated with antibiotics until the cultures are declared negative.

The diagnosis of tuberculous or fungal meningitis should be considered empirically when the CSF reveals a lymphocytic pleiocytosis and decreased glucose. The protein may be normal or slightly elevated. The clinician should be aware that a partially treated bacterial infection may present with a similar profile.

The so-called aseptic profile is commonly seen in viral meningitis or encephalitis. It includes a lymphocytic leukocytosis, a normal CSF sugar, and a normal or only slightly elevated CSF protein. It is important to remember that diabetics and patients suffering from cerebrovascular disease or chronic alcoholism may have a chronically increased CSF protein; unlike patients with meningitis, they have no pleiocytosis.

Causes of Meningitis

Pneumococcal meningitis is the most common form of bacterial meningitis in the adult. It has a sudden onset, and if untreated has a rapid downhill course. Mortality in the pre-

antibiotic era was virtually 100%, and it still remains high. Approximately one-half of all patients present either in coma or with seizures. Parameningeal foci are common. An associated pneumococcal pneumonia is frequently present; the serotypes that most often cause pneumonia are the same ones most frequently found in meningitis. It is therefore possible that the incidence of pneumococcal meningitis will decline if the elderly population is vaccinated against the pneumococcus. Poor prognostic factors in pneumococcal meningitis include old age, the presence of associated diseases, the severity of the meningitis (reflected in a decreased CSF glucose and increased CSF protein), and altered mental status. The extent of the CSF leukocytosis correlates with survival. Neurologic residua, especially deafness, seizure disorders, and pareses are not uncommon.

Meningococcal meningitis is frequently associated with cohort groupings of military recruits. A characteristic skin lesion is seen in 50% of patients. This is a fleeting maculopapular rash that becomes petechial and eventually purpuric. Similar lesions may be caused by staphylococcal septicemia and viral illnesses, especially ECHO virus. The lesions should be scraped and a Gram stain and culture performed, but it is unlikely that meningococcemia will be diagnosed in this manner. Gram stain of a buffy coat smear occasionally demonstrates the characteristic gram-negative cocci. Poor prognostic signs include shock, leukopenia, the early appearance of the rash, and a low or normal erythrocyte sedimentation rate.

Hemophilus influenzae is a common cause of childhood meningitis. Its presence in an adult suggests spread from a parameningeal focus.

Gram-negative meningitis is often seen after trauma or surgery and is being found with increasing frequency in older patients with chronic diseases. At the Detroit Medical Center, *E. coli meningitis* was seen in chronic alcoholics who were on drinking sprees. Both bacteremia and pyuria were frequent associated findings.

In the immunocompromised patient, *cryptococcal* and *listerial meningitides* are common. Cryptococcal meningitis can be diagnosed by an India ink preparation of the CSF, but in practice this is quite difficult, and a culture diagnosis must usually be relied upon. Listeria must be distinguished from diphtheroids.

Tuberculous meningitis is a subacute illness that often presents with cranial nerve involvement. The basal meninges are commonly involved. Although a lymphocytic CSF pleiocytosis is the rule, polymorphonuclear leukocytes can be seen early in the course of disease. Active tuberculosis, especially pulmonary tuberculosis, is usually present. After a bacteremic phase, the meninges are seeded with tubercles that subsequently rupture into the subarachnoid space.

Aseptic or *viral meningitis* is extremely common. The CSF shows a lymphocytic leukocytosis with normal glucose and a normal or slightly elevated protein. No organisms are seen on Gram stain, and cultures are negative. A typical history of an antecedent viral syndrome followed by headache, fever, meningeal signs, and photophobia is frequently elicited. Rashes are common and alterations in consciousness are very mild. Mumps, coxsackievirus, and echoviruses are among the agents most frequently implicated in the syndrome. Hepatitis B may have a meningitic phase prior to the evolution of jaundice.

THERAPY

Therapy for pneumococcal and meningococcal disease consists of high-dose intravenous penicillin. In healthy persons, penicillin does not cross into the CSF, but it passes through inflamed meninges with ease, achieving therapeutic levels when approximately 20 million units per day are given.

Prophylaxis against the meningococcus is required for close household contacts and for medical personnel who have had prolonged contact with the patient (*e.g.*, those who have performed mouth-to-mouth resuscitation). Casual contacts do not need to be treated. Rifampin is an effective prophylactic agent against the meningococcus.

Ampicillin is generally an effective agent against *Hemophilus influenzae*. Cephalosporins do not effectively cross the blood brain barrier even in meningitis and are generally not used to treat meningitis. Chloramphenicol achieves excellent CSF levels and is the drug of choice in patients with penicillin allergy or who have an ampicillin-resistant strain of hemophilus. When gram-negative rods are seen on a CSF Gram stain, intrathecal or intraventricular administration of aminoglycosides may be required.

When bacterial meningitis is suspected, but no organisms are seen on Gram stain, most authorities recommend high-dose penicillin with or without chloramphenicol pending culture results.

After appropriate therapy has been initiated, fever and neurologic signs may persist for several days. After one or two days of treatment, the lumbar puncture should be repeated. While the CSF may still show a leukocytosis and increased protein, no organisms should be found on Gram stain or by culture. Treatment must continue until the patient has been afebrile for five to seven days. Slow resolution of neurologic signs may indicate formation of a brain abscess or intracranial thrombophlebitis. However, dramatic neurologic changes, such as bilateral nerve deafness, may occur suddenly, even during adequate and proper treatment of purulent meningitis. The high-dose penicillin therapy itself may cause seizures.

Patients may require adequate narcotic analgesia for the often severe headache accompanying meningitis. They must be adequately hydrated, and since meningitis is very often associated with inappropriate ADH secretion, electrolytes must be carefully scrutinized daily.

In patients with tuberculous meningitis, acid-fast bacteria are frequently not found on the Ziehl-Neelsen preparation of the CSF, and it is usually necessary to make a presumptive diagnosis and treat accordingly. Isoniazid readily crosses into the CSF and is the mainstay of therapy. Rifampin is usually added, and a three-drug regimen, utilizing either ethambutal or streptomycin, is employed. Ethambutol and streptomycin pass through the meninges only when they are inflamed, and are therefore effective only in the first few weeks of therapy. Corticosteroids may help attenuate cerebral edema, but there is little evidence that mortality is decreased. Although nearly all patients, including those with advanced disease, survive with proper chemotherapy, a large proportion suffer hemiparesis or other permanent neurologic sequelae.

Aseptic meningitis is generally a benign disorder. Treatment is symptomatic, but in some cases a repeat lumbar puncture within 24 hours is prudent to rule out an evolving bacterial infection. Parameningeal infections and inadequately treated bacterial infections can present with an aseptic CSF profile. The clinician should be aware that an aseptic profile may be caused by organisms that are difficult to isolate; such organisms include the tubercle bacillus, the cryptococcus, and *Treponema pallidum* (syphilis). CNS leukemia can also present as aseptic meningitis.

BIBLIOGRAPHY

Berk SL: Meningitis caused by gram-negative bacilli. Ann Intern Med 93:253–260, 1980

Crane LC, Lerner AM: Non-traumatic gram-negative bacillary meningitis in the Detroit Medical Center. Medicine 57:197–209, 1978

Finland M, Barnes MW: Acute bacterial meningitis at Boston City Hospital during 12 selected years, 1935–1972. J Infect Dis 136:400–415, 1977

Swartz MN, Dodge PR: Bacterial meningitis: A review of selected aspects. N Engl J Med 272:725–731, 779–787, 842–848, 898–902, 954–960, 1003–1110, 1965

Weiss W, Figueroa W, Shapiro WH et al: Prognostic factors in pneumococcal meningitis. Arch Intern Med 120:517–524, 1967

52

Acute Infectious Diseases of the Lung: Pneumonia and Acute Bronchitis

An acute lower respiratory infection should be suspected in any patient who develops fever, cough, and respiratory symptoms including dyspnea, sputum production, or chest pain. Unfortunately, there are certain patients with respiratory tract disease who do not display these features. Elderly patients, for example, frequently have few localizing symptoms, and present solely with nonspecific complaints such as confusion. Other patients may present in septic shock.

Respiratory infections are common, and any patient presenting with global deterioration or an exacerbation of an underlying illness (such as congestive heart failure or diabetes) should be investigated for an occult pulmonary infection.

Two types of acute lower respiratory infections are recognized: tracheobronchitis and pneumonia. Their symptoms overlap, and they can be difficult to distinguish purely by history and presenting symptomatology. Occasionally, a physical examination reveals lung consolidation or other evidence of pneumonia, but the key to diagnosis is the chest x-ray. A lower respiratory infection *with* x-ray changes in the lung fields is called a pneumonia; a lower respiratory infection *without* x-ray changes is called a bronchitis. This is a clinical and not a pathologic distinction. Pathologically, a pneumonia represents an infection with consequent inflammation of lung parenchyma (the air spaces and/or alveolar interstitium). A bronchitis represents inflammation of the large airways. If the bronchitic process persists chronically, there may be bronchial thickening and dilatation (bronchiectasis), which may be visible on a chest x-ray.

ACUTE BRONCHITIS

The presentation and course of bronchitis depends to a great extent upon whether underlying lung disease is present. In patients *without* underlying lung disease, bronchitis is usually a viral disease. It is a common presentation of patients with influenza, and is also seen with adenovirus and parainfluenza infections. A prodrome of contitutional symptoms—fever, malaise, myalgias, weakness, and headache—is followed by the development of upper respiratory symptoms, including rhinorrhea and pharyngitis. Chills and rigors may accompany the fever. Within several days, symptoms of lower respiratory tract involvement appear: a nonproductive cough and, frequently, retrosternal pain that is exacerbated by coughing or breathing. These symptoms may persist for a week after the fever has disappeared. Patients generally do not experience dyspnea or respiratory compromise.

In patients *with* underlying lung disease, viral bronchitis is often associated with respiratory deterioration. If the patient's baseline pulmonary function is poor, even a mild infection can precipitate respiratory failure. Patients with chronic lung disease are particularly susceptible to bacterial (or purulent) bronchitis.

Streptococcus pneumoniae (pneumococcus) is responsible for most cases of purulent bronchitis. *Hemophilus influenzae* is also common in patients with chronic obstructive pulmonary disease. In hospitalized patients, especially in those who have taken antibiotics for other reasons, staphylococcus and pseudomonas must be suspected. These latter infections can be especially difficult to eliminate, and pseudomonas bronchitis tends to relapse and persist for months.

Penicillin is the drug of choice for pneumococcal bronchitis. For patients with chronic obstructive pulmonary disease, in whom the incidence of *Hemophilus influenzae* is high, and whenever a Gram stain suggests the possibility of *Hemophilus influenzae*, ampicillin is the drug of choice. When cultures grow staphylococcus or pseudomonas, culture sensitivities will dictate the choice of drugs. Bronchospasm can be significant in patients with bronchitis, and may respond to bronchodilators (Chap. 15).

PNEUMONIA

There are three major types of pneumonias: viral, mycoplasmal, and bacterial. Each is marked by a distinctive symptomatology and course. More exotic causes of pneumonia are usually opportunistic and restricted to immunosuppressed patients. These include fungal infections and infection with *Pneumocystis carinii*.

Viral Pneumonia

Viral pneumonia is usually caused by influenza virus or adenovirus, and typically occurs in community epidemics. The virus spreads from person to person by droplet infections. One to three days after exposure, the new host rapidly evolves a flu-like syndrome with the same symptoms that precede bronchitis. This nonspecific syndrome progresses to pneumonia in up to 5% of affected individuals.

Pneumonia develops one to two days after the generalized symptoms begin. The predominant symptoms are cough and dyspnea. The cough is generally nonproductive, but later in the course a more purulent sputum, representing the sloughing of damaged epithelium, may be produced. No organisms prevail on Gram stain. Patients are hypoxemic, the alveolar-arterial oxygen gradient is elevated, and inspired oxygen frequently fails to correct the hypoxemia, suggesting that shunting of blood past unventilated alveoli may be the cause of the patient's hypoxemia. Patients rarely experience pleuritic chest pain, but cough-related musculoskeletal pain or tracheal pain is not infrequent. The physical examination is generally unremarkable, and rales are usually the only significant finding. Pleural effusions can be seen, but lung consolidation is distinctly unusual.

Within a week, the symptoms usually subside and the fever resolves. Several more weeks pass before the patient feels entirely normal.

Some patients do not recover uneventfully, but develop severe respiratory compromise or failure. The full picture of the adult respiratory distress syndrome may evolve (ARDS, see Chap. 12). Mortality in this group is high.

Many of these patients have underlying respiratory and cardiac disease, and many are elderly. Women in the third trimester of pregnancy are also susceptible to this complication.

Mycoplasmal Pneumonia

Mycoplasmal pneumonia accounts for over one-fourth of community-acquired pneumonias. *Mycoplasma pneumoniae* is a primary respiratory pathogen, but only 10% of mycoplasmal infections produce pneumonia. It is generally a disease of the young, and the incidence declines after the age of 30 to 35. There is often no evidence of epidemic spreads throughout a community, but frequently there is a strong family history of recent infection. The transmission rate among family members may be as high as 40%.

The onset of mycoplasmal pneumonia is more indolent than that of viral pneumonia, and the incubation period is longer than one week. The illness generally includes fever, malaise, coryza, and pharyngitis. A nonproductive cough gradually develops and increases in intensity. Up to 20% of patients complain of pleuritic chest pain. Ear complaints may indicate bullous or hemorrhagic myringitis; this is an unusual accompaniment of mycoplasmal pneumonia, but when present is highly suggestive of the diagnosis.

Viral Versus Mycoplasmal Pneumonia. The distinction between viral and mycoplasmal pneumonia can be difficult to make by history, since both have nonspecific prodromes and follow a similar initial course. The epidemiology may occasionaly prove to be helpful, since influenza is marked by community epidemics, and mycoplasma by family outbreaks.

Chest x-ray findings are similar in viral and mycoplasmal pneumonia. Usually, there is an interstitial pattern without consolidation. Viral pneumonia often presents with bilateral fluffy infiltrates. Mycoplasmal pneumonia appears primarily in the lower lobes and can also be bilateral. Effusions are usually small and transient. They are present in up to 20% of patients with mycoplasmal pneumonia and in a greater percentage of patients with viral pneumonia.

Laboratory findings also offer little help in differentiating between viral and mycoplasmal pneumonia. A significant leukocytosis is unusual in both illnesses. Sixty to seventy percent of patients with mycoplasmal pneumonia have cold agglutinins (serum antibodies that agglutinate human red blood cells when incubated together in the cold). Titers begin to rise during the first week, but do not peak for three to four weeks. Unfortunately, viral pneumonia may also be associated with a nonspecific rise in cold agglutinins. Specific serologic confirmation is available for both mycoplasmal and viral pneumonia, but several days are required to obtain the results.

If the epidemiology and symptomatology cannot convince the physician of the specific etiology, presumptive therapy of mycoplasmal pneumonia should be initiated with erythromycin or tetracycline. It is not clear how effective these drugs are against mycoplasmal pneumonia. Studies suggest that the use of these antibiotics accelerates x-ray clearing and the resolution of symptoms, but the significance of the improvement remains questionable. Nevertheless, until further data are available, the patient with respiratory embarrassment in whom a precise diagnosis cannot be made should be treated with either erythromycin or tetracycline.

Bacterial Pneumonia

The onset of bacterial pneumonia is usually sudden and the patient rapidly becomes toxic. Pleuritic chest pain is common, and the patient develops a cough with sputum production. The sputum is purulent and generally filled with organisms.

A clinically significant prodrome in patients with bacterial pneumonia is unusual. Mild pharyngitis may represent a viral upper respiratory infection that has led to a breakdown of host defenses and allowed the bacteria to gain a foothold. Bacterial pneumonias do not occur in either family or community epidemics.

In patients without any underlying disease, the pneumococcus is the most common cause of bacterial pneumonia. The patient is well until he suddenly develops fever, cough, and pleuritic chest pain. The onset of these symptoms may be preceded by a single episode of rigors, and there are often multiple severe chills early in the course. The initial presentation is typical of most bacterial pneumonias.

Hemophilus influenzae pneumonia may have a more insidious onset, and usually occurs in men with chronic obstructive pulmonary disease or chronic alcoholism. Cough, fever, and malaise predominate, with fewer complaints of rigors and chest pain.

In patients who are already hospitalized, taking antibiotics, or debilitated by underlying disease, staphylococcus and gram-negative aerobes are frequently the infecting pathogens. More than 50% of pneumonias that develop in hospitalized patients are caused by gram-negative organisms. Klebsiella is virtually restricted to males over the age of 50; alcoholism is a common predisposing factor.

Staphylococcus and gram-negative aerobes can cause pneumonia in previously healthy individuals, but there is almost always a history of antecedent viral influenza. These patients, therefore, unlike others with bacterial pneumonia, experience a prodrome. When a patient with influenza pneumonia develops new fever, begins to produce purulent sputum, and experiences clinical deterioration six to ten days after the onset of illness, a secondary bacterial pneumonia must be suspected. The organisms likely to be involved are staphylococcus, gram-negative aerobes, pneumococcus, and *Hemophilus influenzae.*

Although the clinical setting can provide a clue to the specific etiologic diagnosis, a chest x-ray, sputum analysis, and repeated blood cultures are required to identify the organism.

Chest X-Ray Findings. Homogeneous consolidation and air bronchograms can be seen on the chest x-ray of a patient with pneumococcal pneumonia. The majority of pneumococcal pneumonias involve one lobe; the lower and middle lobes predominate (Fig. 52–1). Pleural effusions develop in 10% to 15% of patients and tend to occur late in the course.

Staphylococcal pneumonia usually causes a patchy, nonhomogeneous pneumonia. There are no air bronchograms. Unlike pneumococcal pneumonia, cavitation may develop rapidly. Effusions are present in the majority of patients.

Klebsiella rapidly produces cavitation. Like pneumococcal pneumonia, the chest x-ray shows evidence of an air space pneumonia (air bronchograms). Effusions and loss of lung volume are common, and the pneumonia is more likely to involve several lobes. The most common site of involvement is the right upper lobe. The inflammatory response may be so exuberant that it causes the fissures to bulge away from the consolidated lobe.

Hemophilus influenzae generally produces a patchy bronchopneumonia, but up to one-third of patients have consolidation and a similar number have effusions.

Streptococcus pyogenes is a rare cause of pneumonia in adults, and produces a bronchopneumonia with loss of lung volume. Effusions occur early in the majority of cases.

It must be remembered that typical x-ray findings can be obscured in any patient who has severe underlying lung disease (Fig. 52–2).

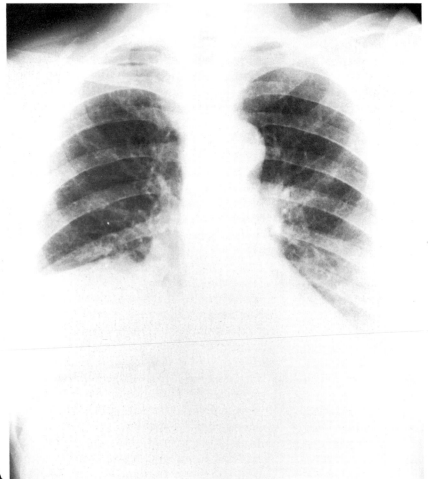

A

FIG. 52–1. Anteroposterior (A) and lateral (B) chest radiographs of a patient with a right middle lobe pneumonia from pneumococcal infection.

Sputum. Because of the rapid destruction of lung tissue caused especially by staphylococcal and gram-negative pneumonias, early diagnosis is essential for prompt intervention. In addition to the chest x-ray, a sputum analysis is the other immediately available diagnostic tool.

In classic descriptions, the pneumococcus is said to produce a rust-colored sputum, Klebsiella a tenacious, brick-red sputum, and staphylococcus a bloody sputum. These distinctions, however, are not very reliable.

It is important to obtain as good a sputum specimen as possible. The most reliable way to obtain sputum for stain and culture is by transtracheal aspiration. In this technique, a needle is passed through the cricothyroid membrane, a catheter inserted and passed into the trachea, and a small volume of (nonbacteriostatic) saline injected and withdrawn. This technique avoids contamination by mouth flora, which, in hospitalized patients,

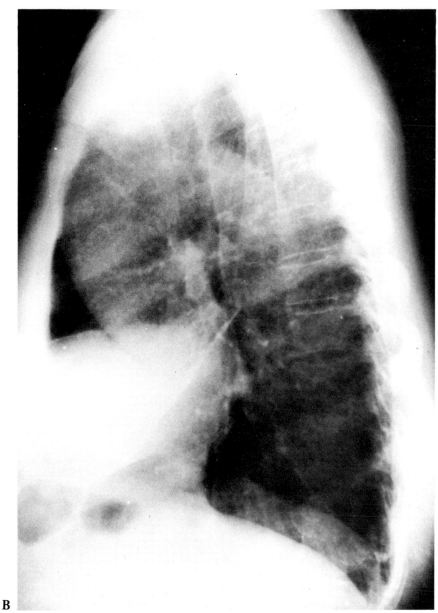

B

FIG. 52–1. (continued)

often includes streptococcus, pneumococcus, *Hemophilus influenzae,* and gram-negative aerobes.

The results of the gram stain support or adjust the tentative diagnoses that are being entertained on the basis of history and chest x-ray. The gram stain is the single most important diagnostic modality, because it allows rapid initiation of appropriate therapy.

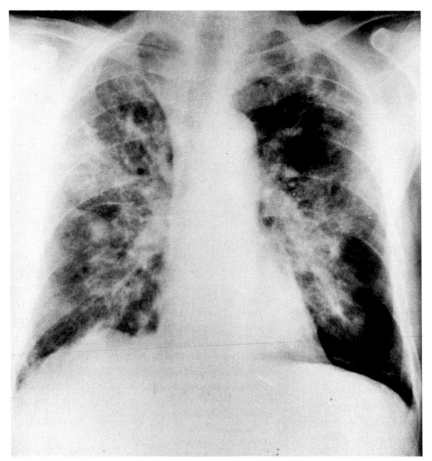

FIG. 52–2. Chest radiograph of a patient with chronic interstitial pneumonia.

The sample must be obtained from sputum coughed from the lung or acquired by transtracheal aspiration. The sputum should not have squamous epithelial cells (which are found in the mouth and therefore indicate oral contamination). Diagnosis is simple if there are sheets of a predominant organism or organisms contained within polymorphonuclear leukocytes. Thus, for example, the finding of sheets of lancet-shaped gram-positive diplococci without other organisms permits a presumptive diagnosis of pneumococcal pneumonia. The presence of small pleomorphic gram-negative cocci suggests *Hemophilus influenzae*. Klebsiella appears as a short, plump, gram-negative rod. An acid-fast stain for *Mycobacterium tuberculosis* should always be performed.

Cultures. A sputum culture takes two to three days to grow, and therapy must be instituted before then. Pneumococcus and *Hemophilus influenzae* often fail to grow from sputum cultures. These are fastidious organisms that can easily be overgrown by mouth flora. In addition, they are distributed unevenly throughout the sputum sample.

Blood cultures and pleural fluid cultures are more reliable. Blood cultures should always be obtained. The pneumococcus can be grown from the blood in up to 35% of patients with pneumococcal pneumonia. Fifteen percent of patients with klebsiella pneumonia have positive blood cultures, and a somewhat smaller percentage of patients with staphylococcal pneumonia have positive cultures. *Hemophilus influenzae* can be grown from the blood in the majority of cases, and a blood culture is probably the most reliable way of making the diagnosis.

Course and Antibiotic Therapy. The course of each type of bacterial pneumonia is distinctive.

Pneumococcal pneumonia generally responds well to low-dose penicillin, and improvement with defervescence occurs within one to two days after therapy has been initiated. The chest x-ray may take up to two months to show clearing, and residual changes may persist even longer. Patients in whom recurrent pneumococcal pneumonia occurs, usually with an insidious onset, and in whom the x-ray picture fails to clear, should be suspected of harboring an endobronchial lesion, with pneumonia occurring secondary to obstruction and the failure of normal clearance mechanisms. Complications of pneumococcal pneumonia, which include empyema, multilobe involvement, and extrathoracic disease, require an increase in the dose of penicillin.

Mortality increases with the patient's age, the existence of underlying disease, and the presence of positive blood cultures. Most deaths occur within the first five days, and the rate of early mortality does not seem to be affected by antibiotics. Patients in this group include the very old, those with serious underlying disease, and those with impaired defenses, such as asplenic individuals. The pneumococcal vaccine, which is effective in immunizing against strains responsible for 85% of pneumococcal infections, is recommended for susceptible high-risk patients.

Staphylococcal pneumonia is a more destructive disease and the patient is usually quite toxic. Response to therapy with high-dose parenteral penicillinase-resistant penicillins is slow. Patients with staphylococcal pneumonia secondary to bacteremia require at least six weeks of antibiotics. Mortality is high, and those who survive are frequently left with residual lung abnormalities due to tissue necrosis.

Gram-negative pneumonias occur in the setting of underlying disease and debilitation, and more than 50% of patients die. Increasing age, leukopenia, and positive blood cultures carry a poor prognosis. Antibiotics are determined by culture identification and sensitivities, and are given parenterally in high doses. An aminoglycoside is generally the drug of choice and should be included in the initial therapy when gram-negative organisms are suspected.

Nonspecific Therapy. Nonspecific measures are important in the therapy of purulent lower tract respiratory infections of any etiology. These measures include hydration and the mobilization of sputum, which may be copious and thick. Chest physical therapy is often used, but there is no evidence that this procedure is of any benefit. A high-humidity face mask and ultrasonic nebulization of high humidity mist have been advocated, but firm data supporting their effectiveness is lacking. Oxygen should be given as needed. Bronchospasm, especially in bronchitis, is often a problem, and bronchodilators may be given parenterally, orally, or by nebulization. These maneuvers may facilitate clearing of the organism and resolution of the infection, and may relieve anxiety.

LEGIONNAIRE'S DISEASE

Legionnaire's disease was first recognized at the American Legion Convention in Philadelphia in 1976. It is now known to be caused by a gram-negative, rod-shaped bacterium. Many aspects of its epidemiology remain unknown.

Legionnaire's disease presents with a constellation of symptoms that share features of both bacterial and nonbacterial acute pneumonias. It is generally a rapidly progressive, severe pneumonia presenting with high, unremitting fevers and recurrent chills. Like bacterial infections, pleuritic chest pain is common, but unlike bacterial pneumonia, the cough is nonproductive and no organisms are seen either in the sputum or in a transtracheal aspirate.

Myalgias and gastrointentinal disturbances are prominent. Patients with Legionnaire's disease are generally very toxic and may even display a toxic encephalopathy.

A chest x-ray usually shows early, unilateral, patchy bronchopneumonia that progresses to consolidation. The majority of patients later develop multilobar changes, with rapid total involvement of an entire lung. Small pleural effusions can be seen in up to 40% of patients.

The diagnosis is ultimately made by observing a rise in specific serum antibody titers. Culture of the organism is difficult and requires special growth media. The pleural fluid may be the best and most accessible source of culture material.

When the diagnosis is suspected, the treatment of choice is erythromycin. Response is often quite rapid, but the patient can relapse if not given a full 3-week course.

BIBLIOGRAPHY

Austrian R, Gold J: Pneumococcal bacteremia with especial reference to bacteremic pneumococcal pneumonia. Ann Intern Med 60:759–776, 1964

Bogart DB, Liu C, Ruth WE et al: Rapid diagnosis of primary influenza pneumonia. Chest 68:513–517, 1975

Briggs DD Jr: Pulmonary infections. Med Clin North Am 61:1163–1183, 1977

Johnson WD, Kaye D, Hood EW: Hemophilus influenzae pneumonia in adults. Am Rev Resp Dis 97:1112–1117, 1968

Lerner AM, Federman MJ: Gram negative bacillary pneumonia. J Infect Dis 124:425–427, 1971

Lerner AM, Jankauskas K: The classical bacterial pneumonias. DM, Feb, 1975

Murray HW, Masur H, Senterfit LB et al: The protean manifestations of mycoplasma pneumonia infection in adults. Am J Med 58:229–242, 1975

Swartz MN: Clinical aspects of Legionnaire's disease. Ann Intern Med 90:492–495, 1979

Tillotson JR, Lerner AM: Pneumonias caused by gram negative bacilli. Medicine 45:65–76, 1966

Winterbauer RA, Bedon GA, Ball WC: Recurrent pneumonia. Ann Intern Med 70:689–700, 1969

53

Tuberculosis

PATHOPHYSIOLOGY

The tubercle bacillus (*Mycobacterium tuberculosis*) can produce an acute illness at the time of infection. More commonly, however, the primary infection is not clinically apparent, and the organism either is eliminated or remains dormant until the host's immunologic defenses are depressed, permitting the infection to reactivate.

Small aerosolized droplets are essentially the only vehicle for tuberculosis transmission. Droplets containing more than three bacilli are too big to reach the alveoli and are cleared from the bronchial surface. Bacilli that do reach the lower air spaces are immediately internalized by alveolar macrophages. The organisms can persist intracellularly and spread to other phagocytes. Eventually, the bacilli can disseminate to local lymph nodes and throughout the body.

The typical pathologic lesion at the earliest stage of infection is the *granuloma*, an intense necrotizing inflammatory reaction that usually destroys the bacilli. Except in those rare instances in which an overwhelming infection occurs at this initial stage of infection, the granulomas eventually heal by scarring and calcification. However, a few bacilli may survive either at the original pulmonary focus or at any metastatic site. If they reactivate, clinical disease may result.

The earliest infection is clinically silent. A month or two later, the PPD skin test (see below) may turn positive while the chest x-ray remains clear. The initial pulmonary focus of infection will evolve in one of four directions:

1. The lesion may heal but still serve as a potential site for reactivation.

2. The mycobacteria may erode into the pleural space or pericardium, producing pleurisy or pericarditis without evidence of parenchymal involvement.

3. The organisms may proliferate locally, producing necrosis and caseation. Erosion into a bronchus may cause pneumonia.

4. The granulomatous reaction may cause erosion into a blood vessel, and the mycobacteria may invade the bloodstream. This is not uncommon, but only rarely is the inoculum large enough to allow establishment of clinically evident tuberculosis infection outside of the lung. If massive amounts of bacteria are released, miliary tuberculosis can result (see later discussion).

In the United States, most tuberculosis in the adult population is evidenced by a positive

399

skin test with or without a small pulmonary scar. If the disease reactivates, it may do so from any site of earlier infection. Most commonly, reactivation occurs from the apex of the lung, although it may occur from a nonpulmonary site, the most common of which is the genitourinary system, including the kidneys, lower urinary tracts, prostate, fallopian tubes, and epididymis. The diagnosis can be subtle but should be suspected in a patient who has a history or radiographic evidence of previous tuberculous infection or who has microscopic pyuria or hematuria. Culture of the urine for routine bacteria will be sterile. An excretory urogram may show cavities, focal strictures, or renal calcification.

Tuberculous meningitis, pleuritis, or pericarditis may occur without evidence of active pulmonary tuberculosis. Tuberculous infection of bone in the adult usually involves the vertebral bodies (Pott's disease). Local destruction may erode the bone and intervening intervertebral disks, causing local tenderness, draining sinuses, collapsed disks, and paraplegia.

Although rare in the United States, tuberculous peritonitis is not uncommon in other countries, particularly Iran. Patients present with fever, abdominal pain, exudative ascites, mass lesions, and, occasionally, bowel obstruction.

DIAGNOSIS

The diagnosis of tuberculosis should be considered when a chest x-ray reveals an upper lobe scar or cavity (Fig. 53–1). However, tuberculosis must also be considered in patients with isolated pleural effusions, lobar pneumonia, or diffuse pneumonia. Miliary tuberculosis may underlie a fever of unknown origin.

Suspicion of tuberculosis should be highest for patients from populations at high risk for tuberculosis. These include the elderly, the malnourished, diabetics, alcoholics, patients afflicted with chronic illnesses or lymphoproliferative diseases, and patients taking corticosteroids or cytotoxic agents. Tuberculosis, sometimes from organisms resistant to standard antituberculosis medications, is a problem in immigrants from endemic regions and veterans of the war in Vietnam. For reasons that are not known, patients who have undergone subtotal gastrectomy or who have advanced silicosis also have an increased risk.

Suspicion of tuberculous infection may be confirmed by skin testing. The skin test is performed by injecting intradermally 0.1 ml of PPD (purified protein derivative), an extract of the tubercle bacillus. Forty-eight to seventy-two hours later, the extent of induration is assessed as a measure of delayed hypersensitivity. The test is considered positive for tuberculosis if the area of induration is more than 10 mm in diameter. A positive reaction implies host sensitization to the tubercle bacillus, but it indicates nothing about the activity of the disease. A positive reaction can also be caused by infection with an atypical strain of mycobacteria.

Once infected, a person may remain PPD positive for life, although there is some waning of skin test reactivity over time. Unfortunately, the skin test may be negative in some patients infected with *M. tuberculosis*. Sometimes this occurs because the patient is anergic to the bacillus. Anergy can occur with widespread disseminated tuberculosis, occasionally with isolated tuberculous pleuritis, in conditions predisposing to anergy (lymphoreticular diseases, sarcoidosis, treatment with immunosuppressive agents), and with viral illnesses. Even more commonly, however, false negative responses are due to poor technique in administering the skin test.

Mycobacterium tuberculosis appears as a thin and beaded organism on Gram stain. On Ziehl-Neelsen stain it is acid-fast (*i.e.*, it re-

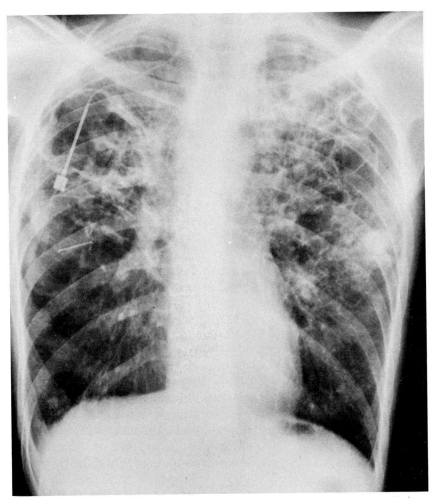

FIG. 53–1. Chest radiograph showing the destruction and cavity formation of tuberculosis.

tains its color after washing with acid alcohol). However, even if the organism is found on direct smear, a culture remains critical to diagnosis; all acid-fast organisms are not *Mycobacterium tuberculosis*, and the existence of drug-resistant strains necessitates determining drug sensitivities.

Diagnosis of active tuberculosis requires culturing the organism from the sputum, infected fluid (pleural, joint, ascitic, or cerebro-spinal), or biopsy tissue. The organisms grow slowly, so cultures rarely become clearly positive in less than two to six weeks.

Miliary Tuberculosis. Massive hematogenous dissemination of mycobacteria can lead to widespread organ involvement. Miliary tuberculosis is characterized on chest x-ray by lungs that are studded with small densities, whose appearance has been likened to scattered millet seeds. The patient typically presents with fever, night sweats, diffuse symptoms of fatigue and weight loss, and splenomegaly. A fundoscopic examination may reveal choroidal tubercles. These are bilateral, pale gray, oblong densities with indistinct edges; occasionally, there is evidence of central caseation.

The diagnosis of miliary tuberculosis can be difficult to make. Although patients are obviously ill and usually febrile, the pulmonary lesions may be below the visible limit of resolution on the chest x-ray, and evidence of specific organ involvement may be lacking. The white blood cell count is frequently normal, but pancytopenia or leukemoid reactions that can be confused with leukemia may also occur. The PPD test result is frequently negative, and cultures of the sputum may fail to grow the mycobacteria. In one-third of patients, a biopsy and culture of the bone marrow reveal tuberculosis. A liver biopsy is less frequently helpful and is occasionally confusing because of the high frequency of nonspecific granulomas that are found in that organ. Miliary tuberculosis is fatal if it remains untreated, but only the most severely ill patients fail to respond to appropriate therapy.

DRUG THERAPY

Many drugs are available for antituberculosis therapy in the United States today. The drugs used most frequently are isoniazid, streptomycin, ethambutol, and rifampin.

Isoniazid (INH) is an oral agent that is bacteriocidal for *Mycobacterium tuberculosis.* The major toxic manifestation is neuritis, which begins as nonspecific nervousness and hyperreflexia and which may culminate in a painful sensory neuritis and a central nervous system picture resembling encephalitis. The neuritis appears to result from interference by INH with pyridoxine metabolism, and can be averted by the dietary addition of pyridoxine. Some populations rapidly acetylate INH and inactivate it. Rapid acetylators (especially prevalent among Oriental and Eskimo populations) seem to carry a higher risk for the other major side-effect of INH—hepatitis. Twenty percent of patients receiving INH have transient elevations in serum transaminases, but this does not require the drug to be discontinued. About 1.5% of patients develop clinical hepatitis, requiring discontinuation of the drug; the frequency increases with the age of the patient. The risk of hepatotoxicity increases when INH is used in combination with rifampin.

Streptomycin is an aminoglycoside given by intramuscular injection. Its major toxic effect is vertigo due to damage to the vestibular part of the eighth cranial nerve. Less frequently, streptomycin causes renal damage and proteinuria.

Ethambutol is an oral agent that can cause a dose-related optic neuritis with loss of color vision and visual acuity. Screening by an ophthalmologist before and during therapy is important. The possibility of developing optic neuritis is slight if the dose is kept within the recommended range.

Rifampin is an expensive oral agent. It is potentially hepatotoxic and can cause a hypersensitivity reaction, especially with intermittent use. However, it is an extremely effective and potent antituberculosis drug.

Treatment Protocols. Because of the slow generation time of the mycobacterium, its tendency to drug resistance, and its ability to persist in a dormant state for many years and then reactivate, combination chemotherapy is necessary for protracted periods of time. Therapy should eliminate viable bacilli within the first 100 days of treatment. Patients should become essentially noninfectious within two weeks of starting the drugs, although some organisms may still be grown. Patients with tuberculosis may be treated at home. There is no need to hospitalize them to protect contacts, because the risk of spread of infection is very small after initiation of effective chemotherapy.

There is much debate about the appropriate drug regimen and the duration of therapy for tuberculosis. Some advocate initiating therapy, especially for those with miliary or disseminated tuberculosis, with three drugs, generally INH, ethambutol, and streptomycin. After 30 to 90 days, treatment is reduced to two drugs (INH and ethambutol) and continued for 18 to 24 months. Others believe that treatment with two bactericidal agents (such as INH and rifampin) is sufficient.

With the recent emphasis on ambulatory therapy for tuberculosis, successful attempts have been made to abbreviate the course of therapy. Such programs are especially attractive for patients who are unlikely to take their medications reliably.

All regimens must be adjusted for patients in whom the organism manifests resistance to the chosen drugs. This is an especially common problem for patients who acquire tuberculosis in Southeast Asia.

Treatment for tuberculosis infection (without evidence of active disease) with INH alone is appropriate only in certain circumstances. These include (1) children who have come into contact with patients with active tuberculosis; (2) persons with documented new conversion to a positive PPD; (3) persons under age 35 with a positive PPD (the risk of hepatotoxicity becomes too great if they are older); (4) persons over 35 with a positive PPD who have chest x-ray evidence of tuberculosis but negative cultures; and (5) patients given inadequate therapy for culture-positive tuberculosis in the past.

BIBLIOGRAPHY

Bentz RR, Dimcheff DG, Nemiroff MJ et al: The incidence of urine cultures positive for mycobacterium tuberculosis in a general tuberculosis patient population. Am Rev Resp Dis 111:647–650, 1975

Glassroth J, Robins AG, Snider DE Jr: Tuberculosis in the 1980s. N Engl J Med 302:1441–1448, 1980

Gunnels JJ, Bates JH, Swindoll H: Infectivity of sputum-positive tuberculosis patients on chemotherapy. Am Rev Resp Dis 109:323–330, 1974

Johnston RF, Wildrick KH: The impact of chemotherapy on the care of patients with tuberculosis. Am Rev Resp Dis 109:636–664, 1974

Sahn SA, Neff TA: Miliary tuberculosis. Am J Med 56:495–505, 1974

Simon HB, Weinstein AJ, Pasternak MS et al: Genitourinary tuberculosis: Clinical features in a general hospital population. Am J Med 63:410–420, 1977

vanScoy RE: Antituberculosis agents. Mayo Clin Proc 52:694–700, 1977

Infection of the lining of the heart is referred to as infectious endocarditis. Most often the focus of infection is one (or more) of the valves of the heart. The patient develops heart murmurs, fever, a bacteremia, and any of a number of manifestations caused by embolism from the lesion, as material breaks free from the vegetations on the valve and seeds distant tissues and organs.

Normal endocardium can be involved in the disease process, but in most instances the establishment of infection requires prior damage of a valve by a previous illness. Prosthetic valves are also the frequent targets of infection.

The combination of a damaged endothelium and turbulent blood flow appears to provide the most fertile setting for endocarditis. Infectious endocarditis is therefore more prevalent on the left side of the heart than the right side, a consequence of the higher pressures in the systemic circulation relative to those of the pulmonary circulation. Turbulent blood flow may also account for the establishment of infection at the impact point of the jet-flow through a ventricular septal defect and in arteriovenous shunts placed for dialysis.

Infectious endocarditis was once a uni-formly fatal disease. Today, however, with the development of antibiotic therapy and cardiac surgery, 65% to 80% of patients survive. There has also been a dramatic shift in the microbiology of the disease. Previously, most cases were caused by relatively noninvasive organisms, such as *Streptococcus viridans*, but now more destructive and invasive organisms, including *Staphylococcus aureus*, *Neisseria gonorrhea*, gram-negative rods, and even fungi are playing an increasing role.

The shifting microbiologic pattern has been due in part to the changing nature of the precipitating injury. In the past, valves damaged by rheumatic heart disease were the most common target for bacterial infection. Today, with the declining incidence of rheumatic fever, two new clinical syndromes of infectious endocarditis have arisen: prosthetic valve endocarditis and endocarditis associated with intravenous drug abuse.

SUBACUTE VERSUS ACUTE ENDOCARDITIS

Subacute infectious endocarditis is a partially compensated disease lasting weeks or months in which the rate of healing never quite equals that of destruction. As the valve is eroded, new murmurs may appear and bits of infective tissue may embolize throughout the body causing metastatic infections or infarcts. The immune system becomes highly activated, and antibody titers, especially of rheumatoid factor, are usually elevated. The classic textbook descriptions of subacute infectious endocarditis do not apply to most cases of the disease seen today. The telltale signs of Roth's spots (small, white lesions surrounded by a rim of hemorrhage, located in the fundus), clubbing of the digits, Osler's nodes (raised, tender skin lesions in the pads of the fingers), and Janeway lesions (hemorrhagic lesions of the palms or soles) are becoming rare.

Streptococcus viridans is still the leading cause of subacute infectious endocarditis. A nidus of infection can form on a damaged valve leaflet or on the wall of a cardiac chamber that is subjected to a high-pressure jet effect. A suitable jet effect can be caused by blood rushing through the narrowed orifice of either a septal wall defect or a stenosed valve. Platelets and fibrin deposit on the damaged tissue, producing a "sticky" area ripe for bacterial invasion when, for example, a transient bacteremia occurs.

Acute infectious endocarditis is usually caused by *Staphylococcus aureus*, an invasive organism that can infect even normal heart valves. Acute endocarditis is characterized by rapid valve destruction, the sudden appearance of new regurgitant murmurs, hemodynamic compromise, and extension of the infection to form myocardial abscesses.

Signs and Symptoms

The signs and symptoms of endocarditis can be divided into three categories: nonspecific, cardiac, and embolic.

Nonspecific Complaints. Most patients complain of malaise, fatigue, and fever. In patients with subacute disease, these symptoms are virtually always present and are often the sole presenting complaints. Backache, arthralgias, and myalgias often accompany these symptoms, and it is therefore not surprising that early endocarditis can be mistaken for a viral illness. Any patient with valvular heart disease who presents with complaints resembling those of a viral syndrome should be evaluated with blood cultures, especially if fever persists for several days.

Cardiac Manifestations. The possibility of endocarditis should be considered whenever a patient presents with new or changing cardiac murmurs or with unexplained congestive heart failure. Murmurs represent either antecedent valvular disease or new valvular destruction caused by the infection. It is rare for endocarditis to occur without murmurs being present, but the murmurs may be soft and difficult to auscultate (*e.g.*, in mitral stenosis or right-sided endocarditis). The presence of changing murmurs, especially the development of new regurgitant murmurs, is an ominous sign.

Embolic Manifestations. An embolic event from vegetations on an infected valve may be the first clinical expression of endocarditis. Pulmonary and splenic emboli are very common and can cause fleeting pulmonary infiltrates and splenomegaly with left upper quadrant abdominal pain. Some of the more familiar signs of endocarditis, including splinter hemorrhages and petechiae, are of embolic origin. Osler's nodes and Janeway lesions may be of embolic or immune etiology. Renal and cerebral emboli can be extremely dangerous and are discussed below.

Diagnosis and Therapy

Any patient with prosthetic or structurally abnormal valves has a risk for developing subacute endocarditis, as are individuals with ventricular septal defects or other congenital heart defects. Surgery performed to ameliorate these defects can leave scars that may form the nidus for future infection. Patients with the click-murmur syndrome (Chap. 5) are at risk, and those with a prior history of endocarditis are susceptible to future infection.

Individuals who inject themselves with illicit drugs are at special risk for developing acute endocarditis. However, since prior injury is not a necessary precursor for infection, anyone experiencing a bacteremia can develop acute endocarditis.

Laboratory testing for endocarditis reveals a normochromic, normocytic anemia, a left-shifted, usually mild leukocytosis (or even a normal white blood cell count), an elevated erythocyte sedimentation rate, and microscopic hematuria. Multiple sequential blood cultures should be drawn and kept for 10 to 14 days. The first two sets of blood cultures will provide the diagnosis in over 80% of cases. Three sets of cultures provide a diagnosis in over 90% of cases, and 6 sets yield a positive diagnosis in virtually all cases in which the organism can be grown. Patients given prior inadequate antibiotic therapy may be culture-negative; the transformation of bacteria to the so-called "L-form" has also been blamed for culture-negative endocarditis. Approximately 10% of all patients with endocarditis are considered culture-negative. These patients have a higher mortality, probably because it is not possible to select the proper antibiotic.

The correct identification of the etiologic organism is critical, and therapy should be delayed for several hours until the six sets of blood cultures can be collected. If, however, the patient's condition is deteriorating or if severe embolic events make urgent therapy necessary, it is prudent to collect three sets of blood cultures over a shorter period. Broad-spectrum antibiotic coverage should be started and later adjusted when the culture results are learned.

The required duration of antibiotic therapy has not been studied prospectively, but most authorities favor four weeks of intravenous therapy followed by another two weeks of oral antibiotics. Prolonged therapy is necessary to eradicate every organism, because normal host defenses are inadequate within the vegetation. Cardiac surgeons should be consulted as soon as the diagnosis is made, since urgent surgery might be required at any time during the course of the disease.

A reduction of the patient's hyperimmune state—especially a falling titer of rheumatoid factor—is a good measure of the success of antibiotic therapy. The best prognostic indicators, however, are a reduction of fever and an improvement in the patient's general sense of well-being. When fever persists, one must consider the possibilities of drug fever, inadequate antibiotic coverage, or the development of myocardial or embolic abscesses.

During the course of antibiotic therapy, the patient must be carefully watched for the major complications of bacterial endocarditis. The clinician should auscultate the chest daily to detect new or changing murmurs, and the electrocardiogram should be repeated regularly. ST elevations may indicate either a new myocardial infarction, resulting from an embolus to a coronary artery, or pericarditis over a site of myocardial abscess.

Special mention should be made of the treatment for staphylococcal endocarditis. Because of the extreme invasiveness of *Staphylococcus aureus*, many physicians have accepted the presence of staphylococcal bacteremia as evidence of endocarditis. Recently, two patterns of *Staphylococcus aureus* septicemia have been delineated, and each syndrome carries a different therapeutic implication. In those patients with an obvious localized and removable focus of infection, such as an infected dialysis shunt or contaminated intravenous device, a short course of antibiotics after removal of the infected source generally suffices. On the other hand, where no clear-cut source of infection can be found, and where numerous localized abscesses appear secondary to bacteremic spread, prolonged therapy for presumed bacterial endocarditis is advised.

Complications

Cardiac Complications. Valvular destruction and myocardial abscesses are most common in acute endocarditis and prosthetic valve endocarditis. Acute destruction of the mitral or aortic valve can lead to fulminant congestive heart failure and necessitate immediate cardiac surgery. Abscesses extend from the valvular ring, and may interrupt the cardiac conducting system, which lies near the valves. Abscesses near the mitral valve may dissect to the A-V node and the bundle of His and can result in complete heart block, Wenckebach block, or junctional tachycardia. Infections of the aortic valve can invade the septum, resulting in new left bundle branch block or bifascicular block.

Renal Complications. Asymptomatic hematuria is the most common manifestation of renal disease associated with endocarditis, but severe renal failure can develop during the course of the illness. There are four potential mechanisms of renal damage:

1. Emboli can lodge in the renal vessels and cause infarction or abscess formation;

2. Immune complexes, which often circulate in endocarditis, can lodge in the glomeruli and bind complement, resulting in a proliferative glomerulonephritis;

3. Antibiotic therapy, such as methicillin or gentamicin, can be toxic to the kidneys;

4. Myocardial complications that lower the cardiac output may reduce renal blood flow and compromise renal function.

Neurologic Complications. Between 25% and 40% of patients manifest neurologic embolic complications, and the risk has not decreased with the introduction of antibiotics. Embolism to the middle cerebral artery is a major neurologic complication, often resulting in a dense hemiplegia. Events similar to transient ischemic attacks have been described in approximately 25% of patients. Bacteremic seeding of the meninges may occur. Septic emboli to the vasa vasorum result in the formation of mycotic aneurysms, especially at arterial bifurcations, and can lead to intracranial hemorrhage. Because of the arteritis produced by these lesions, anticoagulation is contraindicated in subacute endocarditis for fear of inducing hemorrhage. While mycotic aneurysms may heal, the vascular structures remain weakened and are subject to rupture weeks or months after the endocarditis has been successfully treated.

A great range of other neurologic complications can be encountered. An altered level of consciousness without focal findings is frequently described, and has been attributed to a diffuse toxic state, fever, multiple cerebral microemboli or petechial hemorrhages, and uremia. Seizures are not uncommon and are usually the result of stroke, but they may also be caused by penicillin toxicity. Purulent meningitis can be seen in gram-negative, pneumococcal, or staphylococcal infections. Brain abscess is usually a diagnosis made only at postmortem examination. Examination of the cerebrospinal fluid is mandatory in all neurologic events to rule out hemorrhage or purulent meningitis. CT scan is a valuable tool to help evaluate intracranial hemorrhage.

ACUTE ENDOCARDITIS IN THE DRUG ADDICT

Since the 1960's, the drug addict with acute bacterial endocarditis has become a major management problem in large city hospitals. Studies have shown that the organism cultured from the addict's heroin and drug paraphernalia bears little or no relationship to the organism infecting his valve. While the water that addicts use as a diluent (often from public lavatories) may contribute to the infection, it is probable that the bacteria commonly originate from the patient's skin or mucous membranes. For example, in Washington, D.C., where 70% of cases of endocarditis are caused by *Staphylococcus aureus*, drug addicts have a higher staphylococcus carrier rate than occurs in the nonaddict population.

Addicts may develop any type of endocarditis, but they are especially prone to acute staphylococcal endocarditis and to endocarditis of the tricuspid valve. Patients with right-sided endocarditis classically present with a multilobed staphylococcal pneumonia caused by multiple recurrent septic pulmonary emboli originating from the tricuspid valve. Despite adequate therapy, the pneumonia may continue to reappear sporadically in various parts of the lung, especially the lower lobes. Surgical excision of the tricuspid valve, with or without valve replacement, is often necessary.

Although the staphylococcus is the predominant infecting organism in intravenous drug abusers, epidemics of nonstaphylococcal acute bacterial endocarditis have occurred in several cities. In Detroit, pseudomonas endocarditis and enterococcus endocarditis have frequently been seen. In San Francisco, *Serratia marcesens* has been responsible for many cases; investigators have tried to correlate this epidemic with the U.S. Army's aerosol spraying of Serratia over the San Francisco Bay area in the 1950's. Fungal endocarditis is also seen more frequently in the addict population, but it is still a rarity.

PROSTHETIC VALVE ENDOCARDITIS

Endocarditis complicates approximately 1% of valve replacements. Prosthetic valve endocarditis carries a high mortality, exceeding 50% in most institutions. Medical therapy is often ineffective, and surgical valve replacement is frequently necessary.

Two distinct syndromes of prosthetic valve endocarditis have been recognized:

1. *Early prosthetic valve endocarditis* occurs within two months of surgery. It is extremely difficult to treat. *Staphylococcus aureus*, *Staphylococcus epidermidis*, gram-negative rods, and fungi predominate. The organisms are usually resistant to the antibiotics used for routine perioperative prophylaxis. Unfortunately, therapy is sometimes delayed when blood cultures are positive for organisms such as *Staphylococcus epidermidis* or diphtheroids, since these organisms may incorrectly be dismissed as mere contaminants. The source of infection may be contaminated operating room equipment. There have been reports of mycobacterial contamination of porcine valves. Valve dehiscence, congestive heart failure, septic emboli, and myocardial abscess formation are common sequelae; surgical débridement is often unsuccessful.

2. *Late prosthetic valve endocarditis* (occurring more than two months after surgery) has an etiology, presentation, and bacteriology similar to natural-valve subacute bacterial endocarditis, but carries a far worse prognosis, with a higher incidence of myocardial abscess formation. Intravenous therapy should be prolonged, and surgery should be considered for persistent infection. Except for patients with porcine valves or cloth-covered metallic valves, anticoagulation should be continued despite the attendant risk of hemorrhage from

vasculitic cerebral vessels. The prothrombin time should be maintained at only 50% to 75% greater than control in order to minimize the risk of bleeding.

Any patient with a prosthetic valve and an unexplained fever should be suspected of having endocarditis and should be treated appropriately until that diagnosis can be excluded.

PROPHYLAXIS

Patients with structural cardiac abnormalities (prostheses, abnormal valves, and others) face the danger of infectious endocarditis whenever a transient bacteremia occurs. The American Heart Association therefore recommends that parenteral antibiotics be given prior to various medical-surgical procedures as a prophylaxis against the development of endocarditis. Among the high-risk procedures are genitourinary instrumentation and surgery, gastrointestinal biopsies, cardiac surgery, and dental procedures. Patients with prosthetic valves should probably receive prophylaxis during any mildly invasive procedure, such as sigmoidoscopy and GI endoscopy. Prophylaxis regimens usually combine a penicillin with an aminoglycoside; the penicillin protocol used for rheumatic fever prophylaxis is not adequate to prevent the development of endocarditis.

BIBLIOGRAPHY

Garvey GJ, Neu HC: Infective endocarditis: An evolving disease. Medicine 57:105–127, 1978

Hutter AM, Moellering RC: Assessment of the patient with suspected endocarditis. JAMA 235:1603–1605, 1976

Kaye D: Antibiotic treatment of streptococcal endocarditis. Am J Med 69:650–652,1980

Karchmer AW, Dismukes WE, Buckley MJ et al: Late prosthetic valve endocarditis: Clinical features influencing therapy. Am J Med 64:199–206, 1978

Pesanti EL, Smith IM: Infective endocarditis with negative blood cultures: An analysis of 52 cases. Am J Med 66:43–50, 1979

Pruit AA, Rubin RH, Karchmer AW et al: Neurologic complications of bacterial endocarditis. Medicine 57:329–343, 1978

Sande MA, Scheld WM: Combination antibiotic therapy of bacterial endocarditis. Ann Intern Med 92:390–395, 1980

Weinstein L, Schlesinger JJ: Pathoanatomic, pathophysiologic and clinical correlations in endocarditis. N Engl J Med 291:832–837, 1122–1126, 1974

55

**Urinary Tract
Infections**

Bacterial infection is the most common cause of urinary tract disease. Infection can involve the upper urinary tract (pyelonephritis) or the lower urinary tract (cystitis or urethritis). This distinction is important because both the acute and chronic complications of pyelonephritis are more severe than those of cystitis or urethritis, and antibiotic therapy must be adjusted accordingly.

Symptoms

The characteristic symptoms of urinary tract infections are dysuria, frequency of urination, suprapubic tenderness, flank pain, and fever. Of these, only fever is useful in pinpointing a urinary tract infection as upper *versus* lower; fever is a fairly reliable sign that the infection involves the upper urinary tract. In the elderly and in patients with diabetes, a urinary tract infection may present solely with fever or clinical deterioration (*e.g.*, confusion in the elderly and worsening glucose control or even ketoacidosis in diabetics).

Diagnosis

The key to the diagnosis of urinary tract infection is a careful microscopic and bacteriologic examination of a clean-voided specimen of urine. If there is difficulty obtaining a clean-voided specimen, urethral catheterization or a suprapubic percutaneous catheterization should be performed.

Because the urinary tract is normally colonized with bacteria, specific criteria have been delineated to diagnose the presence of infection. These have proven to be most helpful for infections with gram-negative enterobacteria. If a single urine sample reveals more than 10^5 bacteria/ml, the probability of significant infection is 80%. If a second sample duplicates this result, the probability is 95%. In urine with borderline counts of 10^4 to 10^5 bacteria/ml, there is rarely a true infection. With gram-positive or more exotic organisms, bacterial counts of 10^4 organisms/ml may be significant, and the preceding guidelines do not apply.

An estimate of the bacterial count can be made by a Gram stain of the urine prior to sedimentation (unspun urine). If bacteria can be seen, it is likely that there is significant infection and that a urine culture will reveal more than 10^5 organisms/ml. Pyuria can also be seen.

Once an infection has been documented, the next step is to identify the site of infection.

As mentioned above, fever is the most reliable sign of an upper urinary tract infection. In addition, a test that uses immunologic techniques to detect the presence of antibody-coated bacteria can distinguish upper from lower urinary tract disease. Antibody will bind to bacteria in upper urinary tract infections but not in lower tract infections, and a positive result is thus obtained only in patients with pyelonephritis.

Pyelonephritis. A patient who enters the emergency room with severe flank pain, high fever, chills, and evidence of infection on examination of the urine should be presumed to have pyelonephritis and treated with intravenous antibiotics. *E. coli* is responsible for the majority of cases of pyelonephritis; other potential pathogens include proteus, pseudomonas, enterococcus, and staphylococcus.

Even with administration of the correct antibiotic, defervesence is not as dramatic as with other localized bacterial infections (*e.g.,* pneumococcal pneumonia), and spiking fevers may continue for several days. If, however, the patient fails to improve after three or four days, additional complications must be suspected. These include urinary tract obstruction, renal abscess formation, the presence of an organism that is resistant to the antibiotic, drug fever, or a high-grade bacteremia with disseminated infections (*e.g.,* endocarditis). Blood cultures should then be obtained, antibiotic sensitivities determined, and the patient examined for any of the stigmata of endocarditis (Chap. 54). The question of possible ureteral obstruction can often be answered noninvasively with renal ultrasound (Chap. 24).

Urinary Tract Infections in Men. The most common lower tract infections in men are urethritis and prostatitis. *Chronic prostatitis* is quite common, and generally presents with mild symptoms of low back and perineal pain or discomfort. Although there may be pyuria, in most instances organisms are neither seen nor cultured from the urine. Cultures of prostatic secretions can be obtained by prostatic massage and may be positive. *Acute prostatitis* is less common and may present with fever, dysuria, and chills. The urinary sediment is consistent with a urinary tract infection. The prostate is boggy and extremely tender on palpation. Acute prostatitis generally responds rapidly to antibiotics. Chronic prostatitis is more refractory to treatment, and the question of which antibiotic to use and for how long remains unanswered. Currently, trimethoprin-sulfamethoxazole is widely used, and a course of six or more weeks is recommended.

An upper urinary tract infection in males should suggest the possibility of an underlying anatomic abnormality, usually obstruction.

Treatment

More than 80% of urinary tract infections are cured with any of a number of antibiotic regimens. Oral sulfonamides, such as sulfisoxazole or trimethoprin-sulfamethoxazole are the agents of choice. The potential side-effects of sulfa drugs include rash, urticaria, and gastrointestinal disturbances. Most of the failures or relapses occur in upper urinary tract infections. Recently, it has been shown that even a single dose of *amoxicillin* can cure lower urinary tract infections, but approximately 50% of upper infections fail to be cured after ten days of oral therapy. The proper outpatient regimen and duration of therapy for upper tract infections remain undecided.

BIBLIOGRAPHY

Fairly KF, Carson NE, Gutch RC et al: Site of infection in acute urinary-tract infection in general practice. Lancet 2:615–618, 1971

Fang LST, Tolkoff-Rubin NE, Rubin RH: Efficacy of single-dose and conventional amoxicillin therapy in urinary-tract infections localized by the antibody-coated bacteria technic. N Eng J Med 298:413–416, 1978

Jones SR, Smith JW, Sanford JP: Localization of urinary tract infections by detection of antibody-coated bacteria in urine sediment. N Engl J Med 290:591–593, 1974

Kaye D: Host defense mechanisms in the urinary tract. Urol Clin North Am 2:407–422, 1975

Smith JW, et al: Recurrent urinary tract infections in men. Ann Intern Med 91:544–548, 1979

56

Venereal
Disease

Suspicion of venereal disease will naturally arise in any patient who presents with genital skin lesions, a urethral or vaginal discharge, or inguinal adenopathy. The diagnosis may be considerably less obvious, however, in patients in whom the systemic or nongenital manifestations of venereal disease predominate, for example, in the gonococcal arthritis–dermatitis syndrome or with the late skin rashes and destructive gummas of syphilis.

GONORRHEA

Gonorrhea means "semen flow," a name chosen by Galen, who was impressed by the urethral discharge. Three million people contract gonococcal infections each year in the United States, and many will suffer the protracted effects of pelvic inflammatory disease.

Symptoms of gonorrhea begin three to five days after contact, and include urethral discomfort, dysuria, and eventually a purulent urethral discharge. A Gram stain of the discharge reveals Neisseria gonorrhea organisms, appearing as pairs of gram-negative intracellular cocci. The Gram stain has virtually a 100% accuracy in diagnosing acute gonorrhea in males. Diagnosis is often difficult in fe-

males, however, because other neisserial organisms are usually present in the vagina. Identification of N. gonorrhea must be made from cultures of the bacteria that have been grown from swabs of cervical mucus. Vaginal swabs do not suffice, since the organism does not grow in the vagina.

The male almost always has a urethral discharge with N. gonorrhea urethral infection. Diagnosis in the rare asymptomatic male, who has been exposed to a female with gonorrhea, depends upon a urethral smear and culture. Swabs of the pharynx and anal canal should also be taken, since the organism thrives on these mucous membranes as well. The inflammation of gonococcal pharyngitis can resemble a strep throat, and the purulent discharge and anorectal discomfort of gonococcal proctitis can resemble ulcerative colitis.

Two gonococcal syndromes often become serious enough to warrant hospitalization: pelvic inflammatory disease and disseminated gonorrhea.

Pelvic Inflammatory Disease (PID). Ten to seventeen percent of women with cervical gonorrhea develop PID. The gonococci ascend to the uterus and then travel along the fallopian tubes; this route of infection is especially common during menstruation. Tubal pus seeps into the abdomen and causes peritonitis. The patient complains of lower abdominal pain and fever, and leukocytosis is present. The fallopian tube enlarges, especially if it is obstructed and is palpable on pelvic examination. Gonococci can be recovered by culdocentesis. If therapy is inadequate, the tubes may scar, leading to sterility. Recurrences are common and are usually due to reinfection rather than to reactivation; nevertheless, the residua of one bout of PID increase the risk to 30% of developing PID with the next cervical infection.

About 50% of cases of PID are caused by a mixed flora of aerobic and anaerobic organisms rather than by the gonococcus. If cervical cultures in a patient with PID reveal gonorrhea, the gonococcus can safely be assumed to be the responsible agent. Recovery of other organisms is not helpful, because they grow there normally.

Gonococcemia. The gonococcus can invade the bloodstream, often without producing the symptoms of local gonorrhea. Menstruation heightens the risk of gonococcemia. This bacteremic stage is marked by positive blood cultures, fever, polyarthalgias of the knees, wrists, and small joints of the hand, and skin lesions on the distal extremities. The tiny red papules or petechiae may either disappear or evolve into pustules that eventually develop gray necrotic centers. The skin lesions often contain the gonococcus, the joints only rarely. If therapy is delayed, however, septic arthritis may develop and eventually destroy the involved joints. Gonococcal arthritis is probably the most common form of acute arthritis in young adults. Liver function abnormalities and electrocardiographic changes suggestive of hepatitis and pericarditis are common, but the findings are nonspecific and not indicative of infection of the liver or heart. Meningitis

and endocarditis are rare; when present, they are due to active infection at those sites.

Treatment

One injection of procaine penicillin accompanied by oral probenecid is usually sufficient to treat uncomplicated urethral, cervical, rectal, or pharyngeal gonorrhea. Oral ampicillin or tetracycline works almost as well. Patients with disseminated gonorrhea should be hospitalized and treated with parenteral penicillin until symptoms subside. Therapy should be completed with an outpatient course of ampicillin.

Hospitalization for PID is mandatory when there is a question of acute surgical abdominal disease (appendicitis, ectopic pregnancy, diverticulitis, or endometriosis), during pregnancy, or when the patient is too ill to be cared for at home. With gonococcal PID, treatment with high-dose penicillin should be begun immediately. Because of the mixed nature of nongonococcal PID, treatment has not been standardized; chloramphenicol (for *Bacteroides fragilis*) or gentamicin (for gramnegative rods) is often added to penicillin for patients with PID. Tetracycline is sometimes used for outpatient therapy of milder PID.

Nongonococcal Urethritis. Nongonococcal urethritis is becoming increasingly prevalent. Infected patients also experience dysuria and a white discharge, but a stain and culture of the discharge do not reveal gonorrhea. Many cases are thought to be caused by *Chlamydia trachomatis* and some patients respond to tetracycline.

SYPHILIS

Plagues of syphilis swept Europe beginning in Barcelona in 1493, coincident with the return of Columbus from his voyage to Central

America. It remains unclear whether syphilis was a problem in Europe prior to that. In any case, although the origin of the disease cannot be identified, the etiologic organism can.

Treponema pallidum evokes two patterns of tissue damage. One is a *vasculitis,* an obliterative endarteritis with endothelial and fibroblastic proliferation with a surrounding mononuclear infiltrate. The second is a *granuloma* or *gumma,* similar to the lesions of tuberculosis and sarcoidosis, and consisting of a center of coagulative necrosis surrounded by epithelioid cells within a fibroblastic shell. Gummas underlie much of the destruction of late syphilis, destroying large parts of many organs, especially the liver, bones, and testes.

Treponemes enter the body through minute abrasions, usually during sexual intercourse, although sometimes by contact with infectious cutaneous, genital, or mucous membrane lesions. A systemic spirochetemia occurs, but the first lesions of *primary syphilis* do not become apparent for about three weeks. Then a chancre appears at the site of innoculation, usually the penis, vulva, cervix rectum, or mouth. The chancre begins as a papule, and then painlessly erodes to become a shallow ulcer lined on the base by a characteristic obliterative endarteritis. Scrapings of the lesion should reveal the treponemes with either darkfield or phase-contrast microscopy.

Within another three months, just as the untreated chancre is resolving, the second stage begins. Components of *secondary syphilis* include a flu-like illness with lacrimation, headache, sore throat, arthralgias, generalized lymphadenopathy, and a slight fever. A diffuse rash characteristically appears over the skin and mucosal membranes, and has a predilection for the palms and soles. The lesions are discrete and often of a coppery hue; they may be macular, papular, pustular, but not vesicular. Syphilis should be considered in any patient with a diffuse rash involving the palms and soles. Papular lesions filled with spirochetes coalesce in moist regions of the body, and are then referred to as condylomata lata.

Following the second stage, the disease enters a latent phase marked only by positive serologic tests. The disease may (1) eventually subside and all evidence of infection disappear, (2) continue solely with a positive serology, or (3) proceed to tertiary syphilis.

Tertiary syphilis can involve any organ system. It can be divided into three categories: Gummatous syphilis (described above), cardiovascular syphilis, and neurosyphilis.

Cardiovascular Syphilis. An arteritis of the vessels supplying the ascending aorta can eventually produce an aortic aneurysm. Aortic regurgitation is a potential complication. A thin rim of calcification of the ascending aorta, seen on chest x-ray, should suggest the diagnosis.

Neurosyphilis. Neurosyphilis is now a rare complication of syphilis. The symptoms of neurosyphilis derive from chronic meningitis with extension of the inflammation and fibrosis to neighboring parenchymal vessels. Thus, the patient may present with symptoms of meningitis or of focal cerebrovascular accidents. *General paresis* is part of a more global syndrome, beginning with slightly altered behavior and memory loss and progressing to an incapacitating psychosis with dementia, seizures, and tremors; formerly, this syndrome was a common reason for admission to an insane asylum. In *tabes dorsalis,* the destruction of dorsal roots and posterior column neurons causes a loss of position sense and an ataxic, slapping gate. The loss of the sense of pain from joints traumatized by the thumping gate results in destructive arthritis (Charcot joints). Tabes is also associated with lightening pains of the trunk and lower extremities.

Serology

Serologic tests for syphilis measure the antibody produced by the host in response to invasion by *Treponema pallidum*. There are two general types of tests: one measures antibodies not specifically directed against the treponeme, and the other measures the antibodies specifically directed against the organism.

Nonspecific antibodies (reagins) are directed to antigens on the treponeme or antigens that are released by the host–treponeme interaction. Cardiolipin-lecithin antigens are used to measure their production. Because cardiolipin-lecithin antigens are not specific to the treponeme, but are also found in normal tissue, it is not surprising that such tests are plagued by false-positive reactions in as many as 20% of cases. False-positives may occur after immunization, with a variety of infections, with systemic lupus erythematosus or other connective-tissue diseases, with narcotic addiction, and in the elderly. The VDRL (Venereal Disease Research Laboratory slide test) is the test most commonly used.

Specific antibodies are measured by testing the patient's serum on a dried preparation of *Treponema pallidum*. The FTA-ABS test (fluorescent treponemal antibody absorption test) is the one used today. Only rarely is the FTA-ABS test falsely positive, and it is more sensitive than the VDRL. These antibody titers rise earlier in primary syphilis and stay elevated longer into late syphilis than the antibodies measured by the nonspecific tests. The VDRL, however, falls more rapidly after successful therapy, and is therefore more useful for following the course of treatment.

Treatment

Penicillin is used to treat all stages of syphilis. The later stages require higher dosages. The aortic destruction of cardiovascular syphilis does not improve with treatment, but neurosyphilis may respond, and some clinicians recommend hospitalization for the administration of intravenous penicillin for patients with neurosyphilis.

Differential Diagnosis

Because most clinicians today seldom see and hence seldom recognize chancres, a syphilis serology should be checked on any patient with penile, labial, or cervical lesions. Syphilis should also be considered in patients with mucosal or skin lesions elsewhere, especially on the anus or lips, and in patients with diffuse rashes, dementia, and aortic insufficiency.

Several venereal diseases may be confused with syphilis:

Chancroid is caused by *Hemophilus ducreyi*. It produces painful necrotic ulcerations, usually of the genitalia, in contrast to the nonpainful lesions of primary syphilis. Chancroid is wide-spread among urban populations of Africa and Asia, but is less prevalent in the United States. It is diagnosed by biopsy or culture, and is treated with sulfonamide drugs.

Lymphogranuloma venereum is caused by *Chlamydia trachomatis*. It is marked by a fluctuant, pustular, inguinal adenopathy (in males) or by ulcerating vulvar or rectal lesions, which can terminate in fibrotic strictures. The diagnosis is made by a complement fixation test and a skin test. Treatment is also with sulfonamides.

Herpes progenitalis is a genital lesion composed of discrete vesicles on erythematous bases. These lesions may be so painful that the patient requires hospitalization and parenteral analgesia. In rare instances, herpes may disseminate and involve practically any organ; the immunosuppressed host is at special risk of dissemination. Of the 70 known herpes viruses, 5 have been found to infect humans: Herpes simplex virus-1, herpes simplex virus-2, varicella zoster, Epstein-Barr virus, and cytomegalovirus. Herpes simplex virus-2 is the one most commonly associated with sexually transmitted infections. There is no cure at present. This is especially unfortunate because (1) the herpes virus persists after the initial infection and the lesions recur, and (2) herpes can be transmitted to a newborn traversing an infected birth canal. The majority of infants who acquire the infection subsequently die or suffer permanent neurologic or ocular damage. Delivery by cesarean section when cervical herpetic lesions are present prevents this occurrence.

BIBLIOGRAPHY

Eschenbach DA, Buchanan TM, Pollock HM et al: Polymicrobial etiology of acute pelvic inflammatory disease. N Engl J Med 293:166–171, 1975

Fiumara NJ: The sexually transmissible diseases. DM 25, No. 3:1–94, 1978

Handsfield HH, Wiesner J, Holmes K: Treatment of the gonococcal arthritis–dermatitis syndrome. Ann Intern Med 84:661–667, 1976

Kaufman RH: The origin and diagnosis of "nonspecific vaginitis." N Engl J Med 303:637–638, 1980

Nahmias A, Norrild, B: Herpes simplex viruses 1 and 2: Basic and clinical aspects. DM 25, No. 10:1–49, 1980

57

Osteomyelitis and Cellulitis

OSTEOMYELITIS

Osteomyelitis, or inflammation of the bone, can result either from generalized septicemia or from local spread from a nearby locus of infection (*e.g.*, a wound or cellulitis), or an infectious agent may be introduced through surgery. Whereas the early recognition and improved treatment of septicemia have reduced the incidence of septicemia-related osteomyelitis, the expanding use of reconstructive orthopedic surgery has resulted in an increase in the number of patients developing local bone infections. A third category of patients, which includes those who suffer from vascular insufficiency secondary to diabetes or advanced atherosclerosis and persons with sickle cell anemia, also has an increased risk of developing osteomyelitis.

Prior to the onset of puberty, osteomyelitis is likely to develop in the metaphysis of the bone, sparing the epiphysis which is protected by the epiphyseal plate. In the adult, osteomyelitis can involve both the metaphysis and the epiphysis.

Osteomyelitis resulting from septicemia typically involves bones with plentiful blood supply; these include the long bones (humerus, tibia, femur) in children and the vertebral bodies in adults. In approximately one-half of affected patients, *Staphylococcus aureus* is the responsible organism, but an increasing number of cases are now caused by gramnegative organisms and fungi. In patients with an underlying hemoglobinopathy, especially sickle cell anemia, salmonella is frequently implicated, and multiple bone involvement is common. The incidence of tuberculous osteomyelitis is steadily declining.

Patients with osteomyelitis resulting from septicemia may present with the signs and symptoms of sepsis—chills, fever, and leukocytosis—along with evidence of local bone involvement—pain, erythema, swelling, and tenderness. Septic involvement of other tissues may dominate the clinical picture: endocarditis, pericarditis, meningitis, and septic arthritis are frequently encountered in patients with osteomylitis resulting from septicemia. If the vertebral bodies are involved, systemic symptoms are often absent and dull back pain may be the sole presenting complaint. Because of its indolent nature, vertebral osteomyelitis may remain cryptic for a long time. As a result, some of these patients may develop progressive paraplegia.

Staphylococcus aureus is also the predominant organism in patients with osteomyelitis resulting from spread from a local site of infection. In patients with osteomyelitis on the basis of an impaired vascular supply, staphylococcus and streptococcus are the most likely pathogens. Many of these patients have cellulitis or deep ulcers over the site of bone involvement, typically the toes and small bones of the feet.

Osteomyelitis is common in narcotic abusers. The lumbar vertebrae and sacroiliac joints are most often involved. The correct etiologic diagnosis must be diligently sought, because the pathogens in this patient population are not the typical ones encountered in patients with osteomyelitis; pseudomonas, klebsiella, and fungi may be seen.

Diagnosis

The diagnosis of osteomyelitis may occasionally be made by x-ray, but the radiologic changes usually lag several weeks or even months behind the clinical progression of the disease. Radionuclide bone scans are more sensitive, and usually reveal a lesion within 48 hours of the onset of clinical symptoms.

Therapy

Successful therapy for patients with osteomyelitis requires early identification of the etiologic agent. The earlier antibiotic therapy is instituted, the better the prognosis and the less the chances for future recurrences. If wound or blood cultures are negative, a bone biopsy and culture must be performed. These reveal the diagnosis in more than 90% of patients. A long course (4–6 weeks) of antibiotic therapy is then instituted. If no etiologic agent can be identified, an empiric trial of a penicillinase-resistant penicillin derivative may be tried. In many patients, medical therapy alone is effective, but surgery may be required to drain suppurative collections and debride necrotic bone. Recurrences are often

precipitated by local trauma, and must be treated aggressively.

Subacute and Chronic Osteomyelitis

In some patients, osteomyelitis develops insidiously and progresses slowly. This is called subacute pyogenic osteomyelitis. The x-ray may reveal a lucent bone lesion called Brodie's abscess. Fever and pain are the major symptoms, and the causative agent is usually *Staphylococcus aureus*. In a small number of patients, a form of chronic osteomyelitis, usually due to tuberculosis or syphilis, may develop in the hands and feet.

CELLULITIS

Cellulitis, or inflammation of the subcutaneous tissues, is a common disorder usually caused by streptococcus or staphylococcus. Rarely, other organisms may be responsible. A local injury, such as a puncture wound, is frequently the initiating lesion.

Erysipelas

When streptococcus is the cause of cellulitis, the disorder is termed *erysipelas*. The magnitude of the systemic symptoms is always impressive. The onset of erysipelas is generally heralded by a sustained fever of 104 to 105° F and is often accompanied by a shaking chill. Malaise, headache, and nausea are common. The skin eruption may not appear until several hours after the onset of these symptoms. Once the lesion appears, it spreads rapidly. The skin is tender, erythematous, and indurated, and there is often a clear line of demarcation at the advancing edges that can be palpated. Needle aspiration of an advancing edge may reveal the organism, usually a group A streptococcus. The patient develops leukocytosis, blood cultures may be positive, and the antistreptolysin O (ASO) titer often rises over the ensuing one to two weeks. Erysipelas responds promptly to penicillin.

Staphylococcal Cellulitis

Staphylococcal cellulitis does not have as dramatic an array of identifying features as streptococcus cellulitis. The lesion usually spreads less rapidly and without a clearly demarcated border, although in some patients it may be indistinguishable from erysipelas. Many cases of staphylococcal cellulitis are caused by penicillinase-resistant organisms, and if the distinction between staphylococcal and streptococcal cellulitis is at all uncertain, the initial choice of antibiotic should be a penicillinase-resistant derivative of penicillin.

Differential Diagnosis

Cellulitis must be distinguished from deep venous thrombosis (Chap. 17), particularly when the lesion appears on the lower portions of the legs. Both disorders may present with fever and a warm, erythematous skin lesion. The diagnosis can be simplified by finding palpable thrombosed veins (venous cords), which are present only in deep venous thrombosis. Furthermore, because the skin inflammation of deep venous thrombosis directly overlies the venous involvement, the lesion is only seen over the dorsal surface of the calf. Cellulitis may involve either the dorsal or anterior aspects of the leg.

Complications

Local spread from the site of infection is the major complication of cellulitis that must be avoided. Facial cellulitis is especially worrisome; because of the dangers of ocular involvement and spread to the meninges, it warrants immediate treatment with intravenous antibiotics.

Cellulitis may rarely evolve into full-blown sepsis. Diabetics, who have an increased susceptibility to cellulitis, are at an increased risk of developing septic complications.

Patients with facial cellulitis and patients who are extremely ill, regardless of the location of the cellulitis, should be admitted to the hospital. Any patient in whom the infection is likely to pose special risks (e.g., patients with heart valve prostheses, rheumatic valvular disease, diabetes, and others) must be treated promptly and aggressively.

BIBLIOGRAPHY

Duszynski DO, Kuhn JP, Afshani E et al: Early radionuclide diagnosis of acute osteomyelitis. Radiology 117:337–340, 1975

Holzman RS and Bishko F: Osteomyelitis in heroin addicts. Ann Intern Med 75:693–696, 1971

Waldvogel FA, Medoff G, Swartz MN: Osteomyelitis: A review of clinical features, therapeutic considerations and unusual aspects, N Engl J Med 282:198–206, 260–266, 316–322, 1970

Waldvogel FA, Vasey H: Osteomyelitis: The past decade. N Engl J Med 303:360–370, 1980

58

Infections in the Immunosuppressed Host

The hallmark of the immunosuppressed patient is an increased susceptibility to infection. The infections are often persistent, recurrent, resistant to standard antibiotic therapy, and may be due to unusual organisms.

An increased incidence of infection is by no means a sufficient criterion for the diagnosis of immunosuppression. Various anatomic defects and many diseases that do not directly compromise the immune system (*e.g.,* cystic fibrosis and many dermatologic diseases) all predispose to infection, but these are not true cases of immunosuppression. Rather, the term immunosuppression is usually restricted to patients with a deficiency in one or more of the cellular or humoral components of the immune and inflammatory systems.

The number of patients surviving in a state of immunosuppression has been rising for many years, primarily because of continuing advances in medical care:

1. Patients with severe illnesses are surviving longer. Many illnesses are now known to suppress the body's defenses against infection. A major setting for immunosuppression is cancer, especially hematologic malignancies, such as leukemia, Hodgkin's disease, and multiple myeloma. Immunosuppression can also occur in patients with advanced or meta-static solid tumors. Almost any overwhelming inflammatory state, such as systemic lupus erythematosus or disseminated tuberculosis, can also suppress the immune system.

2. Increasingly potent immunosuppressive therapies are being used to treat a widening variety of illnesses. Foremost among these are the corticosteroids, azathioprine, cyclophosphamide, and the many antimitotic and antimetabolite anticancer drugs. These drugs suppress the bone marrow, often producing granulocytopenia, and may inhibit the function of cells of the immune and inflammatory systems.

Different diseases affect the immune system in different ways, and the spectrum of infections to which the patient is susceptible varies accordingly. Antibody plays a key role in protecting against bacterial infections, and patients with multiple myeloma, who are frequently panhypogammaglobulinemic, are susceptible to bacterial infections. On the other hand, patients with depressed cellular immunity, for example, patients with Hodgkin's disease, are susceptible to viral infections.

The spleen, a major component of the reticuloendothelial system, functions to trap and phagocytose opsonized (antibody-coated) pathogens. Splenectomized persons—often young and otherwise healthy—appear to handle most infections normally, but they have an increased risk of developing overwhelming bacterial sepsis that rapidly progresses to shock. Patients with sickle cell anemia, who are functionally asplenic because of repeated splenic infarctions, and patients with congenital splenic aplasia, are also susceptible to sepsis. The most common pathogen in asplenic patients is *Streptococcus pneumoniae* (pneumococcus), but *Hemophilus influenzae*, staphylococcus, and others may also be responsible. Treatment with high-dose intravenous antibiotics must be instituted immediately when sepsis develops. The mortality is high. Because of the high frequency of pneumococcal infections in these patients, prophylactic immunization with pneumococcal vaccine has been advocated for asplenic individuals.

Evaluation of Immunosuppression

The presence of severe, recurrent, or unusual infections in any patient, but especially in a patient with severe underlying illness or who is receiving potentially immunosuppressive therapy, should arouse one's suspicion of immunosuppression. In many patients, lymphopenia or granulocytopenia will be discovered and the source of immune compromise thus revealed. In other patients, a complete blood count may be normal and abnormalities may only be uncovered with more sensitive tests of immune function.

The humoral limb of the immune system can be initially assessed by measuring the levels of each class of immunoglobulin with serum electrophoresis and immunoelectrophoresis (see Chap. 48). Specific antibodies, such as the blood group isoagglutinins and antibodies to previous vaccinations, provide a further measure of humoral immunity; they may be depressed despite normal total immunoglobulin levels.

Cell-mediated immunity can be measured by applying skin tests to elicit delayed hypersensitivity responses. A battery of several skin test antigens is usually employed, and typically includes candida, mumps, tetanus toxoid, streptokinase-streptodornase, purified protein derivative (PPD), and others. Tests are read 24 to 72 hours later, and an area of induration exceeding 10 mm indicates intact cell-mediated immunity.

Course and Management of the Immunosuppressed Patient

The most complete clinical picture of the course of infections in the immunosuppressed host can be drawn from patients who are granulocytopenic. The prototype is the patient with acute leukemia.

Infection is the major cause of death in adults with acute leukemia. The high incidence of infection is primarily the result of neutropenia and is caused by the activity of the disease, by cachexia, and by chemotherapy. An absolute leukocyte count of less than 500 markedly increases the risk of infection. Gram-negative infections are the most common, and include pseudomonas, *E. coli*, and klebsiella. Staphylococcal sepsis is also frequently encountered.

Most infections in granulocytopenic patients are accompanied by fever, and fever in any patient with a leukocyte count of less than 500 should be assumed to be due to infection. Any sudden clinical deterioration, however, even in the absence of fever, should arouse one's suspicion of infection in such patients.

The lung, urinary tract, skin, and perirectal areas are the typical sites of infection, but in many patients the focus of infection cannot be determined. Infectious sites may go unidentified in part because the diminished number of normal white blood cells results in a blunted inflammatory response to infection. Thus, a pneumonic infection may present with only minimal lung infiltrates on x-ray, and the only evidence of infection may be fever or septic shock.

Despite this caveat, rigorous attempts should be made to identify the specific focus of infection. If an abscess is found, drainage can be initiated. Drainage, however, can be risky in immunosuppressed patients. For that matter, any invasive manipulation of the patient, including rectal examinations and bladder catheterization, may induce a bacteremia. In addition, immunosuppressed patients are frequently thrombocytopenic, so that any incision is hazardous, especially in the highly vascular perianal area.

Once infection is suspected, the patient should be carefully examined, a chest x-ray obtained, appropriate cultures taken, and antibiotic sensitivities determined. If meningitis is suspected in a patient with thrombocytopenia, platelet transfusions should be given before a lumbar puncture is performed.

In the febrile and granulocytopenic patient, antibiotics must be instituted immediately, even before a specific organism is identified. Standard coverage includes an aminoglycoside and a semisynthetic penicillin. Many centers routinely add carbenicillin to protect against *Pseudomonas aeruginosa*. When the antibiotic sensitivites are determined, antibiotic coverage should be adjusted accordingly.

Many studies have been performed to compare the effectiveness of various antibiotic regimens but no absolute guidelines have emerged. The advantages of including carbenicillin have not been demonstrated convincingly. Many of the organisms isolated from immunosuppressed patients are sensitive to aminoglycosides, and the inclusion of this class of drugs seems advisable. The aminogly-

cosides have major nephrotoxic and ototoxic side-effects. Cephalothin, a widely used semisynthetic penicillin, may increase the incidence of renal damage when used in combination with gentamicin. The use of granulocyte transfusions (see Chap. 44) offers a promising adjunct to antibiotics in the treatment of infections in severely granulocytopenic patients.

If the patient becomes afebrile, a two-week course of antibiotic therapy is usually adequate. Persistent fever and neutropenia are associated with a high rate of recurrence of sepsis. The nature of the flora may change during therapy, and the antibiotics may have to be readjusted.

Pseudomonas, klebsiella, candida, and multiple bacterial sepsis carry the worst prognoses. If shock supervenes, the prognosis is even more grave.

Fungal infections are becoming increasingly prevalent, and autopsy series show a 25% to 50% incidence of fungal infections in neutropenic patients. In patients with acute leukemia, candida and aspergillus account for almost all fungal infections.

The diagnosis of candidiasis can be difficult. By the time the blood cultures grow candida, the organism is usually disseminated. Candidiasis should be suspected when there are positive cultures from two or more sites (for example, skin, mouth, stool, etc.) or when there are progressively increasing numbers of fungi in the urine. Candida esophagitis is common, but does not necessarily lead to disseminated disease. An esophagogram may show the characteristic shallow esophageal ulcerations.

Aspergillosis is even more difficult to diagnose. It should be suspected when a new pulmonary infiltrate develops in a neutropenic patient who is already receiving antibiotics. A lung biopsy gives the best diagnostic yield, but the sputum should be examined first for hyphae in the hope of avoiding the necessity of the invasive procedure.

Both candida and aspergillus are treated with parenteral amphotericin B. The drug has numerous potentially severe side-effects, including liver toxicity and renal toxicity.

Severely immunosuppressed patients are also susceptible to infections with unusual organisms, such as *Pneumocystis carinii* and various parasites, especially *Toxoplasma gondii*. Patients with pneumocystis infection generally present with an acute interstitial pneumonitis associated with fever, dyspnea, and a nonproductive cough. Therapy includes trimethoprim and sulfamethoxazole. Patients with toxoplasma generally present with disseminated infection or evidence of encephalitis, and are treated with a combination of sulfadiazine and pyrimethamine.

BIBLIOGRAPHY

Edwards JE Jr, Lehrer RI, Stiehm ER et al: Severe candidal infections: Clinical perspective, immune defense mechanisms, and current concepts of therapy. Ann Intern Med 89:91–106 1978

Gurwith MJ, Brunton JL, Lank BA et al: Granulocytopenia in hospitalized patients. I. Prognostic factors and etiology of fever. Am J Med 64:121–126, 1978

Gurwith MJ, Brunton JL, Lank BA, et al: Granulocytopenia in hospitalized patients. II. A prospective comparison of two antibiotic regimens in the empiric therapy of febrile patients. Am J Med 64:127–132, 1978

Ketchel SJ and Rodriquez V: Acute infections in cancer patients. Semin Oncol 5:167–179, 1978

Likhite VV: Immunological impairment and susceptibility to infection after splenectomy. JAMA 236:1376–1377, 1976

Williams DM, Krick JA, and Remington JS: Pulmonary infections in the compromised host. Am Rev Respir Dis 114:359–394, 593–627, 1976

Neurology

59

Coma

Consciousness appears to depend upon the integrity of a structure known as the reticular activating system, which is buried deep in the core of the brainstem. The normal functioning of the reticular activating system can be compromised by expanding intracranial masses or by metabolic or traumatic insults.

Several states of diminished consciousness may precede coma or may appear during recovery from coma. These include (1) delirium, in which the patient is alert, although confused and disoriented, and may be suffering sensory hallucinations, and (2) stupor, in which the patient is unresponsive, but arousable by intense stimuli.

The patient in coma appears to be asleep and is unarousable by any stimuli. In the lightest stages of coma, primitive brain stem and spinal cord reflexes persist. In the deepest stages of coma, these are lost, as are the corneal, pupillary, tendon, and plantar reflexes. Eventually, normal medullary, respiratory, and cardiovascular controls disappear, and the patient dies.

Structural Causes of Coma

A small intracranial lesion can cause coma only by directly impinging upon the brain stem. Central nervous system lesions distant from the brain stem can cause coma indirectly by expanding within the inflexible cranial vault until the brain stem herniates downward or is compressed by the neighboring temporal lobes. This process is called *tentorial herniation.*

The tentorium cerebelli is an inflexible fibrous septum separating the anterior and posterior fossae. It has a hole through which the brain stem passes. The temporal lobes sit on top of the tentorium, abutting the brain stem. Between the temporal lobes and the brain stem pass the oculomotor nerves.

When a supratentorial mass—a tumor, abscess, or hemorrhage—expands, the only place for the temporal lobes to move is over the side of the tentorium and into the tentorial notch, first compressing the oculomotor nerve and then the midbrain. Compression of the oculomotor nerve is responsible for the unilaterally dilated pupil colloquially known as a "blown pupil." It signals the imminent disaster of irreversible brain stem damage.

Diseases of a single hemisphere of the brain do not cause coma unless they expand with consequent herniation. Coma is not caused by the increased pressure *per se*, but rather by the profound structural dislocation of the brain stem.

An appreciation of the clinical course of brain stem dysfunction is essential to the evaluation of coma. Alterations in neurologic function can be assessed by monitoring changes in breathing patterns, pupillary reflexes, oculomotor movement, peripheral motor movements, and posturing.

Breathing. The earliest respiratory change is called *Cheyne-Stokes respiration*, in which periods of rapid and deep breathing are interrupted by apneic pauses. Cheyne-Stokes respiration itself poses no threat to the patient. It results either from (1) central nervous system disease (a massive supratentorial lesion or a metabolic insult), with consequent enhancement of the sensitivity of the carbon dioxide receptor, or (2) congestive heart failure, in which the slowed circulation time causes a delayed transfer of information between the lungs and the carbon dioxide receptor.

With increasing damage to the brain stem, other patterns of breathing may be observed:

1. *Central neurogenic hyperventilation* occurs when there is structural involvement of the lower midbrain and upper pons. The patient hyperventilates continuously.

2. *Apneustic breathing* may indicate a lower pontine lesion. The patient holds his breath for two to three seconds with each inspiration.

3. *Chaotic breathing* suggests medullary involvement, and deteriorates to occasional gasping and eventually to apnea.

Pupillary Response. When structural lesions are responsible for coma, normal pupillary responses are maintained until the pupillary constrictor and dilator regions of the midbrain are compromised; at that time the pupils become fixed and remain at midposition.

Extraocular Movements. Extraocular movements can be elicited in the comatose patient by briskly turning the head from side to side. This is called the *doll's eyes maneuver.* If extraocular movements are preserved, the eyes move conjugately in the direction opposite to the head tilt, indicating that the midbrain and pontine inputs to the third, fourth, and sixth cranial nerves must still be intact. (This can only be elicited in the comatose patient and not in the normal, alert person.) Another test for assessing the integrity of the brain stem involves irrigating an ear with cool water and looking for binocular nystagmus with the rapid phase away from the irrigated ear. Focal lesions may, of course, interrupt specific innervation; thus, for example, abducens nerve palsy produces medial deviation of one eye.

When the brain stem is compressed by temporal lobe herniation, conjugate deviation can no longer be demonstrated.

Peripheral Motor Movements and Posturing. Maintenance of motor movements, such as aimless grasping or picking motions, is an encouraging sign that suggests that the corticospinal tracts are intact. Lesions of the cerebrum may cause *decorticate rigidity,* with flexion of one or both arms and extension of the legs. Disturbances of the lower diencephalic or midbrain structures produce *decerebrate rigidity,* in which both arms and legs are extended and internally rotated. Such posturing can sometimes only be elicited with stimulation. Decerebrate posturing can be caused by certain metabolic disturbances, such as hypoglycemia. Unilateral abnormalities of posture or tendon reflexes suggest that some focal disease is the etiology of the coma. However, evidence of unilateral involvement may be misleading, since severe metabolic disturbances can enhance, or even elicit for the first time, evidence of old, healed unilateral neurologic disease.

Metabolic Causes of Coma

The electrical and metabolic activity of a nerve cell depends critically on its immediate environment, and it is therefore not surprising that coma can follow any severe imbalance in the homeostatic regulation of pH, ionic concentration, or temperature, or the deprivation of critical nutrients such as glucose or oxygen. Toxins which are ingested, injected, or which accumulate because of renal or hepatic failure can depress neural function and produce coma. Reduced cerebral blood flow, either from inadequate cardiac output, peripheral vasodilatation (sepsis), or diffuse small vessel occlusion (systemic lupus erythematosus, disseminated intravascular coagulation) can produce coma.

Several drugs that are capable of inducing coma produce characteristic changes in pupillary size and response: Opiates cause constriction of the pupil to a pinpoint; atropine causes fixed and widely dilated pupils; glutethimide leaves the pupils unreactive and of medium size. In general, however, even the most severe metabolic insults do not affect the normal pupillary response.

With the exception of barbiturates and phenytoin, metabolic disturbances generally also leave conjugate eye movements intact.

Certain generalizations can help to distinguish metabolic causes of coma from structural ones:

1. A period of mental deterioration precedes the onset of metabolic coma. Drowsiness, disorientation regarding time, date, and place, and the loss of awareness may be accompanied by agitation and delirium. Particularly characteristic of this phase are diffuse motor twitchings that include tremors, asterixis, and myoclonus.

2. Certain brainstem functions are preserved despite widespread central nervous system depression that may be severe enough to produce decerebrate posturing and respiratory depression. These include the pupillary light response and, to a lesser degree, conjugate ocular motility. Glutethimide and anoxic brain damage may, however, cause fixed and unequal pupils.

3. Although there are generally no focal neurologic findings in patients with metabolic coma, certain types of metabolic insults can cause stroke-like neurologic findings.

EVALUATION AND TREATMENT OF THE COMATOSE PATIENT

Most cases of coma derive from medical or neurosurgical catastrophes, and can be at least partially remedied if rapidly diagnosed and appropriately treated. The more common causes of coma include (1) shock, from sepsis, hypovolemia, or large myocardial infarctions, (2) hematoma or intracerebral bleed, (3) hypoglycemia, (4) drug and alcohol overdosage, (5) diabetic ketoacidosis, (6) meningitis, (7) hypertensive encephalopathy, (8) uremia, and (9) hepatic encephalopathy. More insidious causes of coma include brain tumors and slow intracerebral bleeds. With the advent of rapid techniques for the detection of drugs in the serum and urine and with the expanding use of computerized axial tomographic (CT) scans, the correct diagnosis can usually be made quickly.

In treating the patient with coma, the first priority should be maintaining a patent airway and providing adequate cardiovascular support. Evidence of trauma, especially to the head and neck, must be sought before moving the patient, in order to avoid the danger of further injuring the spinal cord. Rapid evaluation of brain stem function can be performed while blood and urine samples are obtained for the evaluation of diabetic ketoacidosis, hypoglycemia, hepatic coma, uremia, and poisoning. Immediately after the blood is obtained, naloxone and a bolus of a concentrated

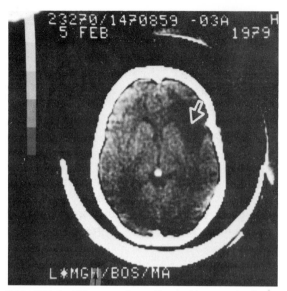

FIG. 59–1. CT scan of a patient with a stroke from a nonhemorrhagic infarct (arrow).

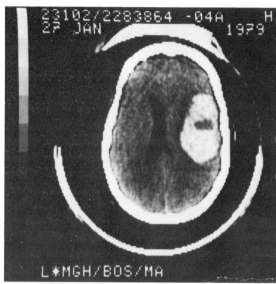

FIG. 59–2. CT scan of a young woman with a hemorrhagic stroke. She was taking anticoagulants at the time. The blood appears as an increased density. Note the fluid level.

FIG. 59–3. CT scan of a patient with a brain metastasis from lung carcinoma. The large metastasis is indicated by the arrow. The enlarged ventricles indicate possible obstructing hydrocephalus, probably caused by another metastasis not visualized in this cut.

FIG. 59–4. CT scan of a man with communicating hydrocephalus. Note how both ventricles are dramatically enlarged.

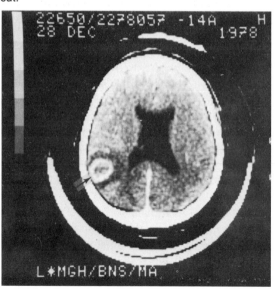

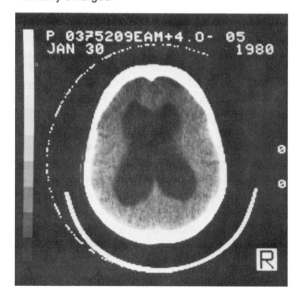

glucose solution are routinely given. Arterial blood gases should be measured to help regulate ventilatory support.

The physical examination may reveal some specific diagnostic hints. For example, a quick perusal of the skin may reveal the cherry red coloration of carbon monoxide poisoning, the rash of meningococcemia, or the pustules of staphylococcal bacteremia. Hypothermia may be due to sepsis, myxedema coma, or barbiturate overdosage; very severe hypothermia is usually the result of exposure. Hypertension may suggest hypertensive encephalopathy. The patient's breath may carry the fruity smell of diabetic ketoacidosis, the musty sweet odor of fetor hepaticus, or the smell of alcohol. Alcohol on the breath does not preclude the possibility that other agents were also ingested.

Lumbar Puncture. In patients with a supratentorial mass lesion, a lumbar puncture may hasten herniation by rapidly lowering the pressure in the lumbar compartment. Fortunately, this complication is rare, and lumbar puncture remains the key diagnostic maneuver in meningitis (Chap. 51). A lumbar puncture is also helpful in diagnosing intracranial hemorrhage or hematoma.

CT Scanning. CT scanning is replacing most invasive diagnostic maneuvers in the emergency diagnosis of intracranial mass lesions. The patient lies in the computerized axial tomographic scanner while the x-ray tube revolves around his head. The computer aligns the images to provide a picture of a thin slice of brain. The quality of the resultant reconstruction, especially if combined with the use of injected contrast agents, has made CT scanning invaluable in the diagnosis of tumors, hemorrhages, abscesses, and hydrocephalus (Fig. 59-1 through 59-4). CT scanning has to a large degree replaced craniotomies in

the initial evaluation of acute head trauma. If a supratentorial mass lesion is suspected, a CT scan should be obtained before a lumbar puncture is performed.

BRAIN DEATH

Brain death means the loss of all cerebral and brain stem function, and does not merely imply a state of prolonged unresponsiveness. The criteria established for brain death have been chosen to correlate with inevitable cardiac death and with irreversible and widespread pathologic destruction of brain tissue. With the emerging need for donor tissues for transplantation, and with the increasingly publicized debates about the proper timing for the withdrawal of life support systems, there have been numerous attempts to outline uniform criteria for brain death.

Before even beginning to consider a patient as having suffered brain death, metabolic causes of coma must be carefully excluded. Thus, for example, both hypothermia and drug intoxication (especially from barbiturate overdosage) may give rise to an isoelectric (flat) electroencephalogram.

At present, the attending physician makes the decision that brain death has occurred. Most agree that brain death has occurred when there is: (1) coma, without any vocal or motor response to external stimuli; (2) apnea, with a reliance upon mechanical ventilations; and (3) loss of brainstem reflexes, with fixed pupils, no ocular movement, and no corneal or pharyngeal reflexes. Spinal cord reflexes may persist. In Europe, confirmation is sometimes obtained by demonstrating a lack of intracranial perfusion on arteriography. In the United States, an isoelectric electroencephalogram is usually used as an adjunct to diagnosis, and is repeated after 24 hours.

BIBLIOGRAPHY

Black PM: Brain Death. N Engl J Med 299:338–344, 393–401, 1978

Fisher CM: The neurological examination of the comatose patient. Acta Neurol Scand (Suppl) 36:45, 1969

Plum F, Posner JB: Diagnosis of Stupor and Coma. Philadelphia, FA Davis, 1980

60

Stroke

If I forget thee, O, Jerusalem,
  Let my right hand forget her cunning.
If I do not remember thee,
  Let my tongue cleave to the roof of my mouth;
If I prefer not Jerusalem above my chief joy.

Psalm 137

During the Babylonian exile, the ancient Hebrews admonished themselves never to forget their spiritual origins under penalty of suffering the devastating consequences of an incapacitating stroke. Today, in the United States, stroke (or cerebrovascular accident, CVA) is the third most common cause of death and contributes greatly to morbidity in the elderly population.

Hypertension and atherosclerosis are the major predisposing factors for most kinds of stroke. For unknown reasons, the incidence of stroke has declined markedly over the past several decades. It is possible that the recent campaigns to lower blood pressure are partly responsible for this decrease. A Veteran's Administration study has shown that treatment of hypertension does diminish the risk of stroke.

A stroke is the clinical manifestation of a vascular lesion that may evolve rapidly over seconds to minutes, or more gradually over a period of days. It is characterized clinically by the abrupt appearance of any new neurologic deficit, excluding seizures (although a seizure disorder may occur as a sequela to a cerebral infarct).

There are three major etiologies of stroke: (1) arterial thrombosis, (2) embolism, and (3) hemorrhage. In most clinical series, thrombosis is the most common cause of stroke, followed by embolism and hemorrhage. The manifestations of these three types of stroke overlap to a large degree, but there are, in addition, certain clinical findings that are characteristic of each of the different etiologies (Table 60-1).

CHRONOLOGY OF A STROKE

The time course of the neurologic changes must be noted in all strokes. A *transient ischemic attack* (TIA) presents as an acute neurologic deficit that is rapid in onset and of short duration. By definition, the deficit must resolve within 24 hours, but most TIAs are completed within 30 minutes.

In a *stroke-in-evolution* (progressing stroke), the severity or the extent of the new neurologic lesion continues to increase after the patient has been placed under medical observation.

In a *completed stroke*, neurologic changes have been stable for 24 to 72 hours.

433

Table 60–1. The Stroke Syndromes

	Stroke Secondary to Cardiac Emboli	Thrombotic and Thromboembolic Stroke	Hypertensive Hemorrhage	Berry Aneurysm
Patient Profile				
Risk factors	Atrial fibrillation Cardiomyopathy Myocardial infarction Endocarditis Mitral valve prolapse	Hypertension Atherosclerosis Diabetes mellitus Advanced age	Hypertension	
Precipitating events	Return to normal sinus rhythm from atrial fibrillation	Hypotension; often occurs during sleep	Hypertension	Exertion where blood pressure is increased
Concomitant disease	Emboli to kidney, spleen, etc.	Diffuse atherosclerosis Carotid bruits	Sequelae of hypertension (renal failure, CHF, etc.)	Polycystic renal disease Coarctation of the aorta
Clinical Course				
Prodrome	TIAs less common, will affect various territories	TIAs very common	None	Usually none—occasionally vague symptoms during week before the stroke
Territory involved	Middle cerebral artery most common; various territories may be affected by repeated emboli	Supplied by a single vessel	Diffuse—by mass effect Putamen most common	Focal signs unusual
Headache	No premonitory headache	Occasionally present	Severe headache and nuchal rigidity common	Sudden & severe nuchal rigidity common
State of alertness	Usually awake	Usually conscious	Usually stuporous May be alert at first	Early coma—may become alert later
Progression	Abrupt; stroke completed within minutes	Develops intermittently Occasional periods of recovery, followed by worsening ("stuttering")	Gradual over minutes to hours	Sudden
Residua & sequelae	Rapid improvement usually within hours to days Appearance of a new seizure focus not uncommon Repeated emboli very common	Gradual improvement over months; considerable deficit often remains	Resolution very slow	Recurrent hemorrhages very common
Laboratory				
CSF	Normal (unless hemorrhage has occurred)	Mild increase in protein Slight pleocytosis No RBCs unless hemorrhage has also occurred	Usually grossly hemorrhagic	Hemorrhagic

These distinctions are important because therapeutic intervention can be effective only for TIAs and strokes-in-evolution (discussion later).

THE STROKE SYNDROMES

The particular neurologic signs and symptoms that a stroke produces reflect the location of the vascular lesion and also provide information about the size of the injured area. A broad array of neurologic syndromes can be seen, ranging from coma and dense paralysis to subtle aphasias and mild weakness.

The various constellations of symptoms comprising the stroke syndromes can be understood by studying the blood supply to the brain.

Strokes of the Internal Carotid System. Each internal carotid artery supplies one cerebral hemisphere. The major branches of the internal carotid include the ophthalmic and anterior choroidal arteries, the middle cerebral artery (which supplies the basal ganglia, large portions of the frontal, parietal, and temporal lobes, and the internal capsule), and the anterior cerebral artery (which supplies portions of the frontal and parietal lobes).

Strokes due to lesions in the internal carotid arterial system are very common. When the *middle cerebral artery* is involved, patients frequently present with contralateral hemiplegia, hemianesthesia, and homonymous hemianopsia (blindness affecting either the right or left half of the visual fields of both eyes). Aphasia (a defect in the comprehension or expression of spoken or written language) may also occur when the dominant hemisphere is affected. If the *anterior cerebral artery* is affected, patients typically have behavioral changes, urinary incontinence, infantile reflexes (*e.g.*, the suck and grasp reflexes), and sensorimotor changes. If the *internal carotid artery* itself is involved, elements of one or both of the above syndromes

may appear. Because the internal carotid artery supplies the optic nerves and retina, a transient monocular blindness is common when the internal carotid artery is occluded.

The amount of collateral blood flow passing between the two internal carotid arteries via the circle of Willis and between the internal and external carotid systems varies from individual to individual. The clinical and pathologic consequences of occlusion of the internal carotid are therefore quite variable. When the collateral supply is substantial, and especially when the occlusion is gradual, a complete occlusion of the internal carotid may even be totally asymptomatic. Collateral circulation is also responsible for the rarity of permanent symptomatology caused by occlusion of the central retinal artery.

Occlusion of the internal carotid is unique among the vascular lesions leading to stroke in that it is accessible to the physical examiner. Diminished blood flow and bruits can frequently be detected in patients with internal carotid disease. In addition, the supratrochlear pulse, which can be palpated on the rim of the superior orbit, is often enhanced on the side of the occlusion, because the vessels serve as collaterals to bypass the occlusion.

Strokes of the Vertebrobasilar Artery System. The brain stem and posterior cortex receive their blood supply via the vertebrobasilar system. The vertebral arteries ascend along the anterior surface of the medulla and enter the posterior fossa through the foramen magnum. These arteries supply the medulla and, via the posterior inferior cerebellar arteries, the inferior portion of the cerebellum.

The two vertebral arteries merge at the level of the pons to form the single basilar artery. Branches of the basilar artery supply the pons and the anterior and superior portions of the cerebellum. The basilar artery then branches into the two posterior cerebral arteries, which supply (1) the occipital lobes (including the visual cortex) and part of the temporal lobes, (2) the thalamus, via perforating thalamic arteries, and (3) the upper brain stem.

The exact pattern of blood supply in the vertebrobasilar system is highly variable. For example, the posterior cerebral arteries frequently receive blood from the circle of Willis via posterior communicating arteries.

The brain stem includes the nuclei for the cranial nerves, the descending motor and ascending sensory tracts, and regions for cardiovascular and respiratory regulation. It is therefore not surprising that, in contrast to most small focal cortical strokes, vertebrobasilar insufficiency can have devastating consequences. Small lesions may compromise the cranial nerves (with consequent extraocular movement discoordination, facial weakness and anesthesia, and loss of normal glottic and gag mechanisms), cause widespread paralysis and sensory loss, or even result in apnea, hypotension, and coma.

Disruption of the vertebrobasilar artery system produces a variety of specific stroke syndromes. The *lateral medullary syndrome*, for example, is generally caused by disruption of the vertebral artery. This stroke syndrome often begins abruptly with the sudden onset of nausea, vomiting, vertigo, and ataxia. Several anatomic regions are affected and produce characteristic symptomatology:

Region of Compromise	Symptoms
Spinothalamic tract	Contralateral loss of pain and heat sensation
Sympathetic tract	Ipsilateral Horner's syndrome (ptosis, meiosis, and anhidrosis)
Vestibular nuclei	Vertigo, nausea, vomiting
Cranial nerves or nerve tracts:	
ninth and tenth	Hoarseness, dysphagia
fifth	Decreased ipsilateral facial sensations
Cerebellar tracts	Ataxia

As is evident from this example, the range of symptoms produced by disruption of the blood supply to the brain stem and cerebellum is extremely varied. Part of the complexity is due to the intricate tapestry of nuclei and ascending and descending tracts in the brain stem.

Thalamic syndromes arise when the perforating thalamic arteries are involved. The hallmark of these stroke syndromes is a varying degree of sensory loss; no motor deficits need accompany the diminished sensation. Most patients gradually recover sensation but may be left with hyperpathia and pain.

Occlusion of the posterior cerebral artery supplying the cortex results in visual loss. This takes the form of a homonymous hemianopsia. Central vision is often maintained because the occipital pole is supplied by the internal carotid system. When both posterior cerebral arteries are compromised, the patient may have cortical blindness due to bilateral homonymous hemianopsia. The optic fundi and pupillary reflexes remain intact, and the patient may even deny being blind.

The Lacunar State. The *lacunar state* is a family of stroke syndromes that occurs in patients who have hypertension and atherosclerosis. This array of syndromes is caused by infarcts of small penetrating arteries. Although postmortem examination reveals the presence of small holes (lacunae), lesions cannot be detected by CT scan or angiography. The clinical syndromes of lacunar stroke include (1) cerebellar ataxia with pyramidal tract signs (due to a midbrain lesion), (2) dysarthria-clumsy hand syndrome (a pontine lesion), (3) isolated hemiplegia (an internal capsule lesion), (4) pure sensory lesions (the lesion may lie in the thalamus), and (5) pseudobulbar palsy, which includes rigidity, a small stepping gait, and uncontrollable laughing and crying (usually the result of multiple lacunae).

DETERMINING THE ETIOLOGY OF STROKE

The cause of a patient's stroke must be determined in order to plan a rational therapeutic regimen.

Thrombotic and Thromboembolic Strokes

Atherosclerosis frequently involves the cerebral arteries. The lumen of the affected vessel is narrowed, and a bruit may be heard over the carotid artery (behind and below the angle of the mandible). These patients are at risk for thrombotic strokes and may experience one or many premonitory transient ischemic attacks (TIAs). There are at least two mechanisms that can cause TIAs in these patients:

1. Thromboembolic TIAs can occur when thrombi break off from friable plaques, course downstream, and finally lodge in a small distal artery and cause ischemia. The resultant neurologic syndrome usually resolves within minutes, although completed strokes can also occur. A white material, thought to be platelet-fibrin emboli or atheromatous material, can often be seen in the vessels on retinal examination during such a TIA.

2. Any hemodynamic insult that produces hypotension can decrease flow through stenotic cerebral arteries and cause ischemia. TIAs can therefore occur in patients with orthostatic hypotension, the sick sinus syndrome, aortic stenosis, or shock.

Not all TIAs herald future strokes. Nearly all thrombotic strokes, however, are preceded by TIAs that usually affect the same region of the brain as the ensuing stroke. Approximately 25% of patients with TIAs suffer a cerebral infarction within five years, often within a month of the first TIA. TIAs affecting the carotid artery system may cause transient monocular blindness (amaurosis fugax) or transient unilateral hemispheral attacks of paresis, numbness, and dysphasias. Vertebro-basilar TIAs are characterized by motor and sensory deficits, dizziness, diplopia, and dysarthria.

Patients who have recently suffered multiple TIAs should be considered to have an impending stroke and should be hospitalized. Hypotension must be avoided. Four-vessel cerebral artery angiography may be appropriate in patients who have had multiple TIAs. The study may reveal an extracranial atherosclerotic stenosis that is amenable to arterial bypass surgery or endarterectomy. Aspirin is effective in decreasing the risk of stroke in men with fibrin-platelet related TIAs, but not in women. Anticoagulants may also prove to be beneficial in decreasing the incidence of future strokes, although data are, at present, conflicting.

The same mechanisms responsible for TIAs can also cause thrombotic or thromboembolic strokes. The stroke often occurs when there is hemorrhage into an atherosclerotic plaque. Platelet and fibrin deposition follow the hemorrhage, resulting in the formation of a thrombus that can occlude the lumen of the vessel. Cerebral infarction may occur instantly, but more often the neurologic deficits occur in a step-wise, "stuttering" fashion over several hours, resulting in a "stroke-in-evolution."

Heparin anticoagulation may be effective in halting the progression of the thrombotic process in patients with a stroke-in-evolution, but once the stroke is completed, anticoagulation will not prove beneficial. Most patients who survive the stroke show mild, gradual improvement over several months.

A major therapeutic problem arises when a patient who has never suffered a TIA or stroke is found to have an asymptomatic carotid bruit on routine physical examination. The potential significance of the bruit should first be evaluated in a noninvasive manner. Carotid phonoangiography can analyze a bruit and pinpoint the site of the lesion. The nature of the lesion can be further explored with carotid Doppler studies and oculoplethys-mography. Cerebral arteriography itself carries the risk of stroke and must be performed only after careful noninvasive examination. In some hospitals, patients with asymptomatic but hemodynamically significant carotid bruits undergo endarterectomy or carotid arterial bypass surgery prior to major noncranial operations (e.g., coronary artery bypass surgery).

Embolic Strokes

The characteristic rapid evolution of neurologic symptoms in embolic strokes is in dramatic contrast to the gradual evolution of symptoms in thrombotic strokes. There are virtually no premonitory signs or symptoms. Embolic strokes often resolve quickly, and improvement in the patient's clinical status may be noted within hours to days. Most cerebral emboli originate from mural thrombi that form within dilated atria, especially in patients with atrial fibrillation. Thrombi can also form in the ventricles of patients with dilated cardiomyopathy or ventricular aneurysms, and during the evolution of a myocardial infarction. Thus, patients with mitral stenosis, who frequently have both dilated atria and atrial fibrillation, have a high incidence of embolic strokes. Valves can also be the source of emboli when fibrin, bacteria, or fungi accumulate on prosthetic valves or on the injured valves of patients with endocarditis. Patients with the click-murmur syndrome are also at an increased risk of suffering an embolic stroke.

An electrocardiogram should be obtained in all patients with suspected stroke, since a silent myocardial infarction can result in arrhythmias and the ejection of emboli.

Emboli usually lodge at a bifurcation of a cerebral artery; the middle cerebral artery is most frequently affected. Embolic strokes occur abruptly, evolve quickly, and are completed rapidly. Most patients suffer repeated embolic events. Patients who experience embolic strokes only infrequently report TIAs. When TIAs do occur, they may cause varying neurologic syndromes reflecting involvement of different cerebral arteries.

The primary therapeutic goal is to halt the thrombotic process in the heart and to prevent the next stroke. Heparin anticoagulation is therefore indicated once the possibility of cerebral hemorrhage has been excluded. Blood cultures must be obtained in all patients who are suspected of having a new embolic stroke in order to exclude the diagnosis of infectious endocarditis.

Future embolic strokes may be prevented if susceptible patients are identified and treated with chronic coumarin therapy. Patients with mitral stenosis and atrial fibrillation should receive anticoagulant therapy, and, in some hospitals, all patients with stable atrial fibrillation or dilated cardiomyopathy are maintained on anticoagulation. The routine use of anticoagulants during acute myocardial infarction remains controversial. Whether the risks of anticoagulation outweigh the benefits must be determined for each patient (see Chap. 17).

Hemorrhagic Strokes

Hypertension is the most common cause of intracerebral bleeding, followed by rupture of saccular (berry) aneurysms (generally of the circle of Willis) and arteriovenous malformations. The rate of evolution of hemorrhagic strokes is variable and probably reflects the rate of bleeding. Although premonitory symptoms may occur, most cerebral hemorrhages are abrupt in onset. They frequently involve the areas supplied by the vertebrobasilar artery system. Most patients are stuporous when first seen, but some are initially alert and may complain of severe headaches and vomit repeatedly. Nuchal rigidity and seizures are more common in this than in other forms of stroke. Most patients die of the stroke within the first month. Among those who survive, resolution of neurologic deficits occurs very slowly.

The most common site of bleeding is the *putamen*, and patients may then develop paralysis, stupor, and coma. Hemorrhages involving the *basal ganglia* often cause seizures and coma, and the prognosis is very poor. A *thalamic hemorrhage* may present with hemiplegia and ocular disturbances; the sensory deficits are usually more dramatic than the motor deficits. A *pontine hemorrhage* can cause total paralysis and coma. Bleeding into the *cerebellum* often presents with occipital headache, vertigo, and vomiting. Lateral eye movements are disturbed, and symptoms of ataxia may not be immediately apparent. These patients deteriorate over hours, becoming stuporous and comatose. The effectiveness of surgical intervention, involving the evacuation of the blood from the posterior fossa, depends upon the expeditious recognition of the possibility of a cerebellar hemorrhage. Prompt diagnosis can thus be lifesaving.

A common cause of stroke in young people is rupture of berry aneurysms that arise from the circle of Willis or its branches. Berry aneurysms can be clearly demonstrated by angiography. Most patients with ruptured berry aneurysms suffer recurrent hemorrhages, and mortality approaches 50% within six months of a rupture. Patients with a ruptured aneurysm require sedation and quiet bed rest for a month or longer. Surgical repair of the aneurysm may be attempted. Epsilon-amino-caproic acid, an antifibrinolytic agent, may successfully retard clot lysis and thereby diminish the extent of the hemorrhage.

Evaluation of Hemorrhage in Strokes

Since the presence of cerebral hemorrhage is a contraindication to the use of anticoagulants in therapy, it is vital to determine whether bleeding has occurred.

Arterial bleeding occurs in a hemorrhagic stroke caused by rupture of a berry aneurysm or small arteriolar microaneurysms, found in patients with chronic hypertension. *Venous bleeding* may occur following cerebral infarction secondary to a thrombotic or embolic stroke when the surrounding brain tissues soften and the veins lose their structural support.

The cranial CT scan is the most reliable method of detecting bleeding, and can identify even small hemorrhages that never reach the subarachnoid space.

In addition to detecting intracerebral hemorrhage, the CT scan can aid in the differential diagnosis of stroke by delineating the presence of a subdural hematoma or an intracranial tumor. Furthermore, the CT scan often localizes the precise site of a cerebrovascular accident.

If anticoagulation is being considered, the cerebrospinal fluid (CSF) should also be examined in an effort to rule out hemorrhage. In a cerebral hemorrhage that communicates with the subarachnoid space, the CSF pressure is elevated and blood is grossly present. The ratio of leukocytes to erythrocytes in the CSF is similar to that in the peripheral blood. Within a few hours, xanthochromia (a yellow hue) is apparent in the supernatant fraction of a centrifuged specimen of CSF.

An incorrect diagnosis of cerebral hemorrhage may be made when the lumbar puncture itself causes local bleeding. When such a "traumatic tap" occurs, the specimens of CSF that are collected earliest contain more red blood cells than later specimens. The sample may clot in the test tube, and xanthochromia is usually absent.

DIFFERENTIAL DIAGNOSIS OF STROKE

A patient with a *subdural hematoma* may also present with altered mentation and paralysis. The global confusion and alteration in mentation, however, are usually more marked than any focal neurologic deficit, and the symptoms typically evolve over a period of days or even weeks. A subdural hematoma must be considered in any patient who has suffered cranial trauma or who has recently fallen. A CT scan usually confirms the diagnosis.

Other diagnostic considerations include *Todd's paralysis*, in which a transient paralysis follows a grand mal seizure. *Migraine headaches* may present with hemianopsia, and *syncope* and *vertigo* can be confused with the symptoms of basilar stroke. *Tumors* and *brain abscesses* can cause paralysis and other symptoms of stroke, although such changes usually occur over many weeks.

THERAPY

The key to therapy for stroke patients is prevention. Hypertension must be aggressively treated early in life. Once a stroke has occurred, the therapeutic options are minimal and generally unsatisfactory.

In addition to the specific measures mentioned above, certain general aspects of care must also be maintained. Many stroke patients are comatose upon presentation, and it is important to maintain a patent airway and provide meticulous pulmonary toilet. Patients should be turned frequently to prevent the development of decubitus ulcers. If the patient is conscious, bed rest should be enforced and hypotension avoided. Several weeks after the stroke is completed, hypertensive patients should have their blood pressure slowly lowered to the normal range.

With a large cerebral infarction, edema may occur within two to three days with consequent tentorial herniation and death. Efforts to reduce cerebral swelling with glucocorticoids or mannitol infusions may be beneficial.

Physical therapy should begin within several days. Passive range of movement exercises can prevent the occurrence of contractures in paralyzed limbs that might otherwise retain the potential for subsequent functional improvement. The close human contact of the physical therapist also provides important psychological support for the patient.

BIBLIOGRAPHY

Barnett HJM, Boughner DR, Taylor DW et al: Further evidence relating mitral-valve prolapse to cerebral ischemic events. N Engl J Med 302:139–144, 1980

Fields WS: The asymptomatic carotid bruit—operate or not? Stroke 9:269–271, 1978

Garrawa WM, Whisnant JP, Furlan AJ et al: The declining incidence of stroke. N Engl J Med 300:449–452, 1979

Genton E, Barnett HJM, Fields WS et al: Cerebral ischemia. XIV. The role of thrombosis and of antithrombotic therapy. Stroke 8:150–175, 1977

Millikan CH: Transient cerebral ischemia: Definition and natural history. Prog Cardiovasc Dis 22:303–308, 1980

Millikan CH, McDowell FH: Treatment of transient ischemic attacks. Stroke 9:299–307, 1978

Pressin MF, Duncan GW, Mohr JP et al: Clinical and angiographic features of carotid transient ischemic attacks. N Engl J Med 296:358–362, 1977

61

Drug and Alcohol Abuse

Drug and alcohol abusers consume an inordinate amount of health services and present medical personnel with an unusual and varying array of difficulties. The 10 million alcoholics in the United States, for example, have a death rate several times that of the general population. It has been estimated that their loss of productivity and increased need for health care cost more than 30 billion dollars each year.

The foremost problem facing the clinician in treating chronic drug and alcohol abusers is the difficulty in initiating a productive dialogue. Drug abusers are often passive, dependent, and demanding, and are thus ready targets for the medical staff's anger and moralizing. The drug abuser is seen as a willful destroyer of his own health, and medical care may be delivered only reluctantly and without appropriate concern and emotional support. The assignment of blame, rather than the well-being of the patient, may become the main objective.

If therapy is to be successful and the patient eventually rehabilitated, the medical staff must learn to deal compassionately with each patient, to treat him as an individual and not merely as a manifestation of social dereliction,

and to recognize the psychological as well as the medical components of his illness.

ALCOHOL

Alcohol abuse leads to a wide array of associated medical illnesses, leaving no organ system unaffected. In conjunction with tobacco smoking, alcohol is considered to be an etiologic co-factor in epidermoid carcinomas of the oral pharynx, larynx, and esophagus. Hepatic cell carcinomas are far more common in patients with cirrhosis than in the general population. The death rate in alcoholics is more than twice that of the normal population of the same age. Many alcoholics die of cirrhosis, and many experience a violent death through accident, homicide, or suicide.

One of the great difficulties in caring for the alcoholic patient is correctly identifying the cause of the patient's altered mental status. The potential etiologies are numerous, and it is not unusual for the alcoholic to be afflicted with several of the following problems simultaneously:

1. Metabolic derangements include alcoholic intoxication, alcoholic hypoglycemia,

441

the alcohol withdrawal syndromes, electrolyte abnormalities, and thiamine deficiency (Wernicke-Korsakoff syndrome).

2. The alcoholic is prone to trauma and serious injury, and the possibility of a subdural hematoma or subarachnoid hemorrhage must always be considered.

3. Hepatic encephalopathy (Chap. 40) and alcohol-induced dementia may cause the organic brain syndrome in the alcoholic.

4. Alcoholics are very susceptible to central nervous system infections. As in any other patient, the co-existence of fever and altered mental status mandates an investigation for infectious meningitis. However, before lumbar puncture or any invasive procedure is performed on an alcoholic patient, clotting parameters must be examined, since liver disease with associated hypoprothrombinemia and marrow suppression with resultant thrombocytopenia are common.

Intoxication

The effects of alcohol intoxication are often considered to be stimulatory: people become boisterous, noisy, and extroverted. In fact, ethanol is a central nervous system (CNS) depressant, and it exerts its excitatory properties by depressing centers of CNS inhibition. With a massive ethanol overdose, central respiratory depression may prove fatal.

The signs of drunkenness need no elaboration. The degree of intoxication is dependent upon the rate of increase of the blood alcohol level. Tolerance to alcohol implies that increased blood alcohol levels are required to produce the intoxicating effects.

Aside from alcohol intoxication, there are two other types of adverse reactions to alcohol. People with *ethanol sensitivity* respond to relatively small doses of alcohol with a syndrome characterized by abdominal pain, muscle weakness, flushing, dizziness, hypotension, and tachycardia.

Pathologic intoxication is an acute idiopathic reaction in which a period of violence and delusions is followed by deep sleep. People who suffer from pathologic intoxication usually do not recall the event when they awaken.

Withdrawal

The appearance of withdrawal symptoms in an alcoholic defines addiction, and is dependent upon the decline in the blood alcohol level. A mere decrease in alcohol consumption can therefore cause withdrawal; total abstinence is not required. Patients can undergo withdrawal even with substantially elevated blood alcohol levels, as long as these levels are lower than those to which the patient has become accustomed. The severity of the withdrawal syndrome depends upon both the amount of alcohol previously consumed and the duration of the binge.

Although the alcohol withdrawal syndromes are usually described as four distinct syndrome complexes, it is more common for patients to have signs and symptoms of two or more stages simultaneously. In addition, the syndromes are often described as occurring in a progressive fashion, one stage leading to the next in an ordered, chronologic manner. It is important to emphasize, however, that not every patient experiences every "stage" of withdrawal.

1. *Tremulousness:* Tremulousness, usually the first sign of withdrawal, appears roughly eight hours after the alcoholic's last drink, often after he awakens from a binge. The tremor increases with activity and may be accompanied by anxiety, tachycardia, and nausea. Relief is often obtained by consuming another alcoholic beverage ("hair of the dog that bit you"); this raises the blood alcohol level, thereby aborting the withdrawal syndrome.

2. *Hallucinosis:* Within the first day of

withdrawal, alcoholics may begin to experience insomnia, severe agitation, and nightmares. Although the total duration of sleeptime is diminished, a higher proportion is REM sleep. Both auditory and visual hallucinations occur. This syndrome may last up to a week.

3. *Alcoholic seizures:* Convulsions are most common within the first 36 hours of withdrawal. Although focal fits with temporal lobe auras do occur, the majority of seizures are *grand mal* and lack premonitory warnings. Single seizures are most common, and the majority of patients have no more than two seizures over a period of several hours. Except for the seizure and the postictal period, the electroencephelogram is normal in most patients who have no associated history of skull trauma or idiopathic epilepsy. Approximately one-third of patients who experience withdrawal seizures progress to full-blown delirium tremens.

4. *Delirium tremens (DTs):* The most severe of the withdrawal syndromes, the DTs typically begin three to five days after abstinence (or after the decline in alcohol consumption), but DTs may commence even 10 to 14 days after abstinence. The DTs occur in up to 5% to 10% of all withdrawal episodes, and mortality ranges from 5% to 20%. Delirium is characterized by a decreased level of cognition and by slowing of the EEG. Agitation, violence, and free-floating anxiety are pronounced. Sleep is greatly diminished, and bizarre thoughts, fantasies, and hallucinations pervade the patient's consciousness. There is marked fluctuation in these symptoms depending upon the patient's immediate surroundings. Autonomic hyperactivity is dramatic: fever, hypertension, tachycardia, and hyperventilation are the cardinal signs. Infections and electrolyte disturbances must be urgently treated. Seizures during the period of DTs, however, are not common. All patients with DTs require hospitalization, constant observation, and quiet surroundings; local detoxification centers are not adequate.

Etiology of Delirium Tremens. The etiology of the DTs is poorly understood. Most research has concentrated upon decreases in serum and total body magnesium. Alcohol consumption increases the urinary excretion of magnesium, and the serum and total body magnesium are frequently low when the alcoholic patient is admitted to the hospital. Serum levels return to normal within the first three days of hospitalization. Magnesium is a divalent cation required for a number of essential enzymes, including the sodium-potassium pump. Without sufficient magnesium, potassium and calcium ions cannot be conserved by the kidney, and body stores of these minerals are depleted. Hypomagnesemia by itself has been associated with photomyoclonus (muscle contractions stimulated by light), fasiculations, chorea, and spontaneous seizures, and the period of alcoholic seizures and neuromuscular instability corresponds with the period of decreased serum magnesium. However, there is *no correlation* between the serum magnesium and the *onset* of DTs. In general, serum magnesium is normal by the time DTs begin, and there is no evidence that magnesium replenishment is a prophylaxis against delirium tremens.

Therapy of Withdrawal Syndromes. There is no evidence that any therapy prevents DTs once the withdrawal syndrome has begun. The main considerations in therapy are rehydration, restoration of normal electrolytes and blood sugar, prevention or treatment of Wernicke's encephalopathy with parenteral thiamine, and proper sedation.

Many patients are dehydrated. In addition to causing an osmotic diuresis, alcohol inhibits ADH secretion. Fluid losses may be further augmented by vomiting and anorexia. Fever and hyperventilation increase the insensible fluid loss. Much of the morbidity of the DTs is secondary to hypotension caused by hypovolemia.

One of the most important questions to consider is why the patient stopped drinking. Hepatitis, pancreatitis, gastrointestinal hemorrhage, injury, or other illness may have made him too disabled to continue to drink. Much of the morbidity and mortality from the DTs can be avoided by treating underlying or concomitant illnesses.

Sedation is an important component of therapy in patients who are withdrawing from alcohol. Drugs such as the benzodiazepines are said to be "cross-tolerant" to alcohol; when they are administered to a patient who has suddenly abstained from alcohol, the withdrawal syndromes can be averted. These medications should therefore be administered to patients who are beginning to demonstrate tremulousness or other early signs of withdrawal. The drug dosage should then be tapered slowly for several days.

Once the DTs have appeared, sedation is required to ameliorate agitation and to calm the delerious patient. One must bear in mind that the DTs last approximately two to three days and that sedation is required throughout.

The drugs most often used in preventing and treating withdrawal are the benzodiazepines (especially diazepam and chlordiazopoxide), paraldehyde, and chloral hydrate. There are indications that the phenothiazines lower the seizure threshold and thereby increase mortality in DTs, and these drugs should not be routinely used in the treatment of withdrawal.

The *benzodiazepines* are poorly and erratically absorbed intramuscularly, and must be given orally or intravenously. Diazepam is metabolized in the liver, and some of its metabolites are also effective sedatives. Since the drug's half-life depends upon hepatic metabolism, patients with liver disease may become oversedated. Intravenous diazepam is extremely effective but also potentially lethal, and countermeasures to treat apnea or severe hypotension must be immediately available whenever the drug is given.

Paraldehyde, often used in conjunction with *chloral hydrate,* has long been a therapeutic mainstay in the treatment of alcohol withdrawal. It is also an excellent anticonvulsant and sedative. It should only be given orally or rectally, since intravenous administration can cause respiratory depression, and intramuscular injections may lead to the formation of sterile abscesses. Paraldehyde is hepatotoxic, and 70% of the drug is metabolized by the liver; a small fraction is eliminated through the lungs. Many alcoholics enjoy the taste of paraldehyde and request it at detoxification centers. In excess, it causes metabolic acidosis.

It is desirable to achieve a level of sedation in which the patient is sleeping lightly but will awaken with mild stimulation. Patients with hepatitis, pancreatitis, or pneumonia often require substantially more medicine to achieve sedation. Since seizures and aspiration are a constant danger, patients should not be given oral feedings. If necessary, the patient should be restrained in a lateral decubitus position.

Mortality. Hypotension, malignant hyperthermia, cardiac arrhythmias, and infections are the most frequent causes of death during alcohol withdrawal. Pneumonia and meningitis may easily be missed. Although hyperpyrexia is part of the withdrawal syndrome, an elevated temperature still mandates a thorough evaluation for the cause of the fever.

It must be remembered that patients in the throes of withdrawal are unlikely to recall recent falls and may not complain of injuries acquired during an alcoholic debauch. The possibility of a potentially lethal subdural hematoma must always be considered.

Metabolic Abnormalities

A number of metabolic abnormalities are liable to complicate the care of the alcoholic patient. *Alcoholic ketoacidosis* is usually seen when the patient is starved and dehydrated. Unlike the situation in diabetic ketoacidosis, the blood sugar in these patients is rarely greater than 300 mg/dl, and may even be lower than normal. Acidosis is usually very mild, and a metabolic alkalosis may be seen if protracted vomiting has been very severe. Most patients with this syndrome are not diabetic, although those who are diabetic may suffer a more profound acidosis. Although the etiology of alcoholic ketoacidosis is not clear, the ketogenic hormones, cortisol and growth hormone, are elevated, and the rate of lipolysis is increased. An element of lactic acidosis may also be present. The ratio of β-hydroxybutyrate to acetoacetate is elevated, and the Acetest tablet may therefore produce a false-negative result (see Chap. 30). Rehydration alone usually reverses the syndrome, but small doses of insulin may occasionally be needed.

Metabolic acidosis with an increased anion gap is also seen in the setting of methanol or ethylene glycol consumption. These substances often provide alternative beverages for impoverished alcoholics. Hypoglycemia can also be seen in this setting.

Hypophosphatemia has only recently been recognized as a major complication of poorly nourished alcoholics. Phosphate is required to activate a number of crucial enzymes, to store energy in the form of adenosine triphosphate (ATP), and, in the form of phospholipids, to ensure the structural integrity of all cells. Because of inadequate diet, vomiting, or diarrhea, half of all hospitalized alcoholics can be expected to have a low total body phosphate. Furthermore, alcohol itself can lead to phosphate wasting: a single drink in a normal subject increases the excretion of urinary phosphate.

Hypophosphatemia usually appears soon after hospitalization, when the patient's diet has been restricted to intravenous glucose; both glycolysis and glycogen formation require phosphate, and glucose feeding without phosphate supplementation therefore results in a large movement of phosphate into the intracellular space. The complications of hypophosphatemia are numerous. Experimental phosphate depletion causes weakness, anorexia, bone pain, joint stiffness, and an intention tremor. Myopathy with pain, stiffness, and weakness, and rhabdomyolysis with serum creatine phosphokinase elevations have been noted when serum phosphate levels fall below 1 mg/dl. Acute respiratory failure and some cases of congestive cardiomyopathy have been attributed to phosphate deficiency. Acute hemolysis may also occur. Many foods, especially dairy products, are rich in phosphate, and replenishment of phosphate is usually readily achieved through a normal hospital diet.

Complications of Alcohol Abuse

Gastrointestinal Disorders. A host of acute and chronic gastrointestinal ailments are among the most common sequelae of alcohol abuse. These include hepatitis, cirrhosis, gastritis, pancreatitis, and gastrointestinal bleeding.

Pulmonary and Cardiovascular Disorders. Aspiration pneumonia is very common, but other bacterial and mycobacterial infections are also frequently seen. Alcohol reduces the ciliary activity of the bronchial epithelium and diminishes the mobility of alveolar macrophages. Since alcoholics have a high carrier rate of gram-negative organisms, especially klebsiella, in their oropharynx, transtracheal aspiration to obtain sputum should be performed in the event of pneumonia.

Chronic alcohol abuse can cause a cardiomyopathy (Chap. 6). Brief alcohol binges can cause a series of cardiac arrhythmias, primarily atrial fibrillation, atrial flutter, and premature ventricular contraction.

Hematologic Disorders. Hematologic abnormalities are nearly always present in the malnourished alcoholic population. Three-quarters of those patients who require hospitalization have been shown to have compromised erythropoiesis, most often as a result of folic acid deficiency. Hemorrhage, usually from gastritis or varices, is another significant, although less frequent, cause of anemia. Examination of a peripheral blood film may show any of several pictures: macrocytosis with hypersegmented neutrophils (with folate deficiency), hypochromic microcytosis (with bleeding and iron deficiency), a dimorphic population (with a mixed nutritional disorder), and normal red blood cells. If liver disease is also present, target cells and spur cells may be seen. These abnormal erythrocytes have increased cholesterol in their cell membranes, the result of an elevated cholesterol/phospholipid ratio caused by a deficiency of hepatic lecithin-cholesterol acyl-transferase activity.

Folic acid deficiency is usually the result of an inadequate diet (Chap. 45). In addition, ethanol inhibits the absorption of folate from the gut and may interfere with folate utilization by the bone marrow. Beer contains adequate folic acid, but the sweet, inexpensive, high-alcohol-content dessert wines favored by many alcoholics have a low concentration of folic acid. The more affluent, better-nourished alcoholics therefore suffer less frequently from vitamin deficiency anemia.

Soon after the patient is hospitalized and vitamin deficiencies are corrected, reticulocytosis begins. The serum iron level, which often is elevated in patients with folate deficiency, decreases. With the formation of newer erythrocytes, the serum potassium and phosphate, which may already be depressed, become further depleted as they are incorporated as intracellular ions. The macrocytosis resolves within one to two weeks, and, in some patients, the red cells become microcytic, indicating the presence of simultaneous iron deficiency.

Alcoholics with cirrhosis may suffer from a chronic, low-grade normochromic normocytic hemolytic anemia associated with hypersplenism. The concurrence of mild hemolytic anemia, jaundice, hyperlipidemia, and alcoholic hepatitis has been termed *Zieve's syndrome.*

Athough ethanol may interfere with vitamin B_{12} absorption from the ileum, pernicious anemia is not seen more frequently in the alcoholic population than in the healthy population. Since the body normally maintains a 3- to 6-year store of vitamin B_{12}, a deficiency due solely to malnutrition is not commonly seen.

Abnormalities of leukocytes and platelets are also encountered in the alcoholic population. Although folate deficiency and hypersplenism may account for the mild neutropenia and thrombocytopenia, ethanol itself suppresses the production of myeloid and megakaryocyte percursors in the marrow. The white blood cell count is usually in the range of 2000 to 4000, and it is often found in association with thrombocytopenia. It resolves spontaneously within ten days of hospitalization. The thrombocytopenia is generally far more severe, and platelet counts below 100,000 are common. Thrombocytopenia is seen in the majority of hospitalized alcoholics, and is frequently the only hematologic abnormality. Within two to three days of hospitalization, the platelet count begins to increase, often rebounding to extremely high levels of 1 million or more before returning to normal.

Sexual and Reproductive Disorders. Chronic alcohol abuse also affects the sexual and reproductive capabilities of the patient. Gynecomastia and testicular atrophy may occur in male alcoholics because of a variety of pathophysiologic alterations, including primary gonadal failure, hypothalamic-pituitary suppression, and the increased hepatic metabolism of testosterone. Increased estrogen synthesis has also been observed.

The chronic consumption of approximately 900 ml of alcohol (6 mixed drinks per day) by pregnant women constitutes a severe risk to the fetus. The fetal alcohol syndrome is associated with a characteristic facies, mental retardation, and other developmental abnormalities.

Neurologic Disorders. The neurologic consequences of chronic alcoholism have been extensively studied. Dementia, with the underlying pathology often graphically depicted on CT scan as severe cortical atrophy and ventricular enlargement, is common even in very young alcoholics.

Thiamine deficiency can present either as *Wernicke's encephalopathy* or, less commonly, as high-output congestive heart failure (beriberi). The administration of glucose to a patient with marginal thiamine reserves may cause acute depletion of those reserves as the glucose is metabolized, resulting in a Wernicke's crisis. Confusion, ataxia, and ophthalmoplegia are the hallmarks of this disease. Polyneuropathy, lethargy, and hypotension may be seen. Since Wernicke's encephalopathy often coincides with alcohol withdrawal, the above signs may be mixed with the protean manifestations of the withdrawal syndromes. The ocular signs are very responsive to thiamine, but the ataxia may not begin to resolve

for several weeks. Many patients are left with permanent disability. Vitamin supplementation should be continued throughout the patient's hospitalization.

Many patients who manifest Wernicke's encephalopathy develop *Korsakoff's psychosis,* an organic brain syndrome characterized by the inability to form new memories or to recall events antecedent to the psychosis. Although not present in all patients, confabulation is the most striking finding on an examination of mental status. Patients invent stories, describe experiences that never occurred, and readily agree to the most outlandish tales suggested by the interviewer.

Rare neurologic consequences of alcohol abuse include cerebellar degeneration, which presents with disturbances of gait and stance, and central pontine myelinolysis, which may cause quadriplegia.

Muscle Abnormalities. Most chronic alcoholics have abnormalities of skeletal muscle when tested by an electromyogram. Rhabdomyolysis and peripheral nerve palsies are seen in alcoholics who have passed out and slept in contorted positions ("Saturday night drunk syndrome"). Alcoholics may also develop severe muscle cramps that are associated with necrosis of myofibers and interstitial inflammation. A chronic myopathy, distinguished by intracellular edema, abnormal mitochondria, and lipid and glycogen storage, may develop after one week of alcohol abuse. Peripheral neuropathies are not uncommon sequelae of alcoholism, and may cause muscle atrophy.

SEDATIVE HYPNOTICS

Benzodiazepines

The benzodiazepines are currently implicated in a majority of drug overdoses. Patients usually combine these drugs with other pharmaceuticals, especially alcohol. Used alone, the benzodiazepines are rarely lethal, but they do potentiate other sedatives when taken together. Although withdrawal syndromes have been described, the very long half-lives of diazepam and chlordiazopoxide make severe withdrawal a truly rare event.

Barbiturates

Though declining in popularity, barbiturates are still commonly used by the elderly. Overdoses of barbiturates may lead to shock and coma. Hypotension, hypothermia, apnea, absent corneal and deep tendon reflexes, and diminished pupillary responses to light are characteristic. The patient may even appear to have electrical brain death, with a nearly flat EEG.

Various skin lesions have been described in barbiturate overdose, including discoid erythematous plaques, tense vesicles, and large clear bullae. Occasionally, sweat gland necrosis is seen on biopsy; these so-called "barb burns" are generally located over pressure areas where physical restraints have been placed. The lesions are not pathognomonic of barbiturate overdosage, and are seen in a variety of comatose states.

Blood levels can be useful in diagnosing and monitoring therapy. A forced diuresis may be helpful, and alkalinization of the urine hastens the clearance of phenobarbital, but not of secobarbital.

Withdrawal symptoms can be expected in most patients who abruptly stop taking barbiturates after having ingested at least 500 mg of short-acting barbiturates per day for one month. With secobarbital, and with hypnotics like methaqualone and meprobamate, withdrawal symptoms begin 12 to 24 hours after the last dose and peak 2 to 3 days after the last dose. Anxiety, anorexia, and tremors herald the beginning of the withdrawal syndrome; these may progress to full-fledged withdrawal,

with seizures and delirium. Treatment is the same as in alcohol withdrawal.

NARCOTIC ADDICTION

The triad of coma, miotic pupils, and hypoventilation is the characteristic presentation of narcotic overdose in the emergency room. With severe overdosage, hypotension, seizures, and noncardiogenic pulmonary edema may occur.

Naloxone, a pure opiate antagonist, rapidly reverses narcotic-induced coma. Given intravenously, naloxone achieves its peak effect within one to 2 minutes, and its duration of action is several hours. Naloxone is generally an extremely safe drug, and should be given along with glucose as a trial to *all* comatose patients. Several injections, repeated at 5-minute intervals, may be required. Patients who have taken an overdose of a long-acting narcotic like methadone may require repeated injections of naloxone every few hours.

Narcotic withdrawal resembles a flu-like syndrome with rhinorrhea, myalgias, arthralgias, fever, nausea, vomiting, and abdominal pain. These symptoms are accompanied by insomnia, yawning, dilated pupils, piloerection, and muscle twitching. Patients not infrequently assume a fetal position. The withdrawal symptoms are usually treated by long-acting narcotics from which the patient is gradually weaned. Experimental evidence suggests that withdrawal symptoms may also be blocked by clonidine, a central α-adrenergic agonist.

Naloxone precipitates a withdrawal syndrome in a patient addicted to narcotics, but narcotic withdrawal is rarely life-threatening. Rapid withdrawal from narcotics, however, is exceedingly unpleasant, and naloxone should never be administered to a noncomatose patient for "detoxification."

After the drug overdose has been treated,

attention must be paid to the myriad other illnesses to which this patient population is especially susceptible. Acute bacterial endocarditis is the most dangerous of these complications, and is discussed in Chapter 54.

The heroin addict frequently develops one or more of several pulmonary ailments. Pulmonary edema of uncertain etiology is seen in acute overdoses. Pneumonia may be caused by aspiration or by septic emboli originating from an infected tricuspid valve. Talc and other impurities in the injected drugs may cause pulmonary fibrosis and granulomas.

A number of immunologic abnormalities have been described in narcotic abusers. An elevated serum IgM and IgG, a false-positive VDRL and latex fixation, and anti-smooth muscle antibody are among the immunologic aberrancies.

Narcotic abuse is also associated with the nephrotic syndrome. In narcotic addicts, focal and segmental glomerulosclerosis is frequently seen on biopsy, and patients may ultimately become uremic.

Musculoskeletal symptoms are very common and can usually be attributed to several causes, including the myalgias of withdrawal, a prodrome of viral hepatitis or bacterial endocarditis, or the pain of osteomyelitis; these symptoms may also arise as a complication of septic arthritis. In patients who inject themselves intramuscularly with pentazocine, the muscle and overlying skin may fibrose and toughen, resulting in a woody hard myopathy.

Addicts who use and share dirty needles have an increased risk of hepatitis, endocarditis, and tetanus. Malaria, one of the earliest consequences of intravenous drug abuse to be recognized, was propagated by shared needles during the Vietnam War era.

The impurities in cut heroin may alter its physical appearance. Recently, so-called "brown heroin" has been blamed for a rash of ITP-like disorders and a musculoskeletal syndrome characterized by fever, myalgias, and periarthritis affecting the knees.

Many addicts steal or engage in heroin trafficking, activities in which the risk of physical injury is high. Since heavily narcotized patients may not complain of pain, the physician must look assiduously for fractures and other consequences of violence.

PHENCYCLIDINE (PCP)

Phencyclidine (angel dust, crystal, hog), originally marketed as an animal tranquilizer, has become one of the most widely abused of the illicit recreational pharmaceuticals. The drug is a white powder and is easily synthesized. It is usually smoked or inhaled (snorted), but can also be taken orally. The drug causes a series of central nervous system effects, beginning with agitation, incoordination, dysarthria, analgesia, and nystagmus, and progresses to vomiting, hypersalivation, myoclonus, and fever. Large doses can cause coma, hypertension, convulsions, and, eventually, death.

Users report a feeling of drunkenness, analgesia, and a state resembling sensory deprivation. Only about 50% of the subjects emphasize positive aspects of the intoxication; euphoria, for example, is a distinctly unusual reaction. On the other hand, negative aspects of the "high" are universally described: users are disturbed by perceptual changes, difficulties with speech, breathlessness, anxiety, and even paranoia. This generally unpleasant response makes it difficult to understand the motivation of the chronic PCP abuser; the fact that the drug is almost always consumed in a group implies that various interpersonal reinforcements may play an important role.

The high from PCP lasts from four to six hours. Overdoses are more common when the drug is taken orally, probably because the longer latency period with the oral approach makes self-titration of the drug dosage difficult. Signs of overdose are nonspecific, but the findings of ataxia, vertical and horizontal nystagmus, and aggressiveness should suggest the diagnosis. Often the patient presents with an acute schizophrenic reaction. The diagnosis ultimately depends upon identification of the drug in the blood, urine, or gastric contents.

Although there are no specific antagonists to PCP, steps can be taken to accelerate the excretion of the drug. PCP becomes positively charged in an acidic environment, and can be trapped and concentrated by acidifying the urine with ammonium chloride. Unfortunately, acid trapping also means that the drug will be secreted from the bloodstream back into the gastric lumen and then reabsorbed in more basic parts of the intestine. This gastroenteric recirculation occurs regardless of the manner of ingestion, and all patients who are suspected of PCP overdose therefore require continuous nasogastric drainage in order to facilitate excretion of the drug. If the patient is comatose, endotracheal intubation should precede gastric lavage. Hyperthermia, severe hypertension, and convulsions may be seen, and should be treated symptomatically. Total excretion of the drug from the body may take several days.

A post-PCP psychosis may ensue, even after a single dose. The psychotic episode, which is often misdiagnosed as schizophrenia, can last for several weeks and is characterized by restlessness and violence. The contribution of the premorbid personality to the character of the psychosis is still being debated.

TRICYCLIC ANTIDEPRESSANT OVERDOSES

Overdoses of tricyclic antidepressants present the emergency medical team with a host of complex clinical decisions. As a general rule, all patients require cardiac monitoring and should be admitted to the hospital.

In therapeutic doses, tricyclic antidepressants may cause mild postural hypotension, tachycardia, and T-wave changes on the EKG. These drugs have both anticholinergic and adrenergic properties, and a number of cardiac arrhythmias have been noted with toxic doses, including sinus tachycardia, sinus bradycardia, atrial fibrillation, ventricular tachycardia, and ventricular fibrillation. A-V blocks and widened QRS complexes are also seen.

Patients with an overdose of tricyclics may manifest signs of atropine poisoning—"red as a beet, dry as a stone, blind as a bat, and mad as a hatter." They may have urinary retention, myoclonic seizures, or they may arrive in coma and require intubation because of hypoventilation.

If the tricyclic overdose has been recent, the patient may appear perfectly well. Since tricyclic antidepressant serum levels are often not immediately available, it may be difficult to gauge the extent of the overdose and thereby estimate the chance of major toxicity occurring several hours thereafter. It has been found, however, that a widened QRS complex of more than 100 milliseconds within the first 24 hours of hospitalization is a reliable index of serious toxicity, and indicates that the blood levels are at least 1000 ng/ml. The half-life of tricyclic antidepressants averages approximately four days, and patients with an overdose of tricyclics will require many days of hospital observation and cardiac monitoring.

When a patient with suspected tricyclic antidepressant overdose is first seen, emesis should be induced only if the patient is awake and alert. If not, intubation should be performed, and the gastric contents removed (the anticholinergic action of the tricyclic antidepressant will have slowed gastric emptying). Activated charcoal should also be given. Urinary retention may necessitate catheterization. Cardiac arrhythmias caused by tricyclic antidepressants should be treated with the same medications normally used for those arrhythmias.

Physostigmine, a centrally acting cholinesterase inhibitor, has been recommended as a specific antidote to tricyclic antidepressant poisoning, especially for those patients who are suffering from cardiac arrhythmias or coma. However, physostigmine should not be used except as a last resort. An analeptic drug, physostigmine is hardly specific, and will awaken patients who have taken, for example, benzodiazepines or phenothiazines. The arousal is only partial and is of very short duration. Like the tricyclic antidepressants, physostigmine may itself cause seizures, especially when given too rapidly. The drug can also cause hypersalivation, and therefore should never be given until the patient is intubated. By potentiating cholinergic effects on the heart, physostigmine may cause asystole.

Because the tricyclic antidepressants are prescribed for severely depressed patients, precisely that segment of the population most likely to commit suicide, the use of tricyclic antidepressants in suicide attempts and suicide gestures is not surprising. The drug should always be dispensed in small quantities, and the use of combination pills that contain benzodiazepines along with tricyclic antidepressants should definitely be avoided.

SALICYLATE OVERDOSE

Salicylate overdose is seen in two clinical circumstances in the adult population: (1) in a younger group who attempt suicide with aspirin, and (2) in an elderly population who inadvertently consume an excessive amount of aspirin that had been prescribed for chronic, usually rheumatologic, illnesses.

The first signs of toxicity are dyspnea, tinnitus, vertigo, and loss of hearing. More profound overdose results in nausea and vomiting, fever, and an array of nonspecific neurologic symptoms, including headache, confusion, excitement, agitation, drowsiness, and hallucinations. Hypoglycemia may also rarely occur. In severe salicylate poisoning, convulsions and coma supervene. The index of suspicion in the elderly population is quite low since neurologic symptoms, tachypnea, and noncardiogenic pulmonary edema are more common in elderly patients. As a result, the diagnosis is often delayed and mortality in this group is high.

In toxic doses, aspirin causes a mixed acid/base disturbance: a respiratory alkalosis combined with a metabolic acidosis. Hyperventilation results from salicylate sensitization of the CNS respiratory center to carbon dioxide, leading to hyperventilation and respiratory alkalosis. With higher doses, salicylate inhibits carbohydrate metabolism, resulting in the abnormal accumulation of organic ions and a metabolic acidosis; the salicylic acid itself may contribute to the metabolic acidosis. Respiratory depression may eventually ensue.

Gastric lavage should be immediately attempted in an acute overdose of aspirin. Further therapy should aim at enhancing renal secretion of aspirin. This can be accomplished by a forced osmotic diuresis, accompanied by alkalinization of the urine. Alkalosis causes the equilibrium to shift to the ionized form of salicylic acid, and this charged form becomes trapped within the renal tubule.

ACETAMINOPHEN OVERDOSE

Acetaminophen (Tylenol) is found in a variety of analgesic-combination, over-the-counter drugs. It is metabolized by the hepatic cytochrome P450 enzyme system into reactive intermediates that are rapidly conjugated to glutathione and then excreted. When the drug is taken in large quantities (greater than 10 grams), the body's store of glutathione may be exhausted, and the reactive metabolites are then free to bind covalently to other constituents of the hepatocytes. Acute centrilobular necrosis and acute liver failure ensue.

Patients who take an overdose of acetaminophen complain of nausea and vomiting soon thereafter, but usually feel much better within 24 hours. However, 24 to 36 hours after the ingestion, the serum aminotransferases start to rise, and by 48 hours many patients experience right upper quadrant discomfort. Fulminant liver failure with hepatic coma may soon follow.

Oral N-acetylcysteine (Mucomyst) is the most promising therapy for acetaminophen poisoning. It must be administered within the first 10 hours after the overdose. N-acetylcysteine is thought to replenish glutathione stores, thereby preventing the toxic matabolites from binding to liver cells.

BIBLIOGRAPHY

Anderson RJ, Potts DE, Gabon PA et al: Unrecognized adult salicylate intoxication. Ann Intern Med 85:745–748, 1976

Cunningham EE, Brentjens JR, Zielezny MA et al: Heroin nephropathy: A clinicopathologic and epidemologic study. Am J Med 68:47–53, 1980

Eichner ER: The hematologic disorders of alcoholism. Am J Med 54:621–630, 1973

Groves JE: Taking care of the hateful patient. N Engl J Med 298:883–887, 1978

Isbell H, Fraser HF, Wikler A et al: An experimental study of the etiology of "rum fits" and delirium tremens. J Stud Alcohol 16:1–33, 1955

Jefferson JW: A review of the cardiovascular effects and toxicity of tricyclic antidepressants. Psychosom Med 37:160–179, 1975

Knochel JP: The pathophysiology and clinical characteristics of severe hypophosphatemia. Arch Intern Med 137:203–220, 1977

Mendelson JH, Mello NK: Biologic concomitants of alcoholism. N Engl J Med 301:912–921, 1979

Sapira JD: The narcotic addict as a medical patient. Am J Med 45:555–588, 1968

Thompson WL: Management of alcohol withdrawal syndromes. Arch Intern Med 138:278–283, 1978

Index